Toronto,

For Joseph Freeman
With compliments

M. Arjer

Induction Chemotherapy

Karl Reinhard Aigner
Frederick O. Stephens

Editors

Induction Chemotherapy

Systemic and Locoregional

Second Edition

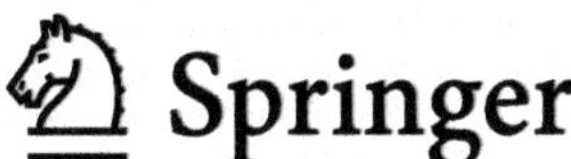

Editors
Karl Reinhard Aigner
Department of Surgical Oncology
Medias Klinikum GmbH & Co KG
Burghausen
Germany

Frederick O. Stephens
Royal Prince Alfred
Sydney Hospitals
Mosman
New South Wales
Australia

ISBN 978-3-319-28771-3   ISBN 978-3-319-28773-7   (eBook)
DOI 10.1007/978-3-319-28773-7

Library of Congress Control Number: 2016936670

Printed on acid-free paper

This Springer imprint is published by Springer Nature
The registered company is Springer International Publishing AG Switzerland

Contents

Introduction: Overview, History, Terminology and Early Clinical Experience

1

Frederick O. Stephens[†]

1.1 History of Modern Cancer Treatments

The history of the search for effective cancer treatment is probably as old as the history of any formal medical practice. However, apart from crude ablative surgery without general anaesthesia, it was not until the discovery of general anaesthesia in the mid-nineteenth century that modern operative surgery, as we know it, could be developed. Thus, safe and painless operative surgery developed as the first significant advance in cancer treatment. Initially, use of operative surgery under general anaesthesia was usually complicated by a very high incidence of wound infection. The problem of wound infection was clarified and largely controlled by the discovery of offending microorganisms by such great pioneers as Semmelweis of Hungary, Pasteur of France, Koch of Germany and the Scot Lister who was working in England [1].

About 50 years later, in the early twentieth century, the second great advance in effective anticancer treatment was the discovery of the effects of gamma irradiation on tissues by Roentgen in Germany and the Curies in France. Radiotherapy thus became the second effective modality for cancer treatment. The third great advance in cancer treatment about mid-twentieth century was the discovery of hormones and chemical agents that could either control or restrain cancer cell production or destroy cancer cells.

Until the mid-twentieth century, most cancer treatment was in the hands of surgeons or radiotherapists. The first discovery of effective hormone treatment was by Dr. George Beatson in Scotland in relation to breast cancer and then by Drs. Huggins and Hodges in America in relation to prostate cancer. Soon after the evidence that

---

[†]Author was deceased at the time of publication.

F.O. Stephens
Department of Surgery, University of Sydney, Inkerman Street 16, 2088 Mosman,
Sydney, NSW, Australia
e-mail: fredstephens@optusnet.com.au

K.R. Aigner, F.O. Stephens (eds.), *Induction Chemotherapy*,
DOI 10.1007/978-3-319-28773-7_1

hormone manipulation could reduce the size and aggressive qualities of some cancers, the first anticancer chemical agents were discovered.

An accidental finding in World War II showed that war gases, nitrogen mustard and related compounds affected dividing cells. Application of these observations by haematologists showed that some haematological malignancies, leukaemias and lymphomas, responded to these agents. This was the beginning of modern chemotherapy for cancer treatment. Thus, historically, haematologists were first to use modern anticancer agents in a clinical situation.

After nitrogen mustard, a number of other anticancer drugs became available including hydroxyurea and methotrexate. These were soon followed by the discovery of more anticancer agents classified according to their different chemical compounds and different biological effects on cancer cells. The first effective anticancer chemical agents were alkylating agents and then followed by different categories of effective anticancer agents, namely, antimetabolites, antimitotics, antibiotics and more recently biological agents such as monoclonal antibodies including Herceptin [1].

Whilst haematologists were the first specialists to use new anticancer agents, surgeons and radiotherapists were next to use the new chemical anticancer agents simply because surgeons and radiotherapists were the traditional carers for people with non-haematological malignancies.

Surgeons and radiotherapists began to use the new anticancer agents in treatment of cancers that were recurrent after initial treatment by operative surgery or radiotherapy. When given as systemic treatment for local recurrence after failed surgery or radiotherapy, results of using the new anticancer agents were disappointing. When given in doses that did not cause unacceptable systemic toxicity, locally recurrent tumour responses were minimal to the agents that were available [2, 3].

Some surgeons rationalised that if the new anticancer agents were given directly into the arteries supplying the cancers with blood, it would increase local concentration of the agents which should affect the local cancer cells more significantly without risking the same degree of systemic toxicity [4–6]. Most head and neck cancers were in a region supplied by the external carotid artery so that most first trials of intra-arterial chemotherapy were in treating locally advanced head and neck cancers [2, 3, 7].

Although logical in theory, the first uses of intra-arterial chemotherapy to treat locally advanced head and neck cancer failed. Most surgeons then lost interest in the then 'new' anticancer agents because they had not been effective in treating their failures, that is, recurrent localised primary cancers.

At the same time, first haematologists and then general physicians recognised the value of systemic chemotherapy in treating not only haematological malignancies but also widespread metastatic cancers, so that the use of these agents was left largely to those clinicians who were treating systemic cancers. Thus, a new speciality to become known as medical oncology developed.

1.2   Origins of Induction Chemotherapy

Meanwhile, it became apparent to some surgeons that most of the first cancers being treated by surgeons using regional chemotherapy had been recurrent cancers after previous surgery and/or radiotherapy had failed. The cancers were recurrent in scarred or poorly vascularised tissues resulting from previous surgical or radiation blood vessel damage. As chemotherapy was taken to the cancer cells in the bloodstream, the dose and concentration reaching cancers in poorly vascularised tissues was less than in well-vascularised tissues.

During surgery, blood vessels are ligated, thus reducing the blood supply to cancers that recur in or near the surgical wound. After radiotherapy, there is also damage to blood vessels. Some surgeons recognised the potential value of anti-cancer drugs in having a significant impact on regional advanced cancers, provided the blood supply had not been compromised by previous surgery or radiotherapy. They also hypothesised that the chemotherapy should have a greater impact if delivered to the cancer in a more concentrated form by direct intra-arterial infusion. Some surgeons renewed their interest in using chemotherapy delivered by direct intra-arterial infusion as initial treatment of locally advanced cancers in a region embraced by one or two arteries that could be safely cannulated and infused [7–9].

Chemotherapy alone rarely cured locally advanced cancers but there was a renewed interest in reducing advanced and doubtfully resectable primary cancers by first treating them with chemotherapy and subsequently using operative surgery and/or radiotherapy to eradicate the residual tumour.

Figure 1.1 is a photomicrograph that shows most of this small previously irradiated artery is blocked leaving only a small central opening for little blood flow. Thus little chemotherapy could flow through this artery to affect a cancer.

The effect of previous radiotherapy on blood flow is shown in Fig. 1.2, which is a photograph of the face of a woman who 2 years previously had radiotherapy for a cancer on her lower lip. Patent blue dye injected into both external carotid arteries showed that the blue flowed into the skin of her face except that part of her face previously in the field of radiotherapy.

Many studies have since confirmed that some locally advanced primary cancers can be reduced in size and aggression by first using chemotherapy. Thus, given as initial treatment, before local surgery or radiotherapy had damaged blood vessels supplying the tumour with blood, chemotherapy would have permeated the tumour

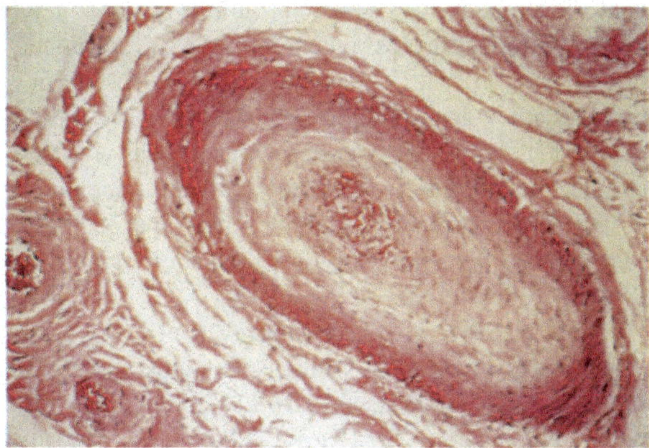

Fig. 1.1 Photomicrograph that shows most of this small previously irradiated artery is blocked leaving only a small central opening for little blood flow. Thus little chemotherapy could flow through this artery to affect a cancer

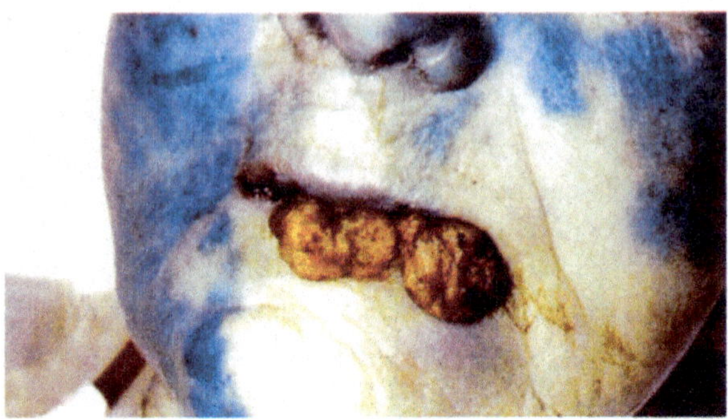

Fig. 1.2 The effect of previous radiotherapy on blood flow is shown in this photograph of the face of a woman who 2 years previously had had radiotherapy for a cancer on her lower lip. Patent blue dye injected into both external carotid arteries showed that the blue flowed into the skin of her face except that part of her face previously in the field of radiotherapy

tissue more effectively and so reduce the size, extent and aggressive qualities of the cancer. The cancer then would very often be reduced to proportions that were curable by following radiotherapy and/or surgery. That chemotherapy to the primary cancer is more effective if administered before radiotherapy or surgery was reported in 1968 from the Christian Medical College in Vellore, India, by Professor Joseph and his colleagues [10].

1.3   Terminology

Many names have been given to such initial chemotherapy administered as first treatment to reduce the tumour, inducing changes to make the cancer more curable by surgery and/or radiotherapy. It has been called *reducing, primary, initial, induction, neoadjuvant* or *basal chemotherapy*.

With reference to the commonly used term *neoadjuvant*, Greek and Latin scholars wonder at the mixture of the Greek prefix 'neo' with the Latin adjective 'adjuvant'. If a mixture of Greek and Latin is acceptable and then the appropriate Greek prefix would be 'protos' meaning initial or forerunner, thus 'proto-adjuvant' would be more appropriate. The prefix 'neo' is Greek for new and this would suggest that this was a new form of adjuvant chemotherapy, which is not true. The term *neoadjuvant* does not fit comfortably with surgeons who first used these agents as 'preoperative' therapy before the term 'adjuvant' chemotherapy was described. The 'new adjuvant' chemotherapy was not a new approach after the term 'adjuvant chemotherapy' had been introduced; it was an old approach being rediscovered by a new group of oncologists.

The term *induction chemotherapy* is probably the most descriptive as the chemotherapy is given to induce changes that make follow-up surgery and/or radiotherapy more likely to be successful [10, 11].

1.4 Early Experience with Intra-arterial Induction Chemotherapy

Some photographic examples of successful application of intra-arterial induction chemotherapy conducted by the Sydney surgical oncology unit from the early 1970s onwards are shown in Figs. 1.3, 1.4, 1.5, 1.6, 1.7, 1.8, 1.9, 1.10, 1.11 and 1.12.

Figure 1.3a is a photograph of a previously untreated SCC growing over the left eye of a 90-year-old woman.

Figure 1.3b is a photograph taken after injection of disulphine blue dye into the external carotid artery. This confirmed that the cancer would get a greater concentration of chemotherapy when it was infused into this artery.

After 4 weeks of continuous intra-arterial chemotherapy (using methotrexate and bleomycin), the cancer was much smaller, and the patient could see again as shown in Fig. 1.3c. She was satisfied with this result as she could see again but, at the age of 90, she declined any further treatment.

Figure 1.4a is a photograph of a man who had neglected a cancer (SCC) destroying his nose.

After 5 weeks of intra-arterial chemotherapy slowly infused into both external carotid arteries, the cancer had regressed considerably to allow following radiotherapy to be very effective as seen in Fig. 1.4b.

After completion of radiotherapy, there was no longer any evidence of residual cancer but quite a deformity of his nose as can be seen in Fig. 1.4c.

After 2 years and no recurrence of his cancer, this man's nose was reconstructed by plastic surgery. When last seen 5 years later, he was well and did not have any evidence of cancer.

In 1974 the man in the photograph in Fig. 1.5a presented with a large cancer of his lower lip, previously untreated.

In Fig. 1.5b it can be seen that the cancer involved the whole of his lower lip and had involved lymph nodes in the right side of his neck.

After 5 weeks of continuous chemotherapy given by slow infusion into both external carotid arteries, the lip cancer was much smaller as shown in Fig. 1.5c. The large lymph nodes in his neck were also smaller.

After a break of 3 weeks, his lower lip was then treated by radiotherapy. The final result, as shown in Fig. 1.5d, showed no evidence of cancer in his lip.

The lymph nodes in the right side of his neck were smaller but still enlarged. The nodes were resected in a block dissection. A small nest of cancer cells was detected in two of the resected lymph nodes. Figure 1.5e shows the scars on his neck 6 months later. There was no evidence of any further cancer.

Like many patients who wait so long to first seek treatment, this man did not keep his follow-up appointments; but I happened to see him at a horserace meeting 12 years later. He remained well. The photograph in Fig. 1.5f was taken.

In August 1981, the lady shown in Fig. 1.6a was referred for treatment of her extensive BCC on her face. She had lived like a hermit in virtual isolation for many years. The extensive carcinoma destroying her nose and involving her right eye and right upper lip had never previously been treated. She presented for treatment

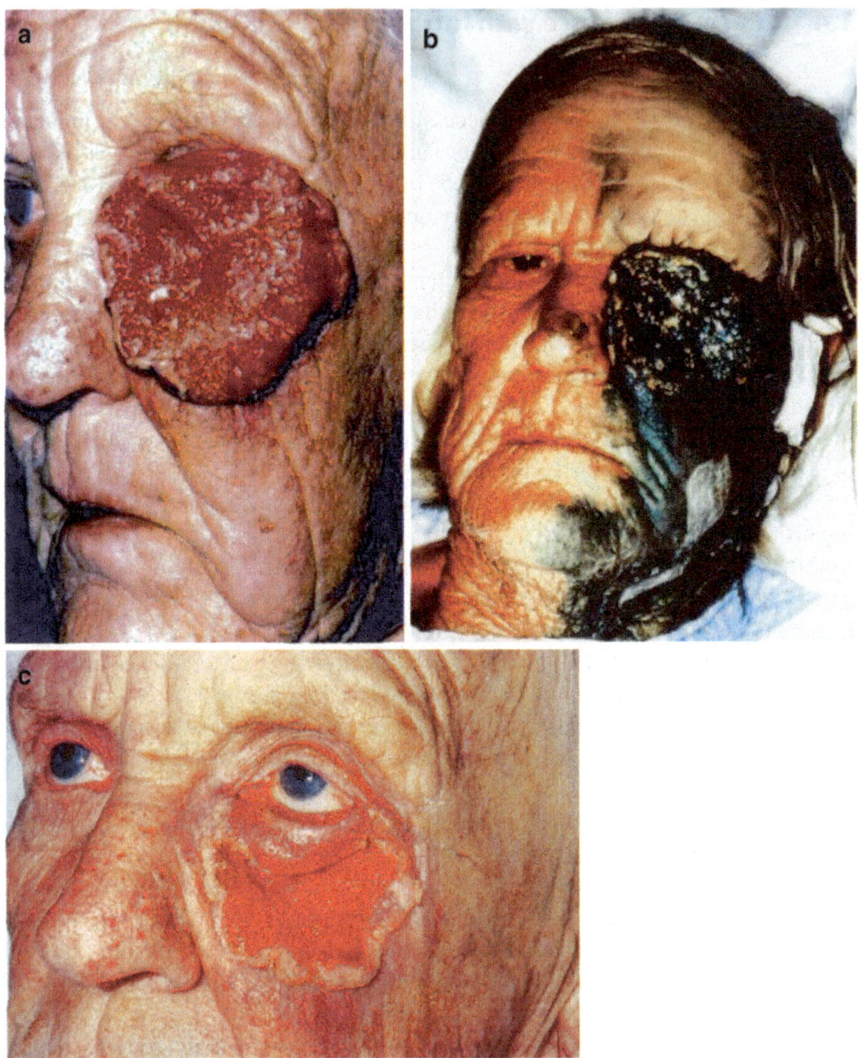

Fig. 1.3 (**a**) is a photograph of a previously untreated SCC growing over the left eye of a 90-year-old woman. (**b**) is a photograph taken after injection of disulphine blue dye into the external carotid artery. This confirmed that the cancer would get a greater concentration of chemotherapy when it was infused into this artery. (**c**) After 4 weeks of continuous intra-arterial chemotherapy (using methotrexate and bleomycin), the cancer was much smaller, and the patient could see again. She was satisfied with this result because she could see again, but at the age of 90, she declined any further treatment

because she was having difficulty with opening her right eye and some difficulty with eating.

She had a fear of surgery but agreed to a trial of chemotherapy. Cannulae were inserted into both external carotid arteries and continuous intra-arterial infusion

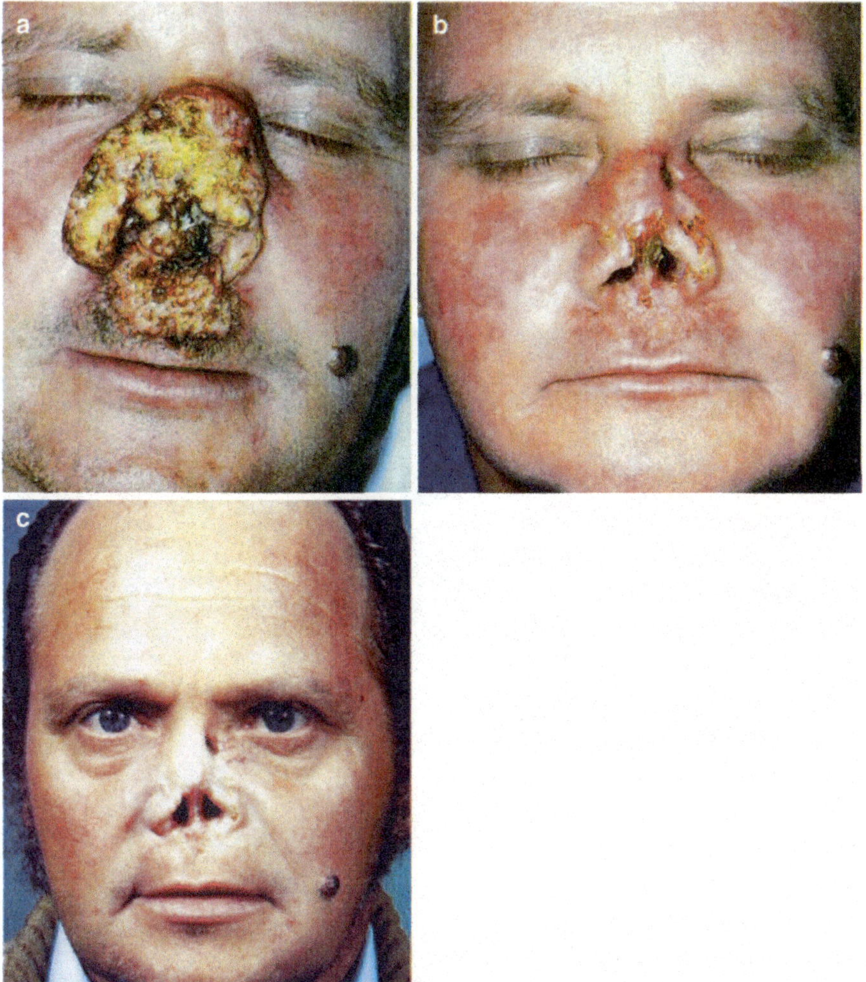

Fig. 1.4 (**a**) is a photograph of a man who had neglected a cancer (SCC) destroying his nose. (**b**) After 5 weeks of intra-arterial chemotherapy slowly infused into both external carotid arteries, the cancer had regressed considerably to allow following radiotherapy to be very effective. (**c**) After completion of radiotherapy, there was no longer any evidence of residual cancer but quite a deformity of his nose as can be seen. After 2 years and no recurrence of his cancer, this man's nose was reconstructed by plastic surgery. When last seen 5 years later, he was well and did not have any evidence of cancer

chemotherapy was administered using methotrexate, bleomycin, vincristine and actinomycin D in daily rotation for 4 weeks.

The BCC resolved and Fig. 1.6b is a photograph taken 2 weeks after completion of the intra-arterial chemotherapy.

As the lady could see and eat better, she was satisfied with the result and declined to have any further treatment.

In 1976, a 56-year-old woman presented with the previously untreated cancer in her right breast shown in Fig. 1.7a.

Because a cancer of this size would be most unlikely to be cured by surgery or by radiotherapy, it was decided to first treat her with continuous chemotherapy administered by slow intra-arterial infusion.

After a cannula had been inserted into the subclavian artery to the origin of the internal mammary artery, blue dye injected into the cannula confirmed that blood flow embraced the cancer and nodes in the axilla as shown in Fig. 1.7b.

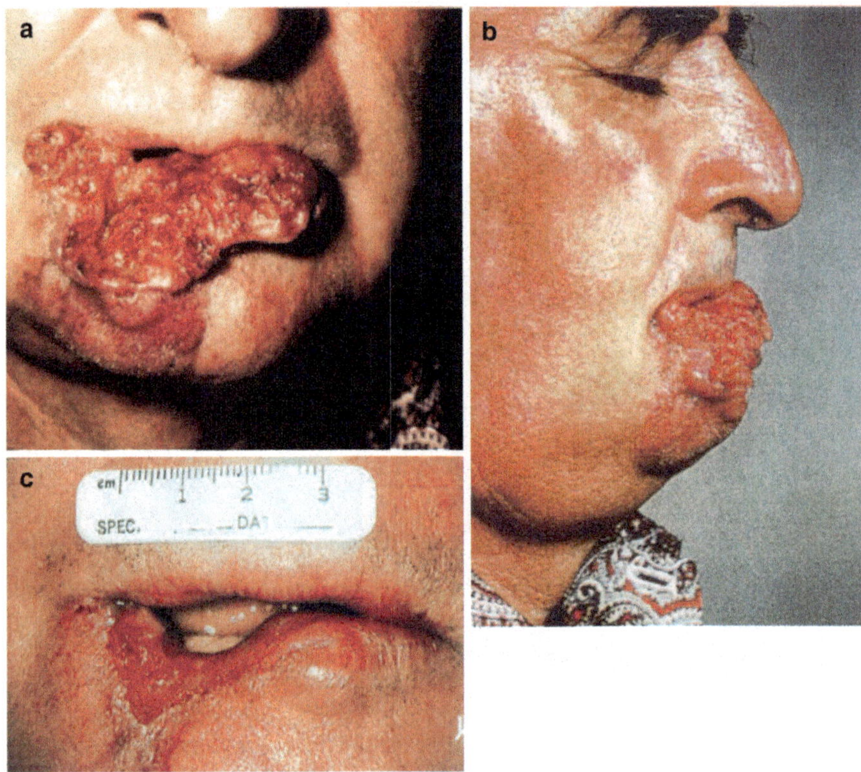

Fig. 1.5 (**a**) In 1974 the man photographed presented with a large cancer of his lower lip, previously untreated. (**b**) In this lateral view, it can be seen that the cancer involved the whole of his lower lip and had involved lymph nodes in the right side of his neck. (**c**) After 5 weeks of continuous chemotherapy given by slow infusion into both external carotid arteries, the lip cancer was much smaller. The large lymph nodes in his neck were also smaller. (**d**) After a break of 3 weeks, his lower lip was then treated by radiotherapy. The final result pictured showed no evidence of cancer in his lip. The lymph nodes in the right side of his neck were smaller but still enlarged. The nodes were resected in a block dissection. A small nest of cancer cells was detected in two of the resected lymph nodes. (**e**) The scars on his neck 6 months later. There was no evidence of any further cancer. (**f**) Like many patients who wait so long to first seek treatment, this man did not keep his follow-up appointments; but I happened to see him at a horserace meeting 12 years later. He remained well. This photograph was taken

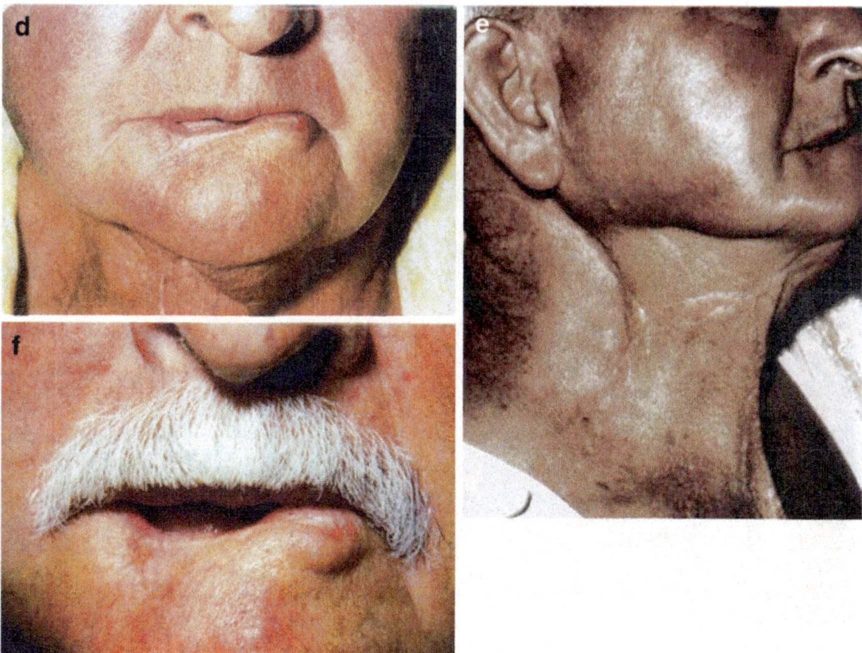

Fig. 1.5 (continued)

The regimen used consisted of Adriamycin, vincristine and methotrexate with intramuscular folinic acid.

After a month of chemotherapy continually infused into the cannula, the cancer had regressed significantly as seen in Fig. 1.7c.

After completion of follow-up radiotherapy that was commenced 3 weeks after finishing chemotherapy, the cancer had completely responded. A scar remained but there was no evidence of residual cancer, as shown in Fig. 1.7d. This lady remained well for 5 years before secondaries in her liver became evident.

To reduce the risk of later recurrence of cancer in the breast, or development of metastases, for apparent stage III breast cancers, we have since always recommended removal of the breast and post-operative systemic 'adjuvant' chemotherapy as routine.

In 1979, the woman shown in Fig. 1.8a, with a huge, bleeding, smelling breast cancer was brought to Sydney Hospital by ambulance. She was an alcoholic and had never before consulted a doctor. A cannula was inserted into her left subclavian artery to the opening of the internal mammary artery and she was treated with intra-arterial chemotherapy.

The regimen used consisted of Adriamycin, vincristine and methotrexate with intramuscular folinic acid. After a month of continuous intra-arterial infusion chemotherapy, the cancer had regressed as can be seen in Fig. 1.8b.

After a break of 3 weeks, this lady was then treated with radiotherapy to her breast and axilla. The result is shown in Fig. 1.8c.

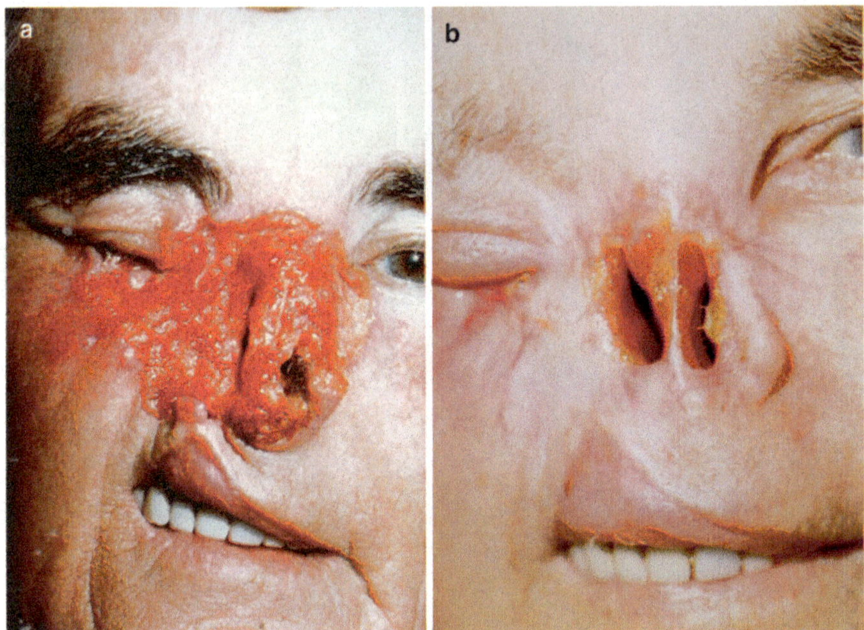

Fig. 1.6 (**a**) In August 1981, this lady was referred for treatment of her extensive BCC on her face. She had lived like a hermit in virtual isolation for many years. The extensive carcinoma destroying her nose and involving her right eye and right upper lip had never previously been treated. She presented for treatment because she was having difficulty with opening her right eye and some difficulty with eating. She had a fear of surgery but agreed to a trial of chemotherapy. Cannulae were inserted into both external carotid arteries and continuous intra-arterial infusion chemotherapy was administered using methotrexate, bleomycin, vincristine and actinomycin D in daily rotation for 4 weeks. (**b**) This is a photograph taken 2 weeks after completion of the intra-arterial chemotherapy. As the lady could see and eat better, she was satisfied with the result and declined to have any further treatment

After completion of treatment, there was no evidence of residual cancer in her breast. However, on admission, she had been found to have small liver metastases but they had not been causing her any symptoms. Her presenting symptoms of breast pain, bleeding and discomfort were relieved by the treatment given but she died 2 years later with liver metastases. At her death, there was no evidence of further recurrence in her breast.

In 1982, a 48-year-old lady presented with a 7 cm inflammatory-type medullary carcinoma in her left breast. The cancer was fixed to overlying red skin and deep tissues. It was treated with a similar regimen as was used in the patient discussed in Fig. 1.7.

The mass much reduced after a month of intra-arterial chemotherapy and further resolved after radiotherapy, but there remained thickened tissue attached to the skin in the region of the original cancer. This tissue was widely resected, and the resulting defect was repaired by a full-thickness rotation flap taken from over her latissimus dorsi muscle. No viable cancer cells were found in the resected fibrous tissue. She was then treated with systemic chemotherapy for 4 months. The photograph

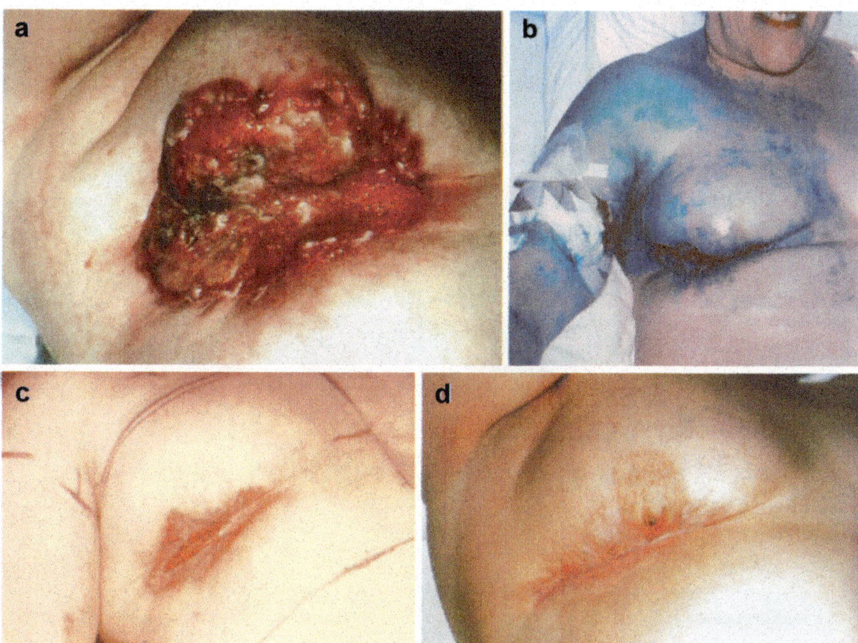

Fig. 1.7 (**a**) In 1976 this 56-year-old woman presented with this previously untreated cancer in her right breast. Because a cancer of this size would be most unlikely to be cured by surgery or by radiotherapy, it was decided to first treat her with continuous chemotherapy administered by slow intra-arterial infusion. (**b**) After a cannula had been inserted into the subclavian artery to the origin of the internal mammary artery, blue dye injected into the cannula confirmed that blood flow embraced the cancer and nodes in the axilla. (**c**) After a month of chemotherapy continually infused into the cannula, the cancer had regressed significantly. (**d**) After completion of follow-up radiotherapy that was commenced 3 weeks after finishing chemotherapy, the cancer had completely responded. A scar remained but there was no evidence of residual cancer. This lady remained well for 5 years before secondaries in her liver became evident. To reduce the risk of later recurrence of cancer in the breast, or development of metastases, for apparent stage III breast cancers, we have since always recommended removal of the breast and post-operative systemic 'adjuvant' chemotherapy as routine

(Fig. 1.9) shows the end result. The patient remains well and free from cancer at the time of writing, which is 27 years after her treatment.

In 1973, a 60-year-old oyster farmer with the previously untreated squamous cell cancer completely surrounding his lower right forearm, as shown in Fig. 1.10a, was referred to our Sydney Hospital Clinic. The forearm mass was fixed and enlarged hard lymph nodes were felt in his right axilla. A surgeon had advised him to have a forequarter amputation but the patient had refused.

A small cannula was inserted surgically into his right subclavian artery. Injection of patent blue dye confirmed that the axilla, arm and forearm were in the field of infusion.

After 6 weeks of continuous, slow chemotherapy infusion, the cancer had regressed, leaving a large but mobile shallow ulcer as seen in Fig. 1.10b. Biopsy

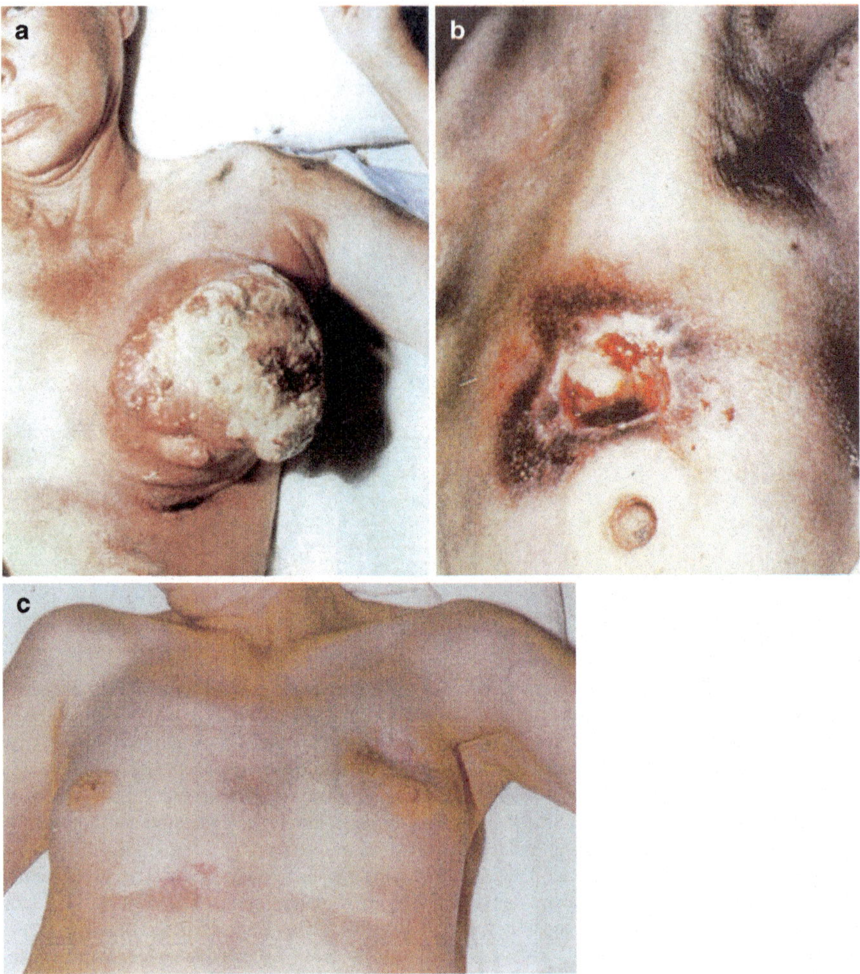

Fig. 1.8 (**a**) In 1979 the woman shown with a huge bleeding, smelling breast cancer was brought to Sydney Hospital by ambulance. She was an alcoholic and had never before consulted a doctor. A cannula was inserted into her left subclavian artery to the opening of the internal mammary artery and she was treated with intra-arterial chemotherapy. The regimen used consisted of Adriamycin, vincristine and methotrexate with intramuscular folinic acid. (**b**) After a month of continuous intra-arterial infusion chemotherapy, the cancer had regressed as can be seen in this photograph. (**c**) After completion of follow-up radiotherapy, there was no evidence of residual cancer in her breast. However on admission, she had been found to have small liver metastases, but they had not been causing her any symptoms. Her presenting symptoms of breast pain, bleeding and discomfort were relieved by the treatment given but she died 2 years later with liver metastases. At her death there was no evidence of cancer in her breast

confirmed that some squamous cancer cells were still present in the wound (the regimen used was bleomycin 15 mg and methotrexate 50 mg on alternate days for 1 week and then methotrexate daily with systemic folinic acid).

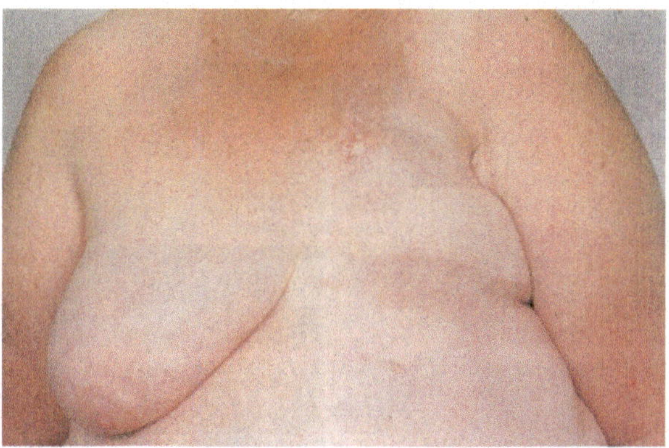

Fig. 1.9 In 1982 a 48-year-old lady presented with a 7 cm inflammatory-type medullary carcinoma in her left breast. The cancer was fixed to overlying red skin and deep tissues. It was treated with a similar regimen as was used in the patient discussed in Fig. 1.7. The mass was much reduced after a month of intra-arterial chemotherapy and further resolved after radiotherapy, but there remained thickened tissue attached to the skin in the region of the original cancer. This tissue was widely resected and the resulting defect was repaired by a full-thickness rotation flap taken from over her latissimus dorsi muscle. No viable cancer cells were found in the resected fibrous tissue. She was then treated with systemic chemotherapy for 4 months. The photograph shows the end result. The patient remains well and free from cancer at the time of writing, which is 27 years after her treatment

After resection of the residual ulcer that still contained some cancer cells, tendons and bone were exposed in the open wound as seen in Fig. 1.10c.

To get full-thickness skin cover with some protective fat, the forearm wound was buried under a bridge of lower abdominal skin as shown in Fig. 1.10d.

A split skin graft was applied to cover the abdominal wound from which the full-thickness skin and subcutaneous tissues had been taken. After 4 weeks, the full-thickness abdominal wall skin was well vascularised and growing over the wound; it was then detached from his abdomen.

The axillary lymph nodes were much smaller but still enlarged. An axillary dissection was completed. Cancer cells were found in two of the resected lymph nodes.

Figure 1.10e shows the final result 1 year later.

For 12 years this man always brought a bucket of oysters when he came for follow-up visits. He claimed that we deserved these not only for saving his arm but for another personal reason. Whenever he went to his local village pub, there was always someone who would want to see his arm covered by abdominal skin and his abdomen with a split skin graft. He was always supplied with free beers. We were sorry to learn that this delightful man died after a heart attack 15 years after his operation, but he had no evidence of residual cancer.

The angiograms shown in Fig. 1.11 show just two of several limb sarcomas treated initially by intra-arterial induction chemotherapy in the Sydney unit. Increasingly, a team approach was developed. Whenever bone had to be resected, and a bone or joint replaced, this was performed by our orthopaedic surgeon colleague (the late Professor William Marsden).

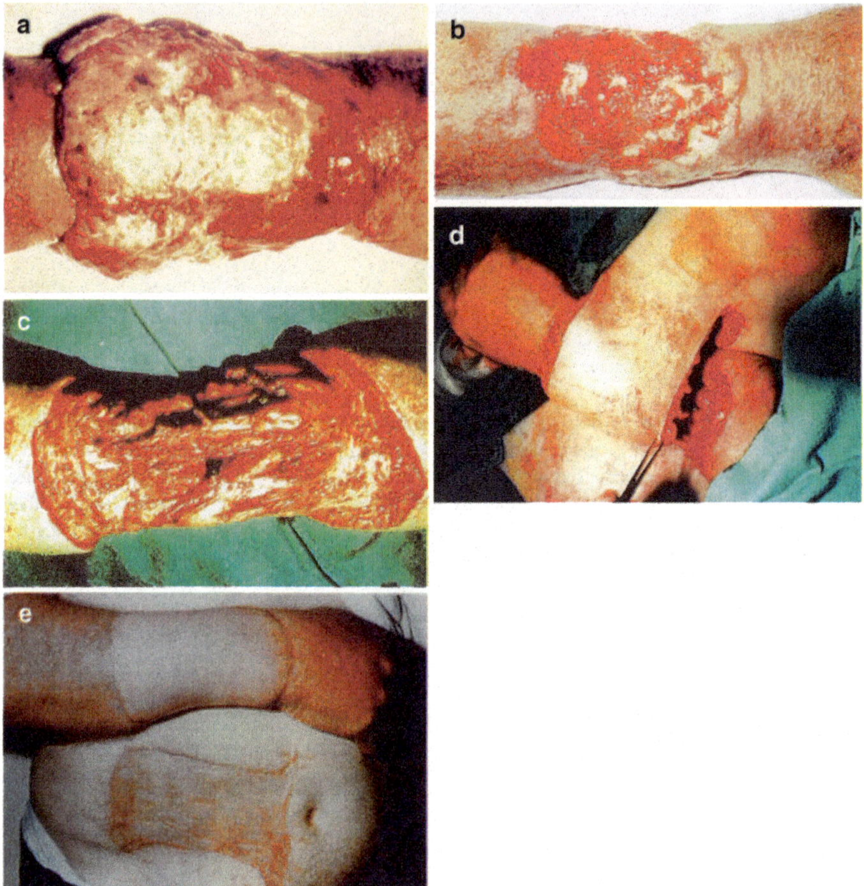

Fig. 1.10 (**a**) In 1973 a 60-year-old oyster farmer presented with this previously untreated squamous cell cancer completely surrounding his lower right forearm, as shown in the photograph. The forearm mass was fixed and enlarged hard lymph nodes were felt in his right axilla. A surgeon had advised him to have a forequarter amputation but the patient had refused. A small cannula was inserted surgically into his right subclavian artery. Injection of patent blue dye confirmed that the axilla, arm and forearm were in the field of infusion. (The regimen used was bleomycin 15 mg and methotrexate 50 mg on alternate days for 6 week and then methotrexate daily with systemic folinic acid.) (**b**) After 6 weeks of continuous, slow chemotherapy infusion, the cancer had regressed, leaving a large but mobile shallow ulcer as seen in this photo. Biopsy confirmed that some squamous cancer cells were still present in the tissue. (**c**) After resection of the residual ulcer that still contained some cancer cells, tendons and bone were exposed in the open wound as seen in this photo. (**d**) To get full-thickness skin cover with some protective fat, the forearm wound was buried under a bridge of lower abdominal skin. A split skin graft was applied to the cover the abdominal wound from which the full-thickness skin and subcutaneous tissues had been taken. After 4 weeks, the full-thickness abdominal wall skin was well vascularised and growing over the wound; it was then detached from his abdomen. The axillary lymph nodes were much smaller but still enlarged. An axillary dissection was completed. Cancer cells were found in two of the resected lymph nodes. (**e**) The final result 1 year later

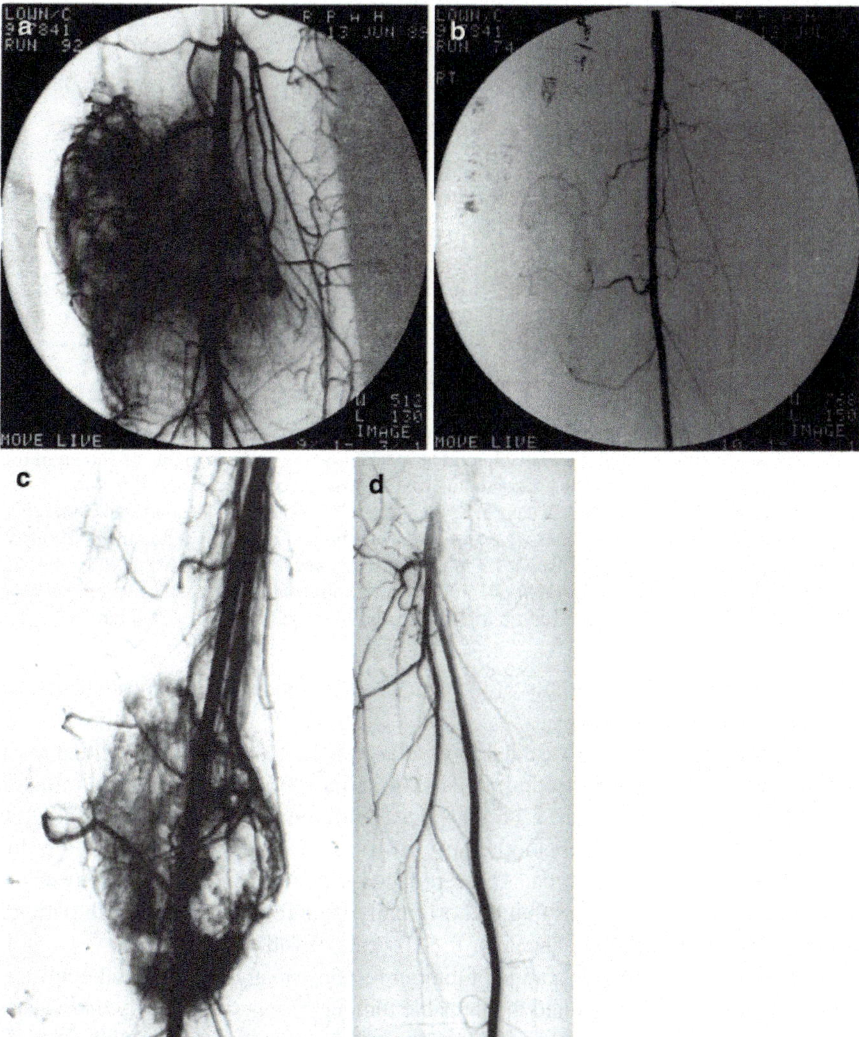

Fig. 1.11 (**a, b**) These illustrations show the vascularity of a large synoviosarcoma of popliteal fossa before and after 4 weeks of continuous slow intra-arterial chemotherapy infusion into the femoral artery. (**c, d**) These illustrations show a similar tumour blush before and after 3 weeks intra-arterial chemotherapy infusion as induction treatment of this malignant fibrous histiocytoma. These reduced cancers were then easily resected without the limb amputations that had originally been recommended. Both patients remained well and without cancer for the 10 years of follow-up

After some years of surgically inserting intra-arterial catheters, a radiological technique of catheter insertion was developed by our vascular radiologist (Dr. Richard Waugh). Closer liaison was developed with our pathologist (Professor Stan

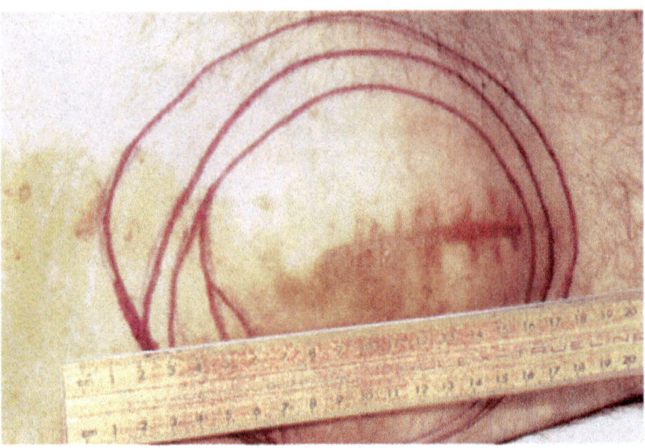

Fig. 1.12 In some cases, another indication of tumour response to regional chemotherapy can be seen by drawing *lines* around the palpable tumour periphery at weekly intervals as shown in this photograph. The *circles* around this liposarcoma were drawn at weekly intervals after commencing intra-arterial chemotherapy. Three weeks after completion of continuous intra-arterial chemotherapy, the residual small necrotic mass was excised. The regimen used was Adriamycin 20 mgm, actinomycin D 0.5 mg and vincristine 0.5 mg on alternate days with oral hydroxyurea 1G and cyclophosphamide 50 mg on day 4. For 6 months systemic adjuvant chemotherapy was given post-operatively. The patient was followed-up for 10 years without evidence of residual tumour

McCarthy) who advised initially of the cancer or sarcoma type and subsequently its response to the chemotherapy.

Figure 1.11a, b show the vascularity of a large synoviosarcoma of popliteal fossa before and after 4 weeks of continuous slow intra-arterial chemotherapy infusion into the femoral artery. Figure 1.11c, d show a similar tumour blush before and after 3 weeks of intra-arterial chemotherapy infusion as induction treatment of this malignant fibrous histiocytoma. These reduced cancers were then easily resected without the limb amputations that had originally been recommended. Both patients remained well and without cancer for the 10 years of follow-up.

In some cases, another indication of tumour response to regional chemotherapy can be seen by drawing lines around the palpable tumour periphery at weekly intervals as shown in Fig. 1.12. The circles around this liposarcoma were drawn at weekly intervals after commencing intra-arterial chemotherapy. Three weeks after completion of continuous intra-arterial chemotherapy, the residual small necrotic mass was excised. The patient was followed-up for 10 years without evidence of residual tumour.

The regimen used was Adriamycin 20 mg, actinomycin D 0.5 mg and vincristine 0.5 mg on alternate days with oral hydroxyurea 1 g and cyclophosphamide 50 mg on day 4.

For 6 months systemic adjuvant chemotherapy was given post-operatively.

CAT scans can also give a good indication of tumour response to chemotherapy in some patients. The CAT scans in Fig. 1.13 show a malignant fibrous histiosarcoma in a thigh before commencing intra-arterial chemotherapy (Fig. 1.13a) and after 3 weeks of continuous chemotherapy when the mass was distinctly smaller (Fig. 1.13b).

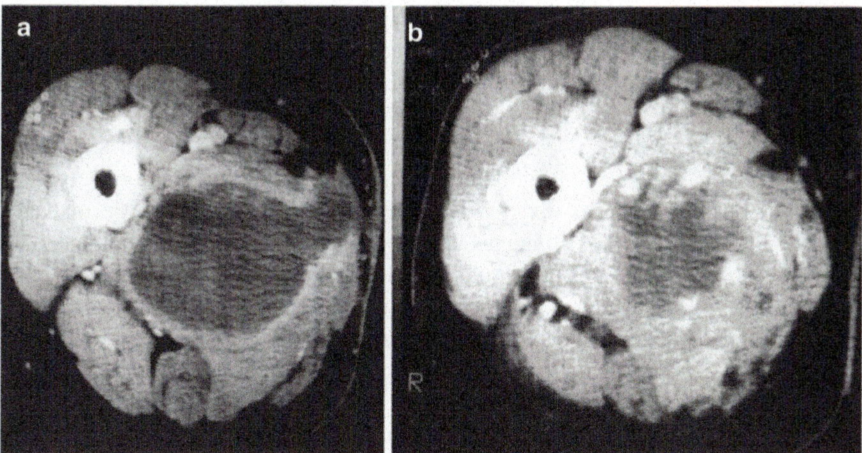

Fig. 1.13 CAT scans can also give a good indication of tumour response to chemotherapy in some patients. These CAT scans show a malignant fibrous histiosarcoma in a thigh before commencing intra-arterial chemotherapy (**a**) and after 3 weeks of continuous chemotherapy when the mass was distinctly smaller (**b**)

1.5   Principles and Practice of Induction Chemotherapy

In summary, it has been established that chemotherapy alone is unlikely to totally eradicate malignant cells in a large or aggressive tumour mass, but in most cases initial *induction chemotherapy* will induce changes in tumour size and aggressive characteristics prior to subsequent management. The residual partly or wholly damaged or necrotic primary tumour can then often be eradicated by operative surgery or radiation therapy or by a combination of both radiotherapy and surgery. It is because at presentation the tumour has a good blood supply, uncompromised by previous radiotherapy or surgery, that chemotherapy, being carried to the tumour by blood, has a greater therapeutic potential in initially treating such locally advanced tumours. Chemotherapy is much less likely to be effective if the tumour blood supply had been compromised by previous operative surgery or irradiation-induced vascular damage [3].

By definition, then induction chemotherapy is chemotherapy used as the first modality of an integrated treatment programme. The simplest and most readily available method of administering induction chemotherapy is by systemic delivery, but in some situations, a greater chemotherapy impact can be achieved by delivering a more concentrated dose of effective anticancer agents more directly to the region containing the cancer. This regional chemotherapy is usually best achieved by delivering the chemotherapy directly into the arterial blood supply of the cancer. However, intra-thoracic, intra-peritoneal or intrathecal delivery may be more appropriate in some situations.

To achieve an advantage by intra-arterial delivery, the tumour must be fully contained in tissue supplied by one or more arteries that can be effectively cannulated and infused. The cancer must also be of a type that will respond better to concentrated doses of anticancer agents over a limited period of possibly up to 4 or 5 weeks and the most appropriate agents to be used must be effective in the state in which they are delivered. Some agents are not active in the state in which they are delivered and do not become active until changed by passage through other tissues, especially the liver. The advantages of intra-arterial delivery must also outweigh any increased risks of regional toxicity. Effective regional delivery can be managed safely only by experienced clinicians with appropriate specialised equipment. This will reduce risk of mistakes that could be made by these more exacting techniques of delivery. Similar results can be achieved using systemic chemotherapy but the doses required will inevitably cause much greater systemic toxicity.

Induction chemotherapy by systemic delivery is most appropriate in treating tumours without a single artery or limited arteries of supply or when the cancers are not contained in a single body cavity. Systemic delivery is also more appropriate when preferred agents are not activated until modified in body tissues (such as cyclophosphamide or DTIC); when satisfactory responses can be achieved more easily by systemic delivery; when technical skills and facilities for regional delivery are not available; or when the patient's general health, poor cooperation or long-term prognosis precludes the additional complexity of regional delivery.

Intra-arterial infusion is most likely to have advantages in treating locally advanced malignancies in regions supplied by a single or perhaps two arteries of supply that can be safely cannulated. These include the head and neck, limbs, some invasive stomach cancers and some breast cancers. Primary liver cancers and some liver metastases, some cancers in the pelvis and some pancreatic malignancies may also respond well to initial direct chemotherapy infusion. These are currently the subject of several studies.

The more complex techniques of isolated perfusion, stop-flow infusion, closed circuit perfusion, chemo-filtration infusion and closed circuit infusion [12–16] are aimed at achieving even greater localised initial tissue concentrations of chemotherapy than simple intra-arterial infusion. These more complex techniques are described in this book but should remain the subject of ongoing studies in highly specialised units.

Malignancies such as melanoma, some sarcomas or pancreatic cancers usually show a poor response to standard safe concentrations of chemotherapy delivered either by standard systemic or intra-arterial delivery but may be made to respond more significantly by the more complex delivery techniques that achieve tumour exposure to more concentrated and higher dose chemotherapy for a short period.

The limitation to dose and concentration of safe chemotherapy given by systemic administration is usually the risk of systemic side effects, especially bone marrow suppression. However, certain conditions are necessary for intra-arterial chemotherapy to be justified. These include:

(a) The primary tumour must be supplied by blood vessels (usually one or two) that can be safely cannulated so allowing the greatest potential impact of dose and concentration of the chemotherapy to be delivered by direct infusion into the artery, or arteries of supply. Unless the whole tumour periphery is effectively infused, the desired impact on the whole tumour mass will not be achieved.

(b) Only those agents that are effective against the tumour in the state in which they are administered can have an enhanced antitumour effect if given by regional delivery. For example, *cyclophosphamide* is not in its active state until it has passed through the liver and become activated. If infused into a peripheral artery before it has become activated by passage through the liver, there would be no additional benefit [17].

(c) With some agents to treat some tumours (e.g. methotrexate used to treat some osteosarcomas in young people), an effective and adequate tumouricidal dose can be safely given by the more simple means of intravenous delivery. There would be no need to deliver such dosage by a more complex intra-arterial delivery system [18].

(d) For some cancers a much greater dose/concentration of agents, than can be given either systemically or by intra-arterial infusion, would be needed to achieve a significant tumour response. It is for these tumours that an even more concentrated regional delivery system has it greatest potential. Melanoma is an example. Melanoma is a highly chemo-resistant malignancy even to more concentrated doses than can be given by intra-arterial infusion. A much more highly concentrated dose of chemotherapy is usually needed to achieve melanoma cell destruction. To achieve such chemotherapy concentration, a closed circuit perfusion or closed circuit infusion technique is required. Closed circuit perfusion or infusion achieves protection of general body tissues with a greatly increased regional chemotherapy concentration. With closed circuit perfusion or closed circuit infusion, the time of exposure must be limited, but the rest of the body is protected from the high concentration and high doses of agents infused [12, 14]. Naturally, regional side effects in infused tissues are inevitable from the more highly concentrated chemotherapy.

(e) Administration of regional chemotherapy requires time, effort, expense, special skills and specialised equipment. It also usually requires prolonged hospital inpatient stay. Although there is likely to be less systemic toxicity, there will be more local toxicity in the region treated. A decision must be made as to whether the patient's likely ultimate long-term survival will justify these more complicated, expensive and time-consuming procedures even if the local regional tumour can be eradicated.

Figures 1.14 and 1.15 illustrate the different impacts on local tissue through intra-arterial delivery.

As was first noticed many years ago, and reported by Klopp [4] and by Bierman [5], there is a greater reaction in the tissues supplied with blood by an artery that had been inadvertently injected with chemotherapy than if the same dose of the drug had been given into a vein. The redness and reaction in this patient's right hand (Fig. 1.14) after accidental injection into the artery in the cubital fossa is greater than in her left hand.

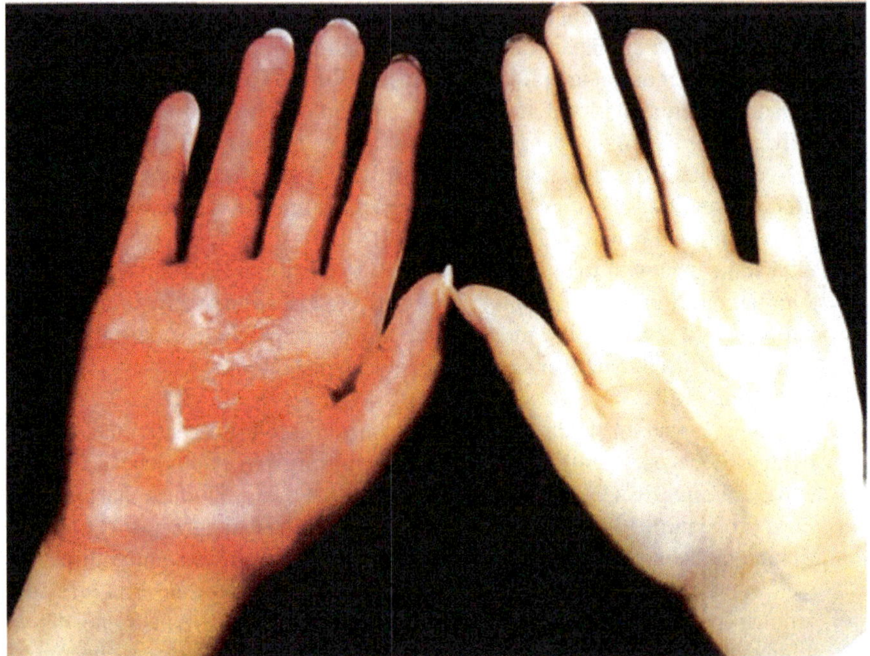

Fig. 1.14 The redness and reaction in this patient's right hand after accidental injection into the artery in the cubital fossa is greater than in her left hand

In treating a cancer on the right side of the face of the man, in Fig. 1.15, by intra-arterial chemotherapy, the chemotherapy infused into the artery supplying blood to the right side of his scalp caused hair loss on the right side of his head. There was also a red reaction in the mucosa of the right side of his mouth and tongue. This confirms that the chemotherapy was more effective in the tissues supplied by the infused artery.

The mucosal reaction soon settles after completion of chemotherapy infusion and hair lost in this way re-grows some weeks later unless follow-up radiotherapy is given to the region.

1.6   Precautions in the Use of Regional Chemotherapy

Some people have used intra-arterial chemotherapy without first learning the importance of keeping a close vigil to be sure the cannula stays in the correct position and does not stream or slip into an artery supplying blood to another tissue not containing the cancer.

The need for very close and diligent supervision otherwise mistakes will be made is illustrated in Fig. 1.16. The damage done to normal tissues in this patient's thigh was because it had not been noticed that the chemotherapy had been flowing

Fig. 1.15 In treating a cancer on the right side of the face of this man by intra-arterial chemotherapy, the chemotherapy infused into the artery supplying blood to the right side of his scalp caused hair loss on the right side of his head. There was also a *red* reaction in the mucosa of the right side of his mouth and tongue. This confirms that the chemotherapy was more effective in the tissues supplied by the infused artery

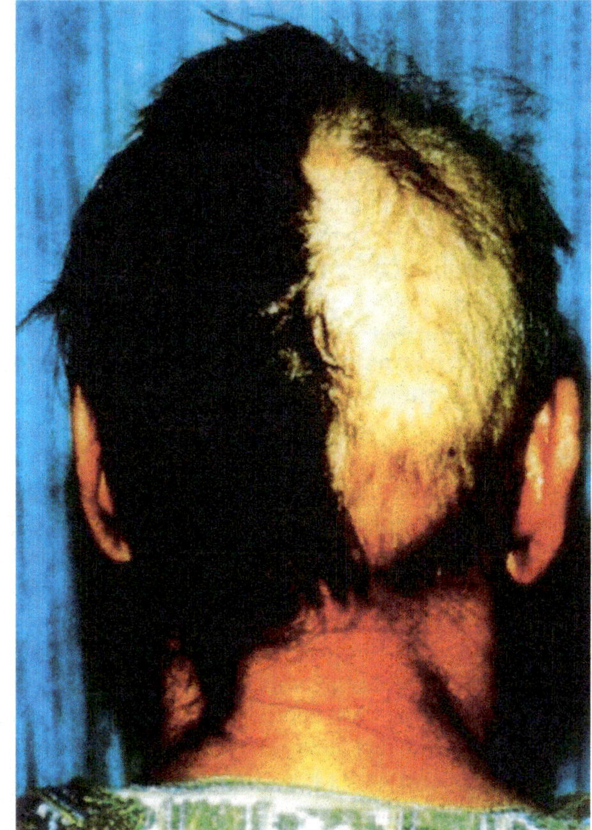

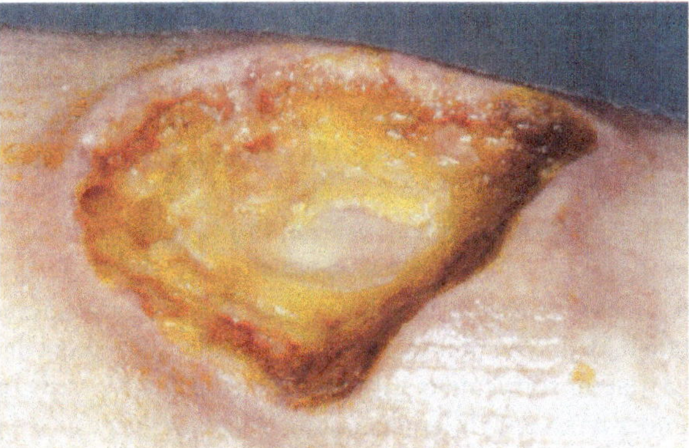

Fig. 1.16 Illustrates the need for very close and diligent supervision otherwise mistakes will be made. The damage done to normal tissues in this patient's thigh was because it had not been noticed that the chemotherapy had been flowing into a branch of the artery into which it had previously been placed. Without the services of well-trained and experienced nurses to constantly watch for such errors, intra-arterial infusions of chemotherapy can cause such problems. This is an example of why intra-arterial chemotherapy is not practised in some cancer clinics without these facilities

into a branch of the artery into which it had previously been placed. A red blush had appeared in the skin of this patient's thigh but the significance of this was not understood. Disulphan blue or patent blue dye injected into the infusion cannula at an early stage would have confirmed that the cannula position needed adjustment before serious tissue damage had occurred.

Without the services of well-trained and experienced nurses to constantly watch for such errors, intra-arterial infusions of chemotherapy can cause such problems. This is an example of why intra-arterial chemotherapy is not practised in some cancer clinics without these facilities.

1.7   Criticisms of Intra-arterial Chemotherapy: Valid and Invalid [19]

Valid

1. It is technically more demanding to administer any form of regional chemotherapy as compared to systemic chemotherapy. Experienced and skilled surgical or vascular radiological staff as well as skilled and experienced nursing-staff are mandatory, otherwise mistakes will be made. The administration and rate of flow of agents requires constant supervision to ensure that the flow is being delivered to the correct region and to detect any early evidence of damaging side effects or misadventure with the infusion.
2. Selection of the most appropriate agents and combination of agents in an integrated regimen and timing and rate of flow for each agent requires special knowledge and experience [20].
3. Cannulation of arteries in any part of the body, particularly in arteriosclerotic or elderly patients, carries some risk of arterial damage. Dislodgement of plaques, thrombosis, aneurisms, bleeding and infection are all possibilities that require constant monitoring.
4. Dislodgement of the catheter or streaming of flow into a branch artery must be constantly and carefully monitored and corrected if necessary.
5. The total cost of treatment is increased requiring special staff and prolonged use of inpatient hospital beds.
6. Selection of patients who best benefit from intra-arterial infusion of chemotherapy requires experienced judgement and skill.
7. Appropriate follow-up treatment and its timing be it radiotherapy, surgery or adjuvant chemotherapy or a combination of these require judgement and experience.
8. Randomised trials are difficult to organise due to the relative rarity of such patients' different tumour types and different circumstances and needs for each patient.

Invalid

1. In treating a locally advanced cancer that may also have systemic lesions, for example, breast cancer, a criticism has been made that chemotherapy needs to circulate throughout the body. The need to circulate systemically is true of course; however, after the first pass of concentrated chemotherapy through the

primary lesion, the flow then does become systemic, but there has been advantage in a more concentrated initial (first pass) chemotherapy impact on the primary lesion. Additional systemic chemotherapy may also be required.

2. Some agents, especially Adriamycin, have been considered too toxic for regional infusion. This is simply a matter of administering an appropriate dosage in this more concentrated infusion.

3. Critics have claimed that randomised studies have shown no advantage in administering intra-arterial chemotherapy to an advanced primary cancer. For reasons stated above, few truly comparable randomised studies have been made, and the majority of those that have been attempted have shown advantage in using regional infusion as induction chemotherapy [19].

After initial scepticism, the principle of additional advantage of delivery of induction chemotherapy by intra-arterial infusion has now been accepted in most comprehensive cancer treatment centres. It is now practised in medical, surgical, radiological, orthopaedic, gynaecological, urological, gastrointestinal and neurological clinics in many countries as will be described in the following chapters. As has been recommended on previous occasions, a team approach involving a medical oncologist, a radiation oncologist, a surgical oncologist and the appropriate system specialist and other experienced nursing or paramedical health contributors should improve results of treatment for people with advanced localised cancers [20, 21].

References

1. Stephens FO, Aigner KR. Basics of oncology. Berlin: Springer; 2009.
2. Helman P, Sealy R, Malkerbe E, Anderson J. The treatment of locally advanced cancer of the head and neck. Lancet. 1965;1:128.
3. Stephens FO. Intra-arterial perfusion of the chemotherapeutic agents methotrexate and epodyl in patients with advanced localised carcinomata recurrent after radiotherapy. Aust N Z J Surg. 1970;39:371–9.
4. Klopp CT, Alford TC, Bateman G, et al. Fractionated intra-arterial chemotherapy with methyl bis amine hydrochloride: a preliminary report. Ann Surg. 1950;132:811–32.
5. Bierman HR, Byron RL, Miller ER, et al. Effects of intra-arterial administration of nitrogen mustard. Am J Med. 1950;8:535.
6. Lundberg WG. In: Becker FF, editor. Cancer – a comprehensive treatise: chemotherapy, vol. 5. New York: Plenum; 1977.
7. Stephens FO. "Crab" care and cancer chemotherapy. Med J Aust. 1976;2:41–6.
8. Jussawalla JD, Shetty PA. Experiences with intra-arterial chemotherapy for head and neck cancer. J Surg Oncol. 1978;10:33–7.
9. Helman P, Bennet MB. Intra-arterial cytotoxic chemotherapy and x-ray therapy for cancer of the breast. Br J Surg. 1968;55:419–23.
10. Von Essen CF, Joseph LBM, Simin GT, Singh AD, Singh SP. Sequential chemotherapy and radiation therapy of buccal mucosa in south India: methods and preliminary results. Am J Roentgenol Radium Ther Nucl Med. 1968;102:530–40.
11. Stephens FO. The case for a name change from neoadjuvant chemotherapy to induction chemotherapy. Cancer. 1989;63(7):1245–6.
12. Creech O, Krementz ET, Ryan RT, Winblad JM. Chemotherapy of cancer: regional perfusion utilizing an extracorporeal circuit. Ann Surg. 1958;148:616.

13. Aigner KR, Gailhofer S. High dose MMC – aortic stop-flow infusion (ASI) with versus without chemo-filtration – a comparison of toxic side effects. Reg Cancer Treat. 1993;6 Suppl 1:3–4.

14. Aigner KR. Intra-arterial infusion: overview and novel approaches. Semin Surg Oncol. 1998;14(3):248–53.

15. Aigner KR, Muller H, Walther H, Link KH. Drug filtration in high-dose chemotherapy. Contrib Oncol. 1988;29:261–80. 6.

16. Thompson JC, Gianotsos M. Isolated limb perfusion form: effectiveness and toxicity of cis-platinum compared with that of melphalan and other drugs. World J Surg. 1992;16(2):227–33.

17. Harker G, Stephens FO. A report on the efficacy of cyclophosphamide administered intra-arterially in sheep bearing epidermal squamous carcinoma. Reg Cancer Treat. 1992;4:170–4.

18. Jaffe N. Comparison of intra-arterial cis-diamminedichloroplatinum II with high-dose methotrexate and citrovorum factor rescue in the treatment of primary osteosarcoma. J Clin Oncol. 1985;3:1102–4.

19. Stephens FO. Intra-arterial induction chemotherapy, objections and difficulties, true and false. Oncol Rep. 1996;3:409–12.

20. Stephens FO. The place of chemotherapy in the treatment of advanced squamous carcinoma in the head and neck and other situations. Med J Aust. 1974;2:587–92.

21. Stephens FO. Developments in surgical oncology: induction (neoadjuvant) chemotherapy – the state of the art. Clin Oncol. 1990;2:168–72.

The Principle of Dose Response in Antineoplastic Drug Delivery

2

Maurie Markman

2.1 Drug Exposure During Active Cycling of Malignant Cells

It is reasonable to state that actively cycling cells (both malignant and normal cell populations) are most vulnerable to the effects of cytotoxic chemotherapeutic agents [1, 2]. Thus, it is not surprising that acute leukemia and high-grade lymphomas are particularly sensitive to such agents, compared to the more slowly dividing and cycling solid tumors (e.g., colon, lung, breast). This phenomenon also explains the sensitivity of bone marrow elements and the mucosa of the gastrointestinal track to these agents, compared to, for example, muscle or fat cells (Table 2.1).

2.2 Adequacy of Drug Delivery by Capillary Flow

Another important principle in this clinical arena is the *essential role of blood supply* in defining the impact of dose. Substantial portions of large poorly vascularized tumor masses, or previously radiated malignant lesions, will almost certainly be exposed to far lower drug concentrations compared to cancer receiving adequate blood supply. Further, in the absence of adequate nutrients, malignant cell populations are less likely to be actively cycling, further decreasing their vulnerability to cytotoxic antineoplastic drugs.

Relevant support for the importance of the adequacy of blood supply in impacting outcome in malignant disease is provided by extensive retrospective experience in women with advanced ovarian cancer [3]. These nonrandomized experiences have documented the benefits of primary surgical resection of advanced epithelial ovarian cancer, in patients with the smallest residual tumor volumes at the initiation

M. Markman
Cancer Treatment Centers of America, Eastern Regional Medical Center,
1331 East Wyoming Avenue, Philadelphia, PA 19124, USA
e-mail: maurie.markman@ctca-hope.com

© Springer-Verlag Berlin Heidelberg 2016
K.R. Aigner, F.O. Stephens (eds.), *Induction Chemotherapy*,
DOI 10.1007/978-3-319-28773-7_2

Table 2.1 Issues influencing the relevance of dose intensity in the delivery of antineoplastic drug therapy

1. Cell cycle specificity of the agents
2. Cell cycling times for particular types of cancer
3. Adequacy of capillary blood flow (and drug delivery) to the site(s) of the cancer
4. Presence of poorly vascularized large tumor masses
5. Relative importance of *peak drug levels* versus *sustained concentrations* (area under the concentration versus time curve) in optimizing the *therapeutic* and increasing the *toxic* effects of the agent
6. Relative importance of *dose* versus *schedule* of individual agents and combination regimens in producing both therapeutic and toxic effects
7. Short-term and long-term side effects of dose-intensive regimens
8. Availability of supportive care medications to prevent or ameliorate toxicity (e.g., emesis, bone marrow suppression) of dose-intensive therapeutic regimens
9. Potential for employing regional dose intensity (designed to minimize systemic side effects while maximizing local drug exposure)

of primary cytotoxic chemotherapy having the greatest opportunity to achieve both a clinically or surgically defined complete response.

Note: In the past, surgical responses were routinely documented in ovarian cancer at the time of a second-look surgical reassessment following the completion of the primary chemotherapy regimen in the setting of no clinical evidence of persistent cancer. This surgery is not routinely performed at the present time due to the absence of data demonstrating the information generated at this invasive procedure that favorably impacts outcome in the malignancy.

The essential argument is that with the removal of large (or even small) volume macroscopic cancer, the residual tumor cells are able to be exposed to adequate concentrations of the cytotoxic chemotherapeutic agents delivered by capillary flow to achieve maximal clinical benefit.

2.3 Drug Delivery and Induction ("Neoadjuvant") Chemotherapy

More recent experiences in several tumor types, including cancers of the breast and ovary, have suggested an alternative approach, initially employing chemotherapy to cytoreduce a large tumor mass (induction or "neoadjuvant" chemotherapy), followed by surgical resection of residual macroscopic lesions, with the subsequent continuation of chemotherapy [4, 5]. In this setting, the first goal of chemotherapy is to reduce the size of malignant masses to permit a more adequate surgical resection.

Again, the ultimate aim of this strategy is to optimize exposure of the tumor to effective concentrations of the antineoplastic drug therapy. Of interest, phase 3 trial data reveal the essential equivalence in outcome associated with either primary surgical cytoreduction versus the induction chemotherapy approach in large volume epithelial ovarian cancer [6].

2.4 Evaluation of the Impact of Dose Intense Cytotoxic Chemotherapy Regimens

Investigators have attempted a variety of strategies to quantify the impact of dose and dose intensity, in favorably influencing outcome in malignant disease. One approach has been to consider the *total concentration of drug delivered over a defined unit of time* (e.g., mg/m^2/week) as a measure of the effect of dose intensity [7, 8]. While in some clinical settings, retrospective evaluations of nonrandomized experiences have suggested improved outcomes associated with greater dose intensity, subsequently conducted phase 3 studies have often failed to confirm the favorable benefits of these strategies [9, 10].

One issue associated with any analysis of a nonrandomized experience is that patients able to receive the most dose-intensive strategies are highly likely to have the most favorable performance status, a clinical factor well known to be independently associated with superior outcomes.

Another issue with these measures of dose intensity is the assumption in the mathematical calculations employed to generate the measurement that all drugs are of equivalent efficacy and that the effect of dose intensity is identical for the several drugs utilized in a particular regimen. In fact, there is unfortunately often little (if any) empirical evidence to support this conclusion, potentially weakening the relevance of such analyses.

2.5 High-Dose Chemotherapy

High-dose chemotherapy programs with bone marrow or peripheral progenitor cell support have been demonstrated to play a major role in the management of hematologic malignancies, including acute leukemia and both Hodgkin's and non-Hodgkin's lymphomas.

Nonrandomized experiences have also suggested the favorable impact of a variety of high-dose chemotherapy regimens in several solid tumors, including cancers of the breast and ovary. However, with the exception of germ cell malignancies, there is currently no solid evidence for the favorable impact of high-dose chemotherapy regimens in the management of the solid tumors [11, 12].

Several reasons can be proposed for the inability of high-dose chemotherapy strategies to improve outcome in this setting, including (as previously noted) the potential inadequacy of drug delivery in the presence of large tumor masses and (perhaps most important) the genuinely modest ability to actually *intensify* the dose of systemically administered antineoplastic drugs without the development of unacceptable toxicity.

In fact, most "high-dose chemotherapy" regimens have only been able to substantially increase the concentration of cytotoxic agents whose dose-limiting side effect is bone marrow suppression (e.g., alkylating agents, etoposide, carboplatin). Where other adverse events' effects predominate (e.g., neuropathy, cardiac, renal toxicity), effective dose intensification is problematic. Further, even where it is possible to increase the dose of an administrated antineoplastic agent, this is generally limited to several fold higher concentrations, as serious side effects other than bone marrow suppression generally appear when these modest escalations are exceeded.

In concluding this section, it is important to note the likely explanation for the frequent favorable reports of high-dose chemotherapy programs in nonrandomized phase 2 trials or retrospective examinations of individual institutional experiences. As previously noted in the setting of dose-intensive strategies not requiring bone marrow support, the patients receiving high-dose chemotherapy regimens almost certainly have a superior performance status and less comorbidity compared to individuals who would *not be selected* to undergo such an intensive therapeutic strategy [13].

Thus, an observed favorable outcome that may appear to result from a particular therapeutic regimen may, in fact, have been due completely (or partially) to *selection bias* in the patients chosen to receive the therapeutic program. With rare exceptions, only data generated from well-designed randomized trials can distinguish genuine clinical benefit from selection bias among the population of individuals managed with a particular strategy. It is also important to note that "selection bias" in the context of documenting the superiority of a dose-intensive therapeutic strategy is appropriately considered "excellent clinical judgment" in the context of the delivery of medical care.

2.6 Optimal Dose Delivery

The general concept of the delivery of a biologically effective concentration of an antineoplastic agent has been highlighted in the discussion of the adequacy of blood supply to the malignant cell population. A related concept is that of the administration of the *optimal dose* in a particular setting. Unfortunately, similar to the situation with defining the necessary dose and concentration to produce a desired cytotoxic effect, it is usually quite difficult to truly determine the optimal dose either for an individual patient or within a population with a specific malignancy.

The optimal dose of an antineoplastic agent can be considered that dose which results in a maximal favorable clinical effect while producing an acceptable degree of toxicity. While one might consider the optimal dose to simply be the highest dose that can be administered with tolerable side effects, in a limited number of settings it has actually been shown that there is a clinically apparent plateau in the degree of tumor cell kill achieved when an individual antineoplastic agent is delivered in a specific setting, and higher concentrations fail to result in further tumor cell kill, but do increase toxicity.

For example, in recurrent ovarian cancer, retrospective data reveal that when single agent carboplatin is administered in the second-line setting, there is an increase in the objective response rate with increasing concentrations up to a calculated carboplatin AUC (area of the concentration versus time curve) of 4 or 5 [14]. Beyond this AUC, the percentage of responding patients does not increase, but hematologic side effects can become severe. Unfortunately, such data regarding individual drugs in specific cancers is uncommon. However, this experience confirms the potential relevance of this issue in routine disease management.

It is also important to note the complexity associated with determining the optimal drug doses for individual agents in a combination chemotherapy regimen, particularly when the drugs produce overlapping toxicities. Further, by reducing the dose of one agent, to permit the administration of a second, the degree of tumor cell kill produced by the first agent may be decreased, potentially substantially.

2.7 Regional Chemotherapy: Dose Intensification with Reduced Systemic Exposure

Following systemic drug administration, it can be reasonably assumed that the extent of exposure to tumor or normal tissue will be principally determined by the extent of blood/capillary flow to these areas and tissues. However, with regional drug delivery (e.g., bladder, cerebrospinal fluid, peritoneal cavity, isolation perfusion of arterial system of an extremity), there is the potential to increase the concentration of the agent in contact with the malignant cell population within a particular body compartment while reducing the degree of exposure to areas outside the compartment and potentially minimizing the risk of serious toxicity.

In several settings (e.g., intrathecal administration of methotrexate in the treatment of meningeal leukemia, intraperitoneal administration of cisplatin in the treatment of small volume advanced ovarian cancer, intravesical delivery of several antineoplastic agents in the treatment of superficial bladder cancer), it has been shown that very high local concentrations of these agents can produce favorable clinical effects with acceptable local and systemic toxicity [15–17]. It is appropriate to note that in each of these settings, the drug concentrations achieved within the body compartments are far greater than could be safely attained following systemic drug administration.

References

1. Frei III E, Canellos GP. Dose: a critical factor in cancer chemotherapy. Am J Med. 1980;69:585–94.
2. Schabel Jr FM, Griswold Jr DP, Corbett TH, Laster Jr WR. Increasing therapeutic response rates to anticancer drugs by applying the basic principles of pharmacology. Pharmacol Ther. 1983;20:283–305.
3. Hennessy BT, Coleman RL, Markman M. Ovarian cancer. Lancet. 2009;374:1371–82.
4. Tan MC, Al MF, Gao F, et al. Predictors of complete pathological response after neoadjuvant systemic therapy for breast cancer. Am J Surg. 2009;198:520–5.
5. Kuhn W, Rutke S, Spathe K, et al. Neoadjuvant chemotherapy followed by tumor debulking prolongs survival for patients with poor prognosis in International Federation of Gynecology and Obstetrics Stage IIIC ovarian carcinoma. Cancer. 2001;92:2585–91.
6. Vergote I, Trope CG, Amant F, et al. Neoadjuvant chemotherapy or primary surgery in stage IIIC or IV ovarian cancer. N Engl J Med. 2010;363:943–53.

7. Hryniuk W, Levine MN. Analysis of dose intensity for adjuvant chemotherapy trials in stage II breast cancer. J Clin Oncol. 1986;4:1162–70.
8. Hryniuk W. Will increases in dose intensity improve outcome: pro. Am J Med. 1995;99:69S–70.
9. McGuire WP, Hoskins WJ, Brady MF, et al. Assessment of dose-intensive therapy in suboptimally debulked ovarian cancer: a Gynecologic Oncology Group study. J Clin Oncol. 1995;13:1589–99.
10. Gore M, Mainwaring P, A'Hern R, et al. Randomized trial of dose-intensity with single-agent carboplatin in patients with epithelial ovarian cancer. London Gynaecological Oncology Group. J Clin Oncol. 1998;16:2426–34.
11. Tallman MS, Gray R, Robert NJ, et al. Conventional adjuvant chemotherapy with or without high-dose chemotherapy and autologous stem-cell transplantation in high-risk breast cancer. N Engl J Med. 2003;349:17–26.
12. Grenman S, Wiklund T, Jalkanen J, et al. A randomised phase III study comparing high-dose chemotherapy to conventionally dosed chemotherapy for stage III ovarian cancer: the Finnish Ovarian Cancer (FINOVA) study. Eur J Cancer. 2006;42:2196–9.
13. Berry DA, Broadwater G, Klein JP, et al. High-dose versus standard chemotherapy in metastatic breast cancer: comparison of Cancer and Leukemia Group B trials with data from the Autologous Blood and Marrow Transplant Registry. J Clin Oncol. 2002;20:743–50.
14. Jodrell DI, Egorin MJ, Canetta RM, et al. Relationships between carboplatin exposure and tumor response and toxicity in patients with ovarian cancer. J Clin Oncol. 1992;10:520–8.
15. Markman M. Regional antineoplastic drug delivery in the management of malignant disease. Baltimore: The Johns Hopkins University Press; 1991.
16. Markman M, Walker JL. Intraperitoneal chemotherapy of ovarian cancer: a review, with a focus on practical aspects of treatment. J Clin Oncol. 2006;24:988–94.
17. Tewari D, Java JJ, Salani R, et al. Long-term survival advantage and prognostic factors associated with intraperitoneal chemotherapy treatment in advanced ovarian cancer: a Gynecologic Oncology Group study. J Clin Oncol. 2015;33:1460–6.

Drug Removal Systems and Induction Chemotherapy

3

James H. Muchmore

3.1 Introduction

Since the advent of cancer chemotherapy in the early 1940s [1–3], multiple drugs, devices, and techniques have been developed for treating advanced solid cancers. The endeavor has been to enhance drug delivery and at the same time to control both local/regional and systemic toxicity. Drug toxicity, the dose-limiting factor for most chemotherapeutic agents, has not been the only impediment to better tumor response rates and patient outcomes. However, drug delivery to the tumor cell within its tumor microenvironment remains one of the more significant factors preventing the complete response of an advanced malignancy.

Advanced hepatic, pancreatic, and pelvic malignancies would be the principal application of induction intra-arterial (IA) chemotherapy plus rapid drug recapture. Only 4 % of those patients with metastatic colorectal cancer to the liver ever achieve a complete response (CR) following preoperative chemotherapy [4]. However, this small cohort of patients can realize a remarkably improved, long-term survival. Similarly, patients with hepatocellular cancer undergoing complete response with regional chemotherapy achieve long-term survival [5]. Improving the CR rate of intra-abdominal hepatic, pancreatic, and pelvic tumors with induction therapy would also be the primary goal of this treatment strategy.

Regional chemotherapy techniques were developed in the 1950s, and these procedures significantly improved local/regional tumor response [6, 7]. Induction chemotherapy for head and neck cancer and hepatic metastatic disease was pioneered by Sullivan et al. of the Lahey Clinic Foundation [8, 9]. His work was important in establishing early treatment regimens using IA antimetabolites for regional cancer treatment [10].

J.H. Muchmore
Department of Surgery, Tulane University School of Medicine,
1430 Tulane Avenue, New Orleans, LA 70112, USA
e-mail: jmuchmo@aol.com; jmuchmo@ad.com

© Springer-Verlag Berlin Heidelberg 2016
K.R. Aigner, F.O. Stephens (eds.), *Induction Chemotherapy*,
DOI 10.1007/978-3-319-28773-7_3

Complete responses then became possible for some head and neck cancers, but most were not complete or durable [11–13]. Also, complete responses for many tumors, that is, melanoma, soft tissue sarcoma, pancreatic cancer, and metastatic colon cancer to the liver, were uncommon, and systemic toxicity remained a persistent dose-limiting factor.

Isolated regional perfusion also developed in the 1950s became the model for induction chemotherapy and resolved some of the drug delivery and toxicity problems [14, 15]. Regional perfusion increases the delivered drug dose to a tumor-bearing region six to ten times over that of systemic chemotherapy [16]. Complete responses were observed for some cases of head and neck cancer, limb melanoma, and sarcoma. Thus, when induction chemotherapy was combined with surgical resection, improved patient survival was then attainable [12, 16–19]. However, the regional perfusion technique requires 4–5 h of operating room time, but in the current era of healthcare cost containment, it remains too expensive for most healthcare systems.

Regional chemotherapy combined with rapid drug retrieval is a less complex regional chemotherapy technique [20–22]. It requires less treatment time and is more cost-effective. Plus this technique can easily be repeated. Drug delivery modeling can be accomplished so as to deliver a truly cytotoxic level of agent to the tumor cell while limiting systemic toxicity by rapidly removing the excess, circulating drug.

There are three principal drug recapture systems – hemodialysis, hemoperfusion, and hemofiltration – that can be used in conjunction with regional chemotherapy. These newer techniques using drug removal systems demonstrate that the combination of induction regional therapies plus surgery can be beneficial in promoting improved patient outcomes [23].

3.2   Regional Therapy Techniques plus Extracorporeal Drug Removal Systems

The drug dose delivered by IA chemotherapy is usually increased two- to fourfold over that of the systemic dose. In 1974, Eckman et al. put together a model describing the potential drug advantage derived from an IA infusion. This regional advantage from IA drug delivery versus systemic chemotherapy is equated to the integral equation of concentration multiplied by time ($C \times T$). The regional advantage, R_d, is then defined as the area under the drug concentration-time curve (AUC) that remains dependent on (1) the drug delivery rate, (2) the regional blood flow, and (3) the total body clearance, Cl_{TB} [24]. Thus, in the tumor-bearing region that metabolizes and clears the infused drug, that is, the liver, the therapeutic advantage is escalated proportionally to the regional drug clearance. The R_d also depends on the fraction of drug, E, extracted during a single pass through the target tissue:

$$R_d = Cl_{TB} / Q(1-E) + 1$$

However, for the region that is not able to clear the infused agent, the R_d remains a function of the regional blood flow (Q_i) and mostly the total body clearance, Cl_{TB}.

$$R_d = Cl_{TB} / Q_i + 1$$

Regional IA chemotherapy plus extracorporeal hemoperfusion or hemofiltration is a strategy devised to expedite the total body drug clearance, Cl_{TB}, allowing the escalation of the regional drug dose. Oldfield and Dedrick et al. in the 1980s first proposed this technique to treat primary brain tumors [20, 25].

Since the earliest report by Hande et al. in the 1970s on employing hemodialysis to rescue patients from the toxicity of chemotherapy, other techniques of extracorporeal drug recapture have replaced hemodialysis [26, 27].

Schreiner and Winchester et al. both from Georgetown University separately reported studies in the 1970s and 1980s on the extracorporeal removal of plant toxins and anticancer agents comparing hemodialysis with charcoal and resin hemoperfusion [28, 29]. Early on, hemoperfusion was recognized as being much more efficient at rapidly recapturing plant toxins and anticancer agents [27].

A variety of problems have confronted these techniques of extracorporeal drug recapture. Initially, problems with coagulopathy and platelet destruction by charcoal hemoperfusion devices restricted the use of these devices [27, 28]. However, the problem with platelet consumption was solved by using drug-specific, adsorbent resins or coated charcoal hemoperfusion devices having improved biocompatibility [27–29].

Drug availability for recapture and drug protein binding are the two remaining limiting factors in utilizing drug removal techniques for chemotherapeutic agents. Only those drugs that remain in the central vascular-plasma compartment can be readily removed using hemodialysis, hemoperfusion, or hemofiltration. However, with lapsed time, drugs will diffuse into various diverse tissue compartments where their release and retrieval from these compartments then depend on multiple factors [26, 28]. Also, red blood cell and protein binding limit the proficiency of drug removal devices to clear a particular drug.

Thus, only those chemotherapeutic agents which have a limited volume of distribution, single compartment kinetics, low endogenous clearance (<4 mL/min/kg), molecular weight <500 Da, soluble in aqueous solutions, and not tightly protein bound can be recaptured from the central vascular compartment. Unfortunately, this leaves only a very limited group of drugs which would be amenable to enhanced elimination using hemodialysis.

Regional drug removal versus systemic drug recapture addresses some of the shortcomings of enhanced elimination by hemodialysis. With catheters placed within the venous effluent of a tumor-bearing region, a significantly greater percentage of drugs can be retrieved. Thus, regionally confined malignancies, that is, hepatic tumors, pancreatic tumors, primary brain tumors, pelvic tumors, and limb malignancies, permit the use of IA chemotherapy plus hemoperfusion or hemofiltration.

Tumor volume versus tissue volume is another aspect of the drug, tissue distribution problem as seen with targeting a small tumor within a large region, that is, pelvic and limb tumors. Large tissue volumes would also limit the capability of the various drug removal systems in adequately detoxifying the venous effluent.

3.3   Drug Removal Devices

Hemodialysis filters and hemofiltration filters are relatively similar in construction, but are considerably different in the manner by which they remove toxins or drugs from the blood. With an extracorporeal, hollow tube hemodialyzer, blood is pumped along one side of a semipermeable membrane, and the opposite side has a counter-current with a crystalloid solution. Hollow fiber dialyzers are composed of different synthetic membrane materials. These materials are used to vary the type of solute to be moved across a semipermeable membrane [30, 31].

Also, where the concentration of a substance to be extracted is zero in the dialysate, it can be removed from the central plasma compartment only up to the point where the drug concentration becomes equivalent on both sides of the membrane [27, 30]. Also, hemodialysis is a technique that excludes drugs which are of higher molecular weight, tightly protein bound, and distributed throughout multiple tissue compartments.

Hemofiltration functions in a different way than that of hemodialysis. In essence, blood under pressure flows down one side of highly permeable membrane permitting, by convection, water, and substances with a molecule weight up to 20,000 Da, to cross the membrane and be collected as an ultrafiltrate. A roller pump generates a constant blood flow creating a transmembrane pressure gradient for ultrafiltration. A post-hemo-filter replacement solution is then used to replace the ultrafiltrate and thus reconstitute the blood [30, 32]. In hemofiltration, drug recapture depends on the rate of ultrafiltra-tion, drug protein binding, and the sieving coefficient of the membrane [32, 33].

High volume hemofiltration with fluid exchange rates greater than 3 L/h is per-formed using a larger 1.2 m^2 hollow tube filter for rapid recapture of regionally infused chemotherapeutic agents [33, 34]. However, with high volume ultrafiltration, the replacement fluid should be added before the hemofilter to prevent clotting. A combi-nation of predilution and postdilution fluid replacement can be used. Also, certain drugs require the use of parallel filters to avoid having the drug clog the filter.

Hemoperfusion is a third type of extracorporeal drug removal. The blood is directed through an extracorporeal circuit containing multiple sorbant-containing capsules arranged in parallel [33, 35]. Coated charcoal hemoperfusion capsules are utilized in most of the larger studies using hepatic arterial infusion with extracorporeal drug recap-ture [36–39]. Also, other resin exchange capsules have been developed for the more lipid soluble drugs. However, the advantage of hemoperfusion is that it can recapture drugs against a transmembrane gradient, whereas hemodialysis and hemofiltration are only efficient in recapturing the peak drug dose. The only disadvantage of this technique is the hemoperfusion capsule often becomes quickly saturated with drug. This problem, however, is easily overcome by using multiple capsules arranged in parallel.

3.4   Intra-arterial Infusion plus Hemoperfusion

This technique was first purposed as an adjunct to regional chemotherapy, and it remains the most applicable in recapturing regionally delivered cytotoxic agents [36, 37]. Like isolated regional perfusion, this technique is most applicable when used as induction chemotherapy to be followed by a surgical resection [23].

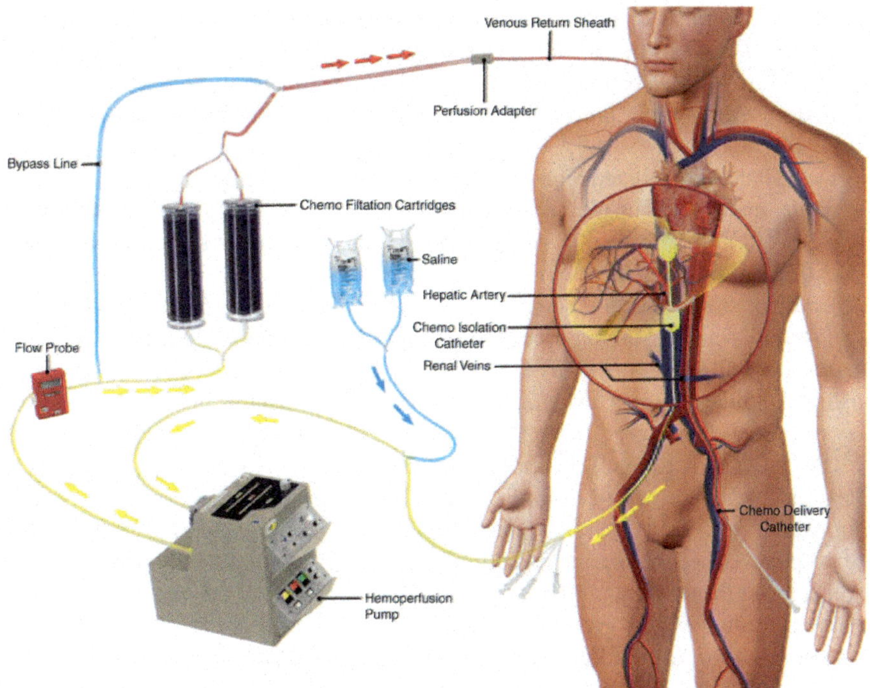

Fig. 3.1 The flow diagram for the Delcath Catheter System (Delcath, Inc., New York, NY). Intra-arterial chemotherapy is injected into the hepatic artery through a percutaneous placed catheter. The hepatic venous effluent is collected via a double lumen catheter positioned in the retrohepatic vena cava. The drug is recaptured from the venous effluent by means of two activated charcoal hemoperfusion capsules

Currently, the most developed drug removal system in the USA is the Yale University School of Medicine or Delcath Catheter System (Delcath Inc., NYC, NY). It is an intra-arterial infusion technique combined with rapid drug recapture of the hepatic venous effluent using percutaneous placed catheters (Fig. 3.1) [23, 38, 39]. Also, Ku et al. in Japan have developed a similar percutaneous isolated liver chemoperfusion (PILP) technique for treating advanced hepatic malignancies [5, 40]. Likewise, recent reports from the Japanese literature confirm the efficacy and advantages of utilizing PILP alone or in combination with a hepatic resection to achieve a complete response and an improved, long-term outcome [41, 42].

Hemoperfusion devices are better than hemodialysis or hemofiltration in recapturing drugs against a transmembrane gradient. Hemoperfusion filter extraction percentages of drug recaptured range from 77 % to 96 % [36, 37]. Thus, the reduction in systemic drug exposure allows the regional drug dose to be escalated approximately up to ten times the systemic drug dose [25, 36, 37].

Several larger studies have been published on the use of hepatic intra-arterial chemotherapy plus charcoal hemoperfusion. A recent review of this technique has established the effectiveness of regional therapy plus hemoperfusion in improving local control of hepatic metastases [5, 23, 39, 40, 42]. The Yale University School of Medicine studies using hepatic IA 5-FU and doxorubicin and a double balloon hepatic catheter positioned in the retrohepatic vena cava showed that this system recaptured 64–91 % of the infused drugs. Thus, with venous hemoperfusion, the drug dose escalation of both 5-FU and doxorubicin could be increased two- to six-fold [38].

A similar study utilized high-dose melphalan (3 mg/kg) to treat a variety of unresectable, metastatic hepatic cancers. However, even though IA dose of melphalan was tenfold greater than a possible systemic dose, the tumor responses were less than that compared to melphalan used in a regional limb perfusion system [39, 43–45]. Other studies using regional IA melphalan plus chemoperfusion for liver metastases from melanoma produced only partial response at best [46]. A recent European multiple center study has evaluated the effectiveness of hepatic, regional melphalan plus hemoperfusion in controlling liver metastases derived from a variety of primary malignancies [47].

The studies of Ku et al. in treating hepatocellular carcinoma using doxorubicin ($60–150$ mg/m^2) produced a significant number of complete responses. A long-term survival of 39.7 % at 5 years was achieved for this group of patients [5, 39]. Eight of 13 patients had undergone repeat treatments [2–4], and of the 28 patients in the study, it was those having repeat treatments who experienced the improved survival. Current studies by this group from Kobe University, Department of Surgery, continue to show improved hepatic responses and outcomes using preoperative PILP followed by hepatic resection [42, 48, 49].

In both the US and Japanese systems, the drug extraction rates for the charcoal hemoperfusion capsules were 85–96 %, and the mean drug clearance fraction was approximately 30 % [5, 38]. Thus, using IA chemotherapy plus venous hemoperfusion, the regional advantage, R_d, is then related to the fraction of drug eliminated, E_r, on the first pass through the tumor-bearing region; the fraction cleared by the liver, E_l; plus, predominantly, the fraction of drug cleared through the hemoperfusion device, E_{hp}:

$$R_d = \mathrm{Cl}_{TB} / Q\left[1-\left(E_r + E_l + E_{hp}\right)\right] + 1$$

Thus, using venous hemoperfusion, the regional drug dose can be escalated up to tenfold over that of the systemically delivered drug dose. Notably, this increase in regional delivered drug dose is similar to that used in regional limb perfusion and infusion systems [43–45]. However, unlike the isolated regional perfusion system, this technique lacks the additive effects of hyperthermia and hyperoxygenation which act to modify the tumor microcirculation and further improve drug delivery.

3.5   Intra-arterial Infusion plus Venous Filtration

Intra-arterial chemotherapy plus hemofiltration was first described by Aigner et al. to modify the pharmacokinetics of a regionally delivered drug dose [21]. Since then several studies of liver, pancreas, and pelvic malignancies treated by regional chemotherapy plus hemofiltration have been published [22, 50–53].

Hemofiltration is most effective in recapturing the peak dose, $C_{max}s$, of an antineoplastic agent, when a steep, drug gradient exists across the filter's semipermeable membrane. However, since hemofiltration clears only the peak dose, this technique recaptures only 20–25 % of the total drug dose [50, 51].

Using IA chemotherapy plus venous filtration, the regional advantage, R_d, is then related to the fraction of drug eliminated, E_r, on the first pass through the tumor-bearing region; the fraction cleared by the liver, E_l; plus, primarily, the fraction of drug cleared through the hemofiltration system, E_{hf} [50, 51]:

$$R_d = Cl_{TB} / Q \left[1 - \left(E_r + E_l + E_{hf} \right) \right] + 1$$

Thus, the regional drug dose can be escalated only approximately three to five times over that of the systemically delivered drug dose. The total drug dose infused, however, is still limited to being only twofold greater than the normal total systemic dose.

As an approach similar to that of Dedrick et al. [20], IA chemotherapy plus hemofiltration was collaboratively modified by Aigner et al. [21] and Muchmore et al. [22] for the treatment of liver metastases, pancreatic cancer, and advanced intra-abdominal malignancies (Fig. 3.2a, b).

For Stage III unresectable pancreatic cancer, response rates over 50 % and a resectability rate of 25 % were achieved using regional IA chemotherapy plus hemofiltration [50]. Aigner and Gailhofer, also, reported a 27 % complete response rate in a group of patients with Stage III unresectable pancreatic cancer using IA chemotherapy with starch microspheres plus hemofiltration [52].

Of the patients with advanced intra-abdominal malignancies, there were 17 in the Tulane series with advanced or recurrent colorectal cancer. Six had liver metastases only and 11 had liver plus peritoneal or pelvic disease [22, 53, unpublished data]. Only one of these patients with metastatic pelvic colorectal cancer achieved long-term survival [22]. This patient had regional IA chemotherapy plus hemofiltration which was then followed by a curative resection. Another patient with peritoneal plus pelvic disease achieved a clinical CR following regional chemotherapy plus hemofiltration and then had a curative resection of his residual disease. The six patients with only liver metastases achieved at best a partial response.

Consequently, the limited improvement in overall survival was essentially only seen in those patients where IA chemotherapy plus hemofiltration was used as induction therapy followed by surgical resection.

3.6   Treating Tumor Microenvironment Using Regional Therapies

The principal target of high-dose regional chemotherapy is the manipulation of the tumor microenvironment, thus enhancing drug delivery to the tumor cell [54, 55]. Regional high-dose chemotherapy can be designed to overcome the multiple peritumoral drug barriers created by the abnormal tumor neovascularity as described by

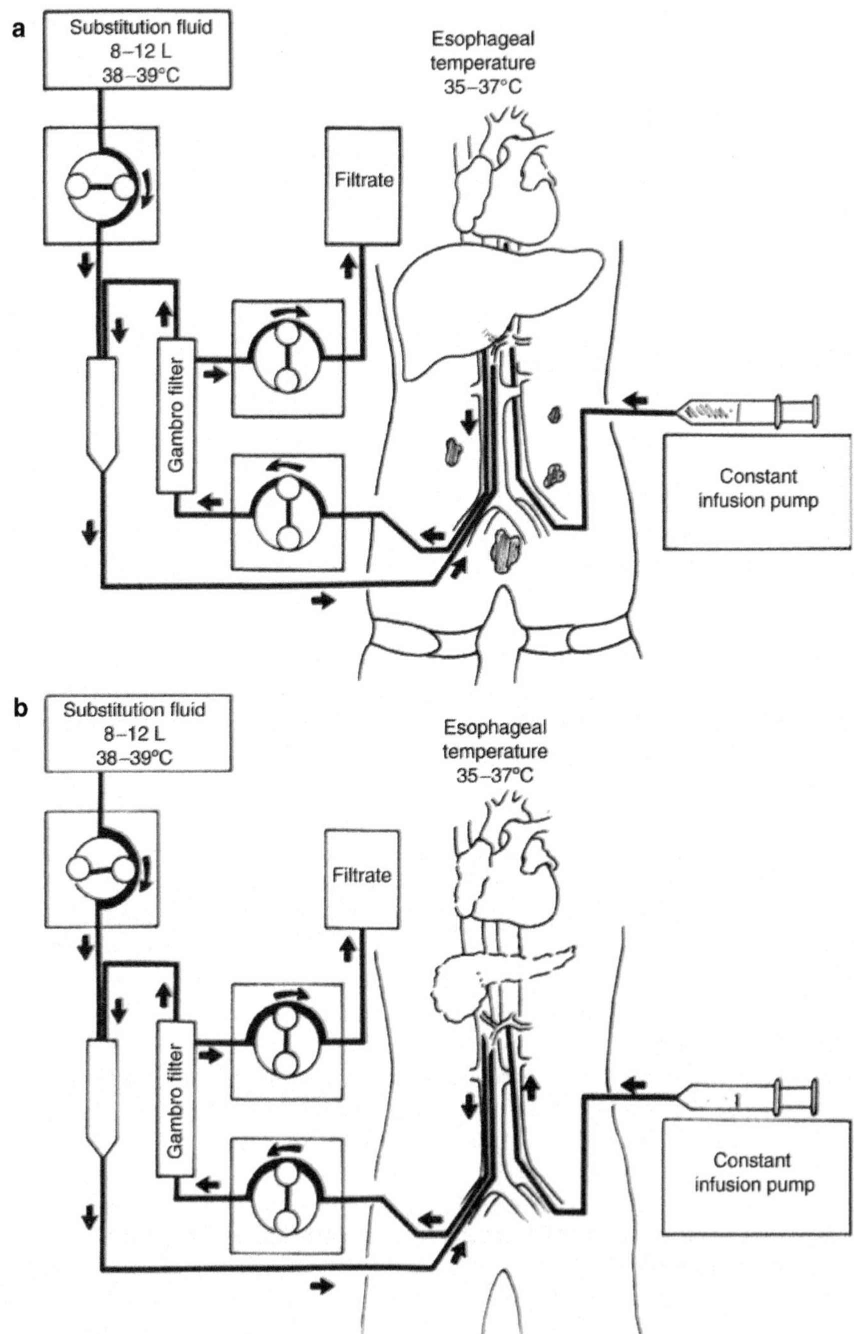
a
Substitution fluid
8–12 L
38–39°C
Esophageal
temperature
35–37°C
Filtrate
Gambro filter
Constant
infusion pump
b
Substitution fluid
8–12 L
38–39°C
Esophageal
temperature
35–37°C
Filtrate
Gambro filter
Constant
infusion pump

Jain and Vaupal. This microenvironment surrounding a tumor nodule thus generates a significant impediment to both systemic and regional cytotoxic drug delivery [56–62]. A similar argument applies to the delivery of all agents, both chemotherapeutic and the newer targeted agents.

The tumor microenvironment effects drug delivery in several ways. The normal blood flow through tissues can be shunted away from the tumor nodule. Tumor neovasularity produces a local capillary leak creating an increased interstitial pressure within the tumor nodule. Then collapse of blood vessels within the central tumor neovasculature results in shunting of the tumor blood flow. Another aspect of blood flow shunting is activation of the inflammatory response causing an overgrowth of fibroblasts resulting in a significant desmoplastic reaction [62]. In pancreatic cancer, this desmoplastic reaction reduces the blood flow through the tumor to half that of the normal, surrounding tissue blood flow [50].

Peritumor edema evolves because 4.5–10.2 % of the perfusing plasma volume of a tumor nodule leaks out into the surrounding tumor interstitium [63]. An elevated interstitial pressure from the peritumoral edema proceeds to then collapse the central tumor neovasculature. Thus within the tumor nodule, there is a central hypoxic and hypovascular zone. Increasing the regional drug dose often then allows an improved delivery of a cytotoxic level of chemotherapy. Mild hyperthermia potentiates the cytotoxic effect of several chemotherapeutic agents plus increasing regional and local blood flow.

However, the locoregional hypoxia within the tumor microenvironment represents the single most important impediment for cytotoxic drug delivery to a malignancy [61]. Tumor cells residing within the edema surrounding a tumor nodule exist and survive in a hypoxic state. These tumor cells remain highly resistant to chemotherapy resultant from decreased drug delivery, upregulation of drug efflux enzyme systems, and decreased intracellular oxygen tension. Like in regional perfusion systems, regional IA chemotherapy plus hemoperfusion can be designed to overcome most or all of these obstacles to cytotoxic drugs, or newer targeted therapies.

High-dose regional chemotherapy is more effective in driving cytotoxic drugs into hypoxic tumor regions, normally not amenable to systemic chemotherapy. Alkylating agents are drugs which are principally concentration dependent for their cytotoxic effect and thus are most fitting for use in regional therapies. Alkylating

Fig. 3.2 (**a**) The flow diagram for high-dose intra-arterial peritoneal chemotherapy with concomitant hemofiltration. After establishing a balanced hemofiltration with a flow rate of 450–500 cc/min and an ultrafiltration rate of 120–150 cc/min, IA chemotherapy is infused through an aortic catheter using a constant infusion pump over 30–35 min. The hemofiltration is continued for 1 h. (**b**) The flow diagram for pancreatic regional chemotherapy in combination with hemofiltration. A balanced hemofiltration is established with a flow rate of 400 mL/min and an ultrafiltration rate of 150 mL/min. The hemofiltration is continued for up to 70 min. The pancreatic intra-arterial chemotherapy is infused by means of a celiac axis arterial catheter or an aortic catheter over the first 30–40 min of the procedure

agents tend to interact rapidly with the DNA and are non-cell-cycle dependent. Their interaction with tumor cells in culture is often potentiated by hyperthermia [66, 67]. Hyperthermia can also have a direct effect on the tumor microcirculation worsening the hypoxia of the tumor, thus increasing the drug cytotoxic effect [67, 68].

Antibiotic chemotherapeutic agents, anthracyclines, and anthracenes are also largely concentration-dependent cytocidal drugs having some time dependence [69]. Thus, theoretically, improved tumor cytotoxicity can be best achieved by significantly escalating the regional drug, peak concentration, as opposed to augmenting the exposure time to a chemotherapeutic agent [69].

Finally, regional chemotherapy plus rapid drug recapture can ideally be limited to a small number of preoperative treatments before a definitive curative surgical procedure. Currently, the better long-term outcomes are now seen when regional therapies plus curative surgery is then followed by adjuvant chemotherapy.

3.7 Summary

Drug removal systems in combination with regional chemotherapy can be a useful technique when applied as induction chemotherapy in treating advanced solid tumors. This treatment strategy would be most applicable for patients with metastatic colorectal cancer to the liver or unresectable hepatocellular cancer. Also, patients with advanced pancreatic and pelvic malignancies would be amenable to this strategy.

Improving the complete response rate of liver metastases or primary hepatic disease with induction chemotherapy IA plus hemoperfusion would have a significant impact on survival of these patients, especially when combined with a curative operative procedure. More recent data suggests that when regional therapies were used in the neoadjuvant setting prior to hepatic resection produced better long-term outcomes [23, 49, 64].

Presently, data in the literature shows that tumor cell resistance mainly resides with the intracellular mechanisms that cause the tumor nodule to be less prone to cytotoxic therapy. However, tumor cells residing within the hypoxic zones would be protected from systemic and even regional chemotherapy. Thus, hypoxia remains one of the principal driving forces generating tumor cell drug resistance. Also, hypoxia acts to drive tumor cells to more malignant phenotypes and to increase their mutation rate to more drug-resistant cell lines [60, 61, 63, 65].

References

1. Gilman A, Philips FS. Biological actions and therapeutic applications of B-chloroethyl amines and sulfides. Science. 1946;103:409–15.
2. Jacobson LO, Spurr CL, Barron ES, et al. Nitrogen mustard therapy; studies on the effect of methyl-bis (beta-chloroethyl) amine hydrochloride on neoplastic disease and allied disorders of hemopoietic system. JAMA. 1946;132:263–71.
3. Rhoads CP. Report on a cooperative study of nitrogen mustard (HN_2) therapy of neoplastic disease. Trans Assoc Am Phys. 1947;60:110–7.

4. Adam R, Wicherts DA, de Haas RJ, Aloia T, Levi F, Paule B, et al. Complete pathologic response after preoperative chemotherapy for colorectal liver metastases: myth or reality? J Clin Oncol. 2008;26:1635–41.
5. Ku Y, Fukumoto T, Tominaga M, Iwasaki T, Maeda I, Kusunoki N, et al. Single catheter technique of hepatic venous isolation and extracorporeal charcoal hemoperfusion for malignant liver tumors. Am J Surg. 1973;173:101–9.
6. Klopp CT, Alford TC, Bateman J, et al. Fractional intra-arterial cancer chemotherapy with methyl-bis-amine hydrochloride. A preliminary report. Ann Surg. 1950;132:811–32.
7. Bierman HR, Shimkin MB, Byron Jr RL, et al. The effects of intra-arterial administration of nitrogen mustard. Paris: Fifth International Cancer Congress; 1950. p. 187–8.
8. Sullivan RD, Norcross JW, Watkins Jr E. Chemotherapy of metastatic liver cancer by prolonged hepatic-artery infusion. N Engl J Med. 1964;270:321–7.
9. Sullivan RD. Chemotherapy in head and neck cancer. JAMA. 1971;217:461–2.
10. Sullivan RD, Miller E, Sykes MP. Antimetabolite-metabolite combination cancer chemotherapy. Effects of intra-arterial methotrexate-intramuscular citrovorum factor therapy in human cancer. Cancer. 1959;12:1248–62.
11. Golomb FM. Perfusion and infusion chemotherapy of the head and neck. In: Fifth national cancer conference proceedings. Philadelphia: JB Lippincott; 1964. p. 561–72.
12. Krementz ET, Kokame GM. Regional chemotherapy of cancer of the head and neck. Laryngoscope. 1966;76:880–92.
13. Stephens FO. CRAB chemotherapy. Med J Aust. 1976;2:41–6.
14. Ryan RF, Krementz ET, Creech O, et al. Selected perfusion of isolated viscera with chemotherapeutic agents using an extracorporeal circuit. Surg Forum. 1957;8:158–61.
15. Creech Jr O, Krementz ET, Ryan RF, Winblad JM. Chemotherapy of cancer: regional perfusion utilizing an extracorporeal circuit. Ann Surg. 1958;148:616–32.
16. Krementz ET. Regional perfusion: current sophistication, what next? Cancer. 1986;57:416–32.
17. Golomb FM, Postel AH, Hall AB, et al. Chemotherapy of human cancer by regional perfusion. Report of 52 perfusions. Cancer. 1962;15:828–45.
18. Austen WA, Monaco AP, Richardson GS, et al. Treatment of malignant pelvic tumors by extracorporeal perfusion with chemotherapeutic agents. N Engl J Med. 1959;261:1045–52.
19. Stehlin JS, Clark RL, White EC, et al. Regional chemotherapy for cancer: experiences with 116 perfusions. Ann Surg. 1960;151:605–19.
20. Dedrick RL, Oldfield EH, Collins JH. Arterial drug infusion with extracorporeal removal. I. Theoretic basis with particular reference to the brain. Cancer Treat Rep. 1984;68:373–80.
21. Aigner KR, Thiller H, Walter H, Link KH. Drug filtration in high-dose regional chemotherapy. Contrib Oncol. 1988;29:261–80.
22. Muchmore JH, Krementz ET, Carter RD, et al. Treatment of abdominal malignant neoplasms using regional chemotherapy with hemofiltration. Arch Surg. 1991;126:1390–6.
23. Magge D, Choudry HA, Zeh 3rd HJ, et al. Outcome analysis of a decade-long experience of isolated hepatic perfusion for unresectable liver metastases at a single institution. Ann Surg. 2014;259:953–9.
24. Eckman WW, Patlak CS, Fenstermacher JD. Critical evaluation of principles governing the advantages of intra-arterial infusions. J Pharmacokinet Biopharm. 1974;2:257–85.
25. Oldfield EH, Dedrick RL, Yeager RL, et al. Reduced systemic drug exposure by combining intra-arterial chemotherapy with hemoperfusion of regional venous drainage. J Neurosurg. 1985;63:726–32.
26. Hande KR, Balow JE, Drake JC, Rosenberg SA, Chabner BA. Methotrexate and hemodialysis [letter]. Ann Intern Med. 1977;87:495–6.
27. Winchester JF, Gelfand MC, Knepshield JH, Schreiner GE. Dialysis and hemoperfusion of poisons and drugs – update. Trans Am Soc Artif Intern Organs. 1977;23:762–827.
28. Winchester JF, Rahman A, Tilstone WJ, Bregman H, Mortensen LM, Gelfand MC, et al. Will hemoperfusion be useful for cancer chemotherapeutic drug removal? Clin Toxicol. 1980;17:557–69.

29. Schreiner GE. Perspectives on the hemoperfusion of drugs and toxins. Biomater Artif Cells Artif Organs. 1987;15:305–21.
30. Forni LG, Hilton PJ. Continuous hemofiltration in the treatment of acute renal failure. N Engl J Med. 1977;336:1303–9.
31. Leypoldt JK, Ronco C. Optimization of high-flux, hollow-fiber artificial kidneys. In: Horl WH, Koch KM, Lindsay RM, Ronco C, Winchester JF, editors. Replacement of renal function by dialysis. 5th ed. Dordrecht: Kluwer Academic; 2004. p. 95–113.
32. Schulman G, Himmelfarb J. Hemodialysis. In: Brenner BM, editor. The kidney. 7th ed. Philadelphia: Saunders; 2004. p. 2563–624.
33. Chang IJ, Fischbach BV, Sile S, Golper TA. Extracorporeal treatment of poisoning. In: Brenner BM, editor. The kidney. 7th ed. Philadelphia: Saunders; 2004. p. 2733–57.
34. Ronco C, Brendolan A, Bellomo R. Dialysis techniques: continuous renal replacement techniques. In: Horl WH, Koch KM, Lindsay RM, Ronco C, Winchester JF, editors. Replacement of renal function by dialysis. 5th ed. Dordrecht: Kluwer Academic; 2004. p. 699–708.
35. Winchester JF. Dialysis techniques: hemoperfusion. In: Horl WH, Koch KM, Lindsay RM, Ronco C, Winchester JF, editors. Replacement of renal function by dialysis. 5th ed. Dordrecht: Kluwer Academic; 2004. p. 725–38.
36. Kihara T, Goya N, Nakazawa H, et al. A pharmacokinetic study of arterial infusion chemotherapy for malignant diseases combined with direct hemoperfusion (DHP). Jpn J Artif Organs. 1986;15:1275–9.
37. Kihara T, Nakazawa H, Agushi T, Honda H. Superiority of selective bolus infusion and simultaneous rapid removal of anticancer agents by charcoal hemoperfusion in cancer treatment. Trans Am Soc Artif Intern Organs. 1988;34:581–4.
38. Ravikumar TS, Pizzorno G, Bodden W, et al. Percutaneous hepatic vein isolation and high-dose hepatic artery infusion chemotherapy for unresectable liver tumors. J Clin Oncol. 1994;12:2733–6.
39. Pinkpank JF, Libutti SK, Chang R, Wood BJ, Neewan Z, Kam AW, et al. Phase I study of hepatic arterial melphalan infusion and hepatic venous hemofiltration using percutaneously placed catheters in patients with unresectable hepatic malignancies. J Clin Oncol. 2005;23:3465–74.
40. Ku Y, Iwasaki T, Fukumoto T, Tominaga M, Muramatsu S, Kusunoki N, et al. Induction of long-term remission in advanced hepatocellular carcinoma with percutaneous isolated liver chemoperfusion. Ann Surg. 1998;227:519–26.
41. Ku Y, Tominaga M, Iwasaki T, et al. Efficay of repeated percutaneous isolated liver chemoperfusion in local control of unresectable hepatocellular carcinoma. Hepatogastroenterology. 1998;45:1961–5.
42. Fukumoto T, Tominaga M, Kido M, et al. Long-term outcomes and prognostic factors with reductive hepatectomy and sequential percutaneous isolated hepatic perfusion for multiple bilobar hepatocellular carcinoma. Ann Surg Oncol. 2014;21:971–8.
43. Krementz ET, Carter RD, Sutherland CM, et al. Regional perfusion of melanoma – a 35 year experience. Ann Surg. 1994;220:520–35.
44. Kroon HM, Moncrieff M, Kam PC, Thompson JF. Outcomes following isolated limb infusion for melanoma. A 14-year experience. Ann Surg Oncol. 2008;15:3003–13.
45. Muchmore JH, Carter RD, Krementz ET. Regional perfusion for malignant melanoma and soft tissue sarcoma: a review. Cancer Invest. 1985;3:129–43.
46. Heusner TA, Antoch G, Wittkowski-Sterczewski A, et al. Transarterial hepatic chemoperfusion of uveal melanoma metastases: survival and response to treatment. Fortschr Röntgenstr. 2011;183:1151–60.
47. Vogl TJ, Zangos SW, Scholtz JE, et al. Chemosaturation with percutaneous hepatic perfusions of melphalan for hepatic metastases: experience from two European centers. Fortschr Röntgenstr. 2014;186:937–44.
48. Urade T, Tanaka M, Fukumoto T, et al. A case of bilobar multiple hepatocellular carcinoma in which complete remission was achieved by preoperative percutaneous isolated hepatic perfusion. Japan J Cancer Chemother. 2012;39:1825–7.

49. Fukumoto T, Komatsu S, Takahashi M, et al. The role of preoperative percutaneous isolated hepatic perfusion and hepatectomy in multidisciplinary treatment. Japan J Cancer Chemother. 2013;40:1822–4.

50. Muchmore JH, Arya J. Regional chemotherapy of cancer of the pancreas. In: Markman M, editor. Current clinical oncology: regional chemotherapy: clinical research and practice. Totowa: Humana Press; 1996. p. 101–25.

51. Muchmore JH. Treatment of advanced pancreatic cancer with regional chemotherapy plus hemofiltration. Semin Surg Oncol. 1995;11:154–67.

52. Aigner KR, Gailhofer S. Celiac axis infusion for locally metastasized pancreatic cancer using spherex/mitoxantrone microembolization and mitomycin C/chemofiltration. Reg Cancer Ther. 1991;4:3.

53. Muchmore JH, Aigner KH, Beg MH. Regional chemotherapy for advanced intraabdominal and pelvic cancer. In: Cohen AM, Winawer SJ, Friedman MA, Gunderson LL, editors. Cancer of the colon, rectum, and anus. New York: McGraw-Hill; 2005. p. 881–9.

54. Watanabe H, Asano M, Tizon X, et al. Eribulin mesylate reduces tumor microenvironment abnormality by vascular remodeling in preclinical human breast cancer models. Cancer Sci. 2014;105:1334–42.

55. Gacche RN, Meshram RJ. Targeting tumor micro-environment for design and development of novel antiangiogenic agents arresting tumor growth. Prog Biophys Mol Biol. 2013;113:333–54.

56. Vaupal P. Hypoxia in neoplastic tissue. Microvasc Res. 1977;13:399–408.

57. Jain RK. Vascular and interstitial barriers to delivery of therapeutic agents in tumors. Cancer Metastasis Rev. 1990;9:253–66.

58. Heldin CH, Rubin K, Pietras K, et al. High interstitial fluid pressure: an obstacle in cancer therapy. Nat Rev Cancer. 2004;4:806–13.

59. Reddy LH. Drug delivery to tumors: recent strategies. J Pharm Pharmacol. 2005;57:1231–42.

60. Jain RK. A new target for tumor therapy. N Engl J Med. 2009;360:2669–71.

61. Rohwer N, Cramer T. Hypoxia-mediated drug resistance: novel insights on the functional interaction of HIFs and cell death pathways. Drug Resist Updat. 2011;14:191–201.

62. Azmi AS, Bao B, Sarkar FH. Exosomes in cancer development, metastasis, and drug resistance: a comprehensive review. Cancer Metastasis Rev. 2013;32:623–42.

63. Curti BD. Physical barriers to drug delivery in tumors. In: Chabner BA, Longo DL, editors. Cancer chemotherapy and biotherapy. 2nd ed. Philadelphia: Lippincott-Raven; 1966. p. 709–19.

64. Agarwala SS, Eggermont AM, O'Day S, Zager JS. Metastatic melanoma to the liver: a contemporary and comprehensive review of surgical, systemic, and regional therapeutic options. Cancer. 2014;120:781–9.

65. Rice GC, Hoy C, Schimke RT. Transient hypoxia enhances the frequency of DHFR gene amplification in Chinese hamster ovary cells. Proc Natl Acad Sci U S A. 1986;83:5978–82. 54*.

66. Komatsu K, Miller RC, Hall EJ. The oncogenic potential of a combination of hyperthermia and chemotherapy agents. Br J Cancer. 1988;57:59–63.

67. Hildebrandt B, Wust P, Ahlers O, et al. The cellular and molecular basis of hyperthermia. Crit Rev Oncol Hematol. 2002;43:33–56.

68. Reinhold HS, van den Berg-Blok A. Enhancement of thermal damage to the microcirculation of 'sandwich' tumours by additional treatment. Eur J Cancer Clin Oncol. 1981;17:781–95.

69. Mitchell RB, Ratain MJ, Vogelzang NJ. Experimental rationale for continuous infusion chemotherapy. In: Lokich JJ, editor. Cancer chemotherapy by infusion. 2nd ed. Chicago: Precept; 1990. p. 3–34.

Cryotherapy

4

Miriam R. Habib and David L. Morris

4.1 The Evolution of Cryotherapy

Some say the world will end in fire,
Some say in ice.
From what I've tasted of desire
I hold with those who favor fire.
But if it had to perish twice,
I think I know enough of hate
To say that for destruction ice
Is also great
And would suffice. [1]

Cryotherapy refers to the application of freezing temperatures to tissues in order to induce cellular necrosis. Its oncological use was first described in 1851 by the physician, James Arnott, who used a mixture of ice and saline to treat advanced breast and cervical cancers [2]. Though not curative, he did achieve a reduction in tumour size and associated symptomatic relief. Such techniques, however, were only suitable for superficial lesions and progress with this modality remained slow until the 1960s. A collaboration at this time between Irving Cooper, a neurosurgeon, and Arnold Lee, an engineer, led to the development of a closed-circuit cryogenic system that could deliver liquid nitrogen to a trochar probe to access deeper lesions [3]. This became the prototype for modern-day cryosurgical apparatus and sparked a renewed interest in the technique.

The 1960s and 1970s saw cryotherapy experimentally utilised in the treatment of benign and malignant prostatic disease [4, 5]. Initial enthusiasm however gave way to concerns about the high complication rate as surgical techniques improved. The development of real-time operative ultrasound technology in the 1980s heralded an important milestone [6, 7]. The ability to visualise the target lesion before treatment

M.R. Habib • D.L. Morris (✉)
Department of Surgery, St George Hospital, The University of New South Wales,
Pitney Building Level 3, Kogarah, NSW 2217, Australia
e-mail: miriam.habib@gmail.com; david.morris@unsw.edu.au

© Springer-Verlag Berlin Heidelberg 2016
K.R. Aigner, F.O. Stephens (eds.), *Induction Chemotherapy*,
DOI 10.1007/978-3-319-28773-7_4

and to monitor the cryolesion during treatment offered a clear advantage over earlier techniques where accuracy of probe placement had been problematic. Gilbert et al. showed excellent correlation between the images seen on ultrasound and the extent of the cryolesion on pathological examination [8]. A further refinement was the use of a urethral warming catheter to prevent cold-mediated urethral injury and stricture [6]. As a result of these developments, cryotherapy has recently become a useful alternative or adjunct to surgical resection for hepatic and prostatic malignancies.

Much of the bulky, early apparatus has now been replaced with smaller devices. These smaller probes use an argon-helium gas combination rather than liquid nitrogen and have been especially favoured for ablation of the prostate, where distances between adjacent viscera are small [9].

4.2 Principles of Cryobiology

The relationship between cooling and cell death is not entirely straightforward. Early in the investigation of cryobiology, Hauschka et al. demonstrated the ability of both normal and neoplastic cells to survive suspension at −78 °C after rewarming [10]. It has since been held that the rate of cooling is the important factor, rather than the absolute temperature reached [11, 12]. When cells are cooled slowly to between −20 and −40 °C, extracellular ice crystals form, creating a hyperosmolar environment. Cells lose water and become dehydrated but may yet survive this insult. Conversely, with rapid cooling, intracellular water freezes before it is able to escape into the extracellular environment.

The next stage of cryonecrosis is the thaw cycle. Upon slow thawing, intracellular ice crystals fuse and expand, resulting in disruption of the cell membrane. Gage and colleagues found the optimal cycle to guarantee cell death to be a rapid freeze followed by a slow thaw [13]. Furthermore, they showed that repetition of the freeze-thaw cycle resulted in maximal cell death.

As well as direct cell damage, microcirculatory injury contributes to the overall tissue response to freezing [14]. Major blood vessels, though, sustain only transient and minor cryoinjury remaining as patent conduits: an important consideration in the approach to highly vascular organs such as the liver and kidney [15].

A third possible response to tissue cryonecrosis is a systemic immune reaction [16, 17]. Although such a response has been postulated, the extent and significance remain elusive. Sporadic reports from early clinical studies described regression of metastatic lesions after cryotherapy of the prostate [18, 19]. Further studies may shed light on this phenomenon and reveal whether this effect may be manipulated to enhance the local effects of cold damage.

4.3 Indications and Technique

The dermatological application of liquid nitrogen to superficial lesions is a well-established practice, and complications arising from such procedures are usually localised and self-limiting. The treatment of deep tissue lesions with cryotherapy has evolved so that it may now be applied to defined patient groups. However, with the rapid development of alternative techniques, the choice of ablative modality is becoming increasingly complex.

Surgical resection is still the gold standard therapy for many cancers. Patients necessarily precluded from this group may benefit from a local ablative strategy with curative intent. In our use of cryotherapy for liver tumours, we consider the following groups of patients eligible:

- Patients with multiple bilobar metastases
- Cirrhotic patients with limited hepatic reserve in whom preservation of liver parenchyma is desirable
- Patients with inadequate margins or residual tumour after surgical resection
- Selected patients with local recurrence after previous surgical resection

Workup prior to the procedure includes blood chemistry, tests of liver function, full blood count and coagulation profile. Patients must undergo computed tomography scanning of the chest, abdomen and pelvis as well as bone scan to exclude extrahepatic disease. It must be remembered that hepatic cryotherapy still largely necessitates laparotomy and bears significant risk; adequate preoperative workup and anaesthetic support is therefore paramount.

Entry to the abdomen is gained through routine rooftop incision, and the extent of disease is confirmed by palpation and operative ultrasound. The liver is then mobilised to optimise access and probe placement. The cryoprobe is placed into the lesion under ultrasound guidance, and iceball formation monitored until a 1 cm margin has been achieved around the lesion. Clamping of the hepatic inflow vessels may be performed to enhance the freezing effect (Fig. 4.1a, b).

The lesion is then allowed to thaw for 1 cm, and the freeze-thaw cycle is repeated.

During the freeze, the edge of the cryolesion is seen on ultrasound as an expanding hyperechoic rim. Upon thawing, this rim recedes leaving a hypoechoic lesion. At termination of the procedure, warm nitrogen gas is circulated through the probe

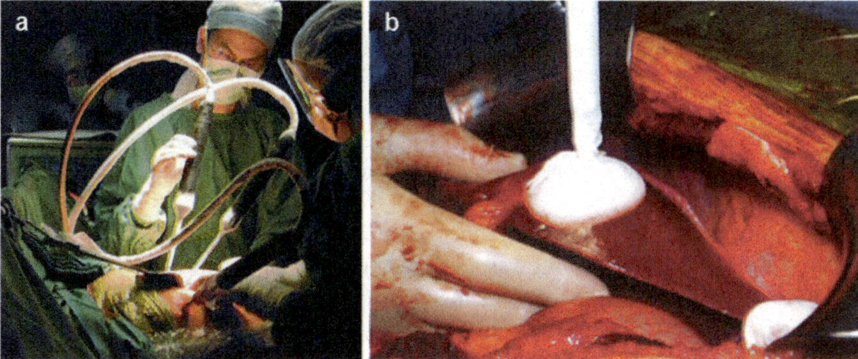

Fig. 4.1 Hepatic cryotherapy. (**a**) Cryoprobes are placed and supported throughout ablation. (**b**) The superficial lesion is seen as an expanding iceball

to allow detachment from liver parenchyma. The probe track is plugged with gelfoam and haemostasis is secured. The cryoprobe may also be used to freeze resection margins after surgical resection where there is concern that adequate tumour clearance has not been obtained. Following cryotherapy, a catheter may be placed in the hepatic artery for delivery of locoregional chemotherapy.

4.4 Complications

Cryotherapy is generally a well-tolerated procedure. Serum chemistry, liver function tests and blood count are monitored after surgery. Complications may be local or generalised and include the following:

4.4.1 Local

- Bleeding: cracking of the ice ball can cause considerable blood loss. In the liver, this may be controlled with the use of liver sutures and abdominal packs.
- Coagulopathy: platelet consumption after hepatic cryotherapy can produce thrombocytopenia, though this is usually self-limiting.
- Local sepsis: abscess formation or fistula into adjacent organs may occur. Due caution should be taken in the vicinity of the extrahepatic bile ducts, urethra and rectum.
- Impotence, urinary incontinence and urethral stricture are risks following prostatic cryotherapy.

4.4.2 Systemic

- Hypothermia: systemic temperature changes depend upon the duration of freeze time and surgery. Given that electrolyte imbalance and disturbances of cardiac conduction are a risk, the risks of hypothermia must be especially minimised through the routine use of warming devices [20, 21].
- Electrolyte disturbance: release of potassium from lysed cells may result in hyperkalaemia and cardiac arrhythmyia, especially in the presence of hypothermia.
- Renal dysfunction: the patient must be kept well hydrated intra- and postoperatively, with attention given to maintenance of fluid balance, blood pressure and good urine output.
- Cryoshock: cryoshock is an infrequent, cytokine-mediated complication characterised by disseminated intravascular coagulation and multiorgan failure. The risk of death is high. The phenomenon was reported to occur in 0.04 % of patients after prostatic cryotherapy and in 1 % after hepatic cryotherapy, though it was responsible for 18.2 % of the deaths from hepatic cryotherapy. Treatment is supportive [22].

4.5   Results of Hepatic Cryotherapy

The approach to malignancies of the liver is frequently multimodal, and there are no randomised controlled trials comparing cryotherapy to alternative or to no treatment for either primary or secondary liver cancers. In 2000, Bilchik and colleagues compared radiofrequency ablation (RFA) with cryotherapy, either alone or in combination and with or without surgical resection [23]. They concluded that RFA resulted in fewer complications but that cryotherapy was more effective for lesions greater than 3 cm in diameter. Combining RFA with cryotherapy reduced cryotherapy-associated complications.

In 2003, Yan and colleagues from our unit performed a retrospective analysis of 146 patients treated for colorectal metastases [24]. They reported a 5-year survival of 19 % using cryotherapy with or without surgery. Morbidity was 27.9 % and included one death from myocardial infarction, as well bleeding and septic complications. More recently, Ruers et al. compared local ablation using RFA or cryotherapy with systemic chemotherapy for unresectable tumours [25]. Although there was no significant survival difference between the two groups (5-year overall survival 27 % and 15 %, respectively), the local ablation group had an improved quality of life. An increasing number of lesions and diameter greater than 4 cm might adversely affect outcome [26]. It is also known that the procedural complication rate is directly related to the volume of tissue frozen [27].

The gold standard treatment for liver metastases is surgical resection, and this achieves 5-year overall survival rates of between 37 % and 58 % [28]. However, of patients with hepatic colorectal metastases, only 10–20 % will be eligible for curative surgery. An important role therefore exists for single or combined therapies to treat patients with inoperable disease, and the aim should be to cure. We have shown that cryotherapy of the resection edge in patients with suboptimal margins can achieve similar outcomes to those with macroscopically clear margins (28 % and 40 % 5-year survival, respectively) [29]. It is unclear which combination of treatments is most effective, and this will no doubt be the subject of future clinical studies.

4.6   The Future

As new technologies are refined and chemotherapeutic options improve, the proportion of tumours deemed untreatable is declining. The ability to downstage tumours with induction (neoadjuvant) chemotherapy, rendering previously untreatable cancers curable, places even more importance on improving local ablative techniques.

Alternatives to cryotherapy include RFA, laser, microwave and high intensity focused ultrasound (HIFU). Given the dearth of evidence in favour of a particular modality, the choice often depends upon the experience of each centre. More trials comparing the efficacy of various energy forms are emerging, as are the varieties of probes and approaches that may be taken.

Limitations of cryotherapy include difficulties using large probes. This necessitates open operation with its associated risks. Even when using smaller probes through a laparoscopic approach, the nature of the ablation risks substantial blood loss through cracking of liver parenchyma. The risk of cryoshock is ever-present, and there is no analogue to this phenomenon with heated ablation devices. Furthermore, there are added costs and logistics of operating theatre time, compared with heated ablation that is frequently performed percutaneously under radiological guidance.

These costs might be partially offset by the ability to resterilise the cryotherapy probes. We have also mentioned the as-yet unconfirmed immunomodulatory effects of cryotherapy. Other factors may come into play in weighing the benefits of cryotherapy over the alternatives. One animal study found cryotherapy to be the least frequently associated with subsequent peritoneal carcinomatosis when compared with RFA and microwave [30], whereas yet another found that cryotherapy triggered the strongest inflammatory response out of RFA or hepatectomy [31].

There is a push towards minimally invasive ablative techniques, and this has been supported by the availability of laparoscopic ultrasound and argon coagulation. Gaseous rather than liquid coolant may be delivered using smaller apparatus and probes. As ablation becomes more finely tuned, the complication rate may also be reduced.

The potentially immunomodulating effects of cryotherapy are yet to be defined. If such an effect is present, chemotherapy might be used to manipulate and create an additive beneficial effect to local tumour destruction. Clearly, further work is needed to improve our understanding of certain aspects of this therapy, as are comparative studies and further refinements in the practicalities of cryosurgical ablation.

References

1. Frost R. Fire and ice. In: New Hampshire. London: Grant Richards Ltd; 1923.
2. Arnott JB. On the treatment of cancer by the regulated application of an anaesthetic temperature. London: J Churchill; 1851. p. 32–54.
3. Cooper IS, Lee A. Cryostatic congelation: a system for producing a limited controlled region of cooling or freezing of biologic tissues. J Nerv Ment Dis. 1961;133:259–63.
4. Gonder MJ, Soanes WA, Shulman S. Cryosurgical treatment of the prostate. Invest Urol. 1966;3:372–8.
5. Flocks RH, Nelson CM, Boatman DL. Perineal cryotherapy for prostatic carcinoma. J Urol. 1972;108:933–5.
6. Onik GM, Cohen JK, Reyes GD, Rubinsky B, Chang Z, Baust J. Transrectal ultrasound guided percutaneous radical cryosurgical ablation of the prostate. Cancer. 1993;72:1291–9.
7. Onik G, Rubinsky B, Zemel R, Weaver L, Kane R. Ultrasound-guided hepatic cryosurgery in the treatment of metastatic colon carcinoma. Preliminary results. Cancer. 1991;67:901–7.
8. Gilbert JC, Onik GM, Hoddick WK, Rubinsky B. Real time ultrasonic monitoring of hepatic cryosurgery. Cryobiology. 1985;22:319–30.
9. Saliken JC, Donnelly BJ, Rewcastle JC. The evolution and state of modern technology for prostate cryosurgery. Urology. 2002;60:26–33.
10. Hauschka TS, Mitchell JT, Niederpruem DJ. A reliable frozen tissue bank: viability and stability of 82 neoplastic and normal cell types after prolonged storage at −78°C. Cancer Res. 1959;19:643–54.

11. Meryman HT. Summary of the panel discussions, symposium on freezing rates. Cryobiology. 1966;24:210–1.
12. Farrant J, Walter CA. The cryobiological basis of cryosurgery. J Dermatol Surg Oncol. 1977;3:403–7.
13. Gage AA, Guest K, Montes M, Caruana JA, Whalen Jr DA. Effect of varying freezing and thawing rates in experimental cryosurgery. Cryobiology. 1985;22:175–82.
14. Bowers Jr WD, Hubbard RW, Daum RC, Ashbaugh P, Nilson E. Ultrastructural studies of muscle cells and vascular endothelium immediately after freeze thaw injury. Cryobiology. 1973;10:9–21.
15. Gage AA, Fazekas G, Riley EE. Freezing injury to large blood vessels in dogs. Surgery. 1967;61:748–54.
16. Johnson JP. Immunologic aspects of cryosurgery: potential modulation of immune recognition and effector cell maturation. Clin Dermatol. 1990;8:39–47.
17. Tanaka S. Immunological aspects of cryosurgery in general surgery. Cryobiology. 1982;19:247–62.
18. Soanes WA, Ablin RJ, Gonder MJ. Remission of metastatic lesions following cryosurgery in prostatic cancer: immunologic considerations. J Urol. 1970;104:154–9.
19. Gursel E, Roberts M, Veenema RJ. Regression of prostatic cancer following sequential cryotherapy to the prostate. J Urol. 1972;108:928–32.
20. Onik GM, Chambers N, Chernus SA, Zemel R, Atkinson D, Weaver ML. Hepatic cryosurgery with and without the Bair Hugger. J Surg Oncol. 1993;52:185–7.
21. Goodie DB, Horton MDA, Morris R, Nagy LS, Morris DL. The anaesthetic experience with hepatic cryotherapy for metastatic colorectal carcinoma. Anaesth Intensive Care. 1992;20:491–6.
22. Seifert JK, Morris DL. World survey on the complications of hepatic and prostate cryotherapy. World J Surg. 1999;23:109–14.
23. Bilchik AJ, Wood TF, Allegra D, Tsioulias GJ, Chung M, Rose M, et al. Cryosurgical ablation and radiofrequency ablation for unresectable hepatic malignant neoplasms: a proposed algorithm. Arch Surg. 2000;135:657–64.
24. Yan DB, Clingan P, Morris DL. Hepatic cryotherapy and regional chemotherapy with or without resection for liver metastases from colorectal carcinoma: how many are too many? Cancer. 2003;98:320–33.
25. Ruers T, Joosten J, Wiering B, Langenhoff BS, Dekker HM, Wobbes T, et al. Comparison between local ablative therapy and chemotherapy for non-resectable colorectal liver metastases: a prospective study. Ann Surg Oncol. 2007;14:1161–9.
26. Seifert JK, Junginger T. Prognostic factors for cryotherapy of colorectal liver metastases. Eur J Surg Oncol. 2004;30:34–40.
27. Sarantou T, Bilchik A, Ramming KP. Complications of hepatic cryosurgery. Semin Surg Oncol. 1998;14:156–62.
28. Abdalla EK, Adam R, Bilchik AJ, Jaeck D, Vauthey JN, Mahvi D. Improving resectability of hepatic colorectal metastases: expert consensus statement. Ann Surg Oncol. 2006;13:1271–80.
29. Hou RM, Chu F, Zhao J, Morris DL. The effects of surgical margin and edge cryotherapy after liver resection for colorectal cancer metastases. HPB. 2007;9:201–7.
30. Ng KK, Lam CM, Poon RT, Shek TW, To JY, Wo YH, et al. Comparison of systemic responses of radiofrequency ablation, cryotherapy, and surgical resection in a porcine liver model. Ann Surg Oncol. 2004;11:650–7.
31. Eichel L, Kim IY, Uribe C, Khonsari S, Basilotte J, Steward E, et al. Comparison of radical nephrectomy, laparoscopic microwave thermotherapy, cryotherapy and radiofrequency ablation for destruction of experimental VX-2 renal tumours in rabbits. J Endourol. 2005;18:1082–7.

Local and Regional Hyperthermia

5

Miriam R. Habib and David L. Morris

5.1 Historical Background

Those diseases which medicines do not cure, iron cures; those which iron cannot cure, fire cures; and those which fire cannot cure, are to be reckoned wholly incurable. [1]

The earliest documented case of cancer originates from ancient Egypt. The Edwin Smith Papyrus describes several cases of breast tumour that were treated with cautery using a 'fire drill'. More than three millennia on, we have gained some understanding of the cellular mechanisms responsible but are still striving to optimise the ways in which hyperthermia is used in cancer.

In 1779, de Kizowitz reported the effects of fever from malaria infection on malignant tumours. Busch added his observations in 1866 after witnessing regression of a sarcoma of the face following high fevers in a patient with erysipelas. He later confirmed this finding by inoculating a patient with sarcoma of the neck with erysipelas, noting transient improvement after the febrile illness. At the end of the nineteenth century, another physician William Coley again induced hyperthermia in cancer patients [2]. Following the injection of *Streptococcus*, he saw a variable tumour response that he initially attributed to differences in tumour biology. Soon after, however, he noted that there was a direct correlation between severity of infection and degree of tumour regression.

Experimentation with local hyperthermia began at the turn of the twentieth century. Byrne used galvanocautery in patients with carcinoma of the cervix and uterus and reported good responses, reduced recurrence and effective palliation [3]. He also observed that cancer cells were more sensitive to heat than normal tissues. Percy supported these findings and commented on the importance of sustained heat

M.R. Habib • D.L. Morris (✉)
Department of Surgery, St George Hospital, The University of New South Wales,
Pitney Building Level 3, Kogarah, NSW 2217, Australia
e-mail: miriam.habib@gmail.com; david.morris@unsw.edu.au

© Springer-Verlag Berlin Heidelberg 2016
K.R. Aigner, F.O. Stephens (eds.), *Induction Chemotherapy*,
DOI 10.1007/978-3-319-28773-7_5

to ensure adequate distribution through diseased tissues [4]. Hot water immersion was another technique used to achieve either local hyperthermia of the extremities or whole-body hyperthermia for disseminated disease.

In 1967, Cavaliere and colleagues reported results from isolated limb perfusion (ILP) in 22 patients [5]. The limbs were perfused for several hours with blood warmed through a heat exchanger, and temperature probes placed within the tumour ensured that the temperature remained above 40 °C. Though there was limited short-term regression in some patients, the complication rate was high and included six deaths and three early amputations.

It has since been felt that hyperthermia as a solitary treatment for cancer is technically challenging and often results in only a transient improvement at the expense of high morbidity and mortality. These studies have however demonstrated that cancer cells are preferentially sensitive to heat, and hyperthermia is now being used in combination with chemotherapy and radiotherapy to target malignant disease.

5.2   Biological Rationale

The cellular and tissue basis for hyperthermic injury has been well studied since the early 1900s and may be summarised as follows:

- Both normal and malignant cells are heat sensitive during the S phase of the cell cycle. Nucleic acid production is reduced and mitosis is arrested. This effect is only transient and proliferation may resume if cells are kept under good growth conditions [6].
- Depression of aerobic metabolism appears to occur preferentially in malignant cells.
- There is increased lysosomal enzyme activity in malignant cells.
- Cellular destruction is enhanced under conditions of hypoxia, poor nutrition and low pH. These conditions may already prevail within the chaotic architecture of a malignant tumour. With the application of heat, microcirculatory changes resulting in stasis of blood flow may occur, further promoting this adverse environment [7].

The optimal temperature to achieve tumour destruction is thought to be between 41 and 42 °C [8]. Above 44 °C, the threshold for injury to normal tissue is exceeded, risking collateral damage to healthy cells. Below 42 °C, the length of time taken to reliably destroy tumour tissue is impractical, and there is a suggestion that at these lower levels of hyperthermia, tumour cell metabolism and spread might actually increase.

A further important phenomenon is that of thermotolerance. Cells exposed to high temperatures may become transiently resistant to repeated heat stress. This response subsides after a week and may be overcome by prolonged heating or heating to a higher temperature than before [9].

5.2.1 Hyperthermia and Radiation Therapy

Heat is a known radiosensitiser, and its efficacy depends upon both the temperature achieved and the duration of exposure at that temperature. As well as a directly cytotoxic effect, heat may transiently improve tumour blood flow and oxygenation [10]. Radiation loses efficacy under hypoxic conditions, and it is by improving this parameter and the cell microenvironment that heat is believed to increase radiosensitivity.

Numerous randomised trials have been conducted to evaluate hyperthermia in combination with radiotherapy [11–13]. Although results have generally been favourable with improved clinical response and survival, uptake of thermoradiotherapy has been slow. This may be due to the technical complexities of delivering and monitoring a reliable dose of thermal energy during radiotherapy.

5.2.2 Hyperthermia and Chemotherapy

There are several mechanisms by which hyperthermia is believed to enhance the efficacy of chemotherapy, although the effect depends upon the agent used and on the timing of heating. Adriamycin, for example, becomes less effective if heat is administered before the drug is given and markedly more effective if the heat and drug are delivered simultaneously [14]. The vinca alkaloids and antimetabolites show limited additional toxicity with heat. Cisplatin, mitomycin C, bleomycin, melphalan and cyclophosphamide work synergistically with heat to supra-additive effect [15–17].

In addition to a temperature-dependent cytotoxicity, hyperthermia may stimulate improved cellular uptake of the drug through an initial improvement in tissue perfusion and increased permeability of the cell membrane. Cellular metabolism may also become altered, with consequences for pharmacokinetics and drug removal.

With the advent of heat-exchange pumps, it has become possible to deliver locoregional chemohyperthermia. This technology is now being used in isolated limb perfusion and intraperitoneal chemotherapy.

5.3 Techniques

5.3.1 Whole-Body Hyperthermia

Building upon the findings of tumour regression after high fevers, various approaches have been taken to induce whole-body hyperthermia. These include total body submersion in hot wax or liquid, encasement in a high-flow water perfusion suit and radiant heat. More recently, venovenous bypass has been trialled for advanced cancers [18].

Such techniques demand specialist skills, facilities and monitoring, and they risk effects of multiorgan dysfunction such as delirium, cardiac arrhythmias and coagulopathy. Surprisingly though, such complications have been rare [19, 20]. Nevertheless, cancer treatments are becoming more organ specific, and it should be possible to direct these techniques to the region of interest to reduce morbidity and cost.

5.3.2 Regional Hyperthermia

5.3.2.1 Isolated Limb Perfusion

In 1958, Creech and colleagues described the use of ILP to treat metastatic melanoma [21]. Blood supply to the limb was isolated using a tourniquet, and the main artery and vein were cannulated. Whole blood, to which phenylalanine mustard (melphalan) was added, was circulated through the limb using an extracorporeal pump. One year after the treatment, the majority of lesions had regressed and no new lesions were seen.

Locoregional chemotherapy is preferable in cases where the disease is confined, enabling the delivery of high-dose therapy whilst limiting systemic side effects. The role of hyperthermia in ILP is twofold. Firstly, heat is necessary to prevent cutaneous vasoconstriction and ensure adequate drug delivery to the area being targeted. Secondly, heat is known to enhance the cytotoxic activity of melphalan [15, 22]. Although this activity is greatest at temperatures higher than 41.5 °C, local toxicity is more likely to occur. Mild hyperthermia in the range of 38–40 °C is therefore chosen as a trade-off between the benefits of heat and the adverse effects of thermochemotherapy [23].

ILP is currently used for the control of locally recurrent or inoperable local melanoma and sarcoma. Isolated limb infusion (ILI) is a similar but minimally invasive procedure that has yielded similar results to ILP [24]. Melphalan is the standard chemotherapy drug and may be used in combination with tumour necrosis factor alpha (TNF-α) and interferon-gamma (IFN-γ). TNF-α acts through direct cytotoxicity and by instigating microvascular damage. It appears to work synergistically with melphalan, and studies have shown an increase in complete response rates from 54 % using melphalan alone to as high as 91 % using both drugs combined [25]. Though its action is enhanced with heat, distal toxicity resulting in amputation has occurred at moderate temperatures [26]. Cost, availability and concerns about side effects remain prohibitive to the widespread addition of TNF-α and IFN-γ to ILP regimes.

5.3.2.2 Heated Intraperitoneal Chemotherapy

Peritoneal carcinomatosis results from the spread of abdominal and pelvic malignancies, mesothelioma or mucinous tumour across the peritoneal cavity. Systemic agents are poorly absorbed across the peritoneal-plasma barrier and are ineffective in treating this type of disease. This isolation, however, makes the peritoneal cavity a suitable vessel for a locoregional approach. There is good evidence that cytoreductive surgery to resect visible tumour, followed by heated intraperitoneal chemotherapy (HIPEC) to treat microscopic disease, results in improved survival in carefully selected patients [27–29].

Perioperative chemotherapy may be administered during surgery or through abdominal catheters early in the postoperative period, and its efficacy is thought to depend upon several factors including timing of chemotherapy, size of residual peritoneal tumour and molecular weight of the chemotherapy agent. Intraoperative chemotherapy allows good exposure of all surfaces within the abdomen and pelvis to the drug at a time when free tumour cells may be circulating after surgery, and administration of HIPEC is associated with significantly improved survival after this type of operation [30].

In 1980, Spratt and colleagues demonstrated that HIPEC was feasible and well tolerated in a patient with pseudomyxoma peritonei [31]. Drugs enter the peritoneal tumour cells by diffusion, and their maximal penetration is up to 3 mm in depth [32]. It is therefore important to remove as much macroscopic tumour as possible prior to the instillation of chemotherapy. The addition of heat improves drug penetration to depths of 5 mm and beyond [33]. Again, local thermal effects on microcirculation and cell membrane permeability are important in propagating the chemotherapeutic effect.

Peritoneal hyperthermia is poorly tolerated and should only be used whilst the patient is under anaesthesia. After all visible disease has been resected and before any anastomosis is created, 2–3 l of dialysis solution containing the chemotherapy agent is warmed to 41 °C and perfused through the abdomen for 90 min. The intraabdominal contents are gently agitated by hand to ensure that all surfaces have good exposure to the drug.

The chosen agent should ideally maintain a high concentration within the peritoneal cavity and penetrate tumour cells without crossing the peritoneal-plasma barrier. Mitomycin C is one such drug. Whilst there is little systemic absorption, it has a synergistic action with moderate hyperthermia and is effective against chemoresistant tumours such a pseudomyxoma peritonei [34]. Similarly, tissue penetration of doxorubicin is markedly increased with hyperthermia of 43 °C without increasing systemic absorption [35].

5.3.3 Local Hyperthermia

Local hyperthermia is being used more and more frequently to treat discrete malignant lesions. The most common mode is radiofrequency ablation (RFA), although other thermal ablative techniques such as microwave, laser and high-intensity focused ultrasound (HIFU) are becoming more widely used.

The approach to local hyperthermia differs from the forms discussed earlier. Since the focus is usually on one or several distinct lesions, the risk of damaging healthy tissue is lessened, and the temperatures that can be created are therefore far higher. During RFA, a probe is inserted into the lesion and an alternating current generates heat at the probe tip. As tissue temperatures rapidly exceed to 60 °C, protein denaturation, the breakdown of nucleic acids and disruption of lipid bilayers result in cell death [36]. An expanding zone of coagulative necrosis is created around the probe as thermal energy is conducted outwards. The extent depends upon the level of RF energy applied and on tissue impedance. The time taken to achieve a 3 cm ablation in the liver is around 10 min.

Microwave ablation uses electromagnetic waves to generate heat. Again, a probe is directed into the tumour under image guidance. Agitation of water molecules produces heat and causes cell death from coagulative necrosis. Expansion of the ablation zone relies on conduction and convection. Interstitial laser ablation is a newer technique where laser fibres are placed into the target tissue to generate cytotoxic hyperthermia.

These techniques are being used to treat primary and metastatic tumours in many tissues including the liver, kidney, bone and lung. They can be performed percutaneously under image guidance or using minimally invasive surgery, and they permit preservation of healthy tissue. Numerous studies have compared these modalities for various cancers. Important future developments will include improved real-time imaging, non-invasive techniques such as HIFU and methods to improve heat distribution across larger tumours such as the use of multiple probes.

5.4 Summary

Hyperthermia is effective at inducing cell death, provided that an optimal temperature between 40 and 42 °C is maintained for sufficient duration. Malignant cells are more susceptible to thermal damage at these temperatures than are normal cells.

A therapeutic elevation in temperature may be achieved through whole-body hyperthermia or locoregional heat, though the latter is preferable. A broader range of therapeutic options has become available to manage locoregional recurrence. Hyperthermia has anecdotally and experimentally demonstrated its ability to downstage disease, but uptake has been slow. Regardless of the method used, specialist equipment and skills are needed to safely perform these procedures. Other limitations include the inability to consistently heat large tumours and to non-invasively monitor tissue temperature during the procedure.

Future studies should aim to clearly define optimal thermal dosimetry as well as to develop the apparatus with which to deliver it. The potential to use gene therapy to potentiate thermal therapy has also been considered [37]. As techniques continue to improve, a complementary pathway in cancer therapy may yet be uncovered by revisiting this ancient remedy.

References

1. Aphorisms by Hippocrates. Translated by Francis Adams. Available at http://classics.mit.edu/Hippocrates/aphorisms.html. Accessed 8 Feb 2010.
2. Coley WB. The treatment of malignant tumours by repeated inoculations of erysipelas with a report of ten original cases. Am J Med Sci. 1893;104:487–511.
3. Byrne J. A digest of 20 years' experience in the treatment of cancer of the uterus by galvanocautery. Am J Obstet Gynecol. 1899;22:1052.
4. Percy JF. Heat the most practical and promising treatment in uterine carcinoma. Calif State J Med. 1921;19:78–81.

5. Cavaliere R, Ciocatto EC, Giovanella BP, Heidelberger C, Johnson RO, Margottini M, et al. Selective heat sensitivity of cancer cells – biochemical and clinical studies. Cancer. 1967;20:1351–81.
6. Overgaard J. Effect of hyperthermia on malignant cells in vivo: a review and a hypothesis. Cancer. 1977;39:2637–46.
7. Dudar TE, Jain RK. Differential response of normal and tumour microcirculation to hyperthermia. Cancer Res. 1984;44:605–12.
8. Dickson JA, Calderwood SK. Temperature range and selective sensitivity of tumours to hyperthermia: a critical review. Ann NY Acad Sci. 1980;335:180–205.
9. Urano M. Kinetics of thermotolerance in normal and tumour tissue: a review. Cancer Res. 1986;46:474–82.
10. Song CW, Park HJ, Lee CK, Griffin R. Implications of increased tumor blood flow and oxygenation caused by mild temperature hyperthermia in tumor treatment. Int J Hyperthermia. 2005;21:761–7.
11. Vernon CC, Hand JW, Field SB, Machin D, Whaley JB, van der Zee J, et al. Radiotherapy with or without hyperthermia in the treatment of superficial localized breast cancer: results from five randomized controlled trials – International Collaborative Hyperthermia Group. Int J Radiat Oncol Biol Phys. 1996;35:731–44.
12. Sneed PK, Stauffer PR, McDermott MW, Diederich CJ, Lamborn KR, Prados MD, et al. Survival benefit of hyperthermia in a prospective randomized trial of brachytherapy boost +/– hyperthermia for glioblastoma multiforme. Int J Radiat Oncol Biol Phys. 1998;40:287–95.
13. De Haas-Kock DFM, Buijsen J, Pijls-Johannesma M, Lutgens L, Lammering G, Mastrigt GAPGV, De Ruysscher DKM, Lambin P, van der Zee J. Concomitant hyperthermia and radiation therapy for treating locally advanced rectal cancer. Cochrane Database Syst. Rev. 2009;(3):CD006269.
14. Hahn GM, Strande DP. Cytotoxic effects of hyperthermia and adriamycin on Chinese hamster cell. J Natl Cancer Inst. 1976;37:1063–7.
15. Hahn GM. Potential for therapy of drugs and hyperthermia. Cancer Res. 1979;39:2264–8.
16. Goldfeder A, Newport S. Thermally-enhanced tumour regression in mice treated with melphalan. Anticancer Res. 1984;4:17–22.
17. Barlogie B, Corry PM, Drewinko B. In vitro thermochemotherapy of human colon cancer cells with cis-dichlorodiammineplatinum(II) and mitomycin C. Cancer Res. 1980;40:1165–8.
18. Zwischenberger JB, Vertrees RA, Bedell EA, McQuitty CK, Chernin JM, Woodson LC. Percutaneous venovenous perfusion-induced systemic hyperthermia for lung cancer: a phase I safety study. Ann Thorac Surg. 2004;77:1916–25.
19. Larkin JM, Edwards WS, Smith DE, Clark PJ. Systemic thermotherapy: description of a method and physiological tolerance in clinical subjects. Cancer. 1977;40:3155–9.
20. Pettigrew RT, Galt JM, Ludgate CM, Smith AN. Clinical effects of whole body hyperthermia in advanced malignancy. Br Med J. 1974;4:679–82.
21. Creech O, Krementz ET, Ryan RF, Winblad JN. Chemotherapy of cancer: regional perfusion utilizing an extracorporeal circuit. Ann Surg. 1958;148:616–32.
22. Urano M, Ling CC. Thermal enhancement of melphalan and oxaliplatin cytotoxicity in vitro. Int J Hyperthermia. 2002;18:307–15.
23. Minor DR, Allen RE, Alberts D, Peng YM, Tardelli G, Hutchinson J. A clinical and pharmacokinetic study of isolated limb perfusion with heat and melphalan for melanoma. Cancer. 1985;55:2638–44.
24. Thompson JF, Kam PC, Waugh RC, Harman CR. Isolated limb infusion with cytotoxic agents: a simple alternative to isolated limb perfusion. Semin Surg Oncol. 1998;14:238–47.
25. Grünhagen DJ, de Wilt JHW, van Geel AN, Eggermont AMM. Isolated limb perfusion for melanoma patients – a review of its indications and the role of tumour necrosis factor-α. Eur J Surg Oncol. 2006;32:371–80.
26. de Wilt JH, Manusama ER, van Tiel ST, van Ijken MG, ten Hagen TL, Eggermont AM. Prerequisites for effective isolated limb perfusion using tumour necrosis factor alpha and melphalan in rats. Br J Cancer. 1999;80:161–6.

27. Esquivel J, Sticca R, Sugarbaker P, Levine E, Yan TD, Alexander R, et al. Cytoreductive surgery and hyperthermic intraperitoneal chemotherapy in the management of peritoneal surface malignancies of colonic origin: a consensus statement. Ann Surg Oncol. 2007;14:128–33.

28. Yan TD, Black D, Savady R, Sugarbaker PH. A systematic review on the efficacy of cytoreductive surgery and perioperative intraperitoneal chemotherapy for pseudomyxoma peritonei. Ann Surg Oncol. 2007;14:484–92.

29. Yano H, Moran BJ, Cecil TD, Murphy EM. Cytoreductive surgery and intraperitoneal chemotherapy for peritoneal mesothelioma. Eur J Surg Oncol. 2009;35:980–5.

30. Yan TD, Deraco M, Baratti D, Kusamura S, Elias D, Glehen O, et al. Cytoreductive surgery and hyperthermic intraperitoneal chemotherapy for malignant peritoneal mesothelioma: multi-institutional experience. J Clin Oncol. 2009;27:6237–42.

31. Spratt JS, Adcock RA, Muscovin M, Sherril W, McKeown J. Clinical delivery system for intraperitoneal hyperthermic chemotherapy. Cancer Res. 1980;40:256–60.

32. Los G, Mutsaers PH, van der Vijgh WJ, Baldew GS, de Graaf PW, McVie JG. Direct diffusion of cis-diamminedichloroplatinum(II) in intraperitoneal rat tumours after intraperitoneal chemotherapy: a comparison with systemic chemotherapy. Cancer Res. 1989;49:3380–4.

33. Van de Vaart PJ, van der Vange N, Zoetmulder FA, van Goethem AR, van Tellingen O, ten Bokkel Huinink WW, et al. Intraperitoneal cisplatin with regional hyperthermia in advanced ovarian cancer: pharmacokinetics and cisplatin-DNA adduct formation in patients and ovarian cancer cell lines. Eur J Cancer. 1998;34:148–54.

34. Witkamp AJ, de Bree E, Kaag MM, van Slooten GW, van Coevorden F, Zoetmulder FAN. Extensive surgical cytoreduction and intraoperative hyperthermic intraperitoneal chemotherapy in patients with pseudomyxoma peritonei. Br J Surg. 2001;88:458–63.

35. Jaquet P, Averbach A, Stuart OA, Chang D, Sugarbaker PH. Hyperthermic intraperitoneal doxorubicin: pharmacokinetics, metabolism and tissue distribution in a art model. Cancer Chemother Pharmacol. 1998;41:147–54.

36. Izzo F. New approaches to hepatic malignancies: other thermal ablation techniques: microwave and interstitial laser ablation of liver tumors. Ann Surg Oncol. 2002;10:491–7.

37. Walther W, Stein U. Heat-responsive gene expression for gene therapy. Adv Drug Deliv Rev. 2009;61:641–9.

The Role of Hypoxia and Hyperthermia in Chemotherapy

6

Giammaria Fiorentini, Maurizio Cantore, Francesco Montagnani, Andrea Mambrini, Michelina D'Alessandro, and Stefano Guadagni

6.1   Introduction

Medical approaches to cancer treatment, primarily radiation therapy and chemotherapy, are almost exclusively based on agents that kill cells. The main problem with these current treatments, however, is that they do not have specificity for cancer cells. In the case of drugs, it is primarily the constant and continuing proliferation of many of the cancer cells that makes them more sensitive to cell killing than their normal cellular counterparts; for radiation therapy, a degree of specificity is achieved by localizing the radiation to the tumor and its immediate surrounding normal tissue. However, both treatments are limited by their toxic effects on normal cells. To achieve greater efficacy, many scientists are attempting to stress differences between normal and malignant cells at the biomolecular properties and cellular milieu. The physiology of solid tumors at the microenvironmental level is sufficiently different from that of the normal tissues from which they arise to provide a selective target for treatment.

6.2   Tumor Hypoxia in Chemotherapy

Tumor hypoxia is an important factor in oncology, since it contributes to tumor progression by the activation of genes associated with those promoting angiogenesis. Moreover, it has profound effects on therapy: Oxygen helps to stabilize

G. Fiorentini (✉) • F. Montagnani • M. D'Alessandro
Department of Oncology, "San Giuseppe" General City Hospital, Empoli, FI, Italy
e-mail: g.fiorentini@iol.it

M. Cantore • A. Mambrini
Department of Oncology, Carrara City Hospital, Massa-Carrara, Italy

S. Guadagni
Department of Surgical Sciences, University of L'Aquila, L'Aquila, Italy

© Springer-Verlag Berlin Heidelberg 2016
K.R. Aigner, F.O. Stephens (eds.), *Induction Chemotherapy*,
DOI 10.1007/978-3-319-28773-7_6

radiation damage in DNA, while hypoxic cells show considerable (about fivefold) resistance to radiotherapy; this is considered the major cause for the failure of radiotherapy in some tumors. Attempts to overcome this effect include the use of hyperthermia, oxygen-mimetic radiosensitizers, and multifractional radiotherapy to allow reoxygenation of tumor tissue. Radiosensitizers are drugs designed to act similarly to oxygen in fixing radiation damage in DNA, but they are less rapidly metabolized and are therefore more widely distributed in tumor tissues.

The first pioneering work of Gray et al. [1] demonstrated that the sensitivity to radiation damage of cells and tissues depends on the presence of oxygen at the time of irradiation. The histological studies on human lung adenocarcinomas by Thomlinson and Gray [2] provided an explanation of the mechanism by which cells could become hypoxic in tumors. They postulated that because of their unrestrained growth, tumor cells would be forced away from vessels, beyond the effective diffusion distance of oxygen in respiring tissue, thereby becoming hypoxic and eventually necrotic.

There are two important further consequences of reducing oxygen concentration: (a) The fraction of proliferating cells and/or the rate of cell proliferation decreases as a function of distance from the vascular supply, a phenomenon that is largely the result of decreasing oxygen levels [3–5]. An important consequence of this hypoxia-induced inhibition of proliferation is that, because most anticancer drugs are primarily effective against constantly and continuously dividing cells, their effectiveness would be expected to fall off as a function of distance from blood vessels. This has been shown experimentally [1–7]. (b) Since hypoxic cells are the ones most distant from blood vessels, they will be exposed to lower concentrations of drug than those adjacent to blood vessels, primarily as a result of the metabolism of such agents through successive cellular layers.

Hypoxia in solid tumors, however, has an important consequence in addition to conferring a direct resistance to radiation and chemotherapy 5–7. Graeber showed that low oxygen levels caused apoptosis in minimally transformed mouse embryo fibroblasts and that this apoptosis depended to a large extent on wild-type *p53* genotype. They further showed, using these same cells growing as solid tumors in immune-deprived mice, that apoptosis co-localized with hypoxic regions in tumors derived from *p53* wild-type mice. In tumors derived from *p53–/–* cells, there was much less apoptosis and no co-localization with tumor hypoxia. These findings provide evidence that hypoxia, by selecting for mutant *p53*, might predispose tumors to a more malignant phenotype.

Clinical data support this conclusion. Studies on both soft tissue sarcomas and on carcinomas of the cervix have shown that hypoxic tumors are more likely to be metastatic.

However, others have proposed that tumor hypoxia can occur in a second way, by temporary obstruction or cessation of tumor blood flow, the so-called acute hypoxia model. Definitive evidence for this type of acute hypoxia arising from fluctuating blood flow has come from elegant studies with transplanted tumors in mice using diffusion-limited fluorescent dyes. Because fluctuating blood flow has also been demonstrated in human tumors, it is likely that this type of hypoxia is also present in human tumors. The consequences of acute hypoxia will be similar to those of the diffusion-limited hypoxia. Any cells surrounding a closed blood vessel will be resistant to radiation killing because of their lack of oxygen at the time of radiation and will be exposed to lower levels of anticancer drugs than those surrounding blood vessels with a normal flow. This would be expected to lead to differences in response to anticancer agents, as has been observed in experimental tumors.

The low oxygen levels in tumors can probably be turned from a disadvantage to an advantage in cancer treatment. Such a possibility was proposed 20 years ago by Lin et al. [8], who reasoned that compounds based on the quinone structure of mitomycin C might be more active in hypoxic tumors. It was known that mitomycin C required metabolic reduction of the benzoquinone ring to produce the cytotoxic bifunctional alkylating agent. Lin reasoned that a lower oxidation reduction (redox) potential for tumor tissue, relative to most normal tissues, could increase reductive activation of these quinone derivatives in tumors. Although this was not the correct mechanism for the increased cytotoxicity of mitomycin C and certain analogues toward hypoxic cells (much lower levels of hypoxia are needed to change cellular redox potential), these studies were important in suggesting the potential of hypoxia-activated drugs and led to the concept of selectively killing the hypoxic cells in solid tumors.

6.3   Hypoxia and Specific Drugs

There are presently four different classes of hypoxia-specific drugs that are in use clinically or are being developed for clinical use. They are the quinone antibiotics, nitroaromatics, and the aliphatic and heteroaromatic N-oxides. All report two peculiarities: They require hypoxia for activation, and this activation is related to the presence of reductases. The most effective drugs have shown the capacity to increase the antitumor efficacy of compounds that kill oxygenated cells, i.e., cytotoxic chemotherapy agents such as cisplatin and cyclophosphamide.

In the quinone class, the three principal agents of current clinical interest are mitomycin C, porfiromycin, and apaziquone (E09). All are structurally similar and require reductive metabolism for activity. Each of them is converted by reductive metabolism to a bifunctional alkylating agent and probably produces its major cytotoxic activity through the formation of DNA interstrand cross-links.

Mitomycin C, considered to be the prototype bioreductive drug, was introduced into clinical use in 1958 and has demonstrated efficacy toward a number of different tumors, in combination with other selective drugs whose toxicity toward hypoxic cells is modest. However, based on this activity, mitomycin C has been combined with radiotherapy in two randomized trials of head and neck cancer, the pooled results of which gave a statistically significant disease-free survival benefit [5–8].

The third drug in this series, E09, is a much more efficient substrate for DT-diaphorase than either mitomycin C or porfiromycin and shows high toxicity to both aerobic and hypoxic cells with high DT-diaphorase levels. Cells with low DT-diaphorase levels are much less susceptible to killing by E09 under aerobic conditions, but this drug shows a high, up to 50-fold, preferential toxicity toward hypoxic cells. However, the pharmacokinetics of this agent works against its clinical utility, and phase I clinical studies have shown little activity of this drug.

A second class of bioreductive agents is that of the nitroimidazoles, the first two of which, metronidazole and misonidazole, have been extensively tested as hypoxic radiosensitizing agents. Further drug development by Adams and Stratford [9] produced a compound, RSU1069, which has been shown to be a highly efficient cytotoxic agent with activity both in vitro and in vivo. RSU1069 has a hypoxic cytotoxicity ratio of some 10–100 for different cell lines in vitro, and it, or its prodrug, RB6145, has shown excellent activity in mouse tumor models when combined with irradiation or agents that induce hypoxia. Unfortunately, however, clinical testing of RB6145 has been aborted due to irreversible cytotoxicity toward retinal cells.

Tirapazamine (TPZ) is the first and, thus far, only representative of the third class of hypoxia-selective cytotoxins [6]. The mechanism for the preferential toxicity of TPZ toward hypoxic cells is the result of an enzymatic reduction that adds an electron to the TPZ molecule, forming a highly reactive radical. This radical is able to cause cell killing by producing DNA damage leading to chromosome aberrations. Moreover, DNA damage occurs only from TPZ metabolism within the nucleus. TPZ produces specific potentiation of cell kill by radiation and cis-platinum. Specifically, the synergistic cytotoxic interaction observed when TPZ and cis-platinum are given in sequence depends on the TPZ exposure being under hypoxic conditions. In fact, there is no interaction when TPZ is given under aerobic conditions. It has also been demonstrated that the cytotoxic activity of TPZ under hypoxia is independent of p53 gene status of tumor cells. This drug has 100-fold differential toxicity toward hypoxic versus aerobic cells.

Based on experimental studies that evaluated the responsiveness of tumor cells under aerobic and hypoxic conditions, Teicher et al. [10] classified chemotherapeutic agents into three groups: (1) preferentially toxic in aerobic conditions (bleomycin, procarbazine, streptonigrin, actinomycin D, vincristine, and melphalan), (2) preferentially toxic under hypoxic conditions (mitomycin C and adriamycin), and (3) no major preferential toxicity to oxygenation (cis-platinum, 5-fluorouracil, and methotrexate).

6.4 Hypoxia and Gene Therapy

Tumor hypoxia also selects for gene mutations in tumor cells. In particular, mutations occurred in genes involved in the process of apoptosis. It could be shown that repeated exposure to low oxygen tension selected for p53 mutations rendered tumor cells resistant to hypoxia-induced apoptosis. It is further well documented that low oxygen tension confers resistance to tumors to irradiation therapy and may thereby contribute to tumor aggressiveness.

The newest direction for exploiting tumor physiology is the field of gene therapy. In this novel approach to anticancer therapy, genetic material is transferred into cells with the ultimate goal of selectively killing cancer cells and sparing normal cells.

Recent studies have regarded the possibility of using the hypoxia-signaling pathway to selectively activate gene expression [11, 12]. Hypoxia induces the expression of a number of genes, principally via the stabilization of members of the bHLH/PAS family of transcription factors that bind to a consensus DNA sequence, the hypoxia response element (HRE). Physiologically regulated expression vector systems, containing HRE sequences, are now under development to target therapeutic gene expression to tumor cells characterized by low oxygen tension [11]. From a clinical point of view, the combination of hyperthermia and hypoxia seems to add activity to intra-arterial chemotherapy [12]. At the same time, the exposure of body regions, such as the pelvis or limbs, to a locally high dose of bioreductive agent such as mitomycin C, in hypoxic conditions, shows activity in refractory cancers [13–16].

Following the study of genes, we understood that there are other ways in which hypoxia might contribute to drug resistance. One is through the amplification of genes, such as dihydrofolate reductase, conferring various glucose-regulated proteins that appear to be responsible for resistance to doxorubicin, etoposide, and camptothecin.

The microenvironment of solid tumors has several characteristics that distinguish it from the corresponding normal tissues. These different aspects are thought to be due to the interaction between the poorly formed tumor vasculature and the physiologic characteristics of the cells within the tumor. The interaction between the cancer cells and vasculature results in three well-known microenvironmental hallmarks of solid tumors: `tension, low extracellular pH, and high interstitial fluid pressure. To overcome this challenge, the new therapy of tumors, particularly renal cell carcinoma (RCC), took a major step forward with the approval of sorafenib and sunitinib in 2005 and 2006. These two multi-targeted tyrosine kinase inhibitors are the first on a growing list of molecularly targeted therapy in RCC. They all share the ability to modulate the hypoxia-inducible factor (HIF)-VEGF-VEGF receptor axis that plays a significant role in the development of many solid tumors [15]. Several aspects of tumor physiology seem to be directly responsive to the low-oxygen environment within the tumor through the activity of the HIF-1 transcription factor. HIF-1 is therefore characterized as responsible for adaptive changes in the hypoxic regions within the tumor. There are many genes that HIF-1 can transactivate, including VEGF, glycolytic enzymes, ion channels, protease regulators, and mitochondrial regulators. The possibility of HIF-1 blockade therefore represents an interesting strategy for modifying the tumor physiology. HIF-1 is part of the loop responsible for the physiologic condition within the tumor. The tumor vasculature leads to hypoxia; this leads to HIF-1 gene expression changes. Several examples of specific HIF-1 target genes fit well into this model of explaining the changes observed in the tumor microenvironment.

6.5 Hyperthermia and Chemotherapy

Preclinical thermo-chemotherapy studies have given valuable information on the schedule of the cytotoxic interaction between the different agents and on the molecular mechanisms responsible for the potentiating effect. Several studies have demonstrated that the cytotoxic activity of various chemotherapeutic agents is enhanced by mild or moderate hyperthermia (40.5–43 °C) [17]. In these investigations, the effect of scheduling on the cytotoxic interaction between hyperthermia and drugs has also been investigated in in vitro experimental systems. There are data regarding doxorubicin, the platinum compounds cisplatin and carboplatin, the bifunctional alkylating agent melphalan, and the antimetabolite methotrexate which indicate that in each case, the maximal cytotoxicity occurs when the drug is administered simultaneously with hyperthermia [17–24].

The mechanisms responsible for the effect of hyperthermia on cell killing by anticancer drugs are not entirely understood. For example, for melphalan, which is widely used in experimental and clinical thermo-chemotherapy studies, different putative mechanisms of potentiation have been suggested including an increase in melphalan influx leading to a higher intracellular drug accumulation [20].

The alteration of DNA quaternary structure favors alkylation; the interference with drug-DNA adduct metabolism and the inhibition of repair [21] induce the stabilization of drug-induced G2 phase cell accumulation [21] through the inhibition of $p32^{ctlc2}$ kinase activity [22, 23]. As regards cisplatin, it has been demonstrated that the cytotoxic activity of this compound, as well as that of the platinum derivatives lobaplatin and oxaliplatin, is increased under hyperthermic conditions as the consequence of an enhanced formation of DNA-platinum adducts [24].

Preclinical studies have also significantly contributed to the proposition of potential cellular determinants of response to individual and combined treatments. The relevance of cell kinetic and DNA ploidy characteristics as indicators of thermoresponsiveness has been determined in primary cultures of human melanoma [25]. Results from this study showed that the median 3 H-thymidine labeling index of sensitive tumors was fourfold that of resistant tumors. Moreover, thermosensitivity was found more frequently in tumors with a diploid nuclear DNA content than in those with DNA aneuploidy.

Since heat and drug sensitivity may be related to the ability of tumor cells to mount a stress response, the relationship between constitutive (and inducible) levels of heat shock proteins (HSPs) and thermosensitivity has been evaluated in the testes and bladder cancer cell lines [26]. No correlation between constitutive levels of HSP90 or HSP72/73 and cellular thermoresponsiveness was found. However, results suggest that low HSP27 expression might contribute to heat sensitivity.

6.6   Hyperthermia and Specific Drugs

The most active agent(s) at elevated temperatures has yet to be determined. Some studies suggest that the drug of choice at elevated temperatures may be different from that at the physiological temperature and that the alkylating agents may be most effective at elevated temperatures. To further investigate these possibilities, the effects of chemotherapeutic agents were compared by Takemoto et al. [27]. He studied these agents: cyclophosphamide, ifosfamide, melphalan, cisplatin, 5-fluorouracil, mitomycin C, and bleomycin. Three tumors (mammary carcinoma, osteosarcoma, and squamous cell carcinoma) were used. They were transplanted into the feet of C3H/He mice. When tumors reached 65 mm, a test agent was injected intraperitoneally.

Tumors were immediately heated at 41.5 °C for 30 min, and the tumor growth (TG) time was studied for each tumor. Using the TG times, the TG-50 (the time required for one-half of the total number of the treated tumors to reach the volume of 800 mm from 65 mm) was calculated. Subsequently, the tumor growth delay time (GDT) and the thermal enhancement ratio (TER) were obtained. The GDT was the difference between the TG-50 of treated tumors and that of non-treated control tumors. The TER was the ratio of the GDT of a group treated with an agent at 41.5 °C to that of a group treated with the agent at room temperature. Results showed that the top three effective agents tested at 41.5 °C were solely alkylating agents: cyclophosphamide, ifosfamide, and melphalan for each kind of tumor. A GDT of cisplatin was smaller than those of the alkylating agents. The smallest TER, 1.1, was observed for 5-fluorouracil, which was given for mammary carcinoma, and for mitomycin C, which was given for squamous cell carcinoma. It could be concluded that the alkylating agents at elevated temperatures might be the drugs of choice for many types of tumors.

6.7 Alkylating Agents and Oxaliplatin

Urano and Ling [28] studied the effects of various agents on animal tumors with different histopathology at elevated temperatures. His studies indicated that alkylating agents were most effective against all tumors at a moderately elevated temperature. Cisplatin was also effective against all tumors, but its effectiveness at 41.5 °C was less than that of alkylating agents. To quantitatively study these findings, the magnitude of thermal enhancement of melphalan, an alkylating agent, and that of oxaliplatin, a new platinum compound, was studied by this author, at 37–44.5 °C by the colony formation assay. The dose of each agent was kept constant, and cell survival was determined as a function of treatment time. The cell survival curve was exponentially related to treatment time at all test temperatures, and the $T(0)$ (the time to reduce survival from 1 to 0.37) decreased with an increasing temperature. These results suggested that the cytotoxic effect of these agents occurred with a constant rate at 37 °C, and the rate was facilitated with an increasing temperature. This suggests that heat can accelerate the cytotoxic chemical reaction, leading to substantial thermal enhancement. The thermal enhancement ratio (TER, the ratio of the $T(0)$ at 37 °C to the $T(0)$ at an elevated temperature) increased with an increase in the temperature. The activation energy for melphalan at moderately elevated temperatures was the largest among the agents tested in the laboratory and that for oxaliplatin was approximately half of the melphalan activation energy. This suggests that the thermal enhancement for the cytotoxicity of melphalan or alkylating agents might be the greatest.

6.8 Taxanes

Recent studies suggest that docetaxel may show improved response at elevated temperatures. Factors that may modify the thermal enhancement of docetaxel were studied by Mohamed et al. [29] to optimize its clinical use with hyperthermia. The tumor studied was an early-generation isotransplant of a spontaneous C3Hf/Sed mouse fibrosarcoma, Fsa-II. Docetaxel was given as a single intraperitoneal injection. Hyperthermia was achieved by immersing the tumor-bearing foot into a constant temperature water bath. Four factors were studied: duration of hyperthermia, sequencing of hyperthermia with docetaxel, intensity of hyperthermia, and tumor size. To study the duration of hyperthermia, tumors were treated at 41.5 °C for 30 or 90 min immediately after intraperitoneal administration of docetaxel. For sequencing of hyperthermia and docetaxel, animals received hyperthermia treatment of tumors for 30 min at 41.5 °C immediately after drug administration, hyperthermia both immediately and 3 h after docetaxel administration, and hyperthermia given only at 3 h after administration of docetaxel. Intensity of hyperthermia was studied using heat treatment of tumors for 30 min at 41.5 °C or 43.5 °C immediately following docetaxel administration. Effect of tumor size was studied by delaying experiments until three times the tumor volume (113 mm^3) was observed. Treatment of tumors lasted for 30 min at 41.5 °C immediately following drug administration. Tumor response was studied using the mean tumor growth time. Hyperthermia in the absence of docetaxel had a small but significant effect on tumor growth time at 43.5 °C but not at 41.5 °C. Hyperthermia at 41.5 °C for 90 min immediately after docetaxel administration significantly increased mean tumor growth time ($P=0.0435$) when compared to tumors treated with docetaxel at room temperature. Treatment for 30 min had no effect. Application of hyperthermia immediately and immediately plus 3 h following docetaxel was effective in delaying tumor growth. Treatment at 3 h only had no effect. No significant difference in mean tumor growth time was observed with docetaxel and one-half hour of hyperthermia at 41.5 °C or 43.5 °C. For larger tumors, hyperthermia alone caused a significant delay in tumor growth time. Docetaxel at 41.5 °C for 30 min did not significantly increase mean tumor growth time compared to large tumors treated with docetaxel at room temperature. Docetaxel shows a moderate increase in antitumor activity with hyperthermia. At 41.5 °C, the thermal enhancement of docetaxel is time dependent if hyperthermia is applied immediately following drug administration. With large tumors, docetaxel alone or docetaxel plus hyperthermia showed the greatest delays in tumor growth time in the experiments.

6.9   Hyperthermia and Gene Therapy

Li et al. reported the activity of adenovirus-mediated heat-activated antisense Ku70 expression radiosensitizers tumor cells in vitro and in vivo [30]. Ku70 is one component of a protein complex, Ku70 and Ku80, that functions as a heterodimer to bind DNA double-strand breaks and activates DNA-dependent protein kinase. The previous study of this group with Ku70−/− and Ku80−/− mice and cell lines has shown that Ku70 and Ku80 deficiency compromises the ability of cells to repair DNA double-strand breaks, increases radiosensitivity of cells, and enhances radiation-induced apoptosis. In this study, Li examined the feasibility of using adenovirus-mediated, heat-activated expression of antisense Ku70 RNA as a gene therapy paradigm to sensitize cells and tumors to ionizing radiation. First, they performed experiments to test the heat inducibility of heat shock protein (hsp) 70 promoter and the efficiency of adenovirus-mediated gene transfer in rodent and human cells. Replication-defective adenovirus vectors were used to introduce a recombinant DNA construct, containing the enhanced green fluorescent protein (EGFP) under the control of an inducible hsp70 promoter, into exponentially growing cells. At 24 h after infection, cells were exposed to heat treatment, and heat-induced EGFP expression at different times was determined by flow cytometry. The data by Li clearly show that heat shock at 42 °C, 43 °C, or 44 °C appears to be equally effective in activating the hsp70 promoter-driven EGFP expression (>300-fold) in various tumor cells. Second, the authors have generated adenovirus vectors containing antisense Ku70 under the control of an inducible hsp70 promoter. Exponentially growing cells were infected with the adenovirus vector, heat shocked 24 h later, and the radiosensitivity determined 12 h after heat shock. Our data show that heat shock induces antisense Ku70 RNA, reduces the endogenous Ku70 level, and significantly increases the radiosensitivity of the cells. Third, the author has performed studies to test whether Ku70 protein level can be downregulated in a solid mouse tumor (FSa-II) and whether this results in enhanced radiosensitivity in vivo, as assessed by in vivo/in vitro colony formation and by the tumor growth delay. Their data demonstrate that heat shock-induced expression of antisense Ku70 RNA attenuates Ku70 protein expression in FSa-II tumors and significantly sensitizes the FSa-II tumors to ionizing radiation. Taken together, these interesting results suggest that adenovirus-mediated, heat-activated antisense Ku70 expression may provide a novel approach to radiosensitize human tumors in combination with hyperthermia.

Guan et al. [31] have examined the safety and efficacy of recombinant adenovirus encoding human p53 tumor suppressor gene (rAd-p53) injection in patients with advanced non-small-cell lung cancer (NSCLC) in the combination with the therapy of bronchial arterial infusion (BAI). A total of 58 patients with advanced NSCLC were enrolled in a non-randomized, two-armed clinical trial. Of which, 19 received a combination treatment of BAI and rAd-p53 (the combo group), while the remaining 39 were treated with only BAI (the control group). Patients were followed up for 12 months, with safety and local response evaluated by the National Cancer Institute's Common Toxicity Criteria and response evaluation criteria in solid tumor (RECIST), respectively. Time to progression (TTP) and survival rates were also analyzed by the Kaplan–Meier method. In the combo group, 19 patients received a total of 49 injections of rAd-p53 and 46 times of BAI, respectively, while 39 patients in the control group received a total of 113 times of BAI. The combination treatment was found to have less adverse events such as anorexia, nausea and emesis, pain, and leukopenia ($P<0.05$) but more arthralgia, fever, influenza-like symptom, and myalgia ($P<0.05$) compared with the control group. The overall response rates (complete response (CR) + partial response (PR)) were 47.3 % and 38.4 % for the combo group and the control group, respectively ($P>0.05$). Patients in the combo group had a longer TTP than those in the control group (a median 7.75 vs 5.5 months, $P=0.018$). However, the combination treatment did not lead to better survival, with survival rates at 3, 6, and 12 months in the combo group being 94.74 %, 89.47 %, and 52.63 %, respectively, compared with 92.31 %, 69.23 %, and 38.83 % in the control group ($P=0.224$). The final results of this work done by Guan YS et al. show that the combination of rAd-p53 and BAI was well tolerated in patients with NSCLC and may have improved the quality of life and delayed the disease progression.

Conclusions

The definition, about 50 years ago, that hypoxic cells are resistant to radiation led to the concept that cancers might be resistant to radiotherapy and chemotherapy because of their poor oxygen supply and subsequent hypoxia. Now, tumor hypoxia is seen as a mechanism of resistance to many antineoplastic drugs, as well as a predisposing factor toward increased malignancy and metastases.

However, tumor hypoxia is a unique target for hyperthermia and cancer bioreductive therapy that could be exploited for therapeutic use. A hypoxic cell is unable to have a stable pH; this increases the permeability of the cell membrane so that antineoplastic agents can easily move through the membrane improving the global concentration of the drug both inside and outside the cell. Hyperthermia seems the best opportunity to enhance these phenomena.

References

1. Gray LH, Conger AD, Ebert M, et al. Concentration of oxygen dissolved in tissue at the time of irradiation as a factor in radiotherapy. Br J Radiol. 1953;26:638–48.
2. Thomlinson RH, Gray LH. The histological structure of some human lung cancers and the possible implications for radiotherapy. Br J Cancer. 1955;9:539–49.
3. Moulder JE, Rockwell S. Tumor hypoxia: its impact on cancer therapy. Cancer Metastasis Rev. 1987;5:313–41.
4. Brown JM. The hypoxic cell: a target for selective cancer therapy. Cancer Res. 1999;59:5863–70.
5. Rauth AM, Melo T, Misra V. Bioreductive therapies: an overview of drugs and their mechanism of action. Int J Radiat Oncol Biol Phys. 1998;42:755–62.
6. Wouters BG, Wang LH, Brown JM. Tirapazamine: a new drug producing tumor specific enhancement of platinum-based chemotherapy in non small cell lung cancer. Ann Oncol. 1999;10 Suppl 5:S29–33.
7. Graeber TG, Osmanian C, Jacks T. Hypoxia-mediated selection of cells with diminished apoptotic potential in solid tumours. Nature. 1996;379:88–91.
8. Lin A, Cosby L, Shansky C, et al. Potential bioreductive alkylating agents. 1. Benzoquinone derivatives. J Med Chem. 1972;15:1247–52.
9. Adams GE, Stratford IJ. Bioreductive drugs for cancer therapy: the search for tumour specificity. Int J Radiat Oncol Biol Phys. 1994;29:231–8.
10. Teicher BA, Holden SA, Al-Achi A, et al. Classification of antineoplastic treatments by their differential toxicity toward putative oxygenated and hypoxic tumor subpopulation in vivo in the FSaIIC murine fibrosarcoma. Cancer Res. 1990;50:3339–44.
11. Binley L, Iqball S, Kingsman S, et al. An adenoviral vector regulated by hypoxia for the treatment of ischaemic disease and cancer. Gene Ther. 1999;6:1721–7.
12. Zaffaroni N, Fiorentini G, De Giorgi U. Hyperthermia and hypoxia: new developments in anticancer chemotherapy. Eur J Surg Oncol. 2001;27:340–2.
13. Guadagni S, Fiorentini G, Palumbo G, et al. Hypoxic pelvic perfusion with mitomycin C using a simplified balloon-occlusion technique in the treatment of patients with unresectable locally recurrent rectal cancer. Arch Surg. 2001;136(1):105–12.

14. Guadagni S, Russo F, Rossi CR, et al. Deliberate hypoxic pelvic and limb chemoperfusion in the treatment of recurrent melanoma. Am J Surg. 2002;183:28–36.
15. Semenza GI. Targeting HIF-1 for cancer therapy. Nat Rev Cancer. 2003;3:721–32.
16. Brown JM, Giacca AJ. The unique physiology of solid tumors: opportunities (and problems) for cancer therapy. Cancer Res. 1998;58:1408–16.
17. Urano M, Kuroda M, Nishimura Y. For the clinical application of thermochemotherapy given at mild temperatures. Int J Hyperthermia. 1999;15:79–107.
18. Zaffaroni N, Villa R, Daidone MG, Vaglini M, Santinami M, Silvestrini R. Antitumor activity of hyperthermia alone or in combination with cisplatin and melphalan in primary cultures of human malignant melanoma. Int J Cell Cloning. 1989;7:385–94.
19. Kusumoto T, Holden SA, Ara G, Teicher BA. Hyperthermia and platinum complexes: time between treatments and synergy in vitro and in vivo. Int J Hyperthermia. 1995;11:575–86.
20. Bates DA, Mackillop WJ. Effect of hyperthermia on the uptake and cytotoxicity of melphalan in Chinese hamster ovary cells. Int J Radiat Oncol Biol Phys. 1998;16:187–91.
21. Zaffaroni N, Villa R, Orlandi L, Vaglini M, Silvestrini R. Effect of hyperthermia on the formation and removal of DNA interstrand cross-links induced by melphalan in primary cultures of human malignant melanoma. Int J Hyperthermia. 1992;8:341–9.
22. Orlandi L, Zaffaroni N, Bearzatto A, Costa A, Supino R, Vaglini M, et al. Effect of melphalan and hyperthermia on cell cycle progression and cyclin B_1 expression in human melanoma cells. Cell Prolif. 1995;28:617–30.
23. Orlandi L, Zaffaroni N, Bearzatto A, Silvestrini R. Effect of melphalan and hyperthermia on p34cdc2 kinase activity in human melanoma cells. Br J Cancer. 1996;74:1924–8.
24. Rietbroek RC, van de Vaart PJ, Haveman J, Blommaert FA, Geerdink A, Bakker PJ, et al. Hyperthermia enhances the cytotoxic activity and platinum-DNA adduct formation of lobaplatin and oxaliplatin in cultured SW 1573 cells. J Cancer Res Clin Oncol. 1997;123:6–12.
25. Orlandi L, Costa A, Zaffaroni N, Villa R, Vaglini M, Silvestrini R. Relevance of cell kinetic and ploidy characteristics for the thermal response of malignant melanoma primary cultures. Int J Oncol. 1993;2:523–6.
26. Richards EH, Hickman JA, Masters JR. Heat shock protein expression in testis and bladder cancer cell lines exhibiting differential sensitivity to heat. Br J Cancer. 1995;72:620–6.
27. Takemoto M, Kuroda M, Urano M, Nishimura Y, Kawasaki S, Kato H, et al. Effect of various chemotherapeutic agents given with mild hyperthermia on different types of tumours. Int J Hyperthermia. 2003;19(2):193–203.
28. Urano M, Ling CC. Thermal enhancement of melphalan and oxaliplatin cytotoxicity in vitro. Int J Hyperthermia. 2002;18(4):307–15.
29. Mohamed F, Stuart OA, Glehen O, Urano M, Sugarbaker PH. Docetaxel and hyperthermia: factors that modify thermal enhancement. J Surg Oncol. 2004;88(1):14–20.
30. Li GC, He F, Shao X, Urano M, Shen L, Kim D, et al. Adenovirus-mediated heat-activated antisense Ku70 expression radiosensitizes tumor cells in vitro and in vivo. Cancer Res. 2003;63(12):3268–74.
31. Guan YS, Liu Y, Zou Q, He Q, La Z, Yang L, et al. Adenovirus-mediated wild-type p53 gene transfer in combination with bronchial arterial infusion for treatment of advanced non-small-cell lung cancer, one year follow-up. J Zhejiang Univ Sci B. 2009;10(5):331–40.

Induction Chemotherapy in Head and Neck Cancers

7

Adorján F. Kovács

7.1 Introduction

7.1.1 Guidelines for Chemotherapy in Head and Neck Cancers

The overwhelming majority of head and neck cancers are squamous cell carcinomas; therefore, other histologies will not be discussed in this chapter. According to the German Cancer Society [1], *the sole usage of (systemic) chemotherapy in head and neck cancer is intended only for palliative use "in case of disease relapses (recurrences) or metastatic tumors."* For head and neck cancers that are not resectable, chemotherapy "is generally combined with a radiation (chemoradiation)," either in parallel or sequentially. Today, the advantage of parallel chemoradiation as compared to a sequential regimen has been established. There has also been a significant superiority of results using concomitant chemoradiation as compared to larger doses of radiotherapy exclusively [2, 3]. Thus, *chemoradiation has now become the "gold standard" of treatment for locally unresectable tumors. In advanced resectable tumors (>T2), surgery with or without adjuvant radiotherapy remains the treatment of choice. In so-called high-risk patients (e.g., positive surgical margins), adjuvant concomitant chemoradiation may be used* [4]. The drugs used mainly are cisplatin or carboplatin, 5-fluorouracil, and/or the taxanes. *Intra-arterial chemotherapy is not even mentioned in those guidelines, whereas in more and more clinics, it is increasingly being used.*

7.1.2 Induction Chemotherapy in Head and Neck Cancers

All in all, surgical treatment of head and neck carcinomas which is the standard for operable cancers shows an increasing tendency to include nonsurgical

A.F. Kovács
Private Practice, Waldstraße 61a, 64569 Nauheim, Germany
e-mail: profkovacs@googlemail.com

© Springer-Verlag Berlin Heidelberg 2016
K.R. Aigner, F.O. Stephens (eds.), *Induction Chemotherapy*,
DOI 10.1007/978-3-319-28773-7_7

modalities [5]. Advanced cancers not curable by surgery alone are submitted to sophisticated multimodality regimens. Thereby, the sequence and temporal integration of the therapeutic modalities becomes essential. More effective integrated combined treatment modalities involve risks of excessive toxicity that may be greater than toxicity of any single therapy alone. If the toxicity of an appropriately increased individual modality can be reduced by a combination therapy as compared to its toxicity in its sole and definitive application, the overall treatment-associated morbidity will possibly be lessened. There is, of course, also a risk of danger of decreased overall effectiveness. An important point of multimodality treatment is, therefore, reduced compliance, be it treatment related (too high toxicity) or patient related (refusal).

Theoretical benefits of using presurgical or preradiation chemotherapy, systemic or regional, include:

- Induction chemotherapy would affect previously untreated tumor cells because of their potentially higher susceptibility to treatment.
- Inhibition of growth or even downsizing of the tumor could reduce the extent of locoregional surgery needed and potentially increase the effectiveness of any subsequent therapy.
- Reduction of tumor aggressiveness and metastatic propensity, especially the sowing of tumor cells during surgical manipulations, could be a welcome effect of an initial therapy.
- A regional treatment could minimize the local recurrence rate which is the main problem with head and neck cancers.

In contrast, radiation or chemoradiation used as induction treatment would have (at least locally) more toxicity, would result in more wound healing problems following surgery, would have problems of dosage because pathological staging is unknown, and could have more patient-related compliance problems.

An important question for the assessment of induction chemotherapy is the definition of success used, as, for example, resectability, local control, disease-free time, or overall survival. Randomized trials and meta-analyses of induction chemotherapy [6–10] offer an undecided picture in this respect.

The second question for correct assessment of the trials which will be discussed in this chapter is whether different regimens and cancer localizations in the head and neck area can be compared. For example, for carcinomas of the pharyngolarynx, the belief of "non-chemocurability of squamous cell carcinoma of the upper aerodigestive tract" has recently been seriously doubted [11]. Other reports on long-term remissions of oral carcinomas after sole chemotherapeutic treatment supported this impression [12]. It is also obvious that degrees of stage and state of different cancers (primary operable, primary inoperable, recurrent, and pretreated cancers) cannot be compared, which makes evaluation of trials and treatments difficult.

7.1.3 Systemic Induction Chemotherapy in Head and Neck Cancers

7.1.3.1 Development

To understand the peculiarity of intra-arterial induction chemotherapy, it is important to have a brief look at the systemic induction chemotherapy in operable patients which was a standard treatment of head and neck cancers practiced since the 1980s. Until recently, a scheme of tricyclic induction chemotherapy with a bolus dose of 100 mg/m^2 cisplatin and a subsequent continuous 120 h infusion of 1,000 mg/m^2 5-fluorouracil (PF), introduced by the Wayne State Group in Detroit, played the largest role [13]. This scheme has proven itself to be most effective in previously untreated patients [14]. Therefore, regimens using other agents for induction did not play a great role; for example, cisplatin with 5-fluorouracil had been shown to be more effective than carboplatin in combination with 5-fluorouracil for induction chemotherapy of stage IV head and neck cancers [15].

For recurrent or metastatic head and neck cancers, it could be shown that combination chemotherapy regimens are superior to monochemotherapy due to the synergism of drug effects [16], but without proven survival benefit, and always with the limitation of potentially greater rates of toxicity. The advantage lay in the control of symptoms.

A study from Italy showed in a subgroup of inoperable patients from a total group of 237 previously untreated patients with head and neck tumors of stages III and IV that PF induction chemotherapy followed by irradiation resulted in a lower local recurrence rate and prolonged survival as compared to radiotherapy alone. *The incidence of the rate of distant metastases would also be reduced*; but for the total group, there was no proven difference in survival [17].

Some other studies with representative objectives and results shall be mentioned in detail: Thyss et al. [18] confirmed the good results achieved with the Wayne-State method. In 108 patients with stages II–IV head and neck carcinomas, after three cycles, there were 87.5 % responses, including 47.5 % complete responses in the primary site. Oro-/hypopharyngeal cancers had best results in contrast to oral cavity cancers. Definitive treatment consisted of radiation or surgery. *Complete responders had a significantly longer survival following definitive treatment as compared to nonresponders.* Wang et al. [19] treated 120 patients with previously untreated head and neck carcinomas stages III and IV with the Wayne-State scheme. The overall response rate was 56 %; *the local response rate depended on the original tumor volume.* Remission rates of up to 81 % and a clinical complete remission rate of 69 % were achieved with PF induction chemotherapy plus leukovorin (PFL) in 102 untreated stages III and IV head and neck cancers [20], where the rate of pathological complete remissions was also very high (84 % of clinical complete remissions). Patients with complete remissions were then irradiated only; the others were operated on plus irradiated. The 5-year survival rate was 52 %. *The need for rescue drugs indicates the high toxicity of such regimens.*

Around the year 2000 with all the early studies of systemic induction chemotherapy combined, it could be concluded:

- That clinical complete remission rates were achieved by 20–70 %.
- That complete pathological remissions were demonstrated in about 66 % of clinical complete remissions and that these patients had a better chance of survival.
- That no increase in surgical or radiation-induced complications was to be feared.
- However, no significant improvement in survival in patients with advanced tumor stages was proven when compared to a sole operation or radiation therapy [7, 9, 21].

Systemic Induction Chemotherapy and Survival Advantage
All of the abovementioned studies suffered from being a mixture of different localizations and/or from the inclusion of both operable and inoperable patients. When these faults were avoided, induction chemotherapy had a much better impact. A French randomized trial used the Wayne-State scheme before a definitive locoregional treatment consisting of either surgery plus radiation or radiation alone. It demonstrated in 318 patients with advanced oropharyngeal cancer that overall survival was significantly better in the induction chemotherapy group than in the control group, with a median survival of 5.1 years versus 3.3 years in the no chemotherapy group [6]. Volling et al. [10] reported the final results of a prospective randomized study using systemic induction chemotherapy prior to surgery and radiotherapy versus surgery and radiotherapy in patients with resectable oral cavity and tonsil cancers T2–3 N0–2 proving a significant survival advantage for the chemotherapy group.

7.1.3.2 Actual Trends and Organ Preservation

In the USA, at the beginning of the twenty-first century, chemoradiation was combined with induction chemotherapy. This nonsurgical concept seemed to become the standard treatment in locally advanced squamous cell carcinomas of the head and neck [22].

This development started in 1991, when the Veterans Affairs Laryngeal Cancer Study Group succeeded in demonstrating [23] that a purely conservative treatment (PF induction chemotherapy followed by radiotherapy with 66–76 Gy for potentially resectable laryngeal cancer) compared with a laryngectomy followed by adjuvant radiotherapy was possible without worsening of overall survival (*organ preservation*). This concept was expanded by addition of chemoradiation. A pioneering study maybe mentioned to measure the compliance and toxicity problems of this modality. Calais et al. [24] accrued 63 patients with stages III and IV oropharyngeal carcinomas prospectively for chemoradiation. Patients of an age over 75 years and those with a Karnofsky index below 60 were excluded, as well as those who lost more than 20 % of their body weight and those with previous or synchronous malignancies. Seventy grays were administered locally, regionally 56 Gy in case of lymph node involvement, and 44 Gy in case of clinically free necks. Patients received concomitant seven cycles of 20 mg/m^2 docetaxel. Eleven percent had to discontinue irradiation; 3 % were not able to finish completely. All seven cycles of chemotherapy were administered to 95 % of patients. Treatment was generally well tolerated; however, 41 % of patients required a temporary gastric tube because of the main acute side effect of mucositis. After 3 years, the calculated total and disease-free survival amounted to 47 % and 39 %; the locoregional control rate was 64 %.

Since inoperable cancer patients had no choice except surgery-sparing treatment, an important question to be answered was whether potentially resectable cancers generally would benefit from organ preservation? During a period of 8 years, Forastiere et al. [25] distributed 517 patients with surgically curable laryngeal cancer, who would have required a total laryngectomy, into three groups, one of which constituted the arm with a chemoradiation. Local radiation dose was 70 Gy, at the neck at least 50 Gy. On days 1, 22, and 43, 100 mg/m^2 cisplatin were given intravenously. The overall survival of this group after 5 years was 54 %, disease-free survival was 36 %. Speaking problems were found in 6 % of patients after 2 years, swallowing problems in 15 %. With radiotherapy of 70 Gy and simultaneous chemotherapy in inoperable, but highly selected patients in the mentioned study of Calais et al. [24], survival rates of 47 % after 3 years could be reached. In the principally surgically curable patients of the mentioned study by Forastiere et al. [25], survival rates were significantly higher. *The concept of "organ preservation" refers, therefore, nowadays mostly to operable patients with laryngeal or hypopharyngeal cancers who are treated nonsurgically from functional reasons.* A distinct look at other single cancer localizations is still rare.

In inoperable patients, another main topic of studies has been the fractionation of definitive chemoradiation [26].

As was previously described, the evolving standard of care has focused on the concurrent use of (adjuvant or definitive) chemotherapy with more aggressive radiotherapy; however, patients' tumors continued to recur locally and/or regionally, albeit at a diminished rate, and distant metastases have become a major site of fatal recurrence, while long-term local and acute systemic toxicities have increased. As a result of these changes in outcomes and a reevaluation of earlier historical data by meta-analyses, interest in PF induction chemotherapy has reemerged and evolved. Early investigations concentrated on the question of which induction therapy would be the best, for example, by adding mitoguazone to PF chemotherapy and customizing definitive treatment according to response [27].

In succession, the Wayne-State scheme was expanded to the most promising systemic induction chemotherapy regimen today, by combining docetaxel, platinum, and fluorouracil (TPF). Most recently, large randomized studies comparing PF with TPF have demonstrated markedly superior survival with the three-drug regimen, as will be delineated. Posner et al. [28] compared TPF plus chemoradiation (weekly carboplatin) versus PF plus chemoradiation in 501 patients with laryngeal, hypopharyngeal, oropharyngeal, and oral stages III and IV cancers which were mainly resectable but had low chance of curability and also unresectable. After minimum follow-up of 2 years, median overall survival was 71 versus 30 months, and toxicity was comparable; these results were confirmed by a follow-up after 5 years (71 versus 35 months) [29]. Subgroup analysis concentrated on laryngeal and hypopharyngeal cancer and confirmed the results (laryngectomy-free survival 52 % versus 32 % [30]).

Induction chemotherapy was also increasingly examined in patients with mainly unresectable head and neck cancer. Ghi et al. [31] compared in 24 patients suffering from stages III and IV M0 carcinomas of the oral cavity, oropharynx, nasopharynx, or hypopharynx chemoradiation with carboplatin and 5-fluorouracil with induction by three cycles of TPF (docetaxel 75 mg/m^2, cisplatin 80 mg/m^2, 5-fluorouracil 800 mg/m^2/day continuous infusion for 96 h) plus chemoradiation of the same regimen. At the end of the study, patients received only two cycles of PF during radiation. At the end of therapy, the complete remission rate was 62.5 % for chemoradiation alone (Group 1) and 80 % for induction TPF followed by chemoradiation (Groups 2 and 3), and toxicity was found to be tolerable. Vermorken et al. [32] carried out a much larger randomized study in 358 patients with stages III and IV unresectable cancer of the larynx, hypopharynx, oropharynx, and oral cavity. TPF plus radiation versus PF plus radiation were compared. The TPF regimen consisted of docetaxel at a dose of 75 mg/m^2, administered as a 1 h infusion on day 1, followed by cisplatin at a dose of 75 mg/m^2, administered as a 1 h infusion on day 1, and 5-fluorouracil at a dose of 750 mg/m^2 per day, administered by continuous infusion on days 1–5. The PF regimen consisted of the Wayne-State scheme. Treatment was administered every 3 weeks. Response to chemotherapy was 54 % (PF) versus 68 % (TPF). Radiation was administered as conventional fractionation or accelerated/hyperfractionated regimens up to 66–74 Gy. After median follow-up of 32.5 months, there was a significant difference in progression-free survival of 11 versus 8.2 months and in overall survival of 18.8 versus 14.5 months. Toxicity was even less in the triple chemotherapy, and quality of life was better. *The valid conclusion of these trials was the acceptance of the combination of docetaxel, cisplatin, and 5-fluorouracil (TPF) as the best polychemotherapy, if systemic induction chemotherapy was considered.* This, however, does not mean that induction chemotherapy with TPF is necessarily the best method for organ preservation treatment.

Figure 7.1 [33] shows the power of such treatment even in problematic cases: a 65-year-old man suffering from T4bN2c cancer of the maxillary sinus with orbital, nasal, cheek, and skull base infiltration who was treated with two cycles of TPF (last one aborted due to general edema) and definitive radiation (without chemotherapy because of liver disease). Treatment resulted in complete remission; the patient died several months later due to concurrent disease.

The described TPF polychemotherapy proved to be feasible with a high rate of treatment compliance with regard to the number of cycles and dose reduction, even in populations of patients with highly advanced cancers and reduced general state. *Toxicity was generally high (up to grade 4 WHO) but comparable in different studies* [33–35]. Deaths during or after TPF polychemotherapy occurred in many studies. Neutropenia with consecutive pneumonia or sepsis which became fatal was the main problem. It is also notable that organizational expense for the therapy and the nursing of the patients is high. Figure 7.2 gives an impression of the high toxicity of both TPF and chemoradiation (mucositis, regional alopecia, dermatitis).

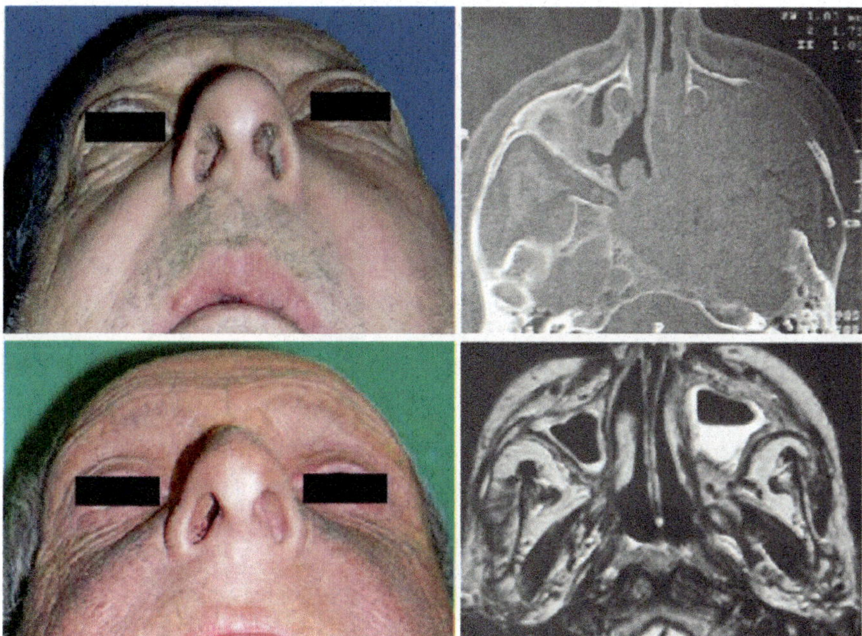

Fig. 7.1 *Top*: Worm's view and CT of a 65-year-old man suffering from T4bN2c cancer of maxillary sinus with orbital, nasal, cheek, and skull base infiltration. *Below*: Complete remission following two cycles of TPF and definitive radiation

TPF is now (2015) considered the standard of care for induction chemotherapy in unresectable disease and in organ preservation, but final judgment is still pending concerning a survival benefit as compared to chemoradiotherapy alone [36]. Induction chemotherapy followed by chemoradiotherapy, known as sequential therapy, has been shown to be rather safe and effective. Both TPF induction and sequential therapy are considered appropriate platforms upon which the new molecularly targeted agents can be tested [37, 38]. Similarly, it is possible to react to the changing epidemiology recognizable by an increasing number of HPV (human papillomavirus) associated cancers which may be accomplished by reduced drug dosages in case of HPV-positive cases [39].

7.2 Intra-arterial Induction Chemotherapy in Head and Neck Cancers

7.2.1 Development of Intra-arterial Chemotherapy in the Head and Neck

Since Klopp et al. [40] observed after an erroneous injection of nitrogen mustard into the brachial artery that the resulting local damage (erythema, blistering and ulcerations on the forearm) healed after a short time, they took courage and for the

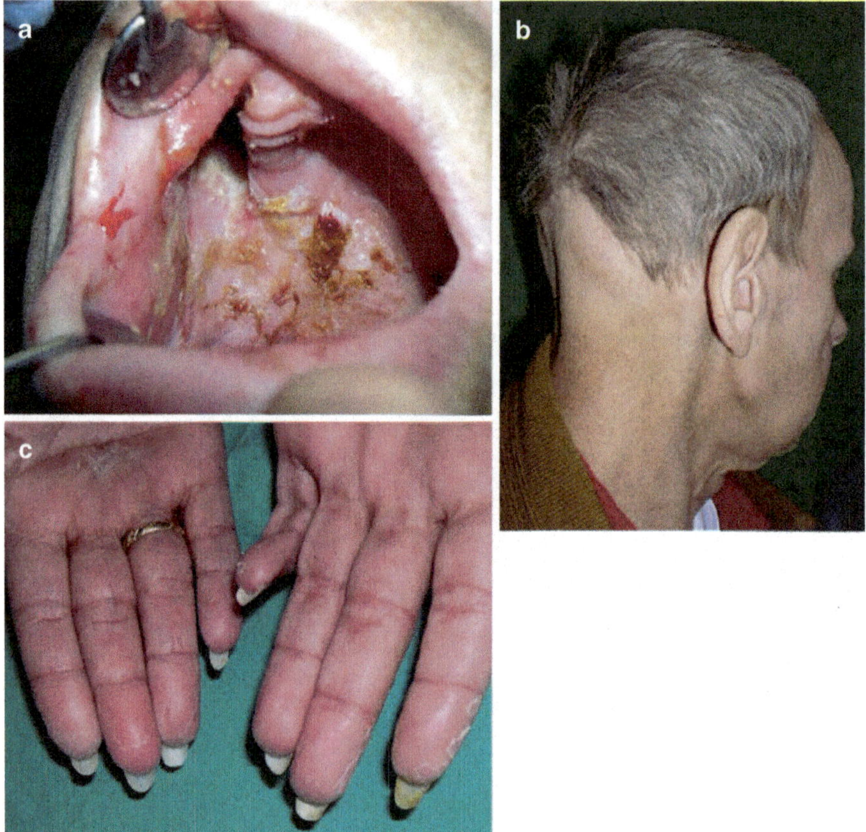

Fig. 7.2 Typical high toxicity of both TPF and chemoradiation ((**a**) mucositis, (**b**) regional alopecia, (**c**) dermatitis)

first time treated oral cancer by intra-arterial infusion of nitrogen mustard into the carotid artery. Sullivan et al. [41] from the National Cancer Institute, New York, carried on the experimental and clinical research, among others through the introduction of methotrexate and folinic acid as a protective factor. A main problem in those early days was the high rate of technical complications and deaths. The complications concerned were mainly arterial thrombosis, malpositioning of the catheters, bleeding, and infection. Most often, an operation was needed for catheterization with exposure of the vessel to be punctured. *Subsequently one of the most common methods was the retrograde insertion of catheters into the external carotid artery through the branches more easily reachable, for example, the superior thyroid or the superficial temporal artery.* The perfusion area was stained with patent blue or disulphan blue as can be seen in Fig. 7.3 [42] where the left lingual artery was aimed at from a retrograde temporal approach in a patient with T4 cancer of the floor of mouth and the alveolar rim; a higher selective chemoperfusion, therefore, was not possible. Adjacent tissue was also perfused via the facial artery, leading to local

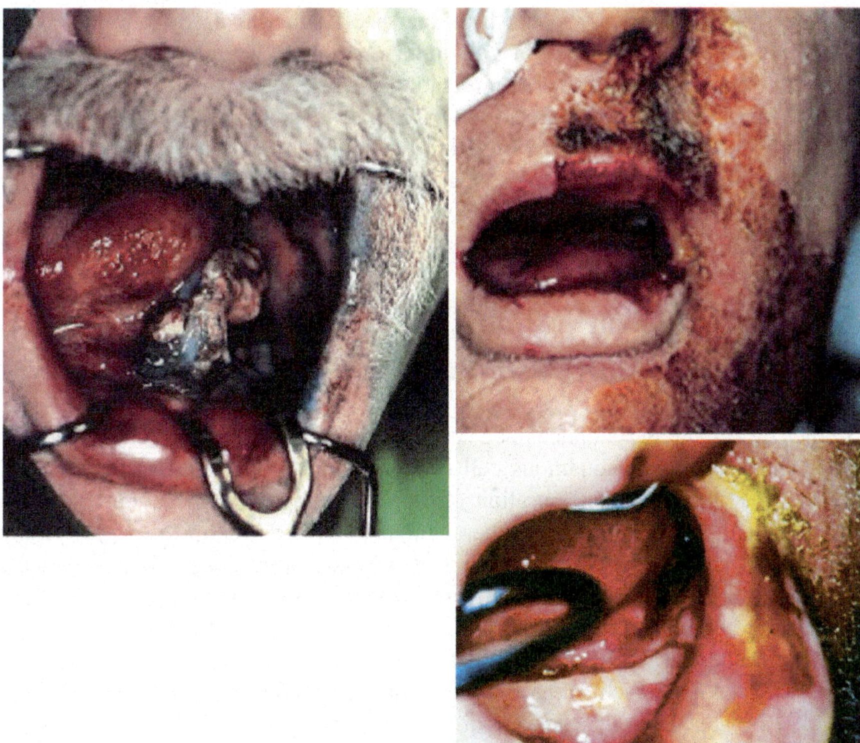

Fig. 7.3 *Left*: Patient with T4 cancer of floor of mouth and alveolar rim during staining of lingual artery from retrograde temporal approach. Note perfusion of adjacent areas via facial artery. *Top right*: Local toxicity (desquamative dermatitis) after intra-arterial bleomycin. *Below right*: Near to complete local response after 1 week

toxicity (desquamative dermatitis) after bleomycin; local response, however, was near to complete after 1 week.

With longer duration of infusion, the catheters had to be fixed or port systems had to be implanted under the skin with subsequent possibilities of dislocation and risk of infection [43]. This required constant supervision, usually as an inpatient, and catheter adjustment if necessary. Even more complex was an incision in the neck with a direct dissection of the external carotid, facial, or lingual artery; to some extent, carotid bypasses with venous grafts, and extensive ligatures of carotid branches not needed were carried out to achieve a higher selective perfusion [44].

As with systemic chemotherapy, combination chemotherapies were used from the end of the 1960s to achieve a dose reduction with greater anticancer effect and to get less toxicity. Here, the combination of methotrexate and bleomycin was one of the most frequently applied [45]. At this time, first experimental investigations were also carried out concerning pharmacokinetic studies to show the superiority of intra-arterial therapy as compared to systemic therapy [46].

Regional chemotherapy in the head and neck area was used by a number of investigators to treat locally advanced tumors, mainly in Germany, Italy, Hungary, Japan, the USA, and Australia. At international symposia organized since 1983 (by Karl Aigner in Germany), progress and problems were discussed. A good overview of the 1997 status was provided by Eckardt [47]. In an International Workshop on Intra-arterial Chemotherapy for Head and Neck Cancer, organized by Tom Robbins in Springfield, IL, in August 2006, investigators from all continents gathered to define the present state of the art of intra-arterial chemotherapy in the head and neck.

7.2.2 Pharmacokinetic Rationale of Intra-arterial Chemotherapy

Studies by Harker and Stephens in a suitable animal model, using a spontaneously occurring keratinizing squamous cell carcinoma on the ear of Australian sheep, showed that a greater concentration of the infused agent in the tumor region is achieved with intra-arterial chemotherapy than by systemic application [48]. At the same time, cisplatin proved to be the chemotherapeutic drug with the greatest response rate as compared to bleomycin, methotrexate, 5-fluorouracil, and cyclophosphamide [49].

Pharmacokinetic justification of intra-arterial chemotherapy can now be summarized as follows: for each antineoplastic chemotherapeutic agent, systemic exposure (i.e., AUC = area under the concentration – time curve) and tumor response (or toxicity) are regulated via the maximally tolerated systemic exposure which is defined by an "acceptable" toxicity with a probability of a certain therapeutic response. The systemic exposure depends on the individual plasma clearance (CL). Regional chemotherapy via a tumor-feeding artery obtains a higher exposure to the drug at the target as compared to a respective systemic exposure and therefore offers the theoretical possibility of a greater therapeutic response without compromising tolerance. Eckman et al. [50] defined the following equation for a therapeutic advantage or "drug targeting index" (DTI), which describes the relative advantage of a selective intra-arterial administration of a drug: DTI = 1+CL/Q(1–E)target(1–E)lung (Q = arterial blood flow to the target tissue, E = extraction of the drug in target tissues and lungs).

The so-called first-pass extraction of the drug in the tumor itself (and in the lungs), that is, a "retention" of the drug at the first passage through the tissue, results in a lower systemic exposure but may play a lesser role in relation to the blood stream [51]. The DTI for various antineoplastic drugs was determined under the assumption of an application in the common carotid artery with a $Q=250$ mL/min and under neglect of the "first-pass extraction." It showed values of, for example, 17 for 5-fluorouracil and 3 for cisplatin [52] or 4,001 for 5-fluorouracil and 401 for cisplatin under assumption of a minimal transport based on a low local flow rate [53]. Both drugs have, as mentioned, a good effect on head and neck squamous cell carcinoma.

The duration of intra-arterial chemotherapy depends, among others, on the phase specificity of the antineoplastic chemotherapeutic drug. While a long-term infusion maybe an important factor for the effectiveness in cell-cycle-specific cytotoxic agents (e.g., 5-fluorouracil), the bolus injection of a certain dose of a cytostatic drug, which is not cell-cycle specific (e.g., cisplatin), is equivalent to the long-term infusion of the same dose. Both methods can be repeated (= chemotherapy cycles).

7.2.3 Modern Intra-arterial Chemotherapy in Head and Neck Cancers

Intra-arterial chemotherapy is established in the treatment of liver metastases, usually from colorectal cancer. During the development of this treatment modality for the liver, the application of high intra-arterial doses of cisplatin was introduced, buffered with systemically administered intravenous sodium thiosulfate [54]. This concept of "two-route" chemotherapy was transferred to the head and neck region.

In patients with head and neck cancer, Robbins et al. [55, 56] found in dose-finding studies a maximally tolerated dose of intra-arterial cisplatin of 150 mg/m^2. This high-dose chemotherapy broke through resistance [57] and led to high biopsy-determined tumor concentrations [58, 59]. Cisplatin, in contrast to other chemotherapeutic agents with theoretically higher DTI, was chosen because sodium thiosulfate, a cisplatin neutralizer [60], can be used as a systemic antagonist. When thiosulfate circulates intravenously, cisplatin is chelated and inactivated reducing the half-life of the drug from 66 to 3.7 min [61, 62]. By this method, the plasma clearance is increased and the DTI is increased. Sensitive areas such as the bone marrow and kidneys are protected from the toxic effects of the drug, and ototoxicity is reduced [63]. *Through the use of advanced catheter systems* via *the percutaneous puncture of the femoral artery, it was possible to infuse the chemotherapeutic agent using coaxial micro-catheters superselectively (mostly in the lingual or facial artery) and safely under angiographic control* [64]. Figure 7.4 [42] demonstrates by images from Frankfurt neuroradiology how accidental perfusion of anastomoses can be avoided and superselectivity achieved.

These small vessels have a lower blood flow (approximately 120 mL/min), which makes the denominator of the above equation smaller and therefore the DTI greater. Therefore, intra-arterial chemotherapy appears to be theoretically ideal for this localization. Moreover, cisplatin was chosen because due to its extensive phase unspecificity, a rapid injection was suitable, which could be repeated. Thus, the sensitivity of the method for complications was further reduced.

By this method, some problems of intra-arterial chemotherapy in the head and neck area have been addressed. However, it was used by Robbins and others in the context of an organ-preservation chemoradiation of advanced and recurrent head and neck cancers of various locations as will be discussed later in this chapter.

7.2.4 Chemoembolization of Head and Neck Cancers

Another method to increase the therapeutic advantage of intra-arterial chemotherapy is the temporary reduction or stop of the intratumoral blood flow using drugs wrapped via *pharmaceutical technology,* that is, microparticulate systems or

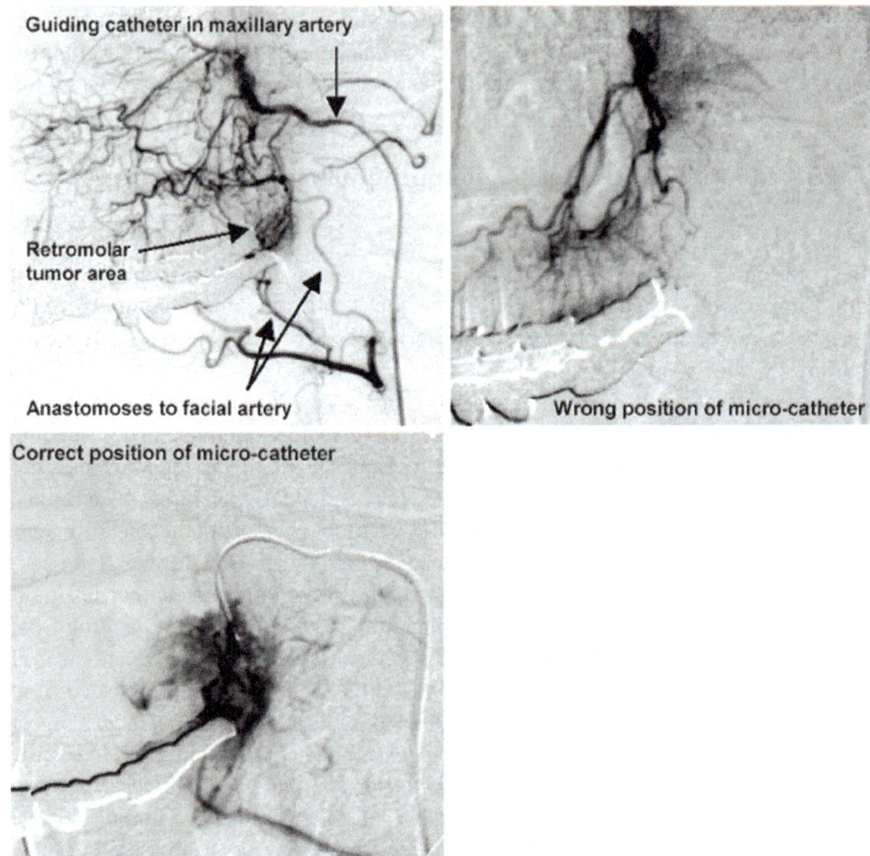

Fig. 7.4 Fluoroscopy images demonstrating achievement of superselectivity in intra-arterial chemotherapy

microcapsules loaded with drugs ("encoated drug microcapsules") [65], *or simultaneously applicated (micro-) embolizing agents such as lipiodol* [66], *which translates into a longer intratumoral length of stay and larger "first-pass extraction" of the drug, and leads to micro-infarctions with a planned consecutive hypoxic necrosis of the tumor.* This method is mainly used in the liver.

The intensification of local chemotherapy by embolization proved in practice to be difficult in the head and neck region, because the vessels are much smaller in diameter and occlude immediately after administration of only a small dose of the embolization agent which may lead to undue necrosis of parts of the face or tongue in case of complete cessation of blood flow and a corresponding risk to the eyes and large nerval ganglions via anastomoses.

Chemoembolization must be distinguished from closure of arteriovenous shunts in advanced and recurrent tumors with microcoils, polyvinyl alcohol, or other substances, in order to prevent early discharge (flowoff) of the agent, as a technical aspect of chemoperfusion to achieve greater selectivity [67]. The occurrence of true shunts, however, is rare, making this technique rarely necessary to employ.

All in all, attempts at embolization of head and neck cancer had been extremely few until Kovács and coworkers introduced a routine method described below in Sect. 7.2.8.

7.2.5 Tumor Platinum Concentrations: A Comparison of Intra-arterial and Systemic Chemotherapy

Platinum-based drugs are now the most commonly used anticancer agents in the treatment of head and neck cancers. They have therefore been appropriately assessed for comparative tumor concentrations. Intratumoral drug levels were assessed mainly *by biopsies*. Okamoto et al. [68, 69] found maximum cisplatin levels from 30 to 150 µg/g wet weight (mainly on the third day) in biopsies performed at 1 h, 3 and 7 days after administration. They were higher than with nonencapsulated intra-arterial cisplatin. Gouyette et al. [70] measured a mean platinum content of 2.72 µg/g after intra-arterial administration of cisplatin over 1 h (total dose 100 mg/m^2) and achieved remission in 20–30 % of oral and oropharyngeal tumors. The amount of the platinum content in this study was lower after intravenous chemotherapy. Sileni et al. [71] found higher intratumoral concentrations of platinum after intravenous 4 h infusions (65.4 µg/g) than after intra-arterial 4 h infusion (17.18 µg/g) and attributed this paradox finding to either a relatively high blood supply to the tumor area, enabling efflux of the surplus free platinum from the tissue, or by the delay between drug infusion and biopsy. The total dose of cisplatin was 100 mg/m^2 but was followed by an infusion of 5-fluorouracil. Biopsies were taken after 48 and 120 h. These platinum levels after intra-arterial and intravenous chemotherapy achieved two complete remissions in six patients with T3/T4 tumors. The optimal duration of the infusion/drug dose has not yet been determined in humans; Jakowatz et al. [72] found in experimental rat models that prolonged arterial infusions (lasting 24 or 48 h) enable a real increase of four to ten times in the concentration of cisplatin in tumor tissues (29 µg/mg tissue for a 48 h intra-arterial infusion and 2.02 µg/mg tissue for a rapid intra-arterial infusion). Los et al. [58] found values between 3.1 and 4.9 µg/g in most tumors with a rapid intra-arterial high-dose cisplatin perfusion (200 or 150 mg/m^2) and concomitant intravenous infusion of sodium thiosulfate (9 g/m^2, followed by an infusion of 12 g/m^2 about 6 h). The levels varied between 0.6 and 50.7 µg/g. The biopsies were taken 24 h after treatment. Very different tumor localizations of the head and neck area were treated. Higher remission correlated with higher platinum levels, but the responses were assessed in most cases after radiotherapy. The rate of complete remission was reported as 92 %. In dose intensity ranges of 75–149 and 150–200 mg/m^2/week, total (partial and complete) response rates were 72.7 % and 100 % [59]. The patients had been administered four cycles with parallel sodium thiosulfate infusion. Tohnai et al. [73] measured in lingual resection specimens of 12 patients shortly after superselective and selective (retrograde) intra-arterial perfusion with 20 mg/m^2 carboplatin, a platinum content of an average of 10.5 or 4.3 µg/g wet weight, respectively. Yoshimura et al. [74] took samples of 0.5 mL blood from the border of the tongue 1 and 10 min after commencing and completing intra-arterial infusion of an unknown dose of carboplatin; the carboplatin concentrations in serum were 1 or 10 min after commencing 496 or 698 µg/dL and to the corresponding time points after the ending of the infusion 52.3 and 14.1 µg/dL.

Tegeder et al. [75] from the Kovács group have compared tumor concentrations of cisplatin *by microdialysis* in ten patients with oral cancer treated with intra-arterial cisplatin perfusion (150 mg/m^2 in 500 mL of 0.9 % sodium chloride) and six patients with oral cancer treated with crystalline cisplatin embolization (150 mg/m^2 in 45–60 ml of 0.9 % sodium chloride), respectively. This method allowed observation of concentrations over time. The microdialysis catheter was placed into the tumor and the intra-arterial catheter into the tumor-feeding artery. Cisplatin was rapidly administered through the intra-arterial catheter. After embolization, cisplatin tumor maximum concentrations were about five times higher than those achieved after intra-arterial perfusion (54.10 µg/mL versus 11.27 µg/mL); they also lasted four times longer. Higher remission correlated with higher platinum levels proving that the effect of chemoembolization was due to the drug and not to hypoxia.

7.2.6 Diagnostic Measures

Before and after intra-arterial chemotherapy (chemoperfusion or chemoembolization), routine staging examinations of the locoregional tumor area such as ultrasound, CT, or MRI are recommended in order to make progress comparisons. Second primaries and foreign metastases must be excluded using panendoscopy, chest x-ray, abdominal ultrasound, and skeletal scintigraphy. The use of "wholebody" PET is increasingly replacing these methods. Before the intervention (be it via open retro-/orthograde or transfemoral approach), a demonstration of the complex vessel anatomy of the head and neck must be defined, usually by DSA (digital subtraction angiography). Perfusion control was carried out with staining of the tissue with patent blue, with scintigraphy using radiolabeled tracers, and mostly with DSA. Recently, a combined CT and angiography system was used which made sophisticated superselectivity possible [76, 77]. A very interesting novelty is the use of magnetic particles which can be used as contrast agents and as a drug carrier system for chemotherapeutics. Thus local cancer therapy is performed with magnetic drug targeting and allows a specific delivery of therapeutic agents to desired targets like tumors, by using a chemotherapeutic substance bound to magnetic particles and focused with an external magnetic field to the tumor after intra-arterial application [78, 79].

7.2.7   Problems of Indications of Intra-arterial Induction Chemotherapy in Head and Neck Cancers

Rationales for induction chemotherapy in head and neck cancers were listed in Sect. 7.1.2. For intra-arterial chemotherapy, there exist some special problems:

- As well as local effects, a consequent systemic effect of systemic chemotherapy is the *eradication of micrometastases* [80]. *Doubts exist about intra-arterial chemotherapy in this regard* [81] although side effects show that free cisplatin reaches the peripheral organs and it is known that intra-arterial chemotherapy without a neutralizing agent can reach similar peripheral cytostatic levels [71]. It is, therefore, a question of objective and respective execution. Recently, clear evidence of a translymphatic chemotherapeutic effect following local perfusion was found [82, 83].
- There is criticism that remission blurs the margins of the tumor and leads to a higher rate of positive surgical margins. Figure 7.5 shows a T2 buccal cancer (left) demonstrating that even in case of complete remission (right) after 150 mg/ m^2 intra-arterial cisplatin, there is a scar which can be seen or palpated guiding the surgeon during resection. The objection was overruled by Kovács [84] by comparing the rates of positive margins in a surgery only group (143 patients; 12 %), a group with postoperative chemotherapy (122 patients; 20 %), and a group with intra-arterial induction high-dose cisplatin (94 patients; 15 %). At the International Workshop on Intra-Arterial Chemotherapy for Head and Neck Cancer, August 20–22, 2006, Springfield, IL, Kovács presented data of 227 oral cancer patients of all stages operated on following intra-arterial induction with at least 2 years follow-up, having a rate of 9 % local recurrences in stages I and II and 15 % in stages III and IV cancers, suggesting that *intra-arterial induction is a local recurrence prophylaxis*. These results were, however, possible only due to radical surgery respecting the original margins.

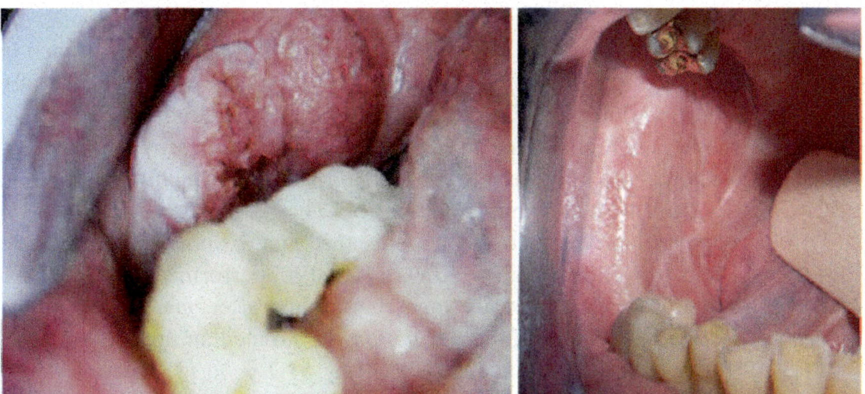

Fig. 7.5 *Left*: T2 buccal cancer. *Right*: Complete remission after 150 mg/m² intra-arterial cisplatin with remaining little visible and palpable scar

- Stephens pointed out in his contribution to the Hanoverian Symposium in 1997 on intra-arterial chemotherapy in the head and neck area that "the original failure of regional chemotherapy in cancer treatment in the head and neck region was because the technique was used predominantly to treat the most difficult regional cancer problems, which in the head and neck, was predominantly recurrent cancer" [85]. Surgical and radiation-induced reduction in vascularization and scars made an impact almost impossible. Therefore, *a preferred application of intra-arterial chemotherapy seemed to be in the absence of any pretreatment.* Moreover, since the initial tumor remission usually was not of long duration, and, therefore, intra-arterial chemotherapy in the rarest of cases could be definitive, embedding in an integrated treatment program with intra-arterial chemotherapy at the beginning (= induction) seemed to be logical. This does not mean that a palliative tumor therapy using intra-arterial chemotherapy may not be possible and meaningful.

- Another big problem was the application of intra-arterial chemotherapy in patients with locally advanced tumors of stages III and IV. The consequence of this patient selection was a relatively lower rate of complete and partial remissions, because the chemotherapy-induced tumor remission is dependent on the tumor mass. Many of these patients have been classified as inoperable, so that the treatment in most cases had to be classified as intended to be non-curative (if not combined with radiation). A demonstrable improvement in survival with induction chemotherapy can only be achieved with inclusion of primarily operable tumor stages. Since, concerning systemic induction chemotherapy, there was a relationship between a response of the tumor to chemotherapy and a favorable prognosis [86], at least 40 % complete remissions by a primary chemotherapy are needed according to statistical projections to be able to demonstrate a chemotherapy-related improvement of treatment results for realistic patient numbers compared to a standard therapy [87]. This rate can be achieved only in tumors of smaller mass [88], so that also this logic necessitates *the involvement of the tumor stages I and II in studies on intra-arterial chemotherapy.* Two volumetric studies should be mentioned in this context. Baghi et al. [89] performed MRI volumetry in 50 patients with advanced head and neck cancer. All patients were to undergo *three cycles of TPF* chemotherapy regimen followed by chemoradiation. They calculated statistically a threshold for pretreatment tumor volume, which was equal to *29.71 cc* for patients with complete remission. They concluded that this could be of prognostic value to stratify patients that may respond completely to systemic induction chemotherapy. Kovács et al. [90] performed CT volumetry in 128 oral cancer patients of all stages before and after *one cycle of intra-arterial cisplatin (150 mg/m2) for induction.* Initial median tumor volume of 11.8 cc (range 0.17–211.7 cc) was reduced by 51.7 % to median post-interventional volume of 5.7 cc (range 0–388.8 cc). Initial volume was reduced in 80.5 % of patients; in 19.5 % post-interventional volume was equal to the initial volume or increased. In mathematical models, prediction of post-interventional volume and the probability of complete radiological remission could be calculated which proved to depend negatively on high initial volume, nonoperability, and, especially, high age. Figure 7.6 shows two of the probability curves demonstrating the dependence between tumor volume in cc and remission.

- In contrast to systemic chemotherapy, the reduction of peripheral toxicity combined with high local efficacy was generally the main aim of intra-arterial chemotherapy [91], especially important in head and neck cancer patients who often suffer from other intercurrent illnesses. *In multimodality treatment regimens for advanced cancers, the actual aim of intra-arterial induction chemotherapy has not necessarily to be complete remission* but to restrain the tumor in its local and possibly metastatic aggressiveness before radical surgery and/or chemoradiation without the very high side effects of systemic chemotherapy so that the following straining definitive modalities can be carried out with a high patient- and treatment-related compliance. Early response even without complete remission in contrast to stable disease might offer the chance to distribute patients to different treatment regimens via use of well-tolerated intra-arterial chemotherapy as *prognostic marker.*

- Furthermore, *it is essential to the meaningful evaluation of results of a cancer treatment that only one tumor entity is investigated.* Under the summary description of "head and neck cancer," a multitude of tumor localizations are hidden. In terms of intra-arterial chemotherapy, it is particularly problematic to compare tumors which have very different volumes within the same tumor classification such as the tongue and larynx. It is immediately apparent that here consistent comparisons cannot be drawn.

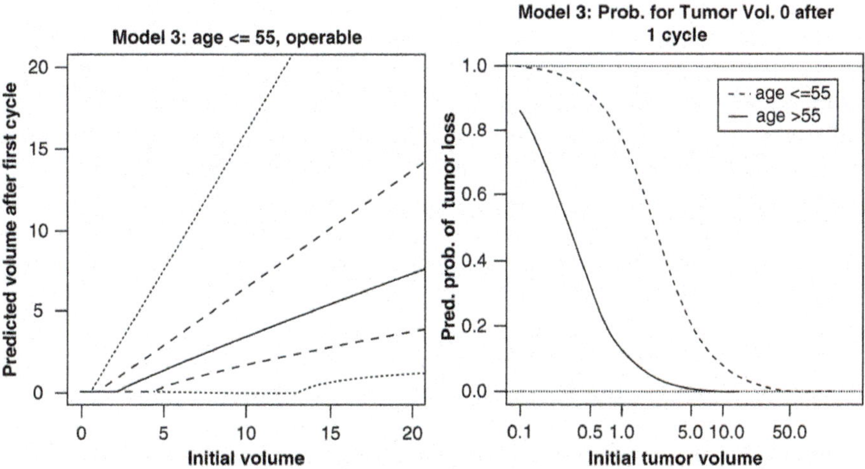

Fig. 7.6 Probability curves demonstrating dependence between tumor volume in cc and remission after 150 mg/m² intra-arterial cisplatin. *Left*: Quantiles (*solid lines*, median; *dashed line*, 0.25- and 0.75-quartiles; *dotted lines*, 0.05- and 0.95-quantiles) for volume. *Right*: Estimated probability of complete radiological remission (tumor volume = 0)

7.2.8 Clinical Trials with Intra-arterial Induction Chemotherapy (Chemo Infusion) in Head and Neck Cancers

Table 7.1 gives a near to exhaustive overview on clinical studies using intra-arterial induction chemotherapy with drug solutions in the head and neck. It can be seen that initially retrograde cannulations of the temporal superficial artery, open catheterizations in the neck with ligatures of the branches of the external carotid artery, or port systems were common to perfuse the tumor region often over extended periods of time when induction use with curative intention was intended. An excellent presentation of catheter-related complications of the continuous infusions of the retrogradely cannulated temporal superficial artery was given by Molinari et al. [125], in whose clinic in Milan, intra-arterial chemotherapy has been used since 1971. Two hundred and sixty-eight patients had been treated with an intra-arterial chemotherapy in 297 attempted cannulations. Eleven percent of cannulations were not successful. Other complications consisted of catheter occlusion or dislocations (8 %), local inflammation (15 %), and neurological disorders (4 %) like a temporary facial paralysis. Interruption of treatment (= continuous infusion) occurred in 20 % of cases. Overall, a "useful" therapy could be achieved in 85 % of cases. Hematological acute side effects were rarely associated with the drugs methotrexate, bleomycin, adriamycin, and cisplatin (2.8 %). Frustaci et al. [126] reported an injury of cranial nerves with an incidence of 6.3 %.

Compared to this approach, the superselective angiography-controlled display and infusion of the tumor-feeding vessel since the late 1970s [127] opened new perspectives in terms of higher response rates through targeted drug delivery and less technical complications. Via transfemoral access and using coaxial microcatheters, chemotherapy could be given safely and without major vascular irritation in a short time. Precondition for a short time of perfusion was the realization that in the most effective chemotherapy drug for head and neck cancer, cisplatin, the bolus administration was possible also in the regional usage, and peripheral neutralization allowed very high doses. In case of multiple arterial pedicles to the tumor, all of them could be reached superselectively by this technique. Administration could be repeated easily.

Table 7.1 shows exactly the drug dosages and administration schemes to give an impression of the width but also somewhat anarchic diversity of clinical investigations. Sixteen (16) trials had less than 50 patients. Randomized studies are listed in bold types.

The mentioned diversity of these clinical trials using intra-arterial induction chemotherapy regimens with respect to the number of patients, whether previously untreated or recurrent cancers, the tumor stages, schemes, drugs, dosages, types of cannulation, and relevant results allows only a few valid conclusions, that is:

- That local clinical response rates of 50–99 % and local clinical complete remission rates of 4–48 % were achieved at the end of a respective intra-arterial induction regimen

Table 7.1 List of reported clinical studies on intra-arterial induction chemotherapy in head and neck cancers in chronological order

Author(s)	Patients	Tumor entities	Chemotherapeutic drugs and doses; application	Definitive treatment	Results
Cruz et al. [92]	40	Head and neck cancers, mainly oropharyngeal carcinomas	5-fluorouracil 15 mg/kg/day, methotrexate 5 mg/day, vinblastine 0.02 mg/kg/day continuously up to 16 days; retrograde	Radiation or surgery	OR 59 %, CR 15 %; 25 % local complications (temporary blindness, facial paralyses, dislocations)
Armstrong and Meeker [93]	15	36 inoperable head and neck, mainly oral and oropharyngeal, carcinomas	5-fluorouracil 15 mg/kg/day, methotrexate 5 mg/day, vinblastine 0.02 mg/kg/day continuously up to 16 days; retrograde	Radiation; compared with radiation alone	OR 93 %; survival 14.1 months versus 9.1 months in comparison group
Curioni and Quadu [94]	47	Stages I–IV oral carcinomas	Vincristine 0.6–1 mg/m² over 1 h day 1–2, methotrexate 80–120 mg/m² over 12 h day 3–4, bleomycin 10–15 mg/m² over 1 h day 5–9, day 11–19, adriamycin 10–20 mg/m² or mitomycin C 2–4 mg/m² over 1 h day 10 and 20; retrograde	Radiation; some responders operated on	OR 61.7 %, CR 19 %; death rate 17 %
Szabó and Kovács [95]	70	126 various head and neck malignomas	Vincristine 0.5 mg intravenously, bleomycin 15 mg day 1, methotrexate 50 mg day 2, elobromol 750 mg per os day 3×3–5; retrograde	70 patients: surgery	PR 98 % (?); thrombosis in two cases
Koch et al. [96]	128	Stages I–IV head and neck carcinomas	Methotrexate 1–1.5 mg/kg over 1 h up to 7 days; retrograde	Radiation	OR 73 %, CR 4 %
Mika [97]	21	Advanced oral and oropharyngeal carcinomas	Vincristine 1–2 mg day 1, methotrexate 240 mg over 20 h day 1, bleomycin 45 mg day 3–5, cisplatin 0.75 mg/kg day 6–7; retrograde	Surgery (16 patients operated on, 15 patients irradiated)	OR 80 %, CR 47 %

(continued)

Table 7.1 (continued)

Author(s)	Patients	Tumor entities	Chemotherapeutic drugs and doses; application	Definitive treatment	Results
Arcangeli et al. [98]	**72**	**142 head and neck carcinomas stages II–IV**	**Methotrexate 3–5 mg/day continuously up to cumulative dose of 90–120 mg; retrograde**	**Radiation; randomized against radiation alone**	**Oral cavity carcinomas: 5-year survival 54 % versus 27 % in comparison group (signif.)**
Molinari et al. [99]	**85**	**Oral cavity carcinomas**	**Methotrexate 500 mg over 10 days; retrograde**	**Radiation or surgery; randomized against bleomycin 95 mg over 13 days**	**Local effectivity of bleomycin better (OR 60 %), catheter-related complications and toxicity higher with methotrexate**
Galmarini et al. [100]	38	Advanced head and neck carcinomas	Bleomycin 20 mg/m^2/day (day 1–2), cisplatin 100 mg/m^2 over 3 h day 3 q3w; retrograde	Surgery or radiation	OR 87 %, CR 29 %; temporary facial paralyses (5 %), anemias (16 %)
Milazzo et al. [101]	12	Oral cavity and oropharyngeal carcinomas stages III and IV	Cisplatin, vinblastine, bleomycin, 5-fluorouracil (doses?); retrograde	Surgery or radiation followed by surgery	OR 67 %; 50 % living after max. 3 years of observation
Inuyama et al. [102]	25	93 head and neck carcinomas stages III and IV (in part pre-treated)	Cisplatin 50 mg/m^2 over 2 h day 1, peplomycin 5 mg/day over 5 h day 2–6; approach?	Chemoradiation (5-fluorouracil); 60 times intravenous application	OR 68 %, CR 26 %; higher response rate in case of intra-arterial application
Mortimer et al. [103]	12	25 inoperable head and neck carcinomas	Cisplatin 100 mg/m^2 q1–3w × 3; transfemoral into external carotid artery	12 patients irradiated	OR 80 %, CR 20 % (locally and lymph nodes); ipsilateral hemialopecia, temporary facial paralyses
Cheung et al. [104]	11	20 oral cavity and oropharyngeal carcinomas stages III and IV	Methotrexate 50 mg/m^2 intravenously, cisplatin 90 mg/m^2 long-time perfusion 1 mg/h; retrograde	11 patients operated on and irradiated	OR 94 %, CR 35 %; 3-year survival 60 %; catheter-related complications 30 %, mortality 5 %

Lee et al. [105]	24	Advanced paranasal sinus carcinomas or sarcomas	Cisplatin 100 mg/m², bleomycin 30 U day 1, 5-fluorouracil 5,000 mg/m² intravenously day 1–5 q3–4w × 2–3; transfemoral superselective	Radiation or surgery; 15 patients irradiated	OR 91 %, CR 48 %; 8 long-time survivors
Claudio et al. [106]	23	40 unresectable oral cavity and oropharyngeal carcinomas and BCC skin	Vincristine 1.5 mg, bleomycin 45 mg, methotrexate 20 mg or cisplatin 50 mg, bleomycin 30 mg, each as long-time infusion (q1w × 5–6); transposed external carotid artery	23 patients operated on	OR 77 %, CR 13 %; pCR 13 patients; 3-year survival 60 %; catheter-related complications 18 %, temporary facial paralyses 10 %
Frustaci et al. [107]	50	Head and neck carcinomas T2–4 N0–1	Cisplatin 20 mg over 4 h, bleomycin 15 mg over 20 h over 8 days; retrograde	39 patients operated on, 13 additionally irradiated, 9 irradiated only	OR 70 %, pCR 16 %; catheter-related complications 8 %, temporary facial paralyses 4 %
Richard et al. [108]	**112**	**222 oral cavity and oropharyngeal carcinomas**	**Vincristine 1 mg day 1, 5, 9, bleomycin 15 mg/day over 8 h over 12 days; retrograde**	**Surgery; randomized against surgery only, oropharyngeal cancers obligatory radiation**	**Oral cavity carcinomas: OR local 48 %, OR lymph nodes 15 %, survival signif. better than comparison group and oropharyngeal carcinomas**
Vieitez et al. [109]	13	Oral cavity and oropharyngeal carcinomas stages III and IV	Carboplatin 400 mg/m² over 4 h day 1–5, 5-fluorouracil 900 mg/m² over 20 h day 1–5; transfemoral superselective	Radiation	OR 84 %, CR 23 %; 3-year survival probability 56 % after median observation time of 18 months; catheter-related complications <7 %
Korogi et al. [110], Hirai et al. [111]	22	Oral cavity carcinomas stages III and IV	Cisplatin 30–50 mg/m² q1w × 2–3; transfemoral superselective	14 patients operated on, 6 irradiated, 1 both	OR 95 %, CR 24 %; 2-year survival probability 70 % after median observation time of 20 months (not significantly better than historical control); 1 death

(continued)

Table 7.1 (continued)

Author(s)	Patients	Tumor entities	Chemotherapeutic drugs and doses; application	Definitive treatment	Results
Scheel et al. [112]	63	Advanced head and neck carcinomas	Long-time infusion up to cumulative dose of 400 mg cisplatin; bypass method	Radiation; only neck operated on; tumor left in place	5-year survival 39 % (adenoid cystic carcinomas 100 %)
Siegel et al. [113], Wilson et al. [114]	32, 43	Advanced head and neck carcinomas	Cisplatin 150 mg/m^2 + STS weekly × 4; transfemoral superselective	Surgery followed by radiation; Wilson et al.: no surgery, only radiation	Siegel et al.: OR 99 %; Wilson et al.: OR 91 %; survival 65 % after median observation of 30 months
Kovács et al. [115]	103	Oral cavity and oropharyngeal carcinomas stages I to IV	Cisplatin 100 mg/m^2 day 1, intravenous 5-fluorouracil 1,000 mg/m^2 day 1–5 in 36 patients; cisplatin 150 mg/m^2 + STS × 1 in 67 patients; transfemoral superselective	67 % and 75 % operated on, respectively, 71 % and 60 % with adjuvant (chemoradiation) (docetaxel)	OR 81 % and 67 %, respectively; survival 61 % (23 months) and 79 % (8 months); 1 apoplexia, no technical problems
Szabó et al. [116]	**47**	**131 sublingual/lingual carcinomas T2–4NXMX**	**Cisplatin 50 mg day 3, 5, 10, 12, epirubicin 60 mg day1, 8; retrograde**	**Surgery; randomized against pre-op radiation**	**5-year survival 38 % versus 31 % in comparison (not significant)**
Benazzo et al. [117], Bertino et al. [118]	46	Head and neck carcinomas stages III and IV	Carboplatin 300–350 mg/m^2 q2w × 3; transfemoral superselective	43 irradiated, 12 patients additionally operated on	OR 78 %, CR 35 %; disease-free survival 50 % after 5 years; no technical problems
Kovács [119]	52	Oral carcinomas stages I–IV	Cisplatin 150 mg/m^2+ STS × 1; transfemoral superselective	All operated on	OR 69 %, pCR 25 %; overall survival 77 % following 5 years of observation and better as compared to a treatment-related prognostic index TPI

Kovács et al. [120]	103	Oral and oropharyngeal carcinomas stages I to IV	Cisplatin 150 mg/m^2 as crystal suspension + STS; transfemoral superselective	83 operated on, 20 radiation or chemoradiation (docetaxel)	OR 73 %, pCR 18.5 %; 3.5 % interventional and 10 % local complications
Damascelli et al. [121, 122]	60	Advanced T3–4 N0–3 oral cavity, oropharyngeal, hypopharyngeal carcinomas	Nanoparticle albumin-bound paclitaxel 150–230 mg/m^2 × 2–4; transfemoral superselective	Subsequent surgery, chemotherapy, radiation or chemoradiation	OR 75 %; 6 temporary facial paralyses
Kovács et al. [123]	40	72 inoperable advanced oral and oropharyngeal carcinomas	150 mg/m^2 cisplatin + STS q4w × 1–3; transfemoral superselective	Radiation or chemoradiation (docetaxel)	OR 57 %, CR 15 %; 2-year overall survival 25 %
Nagai et al. [124]	13	Oral carcinomas	65 mg/ m^2/day S-1 orally over 14 days + 40–50 mg/m^2 docetaxel; approach?	Operation	OR 100 %, CR 69.2 %; neutropenia, cerebral infarct

Q interval between cycles, *W* week, *H* hour, *OR* overall response, *CR* complete remission, *pCR* pathological complete remission, *PR* partial remission, *STS* sodium thiosulfate, *TPI* treatment-dependent prognosis index

- That complete pathological remissions of the tumors were demonstrated in about 16–25 %
- That local and systemic toxicity and complications of the transfemoral superselective approach were extremely few (no measurable toxicity in about 20 % of cases!)
- That compliance was very high (up to 100 %) and no increase in surgical or radiation-induced complications was to be feared

Figure 7.7 shows complete remissions after one course of intra-arterial chemoperfusion with 150 mg/m^2 cisplatin peripherically neutralized with sodium thiosulfate.

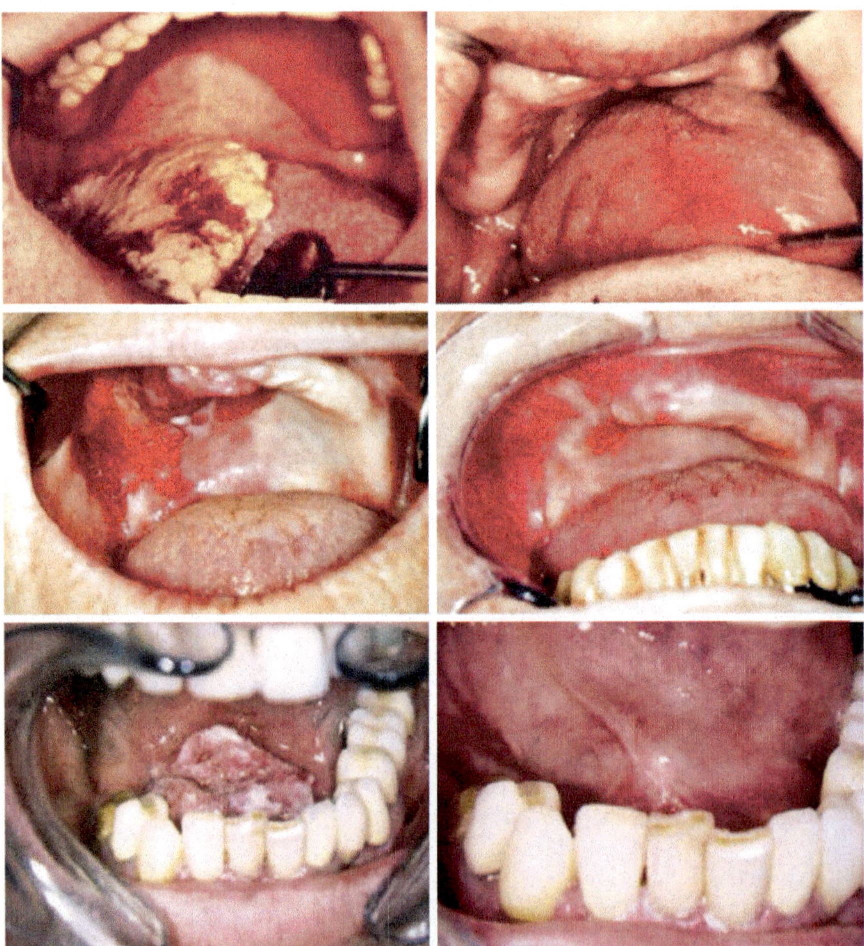

Fig. 7.7 Three examples of complete remissions of oral cavity cancers after one course of intra-arterial chemoperfusion with 150 mg/m^2 cisplatin, respectively. No side effects

Intra-arterial Induction Chemotherapy and Survival Advantage
With respect to survival, randomized studies have to be examined because according to the contemporary conviction, only they can produce level 1 evidence. These demonstrated a survival benefit for oral cancer patients. *Richard* et al. [108] *could demonstrate a survival advantage for 112 operable patients with floor of the mouth cancer after preoperative intra-arterial treatment with bleomycin and vincristine over 12 days*, however, not for patients with oropharyngeal cancer. Only the oropharyngeal cancers got systematically postoperative radiation, the floor of the mouth cancer patients depending on the status of the margins after surgery and the lymph node status. Among the four randomized trials, *in addition to that of Richard* et al. [108], *also Arcangeli* et al. [98] *showed a survival advantage in patients with oral cancer, which have been treated with intra-arterial induction methotrexate prior to definitive radiotherapy*. From these results, the prognostic difference between the different localizations of head and neck tumors clearly emerges.

The difference to preoperative radiation lies in the minimal side effects of intra-arterial chemotherapy and in the preserved possibility of a full-dose radiation. The two modalities were only once compared to each other in a randomized way [116]. The survival rates were practically the same after a preoperative intra-arterial chemotherapy and preoperative irradiation with 46 Gy. The authors nevertheless stressed the higher quality of life after intra-arterial chemotherapy as compared to radiotherapy. Wound healing after surgery was not disturbed, and chronic side effects of radiation like xerostomia were lacking.

Kovács and coworkers [42, 115, 119, 120, 128–130] were the only investigators so far to include consequently also small tumor stages into populations treated with intra-arterial induction chemotherapy and to concentrate on one tumor site (oral cavity, anterior oropharynx). This was a corollary of the abovementioned randomized studies and prerequisites for a successful induction treatment (one tumor localization, tumors of smaller volume, higher rates of complete responses). At the International Workshop on Intra-Arterial Chemotherapy for Head and Neck Cancer, August 20–22, 2006, Springfield, IL, Kovács presented results on 406 patients with previously untreated primary oral and oropharyngeal carcinomas (30 % stages I and II, 70 % stages III and IV), treated between 1997 and 2005 and having an overall response rate of 43 % following one intra-arterial intervention. Patients underwent a complex multimodality regimen starting with intra-arterial chemotherapy, followed by surgery and adjuvant chemoradiation with docetaxel [131, 132]. Allocating patients according to their treatment-related compliance (operability/nonoperability, contraindications to radiation and/or docetaxel) resulted in several groups with multimodality treatment. These were statistically examined and compared [42]. *For the group with all modalities (94 patients), at a median follow-up of 4 years, the 5-year survival rate was 80%, and disease-free survival was 73%. Among patients with advanced disease (stage III and IV), survival was extremely favorable with 83% and 59%, respectively [133]. In 52 patients with resectable cancers of stages I–IV and no adjuvant radiation, the 3-year overall and disease-free survival was 82% and 69%, respectively, and at 5 years 77% and 59%, respectively [119].*

Results were compared favorably with a treatment-dependent prognosis index [134], which is of more value than a historical comparison. Acute and long-term toxicity of intra-arterial induction chemotherapy was insignificant [135]. *However, a new randomized trial comparing intra-arterial induction chemotherapy plus surgery with surgery alone remains to be studied in oral cavity and oropharyngeal cancer, just as randomized studies comparing systemic and intra-arterial induction chemotherapy are lacking.*

Intra-arterial Induction Chemotherapy, Prognosis, and Treatment Stratification

It was unclear until recently, however, whether the assumptions on the relationship of remission and prognosis following systemic induction chemotherapy were true as well for intra-arterial induction chemotherapy. Kovács [136] could prove *a strong prognostic relevance of response to intra-arterial high-dose cisplatin for induction irrespective of stage and consecutive treatment* in 187 unselected consecutive patients with previously untreated oral and oropharyngeal carcinomas. This treatment was followed by surgery and adjuvant concomitant chemoradiation. Thus, induction chemotherapy could help in stratifying further treatment. Figure 7.8 demonstrates the significant difference between overall survival (Kaplan–Meier) compared with degree of response (CR, complete response; PR, partial response; SD, stable disease; PD, progressive disease).

The same idea was followed by Benazzo and Bertino et al. using high-dose carboplatin in advanced cancers [117, 118] who customized their treatment according to the response: Complete responders or partial responders had radiotherapy;

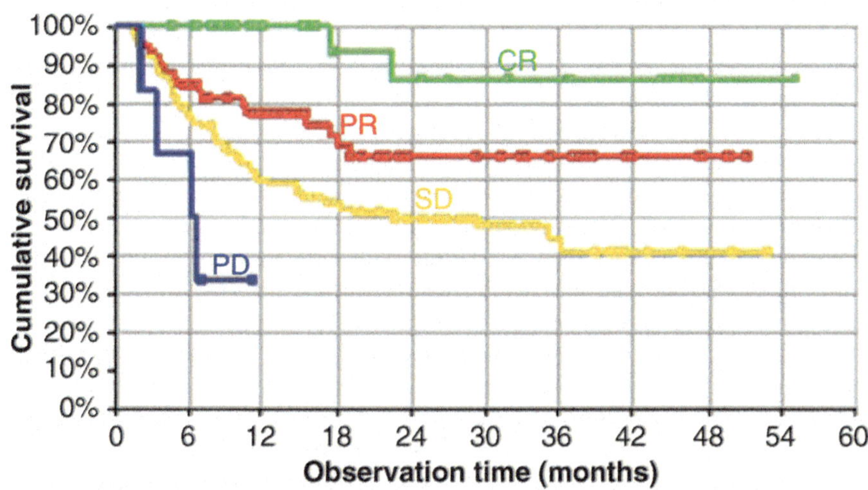

Fig. 7.8 Significant difference between overall survival (Kaplan–Meier) in relation to degree of response (*CR* complete response, *PR* partial response, *SD* stable disease, *PD* progressive disease) after 150 mg/m² intra-arterial cisplatin

nonresponders with resectable disease underwent surgery on the tumor site and/or on the neck nodal metastases followed by radiotherapy; nonresponders with unresectable disease underwent palliative radiotherapy. *Intra-arterial chemotherapy thus functions as selection for organ preservation.* Figure 7.9 [123] shows a 51-year-old patient suffering from a left tongue base cancer T4cN2b (top) who underwent three courses of intra-arterial cisplatin (150 mg/m^2) resulting in local complete remission. Definitive radiation succeeded in 9-year relapse-free survival (below).

Another good example for organ preservation is presented in Fig. 7.10 (courtesy Frankfurt neuroradiology): A 49-year-old woman with histologically proven carcinoma of the left sphenoid sinus (1998, left) was treated with two courses of 150 mg/m^2 intra-arterial cisplatin and remained progression-free for at least 7 years (right).

Recent reports about the intra-arterial treatment of head and neck carcinomas return to long-time continuous infusion by using an improved retrograde approach or an implantable port-catheter system and a portable pump. A Japanese group [137] treated T1/2 lip cancers with intra-arterial chemotherapy via the superficial

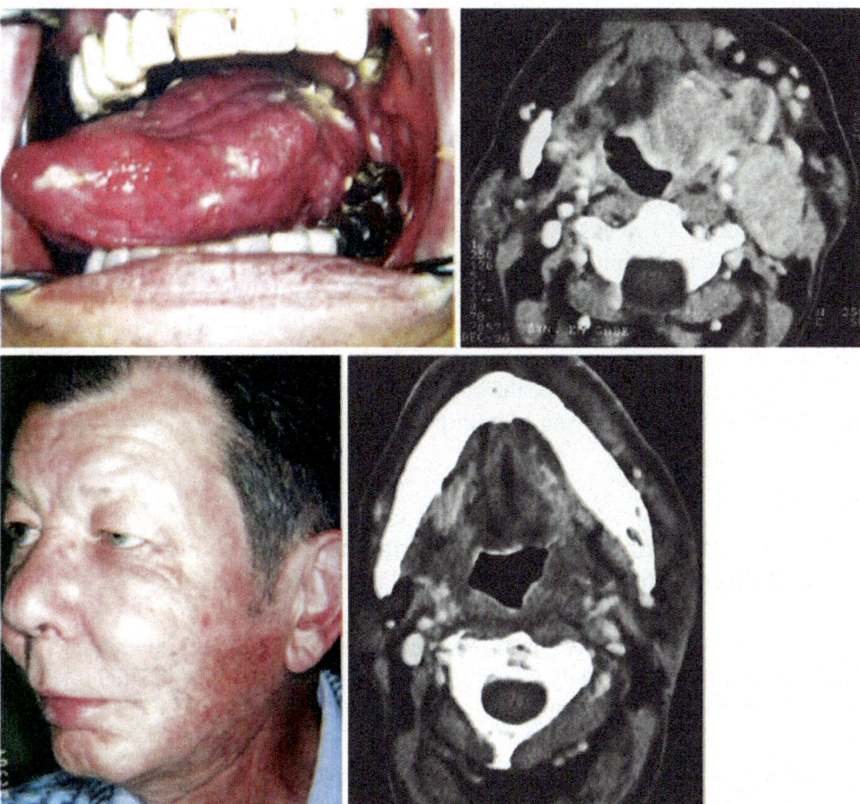

Fig. 7.9 *Top*: Intraoral view and CT of a 51-year-old patient suffering from left tongue base cancer T4cN2b. *Below*: Same patient and CT 9 years later; three courses of 150 mg/m^2 intra-arterial cisplatin and definitive radiation resulted in local complete remission and relapse-free survival

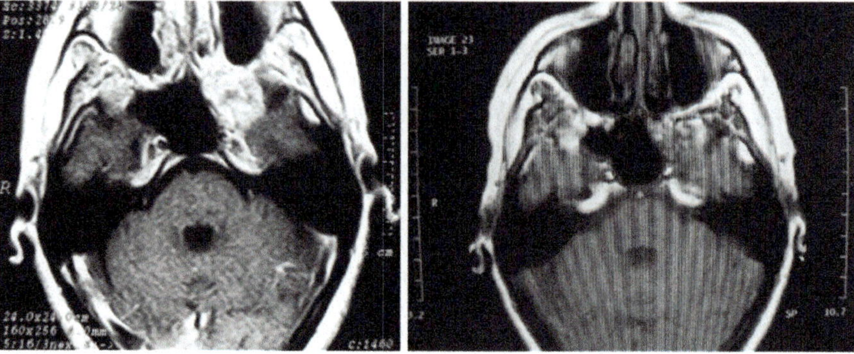

Fig. 7.10 *Left*: CT of a 49-year-old woman with histologically proven carcinoma of left sphenoid sinus. *Right*: CT of same patient 7 years later; complete remission and progression-free survival following two courses of 150 mg/m^2 intra-arterial cisplatin

temporal artery, instead of an operation, so the intention here was similarly surgery-saving as, for example, a photodynamic therapy. The same did Nakasato et al. [138] for all stages of oral cancer (49 patients). Again, the chemotherapy was carried out continuously over time. A superselective catheterization was successful in only 69 % of patients. By a Taiwanese group, methotrexate (50 mg/day) was continuously infused to the external carotid artery for a mean period of about 7 days, followed by weekly bolus of methotrexate (25 mg) via intra-arterial route for a mean period of around 10 weeks. Results were so good with complete long-time remissions of 100 % and minimal to none catheter-related complications or side effects that surgery was avoided (organ preservation) [139, 140]. With better technique for retrograde cannulation succeeding in real superselective drug application, continuous infusions may experience a renaissance. Fuwa et al. [141] used both approaches concluding that the puncture of the superficial temporal artery may be favored by elderly patients. A comparison of multiple-shot and continuous intra-arterial infusions is lacking.

7.2.9 Clinical Trials with Intra-arterial Induction Chemotherapy (Chemoembolization) in Head and Neck Cancers

Table 7.2 gives an exhaustive overview on clinical embolization trials in head and neck cancers. Note the usually very small study groups (less than 50 patients except in two trials). They mostly come from Japan and China.

The type and size of the particles used were as follows. Okamoto et al. [68, 69] administered ethyl cellulose microcapsules with an average size of 396 nm using femoral catheterization to the lingual or maxillary artery. This treatment was given as adjuvant treatment following a combination treatment of preoperative chemoradiation and surgery. In 1998, long-term results were advantageous as compared to combination therapy alone [149]. Kato et al. [65] from the same study group

Table 7.2 List of reported clinical studies on intra-arterial induction chemoembolization in head and neck cancers in chronological order

Authors	Patients	Tumor entities	Particles	Chemotherapeutics	Response	Side effects	Definitive treatment
Okamoto et al. [68, 69]	11	Maxillary sinus, nasal and oral cavity cancers	Ethyl cellulose microcapsules	Cisplatin 40–60 mg	63 %	100 % local pain	Surgery
Kato et al. [65]	28 incl. 11 of Okamoto et al.	Head and neck cancers	Ethyl cellulose microcapsules	Diverse (mainly cisplatin)	28 %	Low toxicity	Surgery
Tomura et al. [142, 143]	19	Head and neck cancers incl. maxillary cancers	Ethyl cellulose microcapsules	Carboplatin 100 mg	20 %	60 % local pain, low systemic toxicity	Surgery
Li et al. [144]	7	Tongue cancers	Albumin microspheres	Cisplatin 13.6 mg	Not reported	Not reported	Surgery
Suvorova et al. [145]	12	Advanced head and neck cancers	Coil fragments	5-fluorouracil 700 mg/m^2 + methotrexate 40 mg/m^2	58 %	Not reported	Radiation
Kovács and Turowski [130]	32 (15 with microspheres)	Oral and oropharyngeal cancers	Starch microspheres	Cisplatin 150 mg/m^2	87 %	One tracheotomy, two temporary facial paralyses	Surgery + adjuvant (chemo)radiation
Li et al. [146]	20	Advanced oral cancers	Gelatin sponge	Cisplatin, adriamycin, mitomycin C	Not reported	Not reported	Surgery

(continued)

Table 7.2 (continued)

Authors	Patients	Tumor entities	Particles	Chemotherapeutics	Response	Side effects	Definitive treatment
Kovács [128]	103	Oral and oropharyngeal cancers	Cisplatin crystal suspension	Cisplatin 150 mg/m^2	73 %	3.5 % interventional and 10 % local complications; 71 % local pain; low systemic toxicity	Surgery + adjuvant (chemo)radiation
He et al. [147]	78	Tongue cancers	Ethyl cellulose microcapsules, meglumine iothalamate suspending liquid	Carboplatin 200–300 mg	100 %(?)	No complications, 100 % local pain	Surgery
Sokurenko et al. [148]	25	Advanced head and neck cancers	Gelatin sponge	Carboplatin 300 mg/m^2 + 5-fluorouracil 1,000 mg/m^2	57 %	Low systemic toxicity	Systemic chemotherapy, radiation

integrated the experience with 1,013 patients from 1978 to 1992, of which 28 were head and neck patients. Various chemotherapeutic agents encapsulated in ethyl cellulose were administered in this period; the maximum size of the capsules was 225 μm. Tomura et al. [142, 143] used carboplatin ethyl cellulose microcapsules of similar size.

One of the Chinese attempts to use chemoembolization in this area was the treatment of tongue cancer with cisplatin-loaded albumin microspheres with an average size of 56 μm administered into the surgically exposed lingual artery [144]. Song et al. [150] reported about diverse treatments including chemoembolization in 11 patients. However, the article is in Chinese, and the abstract does not give sufficient information. Li et al. [146] used transfemoral approach for a polychemotherapy regimen combined with embolization using gelatin sponge which was administered into branches of the external carotid artery. The article mainly dealt with histological changes in the tissue. Interesting are the articles of He et al. [147, 151] who used carboplatin ethyl cellulose microcapsules with an average diameter of 214 μm (range: 40–300 μm) in 78 patients in the period between 1993 and 2006. They examined lingual artery specimens finding an occlusion at the fifth to the sixth branches level of the deep lingual artery. This did not cause complete necrosis of the tongue body; however, as is shown in photographs, large embolized areas of the tongue showed a separation due to necrosis. Russian reports using coils and gelatin sponges treated patients with palliative intention; main rationale was the cessation of tumor bleeding, which succeeded well as reported [145, 148].

According to this body of literature, a total of only 303 head and neck cancer patients have been treated with embolization protocols over a period of nearly 25 years and, out of these, more than 100 patients in the 5 years of 2000–2004. This was possible because Kovács and coworkers succeeded in finding a way to make *chemoembolization a routine procedure in head and neck cancers by creating a cisplatin suspension which has the antineoplastic and embolizing properties combined.* The preparation method is described in several publications [42, 120, 128–130]. Lyophilized cisplatin (maximum 300 mg) was reconstituted with 0.9 % sodium chloride leading to a yellow mixture with a final concentration of 5 mg/mL. This preparation method results in a monocomponent, a highly concentrated aqueous suspension of cisplatin (maximum 60 mL) with precipitation of crystals. The physicochemical properties (e.g., PtPt distances, molecular vibration analyses) of cisplatin crystals which did form in frozen solutions have been previously described elsewhere [152]. The stability of the cisplatin complex is pharmacologically assured in a suspension because of the high concentration of sodium chloride. The resulting fluid is a 5.4 % sodium chloride solution. Hypertonic sodium chloride solutions reportedly do not have an effect on pharmacokinetics of cisplatin [153]. The osmolality is supposedly higher than in an aqueous solution (about 285 mOsm/kg [154]) but cannot be measured exactly because of the presence of crystalline precipitates. Theoretic osmolality of the described suspension as calculated approximately is 2,130 mOsm/kg. Microscopic assessment of particle diameters in the aqueous crystal suspension of cisplatin showed rod-shaped crystals measuring 3×8 μm; regular clumping of these crystals formed particles measuring 30×50 μm.

Ratio of small to large particles was 100/1. In solutions where precipitates did form, redissolution occurred very slowly with warming back to room temperature [155]. At 40 °C, the time of redissolution was about 20–30 min [156]. Due to this formulation, up to 300 mg cisplatin could be administered with extremely high remission rates.

Figure 7.11 [130] demonstrates chemoembolization with the described suspension; a left floor of mouth cancer with blush in fluoroscopy via the sublingual artery (left) cannot be visualized after superselective embolization (right).

Chemoembolization resulted in typical local side effects (pain, swelling) and leukocytosis, that is, clear symptoms of a post-embolization syndrome. This concerned mainly patients with tongue cancer, in whom quite unpredictable swelling of varying degrees could occur in the first post-interventional days. To avoid risk of suffocation, best suited areas for use are the anterior tongue, the floor of mouth, and the mandibular gingiva. In case of anastomoses to the skin, atopic necroses of small skin areas at the chin and cheek occurred. Temporary unilateral facial paralysis had to be included to the severe complications (6 %). Systemic toxicity was negligible.

Figure 7.12 demonstrates typical chances and problems of chemoembolization: a T2 sublingual cancer can be seen (top left); treated via the lingual artery, the tumor typically emerges the third day among small epitheliolyses and necroses before remission due to drug effect starts (top right); below side effects are demonstrated like swelling, atopic skin necroses, and not intended target necroses due to hypoxia in case of very small vessels which nevertheless usually result in good healing and function.

The particle size is of utmost importance for chemoembolization in head and neck cancer because embolization effects are questionable in particle sizes in the nanometer range and, if at all present, only pause briefly [157], so that the intra-arterial administration of paclitaxel–albumin nanoparticles with a size of 150–200 nm in patients with cancer of the head and neck cancer and the anal canal reported by Damascelli et al. [158] has not been described as chemoembolization by the authors.

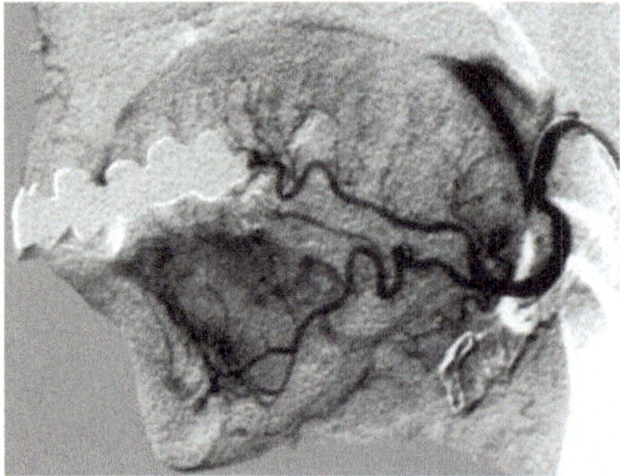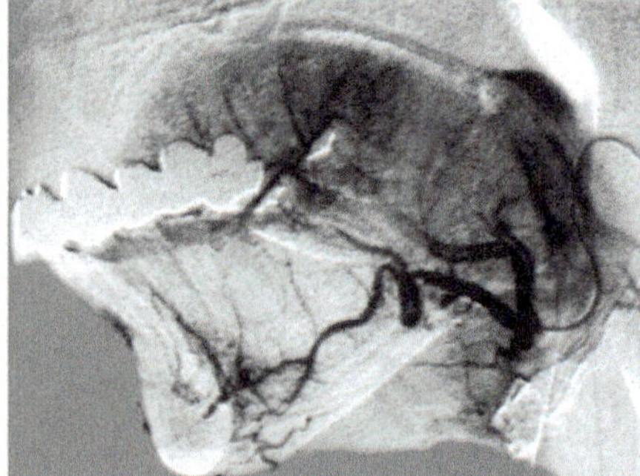

Fig. 7.11 *Left*: Left floor of mouth cancer with blush in fluoroscopy via sublingual artery. *Right*: Same area cannot be visualized after superselective chemoembolization with cisplatin suspension

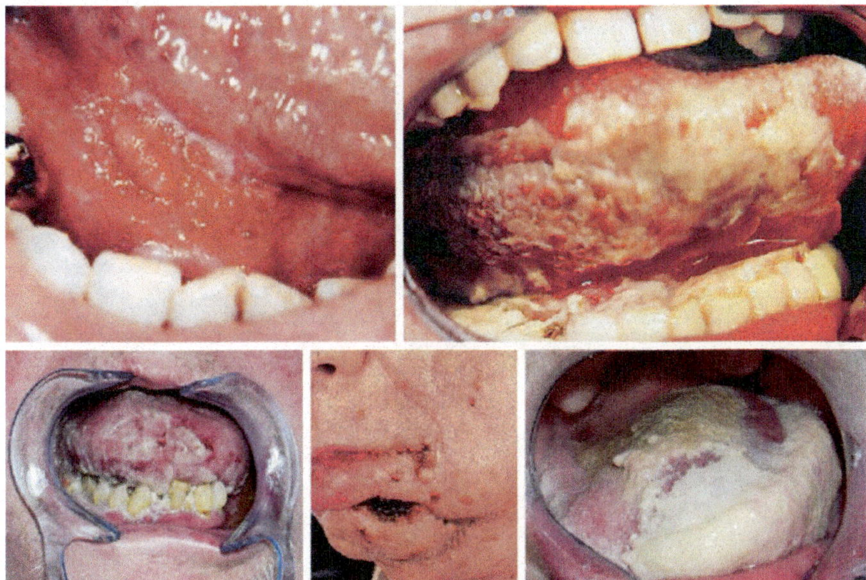

Fig. 7.12 *Top left*: T2 sublingual cancer. *Top right*: Following chemoembolization using cisplatin suspension via lingual artery, small epitheliolyses and necroses can be seen during remission. *Below*: Possible side effects of chemoembolization like swelling, atopic skin necroses, and target necroses due to longer lasting hypoxia (from *left* to *right*)

Only recently it was demonstrated in the rabbit model on VX2 tumors of auricles that particle sizes of between 40 and 60 μm are recommended for the embolization of head and neck cancer [159]. Kovács and Turowski [130] tried an application of a cisplatin/DSM-mix (DSM = "degradable starch microspheres") which led to an early complete vascular blockade by embolization causing increased local swelling and pain. By this method, only between 10 and 25 mg cisplatin could be administered together with DSM; the rest had to be discarded. DSM has a diameter of 45 μm and has been chosen because the risk of extensive necrosis of the tumor surrounding tissue was lower; as other agents, occluding the blood vessels for a long time and being nondegradable such as polyvinyl alcohol appeared to be too dangerous in the oral region. Nevertheless, a limited necrosis of the tumor and surrounding tissue as a result of temporary ischemia was perfectly desirable. The DSM chemoembolization showed no advantage in terms of response and toxicity as compared to the cisplatin crystal suspension and has been abandoned. The trials of He et al. [147, 151] with microcapsules of 214 μm diameter suggest a complete occlusion of vessels with a foremost necrotizing (and not an antineoplastic) effect. Figure 7.13 gives an impression of the embolizing agents used: top left a carboplatin microcapsule (diameter about 150 μm, ×644 [147]), top right degradable starch microspheres (diameter 45 μm, ×1,400, courtesy PharmaCept GmbH Berlin), down left a drop (12×7 mm) of the aqueous cisplatin suspension [42], and down right a microscopy of that suspension [42] showing rod-shaped cisplatin crystals forming precipitate clumps (diameter 30×50 μm, ×400).

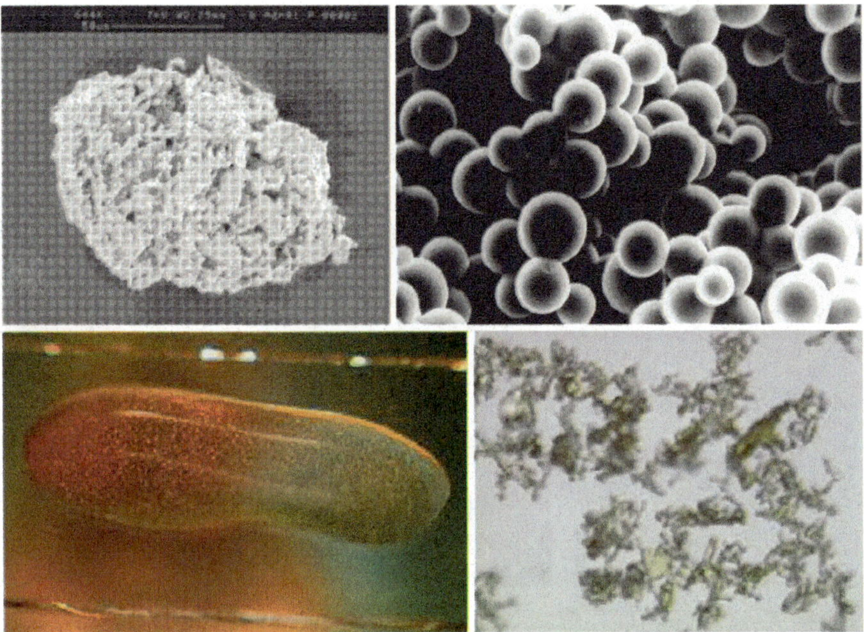

Fig. 7.13 Embolizing agents. *Top left*: Carboplatin microcapsule (diameter about 150 μm, ×644; [147]). *Top right*: Degradable starch microspheres (diameter 45 μm ×1,400, courtesy PharmaCept GmbH Berlin). *Down left*: Drop (12×7 mm) of aqueous cisplatin suspension as described by Kovács [42]. *Down right*: Microscopy of same suspension showing rod-shaped cisplatin crystals forming precipitate clumps (diameter 30×50 μm, ×400)

As compared to monocomponent chemoembolization, the preparation of microcapsules is complicated and expensive. More than 900 % of wrapping material may be necessary in comparison to the antineoplastic agent; the patient's body is stressed with additional substances. Advantages are a good reproducibility of the product with a good control of the particle diameter and a pharmacologically adjusted time of the release of the drug. Other embolization agents such as polyvinyl alcohol and lipiodol or albumin must also be produced first, paid for, and procured and would cause regular uncontrolled necrosis when injected into the facial or lingual artery. Besides that, lipiodol and other viscous substances have little effect outside of the liver because of their viscosity.

7.3   Intra-arterial Chemoradiation in Head and Neck Cancers

Although not induction therapy, the combined use of intra-arterial chemotherapy and radiation should be considered. The idea of combining these two modalities is not new as can be imagined from the initial remarks on systemic chemoradiation. *The idea behind this approach was the presumed higher locoregional impact of this treatment combined with less toxicity.* Table 7.3 gives an overview on 25 years;

Table 7.3 List of reported clinical studies on intra-arterial chemoradiation in head and neck cancers in chronological order

Author(s)	Patients	Tumor entities	Chemotherapeutic drugs and doses application	Radiation, specifics	Results
Szepesi et al. [160]	66	Inoperable head and neck carcinomas	Bleomycin 15 mg/day up to cumulative dose 300 mg, methotrexate 25 mg up to cumulative dose 500 mg, leucovorin 3 mg; retrograde	60–65 Gy	OR 65 %
Scholz et al. [161]	99	134 carcinomas in maxillofacial area	Methotrexate 25 mg/day up to cumulative dose 500 mg, bleomycin 15 mg/day up to cumulative dose 300 mg for 3 w	99 patients irradiated (60 Gy)	OR 68 %, CR 26 %
Imai et al. [162]	26	Head and neck carcinomas	Cisplatin 50 mg/m^2, carboplatin 300 mg/m^2 q4w × 5; transfemoral superselective	60 Gy; 7 patients were operated on	OR 96 %, CR 50 %; no technical problems
Robbins et al. [163]	60	Inoperable head and neck carcinomas	Cisplatin 150 mg/m^2 + STS weekly × 4; transfemoral superselective	66–74 Gy	OR locally and neck 98 %
Kerber et al. [64]	85	Stages III and IV unresectable head and neck carcinomas	Cisplatin 150–200 mg/m^2 + STS weekly × 4; transfemoral superselective	68–74 Gy	One death, six strokes
Oya and Ikemura [164]	15	Oral cavity and oropharyngeal carcinomas stages III and IV	Carboplatin 350 mg/m^2, tegafur 400–600 mg/day (orally); transfemoral superselective	30 Gy; surgery in case of positive biopsy	CR 92 % locally; Leuko-/thrombopenias grade 3–4 53 % and 27 %, respectively, local swelling (33 %)
Fuwa et al. [165]	32	Oral cavity and maxillary sinus carcinomas stages II to IV	Carboplatin 10–20 mg/m^2/day up to cumulative dose 360–500 mg/m^2; retrograde	50–60 Gy	OR 97 %; 3-year survival probability 63 % after median observation time of 3 years
Robbins et al. [166]	213	Surgically or functionally unresectable stages III and IV head and neck cancers	Cisplatin 150 mg/m^2 + STS weekly × 4; transfemoral superselective	68–72 Gy/36–37 fractions/7 w	Local control rate 80 %, regional control rate 61 %, 5-year overall survival 39 %, 5-year local control rate 74 %; treatment-related deaths 3 %

(continued)

Table 7.3 (continued)

Author(s)	Patients	Tumor entities	Chemotherapeutic drugs and doses application	Radiation, specifics	Results
Regine et al. [167]	42	Advanced head and neck carcinomas	Cisplatin 150 mg/m^2 + STS × 2; transfemoral superselective	hyperfractionated radiation (77–82 Gy)	OR 85–88 % locally and neck; 2-year survival probability 57 % after median observation time of 30 months
Balm et al. [168]	79	Unresectable stage IV head and neck cancers	Cisplatin 150 mg/m^2 + STS weekly × 4; transfemoral superselective	70 Gy/35 fractions/7 w	Local control rate 91 %, regional control rate 90 %, 3-year overall survival 43 %, 2-year local control rate 69 %; treatment-related deaths 4 %, PEG necessary 18 %
Homma et al. [169]	43	Resectable and unresectable stages III and IV head and neck carcinomas	Cisplatin 100–120 mg/m^2 + STS weekly × 4; transfemoral superselective	65 Gy/26 fractions/6.5 w	Local control rate 42 %, regional control rate 68 %, 3-year overall survival 54 %, 3-year local control rate 69 %; no treatment-related deaths, 81 % local toxicity
Robbins et al. [170]	67	T4 carcinomas of the oral cavity, oropharynx, hypopharynx, or larynx	Cisplatin 150 mg/m^2 + STS weekly × 4; transfemoral superselective	70 Gy/35 fractions/7 w	Multicenter trial: method feasible; grade 4 and 5 toxicities 14–47 % and 0–4 %, respectively
Spring et al. [171]	24	Unresectable oropharyngeal carcinomas	Cisplatin 150 mg/m^2 + STS w5; transfemoral superselective	Hyperfractionated radiation (77–82 Gy/7 w)	CR locally and neck 88 %; 5-year overall survival 33 %; 58 % of patients with feeding tube in first year
Fuwa et al. [141]	48	134 stage III and IV oral cavity carcinomas	Cisplatin 20–40 mg/m^2 + STS weekly × 4, continuous intravenous 5-fluorouracil 700 mg/m^2 day 1–5 + intravenous cisplatin 85 mg/m^2 over 24 h day 6; retrograde selective	66 Gy	3-year overall survival of all patients 53.9 %

W week, *H* hour, *OR* overall response, *CR* complete remission, *STS* sodium thiosulfate, *Gy* grays

again, the evolution to superselective multiple-shot administration of drugs is as evident as the diversity of treated tumor localizations.

Some trials used this kind of chemoradiation as induction before surgery [162, 164]; again, it cannot be said whether high response rates translate into longer survival time as compared to systemic chemoradiation. The most comprehensive trial sequence of intra-arterial chemoradiation was conducted by Robbins and coworkers [55, 56, 64, 163, 166, 170, 172]. They succeeded in accruing enough patients for valid statistical evaluation and maintained a consistent reproducible method. Results were impressive with regard to all possible end points, even in multicenter studies. Having started as treatment for unresectable patients, intra-arterial chemoradiation was developed as a regimen for organ preservation.

The long-awaited results of the prospective randomized comparison between systemic and intra-arterial chemoradiation carried out by the Netherlands Cancer Institute, however, could not prove a significant advantage of intra-arterial chemoradiation with respect to survival [173, 174]. Although significantly fewer problems with nausea and vomiting occurred in patients treated with intra-arterial chemoradiation [175], the interventional time and effort of intra-arterial chemotherapy as compared to the simple intravenous procedure seems to tip the scales in favor of intravenous chemoradiation. At the International Workshop on Intra-Arterial Chemotherapy for Head and Neck Cancer, August 20–22, 2006, Springfield, IL, procedural divergencies to the original Robbins method were accused to have lessened the impact of intra-arterial chemoradiation. The clinical investigations are still developing. Two interesting alternatives must be mentioned: the use of hyperfractionated radiation [167, 171] and systemic chemotherapy [141] together with intra-arterial chemotherapy. No final conclusion can be made at the moment. With respect to the high response rates, it has to be stressed that they are the result of both radiation and intra-arterial chemotherapy.

Many reports on Japanese trials with other intra-arterial drugs like carboplatin, nedaplatin, pirarubicin, or docetaxel in combination with radiation cannot be judged correctly in most cases due to the language barrier; however, it seems clear that Japan belongs to the countries with the highest experience with intra-arterial chemotherapy [176–182]. There are also variations of the prototypic Robbins method with reduced doses of cisplatin [183, 184]. The diversity of drugs makes an assessment of the methods nearly impossible; there is hope that Japanese investigators will be able to conduct a randomized trial concentrating on one method with respect to intra-arterial drug and dosage and one tumor localization (e.g., maxillary sinus cancer), so that a valid conclusion will be possible. They should also be able to gather large study populations necessary for valid statistics. First attempts to do so are on the way [185].

7.4 Treatment of Recurrent Cancers and Palliation of Head and Neck Cancers with Intra-arterial Chemotherapy

The scientific examination of cancers which have already been treated (recurrences) poses difficulties because of the usual diversity of pretreatment which makes the collection of comparable patient populations nearly impossible. Therefore, reports on intra-arterial chemotherapeutic treatment of recurrent cancers in the head and neck are rare and mixed with treatment of advanced unresectable primary disease [102, 186] or can be pooled with palliation treatment.

Palliation of head and neck cancer patients with intra-arterial chemotherapy must be mentioned because it proved to be extremely effective and useful in the treatment of incurable patients [186–191]. These reports on patient populations between 8 [191] and 64 [186] patients suffering from advanced inoperable primary or recurrent cancers of the head and neck demonstrated high overall response rates between 23 % [189] and 87 % [187] and complete response rates between 9 % [189] and 20 % [187]. In such patients with mainly pretreated recurrent disease, even to stabilize the disease must be counted as a success which is achieved in nearly all cases. Drugs used were methotrexate and bleomycin in the 1970s, mostly with continuous infusion over several days via retrograde approach, and carboplatin plus 5-fluorouracil with port systems and continuous infusion [188] or "two-route" chemotherapy (intra-arterial cisplatin with transfemoral approach and systemic sodium thiosulfate) [186, 191] in the 1990s. Toxicity was very low with this technique which gave the possibility of repeating administrations up to seven times.

The 55-year-old patient in Fig. 7.14 suffered from a cancer of the left maxillary sinus which was operated on but relapsed in the frontoorbital area and the anterior skull base. The aspect, smell, and bleeding of the tumor completely prevented the patient from arranging personal matters.

Three monthly repeated superselective interventions reduced the tumor to 17 % of its volume before commencing palliative treatment. The patient was able to lead a social life free from pain or discomfort.

After the fifth repetition, the tumor started to become refractory and the patient died 9 months after relapse.

In such way, the author could care for patients over several months, sometimes even several years, by administering several interventions in shorter or longer intervals, depending on the speed of progress. Already Donegan and Harris [187] noted that remission lasted for up to 13 months. These remarkably good results of palliation with the "two-route" chemotherapy were confirmed by Yokoyama [192] with repeated weekly administration (preservation of eye and larynx). Russian reports on chemoembolization using coils and gelatin sponges also concerned patients treated with palliative intention to reduce tumor bleeding [145, 148].

Intra-arterial chemotherapy used with palliative intent can be considered inductive when followed by additive treatment (most often radiation). Two clinical studies on patients with unresectable head and neck cancer [93, 103] have already been presented in the section on induction chemotherapy. Rohde et al. [186] from the Kovács group also added radiation in 33 of 64 incurable patients whose general physical condition was good enough. Kaplan–Meier analysis revealed 1-year survival rates of 41 % for patients with combined treatment and 21 % after intra-arterial chemotherapy alone ($P<0.05$) and 2-year survival of 25 % versus 14 %, respectively (nonsignificant).

It cannot be stressed enough that intra-arterial chemotherapy should be considered whenever possible in recurrent cancers already treated by surgery or radiation. For 10–20 % of patients, a long-lasting remission can be achieved.

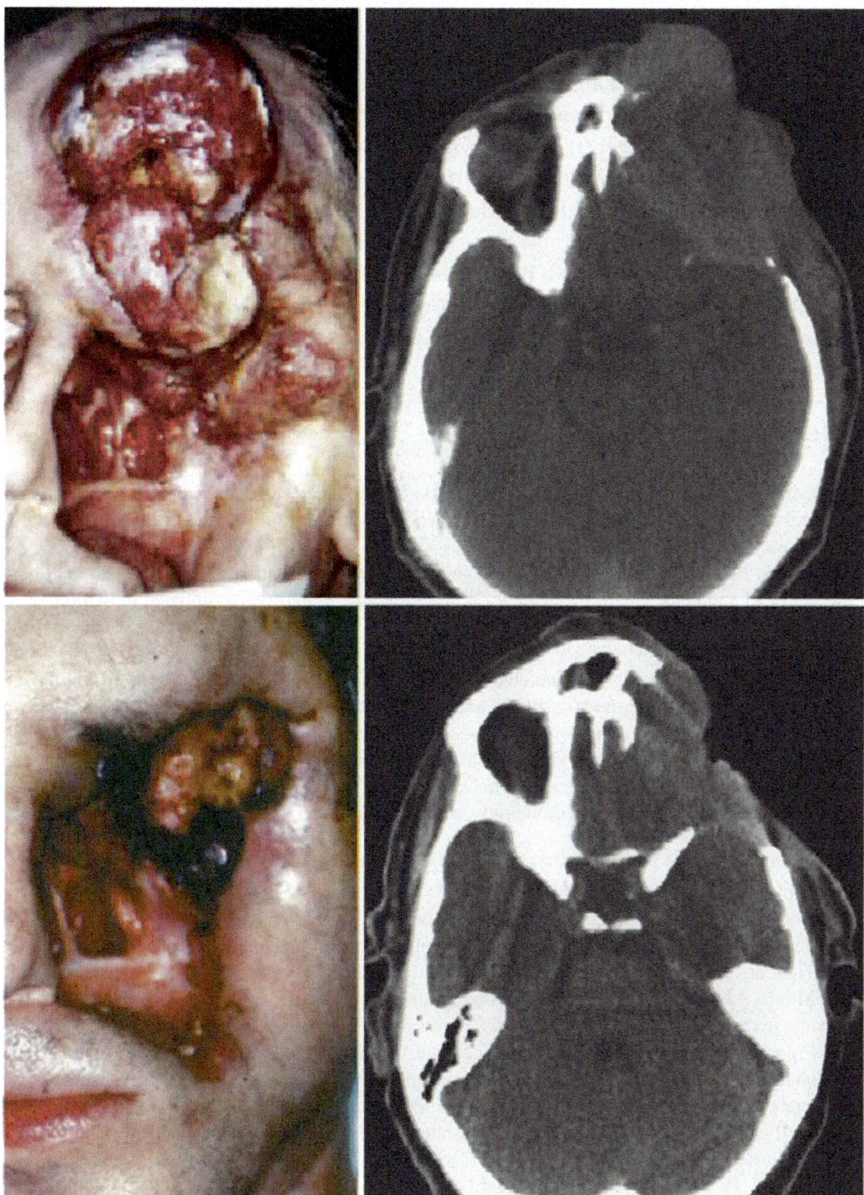

Fig. 7.14 *Top*: A 55-year-old patient suffering from a relapse of cancer of left maxillary sinus in frontoorbital area and anterior skull base. *Below*: Three monthly repeated super-selective interventions (150 mg/m² intra-arterial cisplatin) reduced tumor to 17 % of its volume

Conclusion

While systemic induction chemotherapy has proven an advantage in large trials for unresectable head and neck cancer and in case of larynx preservation, intra-arterial chemotherapy should have an even greater potential, but this has not yet been proven. However, it has known high merits in palliation of advanced and recurrent cancers but is used much too rarely, and available data indicate that it should now be considered for induction of resectable cancers of the oral cavity and anterior oropharynx. Intra-arterial chemoradiation is as effective as systemic chemoradiation and offers a better quality of life. As an important and carefully examined part in the armamentarium of anticancer tools, intra-arterial chemotherapy should be used in daily routine and considered for future trials.

References

1. German Cancer Society, Head-Neck-Tumors, Treatment [Deutsche Krebsgesellschaft, Kopf-Hals-Tumoren, Therapie 2009]. 2009. (http://www.krebsgesellschaft.de/pat_ka_kopf_hals_tumor_therapie,108203.html).
2. Pignon JP, Bourhis J, Domenge C, Designe L. Chemotherapy added to locoregional treatment for head and neck squamous-cell carcinoma: three meta-analyses of updated individual data. MACH-NC Collaborative Group. Meta-analysis of chemotherapy on head and neck cancer. Lancet. 2000;355:949–55.
3. Taylor 4th SG, Murthy AK, Vannetzel JM, Colin P, Dray M, Caldarelli DD, et al. Randomized comparison of neoadjuvant cisplatin and fluorouracil infusion followed by radiation versus concomitant treatment in advanced head and neck cancer. J Clin Oncol. 1994;12:385–95.
4. Bernier J, Cooper JS, Pajak TF, van Glabbeke M, Bourhis J, Forastiere A, et al. Defining risk levels in locally advanced head and neck cancers: a comparative analysis of concurrent postoperative radiation plus chemotherapy trials of the EORTC (#22931) and RTOG (#9501). Head Neck. 2005;27:843–50.
5. Robbins KT. The evolving role of combined modality therapy in head and neck cancer. Arch Otolaryngol Head Neck Surg. 2000;126:265–9.
6. Domenge C, Hill C, Lefebvre JL, De Raucourt D, Rhein B, Wibault P, et al. Randomized trial of neoadjuvant chemotherapy in oropharyngeal carcinoma. French Groupe d'Etude des Tumeurs de la Tête et du Cou (GETTEC). Br J Cancer. 2000;83:1594–8.
7. Munro AJ. An overview of randomised controlled trials of adjuvant chemotherapy in head and neck cancer. Br J Cancer. 1995;71:83–91.
8. Pignon JP, le Maître A, Maillard E, Bourhis J, Collaborative Group MACH-NC. Meta-analysis of chemotherapy in head and neck cancer (MACH-NC): an update on 93 randomised trials and 17,346 patients. Radiother Oncol. 2009;92:4–14.
9. Stell PM, Rawson NS. Adjuvant chemotherapy in head and neck cancer. Br J Cancer. 1990;61:779–87.
10. Volling P, Schröder M, Eckel H, Ebeling O, Stennert E. Primäre Chemotherapie bei Mundhöhlen- und Tonsillenkarzinomen. Ergebnisse einer prospektiv randomisierten Studie [Results of a prospective randomized trial with induction chemotherapy for cancer of the oral cavity and tonsils]. HNO. 1999;47:899–906.
11. Laccourreye O, Veivers D, Hans S, Ménard M, Brasnu D, Laccourreye H. Chemotherapy alone with curative intent in patients with invasive squamous cell carcinoma of the pharyngo-larynx classified as T1-T4N0M0 complete clinical responders. Cancer. 2001;92:1504–11.
12. Kovács AF, Grüterich G, Wagner M. Long-term complete remission of oral cancer after antineoplastic chemotherapy as single treatment modality: role of local chemotherapy. J Chemother. 2002;14:95–101.

13. Weaver A, Fleming S, Vandenberg H, Drelichman A, Jacobs J, Kinzie J, et al. Cis-platinum and 5-fluorouracil as initial therapy in advanced epidermoid cancers of the head and neck. Head Neck Surg. 1982;4:370–3.
14. Dimery IW, Hong WK. Overview of combined modality therapies for head and neck cancer. J Natl Cancer Inst. 1993;85:95–111.
15. De Andres L, Brunet J, Lopez-Pousa A, Burgues J, Vega M, Tabernero JM, et al. Randomized trial of neoadjuvant cisplatin and fluorouracil versus carboplatin and fluorouracil in patients with stage IV-M0 head and neck cancer. J Clin Oncol. 1995;13:1493–500.
16. Jacobs C, Lyman G, Velez-Garcia E, Sridhar KS, Knight W, Hochster H, et al. A phase III randomized study comparing cisplatin and fluorouracil as single agents and in combination for advanced squamous cell carcinoma of the head and neck. J Clin Oncol. 1992;10:257–63.
17. Paccagnella A, Orlando A, Marchiori C, Zorat PL, Cavaniglia G, Sileni VC, et al. Phase III trial of initial chemotherapy in stage III or IV head and neck cancers: a study by the Gruppo di Studio sui Tumori della Testa e del Collo. J Natl Cancer Inst. 1994;86:265–72.
18. Thyss A, Schneider M, Santini J, Caldani C, Vallicioni J, Chauvel P, et al. Induction chemotherapy with cis-platinum and 5-fluorouracil for squamous cell carcinoma of the head and neck. Br J Cancer. 1986;54:755–60.
19. Wang HM, Wang CH, Chen JS, Chang HK, Kiu MC, Liaw CC, et al. Cisplatin and 5-fluorouracil as neoadjuvant chemotherapy: predicting response in head and neck squamous cell cancer. J Formos Med Assoc. 1995;94:87–94.
20. Clark JR, Busse PM, Norris Jr CM, Andersen JW, Dreyfuss AI, Rossi RM, et al. Induction chemotherapy with cisplatin, fluorouracil, and high-dose leucovorin for squamous cell carcinoma of the head and neck: long-term results. J Clin Oncol. 1997;15:3100–10.
21. El-Sayed S, Nelson N. Adjuvant and adjunctive chemotherapy in the management of squamous cell carcinoma of the head and neck region. A meta-analysis of prospective and randomized trials. J Clin Oncol. 1996;14:838–47.
22. Posner MR, Colevas AD, Tishler RB. The role of induction chemotherapy in the curative treatment of squamous cell cancer of the head and neck. Semin Oncol. 2000;27 Suppl 8:13–24.
23. Department of Veterans Affairs Laryngeal Cancer Study Group. Induction chemotherapy plus radiation compared with surgery plus radiation in patients with advanced laryngeal cancer. N Engl J Med. 1991;324:1685–90.
24. Calais G, Bardet E, Sire C, Alfonsi M, Bourhis J, Rhein B, et al. Radiotherapy with concomitant weekly docetaxel for stages III/IV oropharynx carcinoma. Results of the 98–02 GORTEC Phase II trial. Int J Radiat Oncol Biol Phys. 2004;58:161–6.
25. Forastiere AA, Goepfert H, Maor M, Pajak TF, Weber R, Morrison W, et al. Concurrent chemotherapy and radiotherapy for organ preservation in advanced laryngeal cancer. N Engl J Med. 2003;349:2091–8.
26. Bourhis J, Lapeyre M, Tortochaux J, Rives M, Aghili M, Bourdin S, et al. Phase III randomized trial of very accelerated radiation therapy compared with conventional radiation therapy in squamous cell head and neck cancer: a GORTEC trial. J Clin Oncol. 2006;24:2873–8.
27. Urba SG, Forastiere AA, Wolf GT, Esclamado RM, McLaughlin PW, Thornton AF. Intensive induction chemotherapy and radiation for organ preservation in patients with advanced resectable head and neck carcinoma. J Clin Oncol. 1994;12:946–53.
28. Posner MR, Hershock DM, Blajman CR, Mickiewicz E, Winquist E, Gorbounova V, et al. Cisplatin and fluorouracil alone or with docetaxel in head and neck cancer. N Engl J Med. 2007;357:1705–15.
29. Lorch JH, Goloubeva O, Haddad RI, Cullen K, Sarlis N, Tishler R, et al. Induction chemotherapy with cisplatin and fluorouracil alone or in combination with docetaxel in locally advanced squamous-cell cancer of the head and neck: long-term results of the TAX 324 randomised phase 3 trial. Lancet Oncol. 2011;12:153–9.
30. Posner MR, Norris CM, Wirth LJ, Shin DM, Cullen KJ, Winquist EW, et al. Sequential therapy for the locally advanced larynx and hypopharynx cancer subgroup in TAX 324: survival, surgery, and organ preservation. Ann Oncol. 2009;20:921–7.

31. Ghi MG, Paccagnella A, D'Amanzo P, Mione CA, Fasan S, Paro S, et al. Neoadjuvant docetaxel, cisplatin, 5-fluorouracil before concurrent chemoradiotherapy in locally advanced squamous cell carcinoma of the head and neck versus concomitant chemoradiotherapy: a phase II feasibility study. Int J Radiat Oncol Biol Phys. 2004;59:481–7.
32. Vermorken JB, Remenar E, van Herpen C, Gorlia T, Mesia R, Degardin M, et al. Cisplatin, fluorouracil, and docetaxel in unresectable head and neck cancer. N Engl J Med. 2007;357:1695–704.
33. Kovács AF, Eberlein K, Hülsmann T. Organ preservation treatment using TPF-a pilot study in patients with advanced primary and recurrent cancer of the oral cavity and the maxillary sinus. Oral Maxillofac Surg. 2009;13:87–93.
34. Baghi M, Hambek M, Wagenblast J, May A, Gstoettner W, Knecht R. A phase II trial of docetaxel, cisplatin and 5-fluorouracil in patients with recurrent squamous cell carcinoma of the head and neck (SCCHN). Anticancer Res. 2006;26:585–90.
35. Rapidis AD, Trichas M, Stavrinidis E, Roupakia A, Ioannidou G, Kritselis G, et al. Induction chemotherapy followed by concurrent chemoradiation in advanced squamous cell carcinoma of the head and neck: final results from a phase II study with docetaxel, cisplatin and 5-fluorouracil with a four-year follow-up. Oral Oncol. 2006;42:675–84.
36. Hitt R, Grau JJ, López-Pousa A, Berrocal A, García-Girón C, Irigoyen A, Spanish Head and Neck Cancer Cooperative Group (TTCC), et al. A randomized phase III trial comparing induction chemotherapy followed by chemoradiotherapy versus chemoradiotherapy alone as treatment of unresectable head and neck cancer. Ann Oncol. 2014;25:216–25.
37. Posner M, Vermorken JB. Induction therapy in the modern era of combined-modality therapy for locally advanced head and neck cancer. Semin Oncol. 2008;35:221–8.
38. Vermorken JB, Mesia R, Rivera F, Remenar E, Kawecki A, Rottey S, et al. Platinum-based chemotherapy plus cetuximab in head and neck cancer. N Engl J Med. 2008;359:1116–27.
39. Posner MR, Lorch JH, Goloubeva O, Tan M, Schumaker LM, Sarlis NJ, et al. Survival and human papillomavirus in oropharynx cancer in TAX 324: a subset analysis from an international phase III trial. Ann Oncol. 2011;22:1071–7.
40. Klopp CT, Alford TC, Bateman J, Berry GN, Winship T. Fractionated intra-arterial cancer chemotherapy with methyl bis amine hydrochloride: a preliminary report. Ann Surg. 1950;132:811–32.
41. Sullivan RD, Jones R, Schnabel TG, Shorey J. The treatment of human cancer with intraarterial nitrogen mustard utilizing a simplified catheter technique. Cancer. 1953;6:121–4.
42. Kovács AF. Mundhöhlen- und Oropharynxkarzinome: neue Mittel und Wege der Therapie. Norderstedt: Books on demand; 2003.
43. Eckardt A, Kelber A. Palliative, intraarterial chemotherapy for advanced head and neck cancer using an implantable port system. J Oral Maxillofac Surg. 1994;52:1243–6.
44. Mees K, Lauterjung L, Kastenbauer E, Riederer A. Unsere Katheterführung zur intraarteriellen Chemotherapie bei Kopf- und Hals-Karzinomen [Personal catheter technic for intraarterial chemotherapy in cancers of the head and neck]. Laryngol Rhinol Otol (Stuttg). 1987;66:460–4.
45. Bitter K. Erste Ergebnisse der zytostatischen Behandlung von Plattenepithelkarzinomen der Mundhöhle mit einer Kombination von Methotrexat und Bleomycin [Initial results of cytostatic therapy of squamous cell carcinoma of the oral cavity using a combination of methotrexate and bleomycin]. Dtsch Zahn Mund Kieferheilkd. 1973;60:81–93.
46. Bitter K. Pharmacokinetic behaviour of bleomycin-cobalt-57 with special regard to intraarterial perfusion of the maxillo-facial region. J Maxillofac Surg. 1976;4:226–31.
47. Eckardt A, editor. Intra-arterial chemotherapy in head and neck cancer – current results and future perspectives. Reinbek: Einhorn-Presse Verlag; 1999.
48. Harker GJS, Stephens FO. Comparison of intra-arterial versus intravenous 5-fluorouracil in sheep bearing epidermal squamous carcinoma. Eur J Cancer. 1992;28:1437–41.
49. Harker GJS. Intra-arterial infusion chemotherapy in a sheep squamous cell carcinoma model. In: Eckardt A, editor. Intra-arterial chemotherapy in head and neck cancer – current results and future perspectives. Reinbek: Einhorn-Presse Verlag; 1999.

50. Eckman WW, Patlack CS, Fenstermacher JD. A critical evaluation of the principles governing the advantages of intra-arterial infusions. J Pharmacokinet Biopharm. 1974;2:257–85.
51. Campbell TN, Howell SB, Pfeifle CE, Wung WE, Bookstein J. Clinical pharmacokinetics of intraarterial cisplatin in humans. J Clin Oncol. 1983;1:755–62.
52. Weiss M. Pharmacokinetic rationale for arterial drug infusion. In: Eckardt A, editor. Intra-arterial chemotherapy in head and neck cancer – current results and future perspectives. Reinbek: Einhorn-Presse Verlag; 1999.
53. Collins JM. Pharmacologic rationale for regional drug delivery. J Clin Oncol. 1984;2:498–504.
54. Abe R, Akiyoshi T, Koba F, Tsuji H, Baba T. 'Two-route chemotherapy' using intra-arterial cisplatin and intravenous sodium thiosulfate, its neutralizing agent, for hepatic malignancies. Eur J Cancer Clin Oncol. 1988;24:1671–4.
55. Robbins KT, Storniolo AM, Kerber C, Seagren S, Berson A, Howell SB. Rapid superselective high-dose cisplatin infusion for advanced head and neck malignancies. Head Neck. 1992;14:364–71.
56. Robbins KT, Storniolo AM, Kerber C, Vicario D, Seagren S, Shea M, et al. Phase I study of highly selective supradose cisplatin infusions for advanced head and neck cancer. J Clin Oncol. 1994;12:2113–20.
57. Teicher BA, Holden SA, Kelley MJ, Shea TC, Cucchi CA, Rosowsky A, et al. Characterization of a human squamous carcinoma cell line resistant to cisdiamminedichloroplatinum(II). Cancer Res. 1987;47:388–93.
58. Los G, Blommaert FA, Barton R, Heath DD, den Engelse L, Hanchett C, et al. Selective intra-arterial infusion of high-dose cisplatin in patients with advanced head and neck cancer results in high tumor platinum concentrations and cisplatin-DNA adduct formation. Cancer Chemother Pharmacol. 1995;37:150–4.
59. Robbins KT, Storniolo AM, Hryniuk WM, Howell SB. "Decadose" effects of cisplatin on squamous cell carcinoma of the upper aerodigestive tract. II. Clinical studies. Laryngoscope. 1996;106:37–42.
60. Shea M, Koziol JA, Howell SB. Kinetics of sodium thiosulfate, a cisplatin neutralizer. Clin Pharmacol Ther. 1984;35:419–25.
61. Goel R, Cleary SM, Horton C, Kirmani S, Abramson I, Kelly C, et al. Effect of sodium thiosulfate on the pharmacokinetics and toxicity of cisplatin. J Natl Cancer Inst. 1989;81:1552–60.
62. Pfeifle CE, Howell SB, Felthouse RD, Woliver TB, Andrews PA, Markman M, et al. High-dose cisplatin with sodium thiosulfate protection. J Clin Oncol. 1985;3:237–44.
63. Muldoon LL, Pagel MA, Kroll RA, Brummett RE, Doolittle ND, Zuhowski EG, et al. Delayed administration of sodium thiosulfate in animal models reduces platinum ototoxicity without reduction of antitumor activity. Clin Cancer Res. 2000;6:309–15.
64. Kerber CW, Wong WH, Howell SB, Hanchett K, Robbins KT. An organ-preserving selective arterial chemotherapy strategy for head and neck cancer. AJNR Am J Neuroradiol. 1998;19:935–41.
65. Kato T, Sato K, Sasaki R, Kakinuma H, Moriyama M. Targeted cancer chemotherapy with arterial microcapsule chemoembolization: review of 1013 patients. Cancer Chemother Pharmacol. 1996;37:289–96.
66. Araki T, Hihara T, Kachi K, Matsusako M, Ito M, Kohno K, et al. Newly developed transarterial chemoembolization material: CDDP-lipiodol suspension. Gastrointest Radiol. 1989;14:46–8.
67. Brassel F. Technical aspects of superselective chemotherapy in head and neck cancer. In: Eckardt A, editor. Intra-arterial chemotherapy in head and neck cancer – current results and future perspectives. Reinbek: Einhorn-Presse Verlag; 1999.
68. Okamoto Y, Konno A, Togawa K, Kato T, Amano Y. Microcapsule chemoembolization for head and neck cancer. Arch Otorhinolaryngol. 1985;242:105–11.
69. Okamoto Y, Konno A, Togawa K, Kato T, Tamakawa Y, Amano Y. Arterial chemoembolization with cisplatin microcapsules. Br J Cancer. 1986;53:369–75.

70. Gouyette A, Apchin A, Foka M, Richard JM. Pharmacokinetics of intra-arterial and intravenous cisplatin in head and neck cancer patients. Eur J Cancer Clin Oncol. 1986;22:257–63.

71. Sileni VC, Fosser V, Maggian P, Padula E, Beltrame M, Nicolini M, et al. Pharmacokinetics and tumor concentration of intraarterial and intravenous cisplatin in patients with head and neck squamous cancer. Cancer Chemother Pharmacol. 1992;30:221–5.

72. Jakowatz JG, Ginn GE, Snyder LM, Dieffenbach KW, Wile AG. Increased cisplatin tissue levels with prolonged arterial infusion in the rat. Cancer. 1991;67:2828–32.

73. Tohnai I, Fuwa N, Hayashi Y, Kaneko R, Tomaru Y, Hibino Y, et al. New superselective intra-arterial infusion via superficial temporal artery for cancer of the tongue and tumour tissue platinum concentration after carboplatin (CBDCA) infusion. Oral Oncol. 1998;34:387–90.

74. Yoshimura H, Mishima K, Nariai Y, Sugihara M, Yoshimura Y. Targetting intraarterial infusion chemotherapy for oral cancers using Seldinger technique. In: Varma AK, Roodenburg JLN, editors. Oral oncology, vol. VII. New Delhi: Macmillan India; 2001.

75. Tegeder I, Bräutigam L, Seegel M, Al-Dam A, Turowski B, Geisslinger G, et al. Cisplatin tumor concentrations after intra-arterial cisplatin infusion or embolization in patients with oral cancer. Clin Pharmacol Ther. 2003;73:417–26.

76. Iida E, Okada M, Mita T, Furukawa M, Ito K, Matsunaga N. Superselective intra-arterial chemotherapy for advanced maxillary sinus cancer: an evaluation of arterial perfusion with computed tomographic arteriography and of tumor response. J Comput Assist Tomogr. 2008;32:397–402.

77. Ishii A, Korogi Y, Nishimura R, Kawanaka K, Yamura M, Ikushima I, et al. Intraarterial infusion chemotherapy for head and neck cancers: evaluation of tumor perfusion with intraarterial CT during carotid arteriography. Radiat Med. 2004;22:254–9.

78. Alexiou C, Jurgons R, Schmid RJ, Bergemann C, Henke J, Erhardt W, et al. Magnetic drug targeting-biodistribution of the magnetic carrier and the chemotherapeutic agent mitoxantrone after locoregional cancer treatment. J Drug Target. 2003;11:139–49.

79. Alexiou C, Jurgons R, Seliger C, Brunke O, Iro H, Odenbach S. Delivery of superparamagnetic nanoparticles for local chemotherapy after intraarterial infusion and magnetic drug targeting. Anticancer Res. 2007;27:2019–22.

80. Jaulerry C, Rodriguez J, Brunin F, Jouve M, Mosseri V, Point D, et al. Induction chemotherapy in advanced head and neck tumors: results of two randomised trials. Int J Radiat Oncol Biol Phys. 1992;23:483–9.

81. Forastiere AA, Baker SR, Wheeler R, Medvec BR. Intra-arterial cisplatin and FUDR in advanced malignancies confined to the head and neck. J Clin Oncol. 1987;5:1601–6.

82. Kovács AF, Döbert N, Engels K. The effect of intraarterial high-dose cisplatin on lymph nodes in oral and oropharyngeal cancer. Indian J Cancer. 2012;49:230–5.

83. Yokoyama J, Ohba S, Ito S, Fujimaki M, Shimoji K, Kojima M, et al. Impact of lymphatic chemotherapy targeting metastatic lymph nodes in patients with tongue cancer (cT3N2bM0) using intra-arterial chemotherapy. Head Neck Oncol. 2012;4:64.

84. Kovács AF. Relevance of positive margins in case of adjuvant therapy of oral cancer. Int J Oral Maxillofac Surg. 2004;33:447–53.

85. Stephens FO. Intra-arterial chemotherapy in head and neck cancer. Historical perspectives – important developments, contributors and contributions. In: Eckardt A, editor. Intra-arterial chemotherapy in head and neck cancer – current results and future perspectives. Reinbek: Einhorn-Presse Verlag; 1999.

86. Ervin TJ, Clark JR, Weichselbaum RR, Fallon BG, Miller D, Fabian RL, et al. An analysis of induction and adjuvant chemotherapy in the multidisciplinary treatment of squamous-cell carcinoma of the head and neck. J Clin Oncol. 1987;5:10–20.

87. Frei E, Clark JR, Fallon BG. Guidelines, regulations and clinical research. J Clin Oncol. 1986;4:1026–30.

88. Volling P, Schröder M. Vorläufige Ergebnisse einer prospektiv randomisierten Studie zur primären Chemotherapie bei Mundhöhlen- und Pharynxkarzinomen [Preliminary results of a prospective randomized study of primary chemotherapy in carcinoma of the oral cavity and pharynx]. HNO. 1995;43:58–64.

89. Baghi M, Mack MG, Hambek M, Bisdas S, Muerthel R, Wagenblast J, et al. Usefulness of MRI volumetric evaluation in patients with squamous cell cancer of the head and neck treated with neoadjuvant chemotherapy. Head Neck. 2007;29:104–8.
90. Kovács AF, Turowski B, Stefenelli U, Metzler D. Primary tumor volume as predicitive parameter for remission after intraarterial high-dose cisplatin in oral and oropharyngeal cancer: a mathematical model analysis. Chir Czaszkowo Szczękowo Twarzowa I Ortop Szczękowa Cranio Maxillofac Surg Orthodont. 2008;3:174–86.
91. Baker SR, Wheeler RH. Intraarterial chemotherapy for head and neck cancer: part I. Theoretical considerations and drug delivery systems. Head Neck Surg. 1983;6:664–82.
92. Cruz Jr AB, McInnis WD, Aust JB. Triple drug intra-arterial infusion combined with x-ray therapy and surgery for head and neck cancer. Am J Surg. 1974;128:573–9.
93. Armstrong AL, Meeker WR. Palliation of inoperable head and neck cancer: combined intra-arterial infusion chemotherapy and irradiation. South Med J. 1978;71:1228–31.
94. Curioni C, Quadu G. Clinical trial of intra-arterial polychemotherapy in the treatment of carcinoma of the oral cavity. J Maxillofac Surg. 1978;6:207–16.
95. Szabó G, Kovács Á. Possibilities of enhancing the effectiveness of intra-arterial chemotherapy. Int J Oral Surg. 1980;9:33–44.
96. Koch U, Straehler-Pohl HJ, Helpap B, Frommhold H. Intraarterielle Chemotherapie bei Karzinomen der oberen Speisewege (Erfahrungsbericht über 128 Patienten) [Intraarterial chemotherapy in carcinomas of the oral cavity, oro- and hypopharynx]. Laryngol Rhinol Otol (Stuttg). 1981;60:71–6.
97. Mika H. Die Remission ausgedehnter Karzinome der Mundhöhle und des Oropharynx unter intraarterieller Polychemotherapie mit Vincristin, Methotrexat, Bleomycin, Cisplatin (VMBP) [The remission of extensive cancers of the mouth and oropharynx with intra-arterial polychemotherapy with vincristine, methotrexate, bleomycin, cisplatin (VMBP)]. Laryngol Rhinol Otol (Stuttg). 1982;61:520–3.
98. Arcangeli G, Nervi C, Righini R, Creton G, Mirri MA, Guerra A. Combined radiation and drugs: the effect of intra-arterial chemotherapy followed by radiotherapy in head and neck cancer. Radiother Oncol. 1983;1:101–7.
99. Molinari R, Jortay A, Sancho-Garnier H, Brugere J, Demard M, Desaulty A, et al. A randomized EORTC trial comparing intra-arterial infusion with methotrexate vs bleomycin as initial therapy in carcinoma of the oral cavity. Eur J Cancer Clin Oncol. 1982;18:807–12.
100. Galmarini FC, Yoel J, Nakasone J, Molina CM. Intraarterial association of cis-platinum and bleomycin in head and neck cancer. Auris Nasus Larynx. 1985;12 Suppl 2:S234–8.
101. Milazzo J, Mohit-Tabatabai MA, Hill GJ, Raina S, Swaminathan A, Cheung NK, et al. Preoperative intra-arterial infusion chemotherapy for advanced squamous cell carcinoma of the mouth and oropharynx. Cancer. 1985;56:1014–7.
102. Inuyama Y, Fujii M, Tanaka J, Takaoka T, Hosoda H, Kohno N, et al. Combination chemotherapy with cisplatin and peplomycin in squamous cell carcinoma of the head and neck. Auris Nasus Larynx. 1986;13:191–8.
103. Mortimer JE, Taylor ME, Schulman S, Cummings C, Weymuller Jr E, Laramore G. Feasibility and efficacy of weekly intraarterial cisplatin in locally advanced (stage III and IV) head and neck cancers. J Clin Oncol. 1988;6:969–75.
104. Cheung DK, Regan J, Savin M, Gibberman V, Woessner W. A pilot study of intraarterial chemotherapy with cisplatin in locally advanced head and neck cancers. Cancer. 1988;61:903–8.
105. Lee YY, Dimery IW, Van Tassel P, De Pena C, Blacklock JB, Goepfert H. Superselective intra-arterial chemotherapy of advanced paranasal sinus tumors. Arch Otolaryngol Head Neck Surg. 1989;115:503–11.
106. Claudio F, Cacace F, Comella G, Coucourde F, Claudio L, Bevilacqua AM, et al. Intraarterial chemotherapy through carotid transposition in advanced head and neck cancer. Cancer. 1990;65:1465–71.
107. Frustaci S, Barzan L, Caruso G, Ghirardo R, Foladore S, Carbone A, et al. Induction intra-arterial cisplatin and bleomycin in head and neck cancer. Head Neck. 1991;13:291–7.

108. Richard JM, Kramar A, Molinari R, Lefèbvre JL, Blanchet F, Jortay A, et al. Randomised EORTC head and neck cooperative group trial of preoperative intra-arterial chemotherapy in oral cavity and oropharynx carcinoma. Eur J Cancer. 1991;27:821–7.
109. Vieitez JM, Bilbao JI, Hidalgo OF, Martin S, Manzano RG, Tangco E. Intra-arterial chemotherapy with carboplatin and 5-fluorouracil in epidermoid cancer of the oropharynx and oral cavity. Reg Cancer Treat. 1991;4:152–5.
110. Hirai T, Korogi Y, Hamatake S, Nishimura R, Baba Y, Takahashi M, et al. Stages III and IV squamous cell carcinoma of the mouth: three-year experience with superselective intraarterial chemotherapy using cisplatin prior to definitive treatment. Cardiovasc Intervent Radiol. 1999;22:201–5.
111. Korogi Y, Hirai T, Nishimura R, Hamatake S, Sakamoto Y, Murakami R, et al. Superselective intraarterial infusion of cisplatin for squamous cell carcinoma of the mouth: preliminary clinical experience. Am J Roentgenol. 1995;165:1269–72.
112. Scheel JV, Schilling V, Kastenbauer E, Knöbber D, Böhringer W. Cisplatin intraarteriell und sequentielle Bestrahlung. Langzeitergebnisse [Intra-arterial cisplatin and sequential radiotherapy. Long-term follow-up]. Laryngorhinootologie. 1996;75:38–42.
113. Siegel RS, Bank WO, Maung CC, Harisiadis L, Wilson WR. Assessment of efficacy and tolerance of high-dose intra-arterial cisplatin in advanced head and neck tumors. Proc Am Soc Clin Oncol 1998;17 (Abstract 1582).
114. Wilson WR, Siegel RS, Harisiadis LA, Davis DO, Nguyen HH, Bank WO. High-dose intra-arterial cisplatin therapy followed by radiation therapy for advanced squamous cell carcinoma of the head and neck. Arch Otolaryngol Head Neck Surg. 2001;127:809–12.
115. Kovács AF, Turowski B, Ghahremani TM, Loitz M. Intraarterial chemotherapy as neoadjuvant treatment of oral cancer. J Craniomaxillofac Surg. 1999;27:302–7.
116. Szabó G, Kreidler J, Hollmann K, Kovács Á, Németh G, Németh Z, et al. Intra-arterial preoperative cytostatic treatment versus preoperative irradiation: a prospective, randomized study of lingual and sublingual carcinomas. Cancer. 1999;86:1381–6.
117. Benazzo M, Caracciolo G, Zappoli F, Bernardo G, Mira E. Induction chemotherapy by superselective intra-arterial high-dose carboplatin infusion for head and neck cancer. Eur Arch Otorhinolaryngol. 2000;257:279–82.
118. Bertino G, Benazzo M, Gatti P, Bernardo G, Corbella F, Tinelli C, et al. Curative and organ-preserving treatment with intra-arterial carboplatin induction followed by surgery and/or radiotherapy for advanced head and neck cancer: single-center five-year results. BMC Cancer. 2007;7:62.
119. Kovács AF. Intra-arterial induction high-dose chemotherapy with cisplatin for oral and oropharyngeal cancer: long-term results. Br J Cancer. 2004;90:1323–8.
120. Kovács AF, Obitz P, Wagner M. Monocomponent chemoembolization in oral and oropharyngeal cancer using an aqueous crystal suspension of cisplatin. Br J Cancer. 2002;86:196–202.
121. Damascelli B, Patelli GL, Lanocita R, Di Tolla G, Frigerio LF, Marchianò A, et al. A novel intraarterial chemotherapy using paclitaxel in albumin nanoparticles to treat advanced squamous cell carcinoma of the tongue: preliminary findings. AJR Am J Roentgenol. 2003;181:253–60.
122. Damascelli B, Patelli G, Tichá V, Di Tolla G, Frigerio LF, Garbagnati F, et al. Feasibility and efficacy of percutaneous transcatheter intraarterial chemotherapy with paclitaxel in albumin nanoparticles for advanced squamous-cell carcinoma of the oral cavity, oropharynx, and hypopharynx. J Vasc Interv Radiol. 2007;18:1395–403.
123. Kovács AF, Eberlein K, Smolarz A, Weidauer S, Rohde S. Organerhaltende Therapie bei inoperablen Patienten mit primären Mundhöhlen- und Oropharynxkarzinomen. Möglichkeiten und Grenzen [Organ-preserving treatment in inoperable patients with primary oral and oropharyngeal carcinoma: chances and limitations]. Mund Kiefer Gesichtschir. 2006;10:168–77.
124. Nagai H, Takamaru N, Ohe G, Uchida D, Tamatani T, Fujisawa K, et al. Evaluation of combination chemotherapy with oral S-1 administration followed by docetaxel by superselective

intra-arterial infusion for patients with oral squamous cell carcinomas. Gan To Kagaku Ryoho. 2011;38:777–81.

125. Molinari R, Chiesa F, Cantù G, Costa L, Grandi C, Sala L. Prognostic factors in cancer of the oral cavity and anterior oropharynx treated with preliminary neoadjuvant intra-arterial chemotherapy followed by surgery. In: Eckardt A, editor. Intra-arterial chemotherapy in head and neck cancer – current results and future perspectives. Reinbek: Einhorn-Presse Verlag; 1999.

126. Frustaci S, Barzan L, Comoretto R, Tumolo S, Lo Re G, Monfardini S. Local neurotoxicity after intra-arterial cisplatin in head and neck cancer. Cancer Treat Rep. 1987;71:257–9.

127. Andersson T, Andreasson L, Björklund A, Brismar J, Elner A, Eneroth CM, et al. Intra-arterial chemotherapy of malignant head and neck tumours with superselective angiographic technique. Acta Otolaryngol Suppl. 1979;360:167–70.

128. Kovács AF. Chemoembolization using cisplatin crystals as neoadjuvant treatment of oral cancer. Cancer Biother Radiopharm. 2005;20:267–79.

129. Kovács AF. Intraarterial chemotherapy and chemoembolization in head and neck cancer. Establishment as a neoadjuvant routine method. Cancer Ther. 2003;1:1–9.

130. Kovács AF, Turowski B. Chemoembolization of oral and oropharyngeal cancer using a high-dose cisplatin crystal suspension and degradable starch microspheres. Oral Oncol. 2002;38:87–95.

131. Kovács AF. Maximized combined modality treatment of an unselected population of oral and oropharyngeal cancer patients. Final results of a pilot study compared with a treatment-dependent prognosis index. J Craniomaxillofac Surg. 2006;34:74–84.

132. Kovács AF, Schiemann M, Turowski B. Combined modality treatment of oral and oropharyngeal cancer including neoadjuvant intraarterial cisplatin and radical surgery followed by concurrent radiation and chemotherapy with weekly docetaxel – three year results of a pilot study. J Craniomaxillofac Surg. 2002;30:112–20.

133. Kovács AF, Mose S, Böttcher HD, Bitter K. Multimodality treatment including postoperative radiation and concurrent chemotherapy with weekly docetaxel is feasible and effective in patients with oral and oropharyngeal cancer. Strahlenther Onkol. 2005;181:26–34.

134. Platz H, Fries R, Hudec M. Computer-aided individual prognoses of squamous cell carcinomas of the lips, oral cavity and oropharynx. Int J Oral Maxillofac Surg. 1992;21:150–5.

135. Kovács AF, Stefenelli U, Thorn G. Long-term quality of life after intensified multi-modality treatment of oral cancer including intra-arterial induction chemotherapy and adjuvant chemoradiation with docetaxel – a cross-sectional study. Ann Maxillofac Surg. 2015;5:26–31.

136. Kovács AF. Response to intraarterial induction chemotherapy: a prognostic parameter in oral and oropharyngeal cancer. Head Neck. 2006;28:678–88.

137. Kishi K, Matsunaka M, Sato M, Sonomura T, Sakurane M, Uede K. T1 and T2 lip cancer: a superselective method of facial arterial infusion therapy – preliminary experience. Radiology. 1999;213:173–9.

138. Nakasato T, Katoh K, Sone M, Ehara S, Tamakawa Y, Hoshi H, et al. Superselective continuous arterial infusion chemotherapy through the superficial temporal artery for oral cavity tumors. AJNR Am J Neuroradiol. 2000;21:1917–22.

139. Wu CF, Chen CM, Chen CH, Shieh TY, Sheen MC. Continuous intraarterial infusion chemotherapy for early lip cancer. Oral Oncol. 2007;43:825–30.

140. Wu CF, Chen CM, Shen YS, Huang IY, Chen CH, Chen CY, et al. Effective eradication of oral verrucous carcinoma with continuous intraarterial infusion chemotherapy. Head Neck. 2008;30:611–7.

141. Fuwa N, Kodaira T, Furutani K, Tachibana H, Nakamura T, Nakahara R, et al. Intra-arterial chemoradiotherapy for locally advanced oral cavity cancer: analysis of therapeutic results in 134 cases. Br J Cancer. 2008;98:1039–45.

142. Tomura N, Kobayashi M, Hirano J, Watarai J, Okamoto Y, Togawa K, et al. Chemoembolization of head and neck cancer with carboplatine microcapsules. Acta Radiol. 1996;37:52–6.

143. Tomura N, Kato K, Hirano H, Hirano Y, Watarai J. Chemoembolization of maxillary tumors via the superficial temporal artery using a coaxial catheter system. Radiat Med. 1998;16:157–60.

144. Li H, Wang C, Wen Y, Wu H. Treatment of squamous cell carcinoma of the tongue using arterial embolism with cisplatin-loaded albumin microspheres: a microstructural and ultrastructural investigation. Chin J Dent Res. 1999;2:61–6.
145. Suvorova IV, Tarazov PG, Korytova LI, Sokurenko VP, Khazova TV. Arterial chemoembolization in the combined treatment of malignant tumors of the tongue and maxilla: preliminary results. Vestn Rentgenol Radiol. 2002;2:23–8.
146. Li WZ, Ma ZB, Zhao T. Transcatheter arterial chemoembolization of oral squamous-cell carcinoma: a clinicopathological observation. Di Yi Jun Yi Da Xue Xue Bao. 2004;24:614–8.
147. He H, Huang J, Ping F, Chen G, Zhang S, Dong Y. Anatomical and clinical study of lingual arterial chemoembolization for tongue carcinoma. Oral Surg Oral Med Oral Pathol Oral Radiol Endod. 2007;103:e1–5.
148. Sokurenko VP, Korytova LI, Tarazov PG, Suvorova IV. Intra-arterial chemotherapy and chemoembolization in the combined treatment for locally advanced carcinoma of the head and neck. Vopr Onkol. 2008;54:625–30.
149. Konno A, Ishikawa K, Terada N, Numata T, Nagata H, Okamoto Y. Analysis of long-term results of our combination therapy for squamous cell cancer of the maxillary sinus. Acta Otolaryngol Suppl. 1998;537:57–66.
150. Song M, Chen FJ, Zeng ZY, Wu GH, Wei MW, Guo ZM, et al. Clinical value of inducing chemotherapy for patients with advanced tongue cancer. Ai Zheng. 2002;21:68–70.
151. He H, Ping F, Chen G, Zhang S. Chemoembolization of tongue carcinoma with ethylcellulose microcapsuled carboplatinum and its basic study. Artif Cells Blood Substit Immobil Biotechnol. 2008;36:114–22.
152. Milburn GHW, Truter MR. The crystal structures of cis- and trans-dichlorodiammineplatinum (II). Inorg Phys Theor J Chem Soc (A). 1966;11:1609–16.
153. Medac, editor. Professional information Medac Cisplatin Medac [in German. Hamburg: Medac; 2000.
154. McEvoy GK, editor. American hospital formulary service drug information, vol. 91. Bethesda: American Society of Hospital Pharmacists; 1991.
155. Greene RF, Chatterji DC, Hiranaka PK, Gallelli JF. Stability of cisplatin in aqueous solution. Am J Hosp Pharm. 1979;36:38–43.
156. Kristjansson F, Sternson LA, Lindenbaum S. An investigation on possible oligomer formation in pharmaceutical formulations of cisplatin. Int J Pharm. 1988;41:67–74.
157. Bastian P, Kissel T, Bartkowski R. Maligne Lebererkrankungen: Arterielle Chemo- und Embolisationstherapie mit Hilfe von Trägersystemen. PZ Prisma. 1999;6:235–48.
158. Damascelli B, Cantù G, Mattavelli F, Tamplenizza P, Bidoli P, Leo E, et al. Intraarterial chemotherapy with polyoxyethylated castor oil free paclitaxel, incorporated in albumin nanoparticles (ABI-007): phase II study of patients with squamous cell carcinoma of the head and neck and anal canal: preliminary evidence of clinical activity. Cancer. 2001;92:2592–602.
159. van Es RJ, Nijsen JF, Dullens HF, Kicken M, van der Bilt A, Hennink W, et al. Tumour embolization of the Vx2 rabbit head and neck cancer model with Dextran hydrogel and Holmium-poly(L-lactic acid) microspheres: a radionuclide and histological pilot study. J Craniomaxillofac Surg. 2001;29:289–97.
160. Szepesi T, Stadler B, Hohenberg G, Hollmann K, Kühböck J, Mailath G. Prognostische Faktoren bei der Behandlung inoperabler orofazialer Malignome mit simultaner Radio- und Chemotherapie [Prognostic factors in the treatment of inoperable orofacial tumors with simultaneous radiotherapy and intra-arterial chemotherapy]. Strahlentherapie. 1985;161:299–307.
161. Scholz F, Scholz R, Schratter A, Hollmann K. Intraarterielle Chemotherapie bei Tumoren im maxillo-facialen Bereich. In: Vinzenz K, Waclawiczek HW, editors. Chirurgische Therapie von Kopf-Hals-Karzinomen. New York: Springer; 1992.
162. Imai S, Kajihara Y, Munemori O, Kamei T, Mori T, Handa T, et al. Superselective cisplatin (CDDP)-carboplatin (CBDCA) combined infusion for head and neck cancers. Eur J Radiol. 1995;21:94–9.

163. Robbins KT, Kumar P, Regine WF, Wong FS, Weir 3rd AB, Flick P, et al. Efficacy of targeted supradose cisplatin and concomitant radiation therapy for advanced head and neck cancer: the Memphis experience. Int J Radiat Oncol Biol Phys. 1997;38:263–71.
164. Oya R, Ikemura K. Targeted intra-arterial carboplatin infusion with concurrent radiotherapy and administration of tegafur for advanced squamous cell carcinoma of the oral cavity and oropharynx. In: Eckardt A, editor. Intra-arterial chemotherapy in head and neck cancer – current results and future perspectives. Reinbek: Einhorn-Presse Verlag; 1999.
165. Fuwa N, Ito Y, Matsumoto A, Kamata M, Kodaira T, Furutani K, et al. A combination therapy of continuous superselective intraarterial carboplatin infusion and radiation therapy for locally advanced head and neck carcinoma. Phase I study. Cancer. 2000;89:2099–105.
166. Robbins KT, Kumar P, Wong FS, Hartsell WF, Flick P, Palmer R, et al. Targeted chemoradiation for advanced head and neck cancer: analysis of 213 patients. Head Neck. 2000;22:687–93.
167. Regine WF, Valentino J, Arnold SM, Haydon RC, Sloan D, Kenady D, et al. High-dose intra-arterial cisplatin boost with hyperfractionated radiation therapy for advanced squamous cell carcinoma of the head and neck. J Clin Oncol. 2001;19:3333–9.
168. Balm AJ, Rasch CR, Schornagel JH, Hilgers FJ, Keus RB, Schultze-Kool L, et al. High-dose superselective intra-arterial cisplatin and concomitant radiation (RADPLAT) for advanced head and neck cancer. Head Neck. 2004;26:485–93.
169. Homma A, Furuta Y, Suzuki F, Oridate N, Hatakeyama H, Nahahashi T, et al. Rapid superselective high-dose cisplatin infusion with concomitant radiotherapy for advanced head and neck cancer. Head Neck. 2005;27:65–71.
170. Robbins KT, Kumar P, Harris J, McCulloch T, Cmelak A, Sofferman R, et al. Supradose intra-arterial cisplatin and concurrent radiation therapy for the treatment of stage IV head and neck squamous cell carcinoma is feasible and efficacious in a multi-institutional setting: results of Radiation Therapy Oncology Group Trial 9615. J Clin Oncol. 2005;23:1447–54.
171. Spring PM, Valentino J, Arnold SM, Sloan D, Kenady D, Kudrimoti M, et al. Long-term results of hyperfractionated radiation and high-dose intraarterial cisplatin for unresectable oropharyngeal carcinoma. Cancer. 2005;104:1765–71.
172. Robbins KT, Vicario D, Seagren S, Weisman R, Pellitteri P, Kerber C, et al. A targeted supradose cisplatin chemoradiation protocol for advanced head and neck cancer. Am J Surg. 1994;168:419–22.
173. Rasch CRN, Hauptmann M, Schornagel J, Wijers O, Buter J, Gregor T, et al. Intra-arterial versus intravenous chemoradiation for advanced head and neck cancer: results of a randomized phase III trial. Cancer. 2010;116:2159–65.
174. Heukelom J, Lopez-Yurda M, Balm AJ, Wijers OB, Buter J, Gregor T, et al. Late follow-up of the randomized radiation and concomitant high-dose intra-arterial or intravenous cisplatin (RADPLAT) trial for advanced head and neck cancer. Head Neck. 2015. doi:10.1002/hed.24023.
175. Ackerstaff AH, Balm AJ, Rasch CR, de Boer JP, Wiggenraad R, Rietveld DH, et al. First-year quality of life assessment of an intra-arterial (RADPLAT) versus intravenous chemoradiation phase III trial. Head Neck. 2009;31:77–84.
176. Endo S, Suzuki S, Tsuji K, Niwa H, Noguchi Y, Yoshida K, et al. Intraarterial concomitant chemoradiation for tongue cancer: analysis of 20 patients. Nippon Jibiinkoka Gakkai Kaiho. 2005;108:689–93.
177. Iguchi H, Kusuki M, Nakamura A, Nishiura H, Kanazawa A, Takayama M, et al. Concurrent chemoradiotherapy with pirarubicin and 5-fluorouracil for resectable oral and maxillary carcinoma. Acta Otolaryngol Suppl. 2004;554:55–61.
178. Iguchi H, Kusuki M, Nakamura A, Kanazawa A, Hachiya K, Yamane H. Outcome of preoperative concurrent chemoradiotherapy and surgery for resectable lingual squamous cell carcinoma greater than 3 cm: the possibility of less extensive surgery. Oral Oncol. 2006;42:391–7.
179. Ishii A, Korogi Y, Hirai T, Nishimura R, Murakami R, Ikushima I, et al. Intraarterial infusion chemotherapy and conformal radiotherapy for cancer of the mouth: prediction of the histological response to therapy with magnetic resonance imaging. Acta Radiol. 2007;48:900–6.

180. Ito K, Shiba H, Fujiwara K, Kunimoto Y, Tanimoto S, Higami Y, et al. Superselective intra-arterial chemotherapy using low dose CBDCA and Pirarubicin with concurrent radiotherapy for head and neck cancer. Nippon Jibiinkoka Gakkai Kaiho. 2005;108:195–201.
181. Yamashita Y, Goto M, Katsuki T. Chemotherapy by superselective intraarterial infusion of nedaplatin combined with radiotherapy for oral cancer. Gan To Kagaku Ryoho. 2002;29:905–9.
182. Yamashita Y, Shikimori M, Goto M. Clinical trial of chemotherapy by superselective intra-arterial infusion of nedaplatin combined with radiotherapy for advanced oral cancer. Gan To Kagaku Ryoho. 2005;32:1267–71.
183. Homma A, Oridate N, Suzuki F, Taki S, Asano T, Yoshida D, et al. Superselective high-dose cisplatin infusion with concomitant radiotherapy in patients with advanced cancer of the nasal cavity and paranasal sinuses: a single institution experience. Cancer. 2009;115:4705–14.
184. Ikushima I, Korogi Y, Ishii A, Hirai T, Yamura M, Nishimura R, et al. Superselective intra-arterial infusion chemotherapy for stage III/IV squamous cell carcinomas of the oral cavity: midterm results. Eur J Radiol. 2008;66:7–12.
185. Homma A, Nakamura K, Matsuura K, Mizusawa J, Onimaru R, Fukuda H, et al. Dose-finding and efficacy confirmation trial of superselective intra-arterial infusion of cisplatin and concomitant radiotherapy for patients with locally advanced maxillary sinus cancer (JCOG1212, RADPLAT-MSC). Jpn J Clin Oncol. 2015;45(1):119–22. doi:10.1093/jjco/hyu169.
186. Rohde S, Kovács AF, Turowski B, Yan B, Zanella F, Berkefeld J. Intra-arterial high-dose chemotherapy with cisplatin as part of a palliative treatment concept in oral cancer. AJNR Am J Neuroradiol. 2005;26:1804–9.
187. Donegan WL, Harris P. Regional chemotherapy with combined drugs in cancer of the head and neck. Cancer. 1976;38:1479–83.
188. Eckardt A, Kelber A, Pytlik C. Palliative intra-arterial (i.a.) chemotherapy with carboplatin (CBDCA) and 5-FU in unresectable advanced (stage III and IV) head and neck cancer using implantable port-systems. Eur J Surg Oncol. 1995;21:486–9.
189. Huntington MC, DuPriest RW, Fletcher WS. Intra-arterial bleomycin therapy in inoperable squamous cell carcinomas. Cancer. 1973;31:153–8.
190. Matras H, Bürkle K, Watzek G, Kühböck J, Pötzi P, Dimopoulos J. Concept of cytostatic therapy in advanced tumours of the head and neck. J Maxillofac Surg. 1979;7:150–4.
191. Teymoortash A, Bien S, Dalchow C, Sesterhenn A, Lippert BM, Werner JA. Selective high-dose intra-arterial cisplatin as palliative treatment for incurable head and neck cancer. Onkologie. 2004;27:547–51.
192. Yokoyama J. Present role and future prospect of superselective intra-arterial infusion chemotherapy for head and neck cancer. Gan To Kagaku Ryoho. 2002;29:169–75.

Isolated Thoracic Perfusion with Carotid Artery Infusion for Advanced and Chemoresistant Tumors of the Parotid Gland and Tonsils

Karl Reinhard Aigner, Emir Selak, and Rita Schlaf

8.1 Introduction

Although only few patients with advanced cancers of the parotid gland and tonsils are described in this chapter, the results of the new approach in using regional chemotherapy have been so dramatic and encouraging that this limited experience is included in this book.

Regional chemotherapy has many facets and implies that the adequate mode of application is performed. Good results are jeopardized when intra-arterial infusions are performed after the vascular supply has been interrupted or extremely reduced by scars from prior surgery or connective tissue and vascular fibrosis from irradiation [1] or when the tumor had invaded tissues beyond the territory of selective or superselective catheterization.

The theoretical advantage of intra-arterial drug delivery is most evident [2, 3] clinically; it was investigated in numerous clinical studies [1, 4–11]. In the last two decades, chemoradiation gained a firm position in treatment protocols [12–15], and supradose intra-arterial cisplatin infusion achieves a fundamental improvement with regard to increased drug exposure. Actually, the best results in terms of local tumor control have been achieved when chemotherapy has been applied concomitantly with irradiation although there is increased risk of intensified damage to adjacent tissues. In extremely huge tumors, however, irradiation can hardly be applied, and chemotherapy alone is not efficient enough to induce substantial remission. Since in intra-arterial chemotherapy all of the advantages occur within the time of the first pass through the tumor bed, as once the drug is diluted in the venous drainage of the tumor area, subsequent tumor exposure of the recirculating blood will be equivalent to systemic administration. A reduction of the circulating blood volume,

K.R. Aigner, MD (✉) • E. Selak • R. Schlaf
Department of Surgical Oncology, Medias Klinikum GmbH & Co. KG,
Krankenhausstrasse 3a, Burghausen 84489, Germany
e-mail: info@prof-aigner.de; prof-aigner@medias-klinikum.de

© Springer-Verlag Berlin Heidelberg 2016
K.R. Aigner, F.O. Stephens (eds.), *Induction Chemotherapy*,
DOI 10.1007/978-3-319-28773-7_8

however, may further increase the overall local drug exposure. The question is whether it is possible to induce optimal immediate and long-term results and good quality of life without mutilating side effects.

8.2 Material and Methods

The method described herein is performed as ultimate ratio in patients with huge and non-resectable tumors of the head and neck area that are no longer responsive and are in progression after or during systemic chemotherapy or where the only remaining option was mutilating surgery and irradiation.

The isolated thoracic perfusion (ITP) technique that is applied can be considered a segmental intra-arterial chemotherapy of the isolated head and neck and chest area with a reduced blood volume of one-third or one-fourth of the total body blood volume. Reduction of the circulating blood volume is achieved by means of balloon blocking of aorta and vena cava at the level of the diaphragm. The three-channel balloon catheters are introduced after exposing the femoral artery and vein in the groin. The patient is fully heparinized. For administration of chemotherapeutics, an angiographic sidewinder catheter is proceeded in Seldinger's technique from the contralateral femoral artery into the tumor feeding common carotid artery. Both upper arms are blocked with pneumatic cuffs. After correct positioning of the angiographic catheter, the vena cava balloon is blocked first in order to further reduce the intrathoracic blood volume. Under continuous monitoring of the aortic blood pressure, the aorta is blocked at a pressure of 75–80 mmHg, which immediately adapts and rises to some 100 mmHg shortly after the aorta has been blocked (Figs. 8.1 and 8.2).

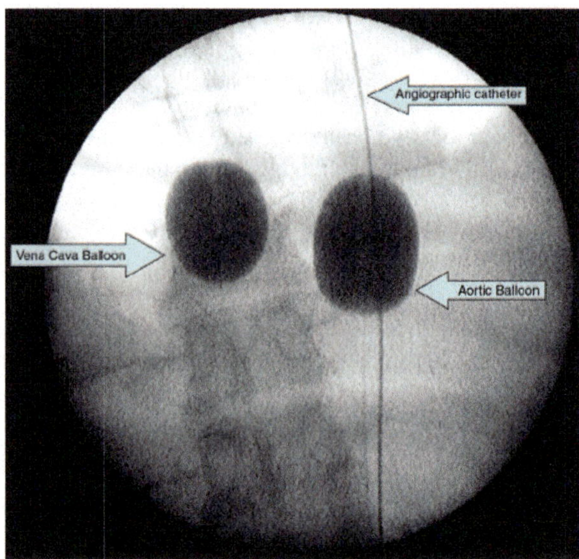

Fig. 8.1 Balloon blocking of aorta and vena cava

Chemotherapeutics are infused over 5–10 min, depending on the total dose, into the carotid artery. Vascular isolation of the chest is maintained over 15 min. Subsequently, the vena cava and aortic balloon are deflated first and the upper arm cuffs thereafter. At this point, chemofiltration is started at a flow rate of 500 mL/min with a filtrate flow of 80–150 mL/min (median 100 mL/min). After substitution of 4 L of filtrate, the catheters are removed and the vessels repaired with running sutures.

8.3   Patients

Two patients with huge cancers of the parotid gland that were in progression during systemic chemotherapy and one patient with advanced cancer of the tonsil and mediastinal lymph node metastases underwent isolated thoracic perfusion with carotid artery infusion.

The first patient was referred because of repeated bleedings of an advanced chemoresistant tumor of the right parotid gland (Fig. 8.3). He received a total of three courses of isolated thoracic perfusion with subsequent chemofiltration (ITP-F), where the drugs were infused through the angiographic carotid artery catheter. The total dose administered with each cycle was 100 mg of cisplatin and 20 mg of mitomycin at an infusion time of 7 min each. Thoracic isolation perfusion time was 15 min. The tumor responded clearly to the first course of isolated chemotherapy, revealing substantial shrinkage (Fig. 8.4). After three therapies in 3-week intervals, the residual tumor was resected (Fig. 8.5).

The second patient suffered from a left-side parotid gland cancer with a bulky metastasis on the left side of the face. He was in progression after systemic chemotherapy with 5-FU and docetaxel (Fig. 8.6). In addition, there were disseminated lung metastases. After three cycles of isolated thoracic perfusion (ITP-F) with carotid artery infusion of 100 mg of cisplatin and 30 mg of mitomycin, the residual tumor was resected. Nine months after regional chemotherapy, there was local relapse but no progression of lung metastases (Fig. 8.7).

The third patient suffered from an advanced cancer of the left tonsil (Fig. 8.8) with a bulky and prominent local lymph node metastasis at the neck, adjacent to the primary tumor. In addition, there were three suspicious lesions in the mediastinum. The entire soft palate was rigid and immobile. As a professional musician, he was unable to play on his saxophone because of escaping air via the immobile, not closing soft palate. After implantation of a Jet Port Allround catheter (PfM Cologne, FRG) in both carotid arteries, a total of four isolated thoracic perfusions with chemofiltration (ITP-F) were performed in 4-week intervals each. The drug combination infused via the Jet Ports in 7 min each during isolation perfusion consisted of 100 mg of cisplatin and 20 mg mitomycin. Two weeks after the first isolated perfusion, the patient started to play his instrument again. After four cycles, he was in a complete remission (Fig. 8.9), actually completing 5 years without relapse or complaints. He never suffered toxicity or side effects.

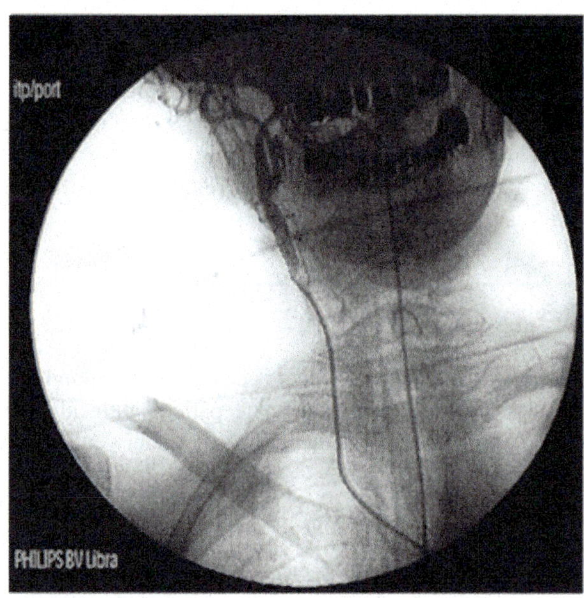

Fig. 8.2 Sidewinder catheter in common carotid artery

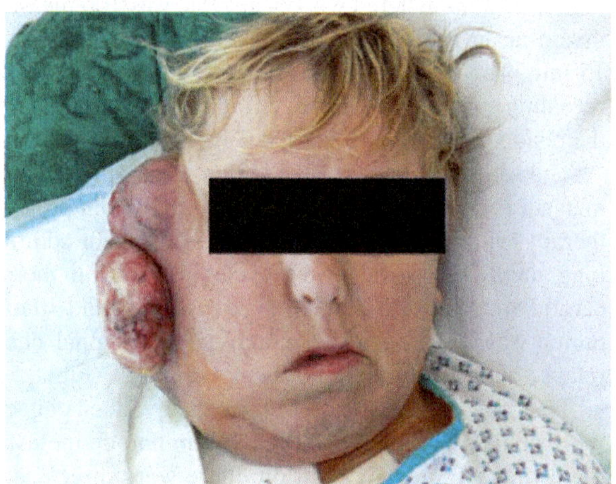

Fig. 8.3 Advanced chemoresistant tumor of the right parotid gland

8.4 Discussion

Because the term "regional chemotherapy" is used to describe a number of different approaches, it is important that details of the particular approach used are made clear. Whether or not the result is positive in terms of response and survival time or whether pitfalls and failures are encountered strongly depends on how the treatment has been carried out [1]. The type of catheters, technique of catheter placement, selection of the arterial access, drug exposure in terms of dosage, drug concentration, and infusion time may promote or jeopardize the outcome.

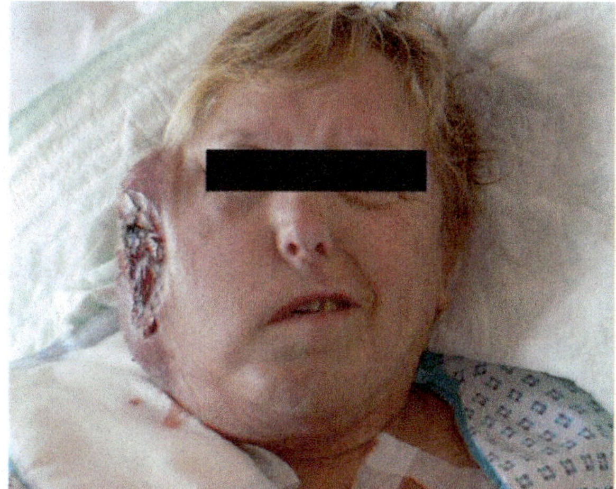

Fig. 8.4 Same tumor 3 weeks after first isolated thoracic perfusion with common carotid artery infusion of CDDP and mitomycin

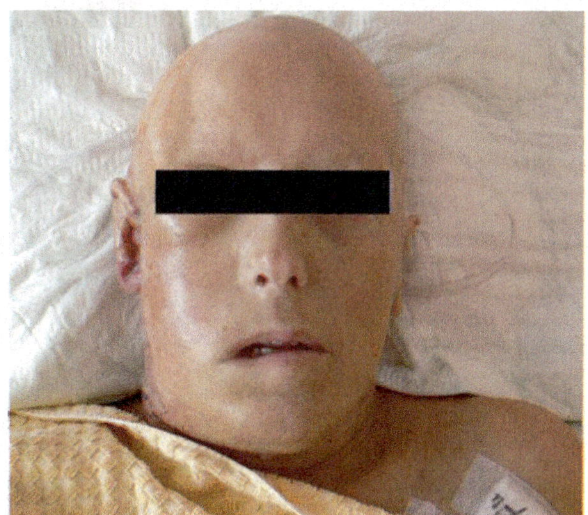

Fig. 8.5 Resection of residual tumor after three courses of isolated thoracic perfusion

In the three cases reported herein, isolated thoracic perfusion was chosen from the clinical aspect because one patient already had lung metastases and one had lymph node metastases in the mediastinum. In the other case, lung metastases could not be entirely excluded, and from the pharmacodynamic aspect, isolated thoracic perfusion was chosen in order to reduce the circulating blood volume and therefore create a better second- and third-pass effect with prolonged augmented drug exposure. In the treatment of advanced and nonoperable lung cancer (NSCLC), isolated thoracic perfusion is a technically safe and well-established method with predictable outcome. In far advanced cancers of the head and neck, however, large studies are still to come. In single cases, there has been a high incidence of good palliation, but as long as there is no controlled study with a larger number of patients providing

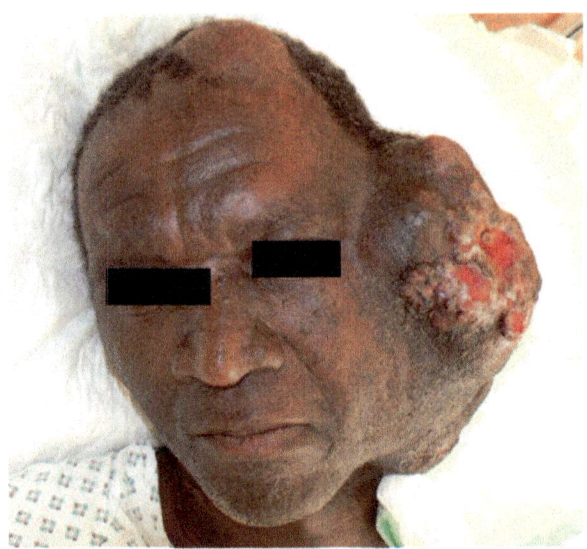

Fig. 8.6 Bulky tumor of the left parotid gland in progression after systemic chemotherapy with 5-FU and docetaxel

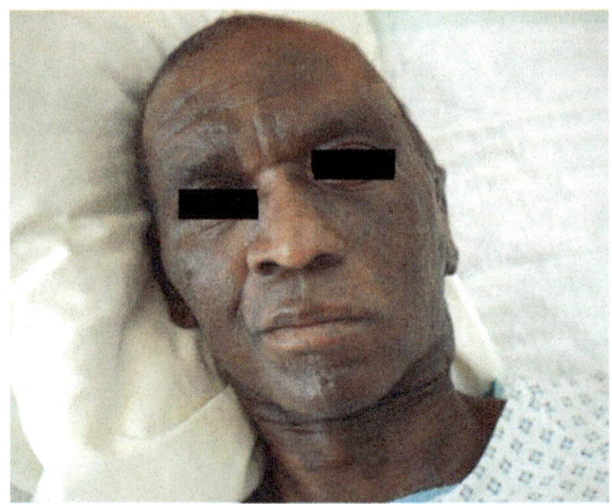

Fig. 8.7 Same patient 3 months after tumor resection, 6 months after start therapy

reliable data on response and overall survival, the method will further on be considered experimental. However, taking into account the patients presented here lacked any chance of cure, and there was no alternative therapeutic option that offered them good local palliation without those extreme toxic side effects like nerve damage, dry mouth, long-term dysphagia, and aspiration. When chemotherapeutics are infused via the common carotid artery, drug streaming with skin and soft tissue burns was not observed. Drug concentrations at the target site during a 5–10 min short-term intra-arterial infusion most obviously are sufficient to generate effective drug exposure that may induce substantial visible remission. Superselective techniques, however, due to low blood flow and exceeded drug concentration may lead to identical

Fig. 8.8 Patient before isolated thoracic perfusion with chemofiltration (ITP-F)

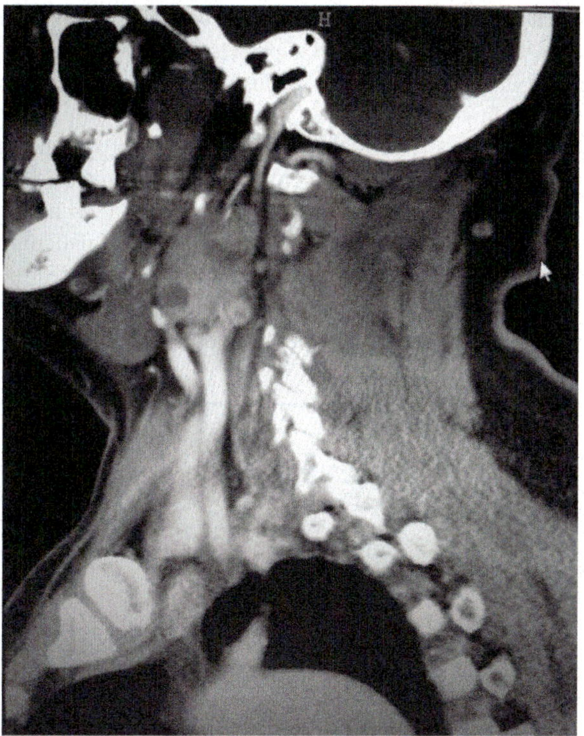

Fig. 8.9 Patient 4 weeks after isolated thoracic perfusion (ITP-F)

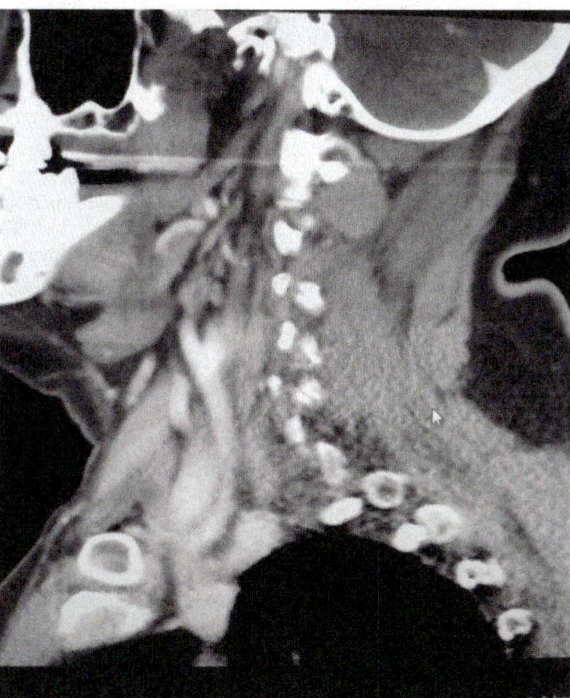

local toxic side effects as are observed with drug streaming [1]. Another complication that may occur with superselective arterial infusion has been intimal damage with subsequent vascular occlusion. This was never observed after common carotid artery infusion.

Most importantly, there was no essential systemic toxicity because of the systemic detoxification by chemofiltration. Therefore, in patients who have no chance of cure and who already suffer enough from their tumor and face a dismal outcome, every effort should be made to achieve good palliation without causing unacceptable toxicity. These three patients tolerated the treatments without any remarkable side effects. One of them can be considered a disease-free long-term survivor, and in case of relapse, the treatment can easily be repeated.

References

1. Stephens FO. Why use regional chemotherapy? Principles and pharmacokinetics. Reg Cancer Treat. 1988;1:4–10.
2. Howell SB. Pharmacokinetic principles of regional chemotherapy. Contrib Oncol. 1988;29:1–8.
3. Howell SB. Editorial: improving the therapeutic index of intra-arterial cisplatin chemotherapy. Eur J Cancer Clin Oncol. 1989;25:775–6.
4. Stephens FO. Intra-arterial chemotherapy in head and neck cancer. Historical perspectives – important developments, contributors and contributions. In: Eckardt A, editor. Intra-arterial chemotherapy in head and neck cancer – current results and future perspectives. Reinbek: Einhorn-Presse Verlag; 1999.
5. Wolpert SM, Kwan ES, Heros D, et al. Selective delivery of chemotherapeutic agents with a new catheter system. Radiology. 1988;166:547–9.
6. Forastiere AA, Baker SR, Wheeler R, et al. Intra-arterial cisplatin and FUDR in advanced malignancies confined to the head and neck. J Clin Oncol. 1987;5:1601–6.
7. Cheung DK, Regan J, Savin M, et al. A pilot study of intra-arterial chemotherapy with cisplatin in locally advanced head and neck cancers. Cancer. 1988;61:903–8.
8. Lee YY, Dimery IW, Van Tassel P, et al. Superselective intra-arterial chemotherapy of advanced paranasal sinus tumors. Arch Otolaryngol Head Neck Surg. 1989;115:503–11.
9. Robbins KT, Storniolo AM, Kerber C, et al. Rapid superselective high dose cisplatin infusion for advanced head and neck malignancies. Head Neck. 1992;14:364–71.
10. Kovacs AF. Intra-arterial induction high-dose chemotherapy with cisplatin for oral and oropharyngeal cancer: long-term results. Br J Cancer. 2004;90:1323–8.
11. Kovacs AF. Response to intraarterial induction chemotherapy: a prognostic parameter in oral and oropharyngeal cancer. Head Neck. 2006;28:678–88.
12. Robbins KT, Vicario D, Seagren S, et al. A targeted supradose cisplatin chemoradiation protocol for advanced head and neck cancer. Am J Surg. 1994;168:419–22.
13. Robbins KT, Kumar P, Regine WF, et al. Efficacy of supradose intra-arterial targeted (SIT) cisplatin (P) and concurrent radiation therapy (RT) in the treatment of unresectable stage III-IV head and neck carcinoma: the Memphis experience. Int J Radiat Oncol Biol Phys. 1997;38:263–71.
14. Robbins KT, Kumar P, Wong FS, et al. Targeted chemoradiation for advanced head and neck cancer: analysis of 213 patients. Head Neck. 2000;22(7):687–93.
15. Robbins KT, Kumar P, Harris J, et al. Supradose intra-arterial cisplatin and concurrent radiation therapy for the treatment of stage IV head and neck squamous cell carcinoma is feasible and efficacious in a multi-institutional setting: results of Radiation Therapy Oncology Group Trial 9615. J Clin Oncol. 2005;23(7):1447–54.

Induction Chemotherapy for Breast Cancer

François-Michel Delgado, Maria Angeles Gil-Delgado, and David Khayat

9.1 Introduction and Rationale

Breast cancer is a major public health problem for women throughout the world. Breast cancer represents the second most common cancer in the world and the most frequent cancer among women, with 1.67 million new cases diagnosed in 2012 according to GLOBOCAN data. Breast cancer alone represents 25 % of all cancer cases and 15 % of all cancer deaths among females (521,900 deaths in 2012). More developed countries account for about one-half of all breast cancer cases and 38 % of deaths [1, 2].

In the European Union, breast cancer remains the most frequent cancer in women and the second most frequent cause of cancer death. As a result, 456,000 new cases (29 % of female cancer and 12 % of the total) of invasive breast cancer were diagnosed and 131,000 women died of breast cancer in 2012 (17 % of female deaths and 7 % of the total) [3, 4]. Nevertheless, since 1990, the death rate from breast cancer has decreased in the USA by 24 % and similar reductions have been observed in Europe and in other countries [5]. Mathematical models suggest that both the adoption of screening mammography and the availability of induction chemotherapy, targeted therapy (hormonal, monoclonal antibodies and small molecules), and molecular biology have contributed approximately equally to this improvement [6, 7]. Although breast cancer has traditionally been less common in non-industrialised nations, its incidence in these areas is increasing [1, 2].

The tumour size, axillary node status, histological grade and the existence of micrometastasis and molecular biology features all have an important impact in breast cancer prognosis as well as the addition of recent new criteria such HER-2 overexpression. These prognostic markers have led, since the early 1970s, to

F.-M. Delgado (✉) • M.A. Gil-Delgado • D. Khayat
Service d'Oncologie Médicale, Groupe Hospitalier Pitié Salpêtrière,
47 Boulevard de l'Hôpital, Paris 75013, France
e-mail: delgadofm@orange.fr; marian.gil-delgado@psl.ap-hop-paris.fr

© Springer-Verlag Berlin Heidelberg 2016
K.R. Aigner, F.O. Stephens (eds.), *Induction Chemotherapy*,
DOI 10.1007/978-3-319-28773-7_9

numerous studies with adjuvant chemotherapy, which have as their main objective the intention to modify the natural history of breast cancer. The data provided by Nissen-Meyer, Fisher, Mansour and Bonadonna [8, 9] have all demonstrated that chemotherapy or hormonal therapy could improve the outcome. The Early Breast Cancer Trialists' Collaborative Group established a database of all randomised clinical trials of primary breast cancer [10, 11]. These meta-analyses have been conducted at 5-year intervals, starting in 1985, and have contributed immensely to the general acceptance of various forms of adjuvant therapy as standard treatment. However, some of the conclusions of the meta-analyses have been questioned based on biological mechanisms, whereas others were in conflict with the results of some of the largest multicentre clinical trials [12] and this has led investigators to question this approach.

The concept of induction (also known as primary, preoperative or neoadjuvant) chemotherapy started as an alternative for the management of patients with large clinical stage IIA, stage IIB and T3N1M0 breast cancers [13]. Such treatment is administered with the aim to downstage the primary tumour, to increase the likelihood of breast conservation and to abolish occult systemic metastases in order to improve survival and eventually to test the tumour's chemosensitivity [13]. This approach was enhanced with a large pioneer trial conducted by Jacquillat et al. in the beginning of the 1980s [14], in which 250 patients underwent induction chemotherapy. They received the combination of vinblastine, thiotepa, methotrexate and 5-fluorouracil with or without doxorubicin, followed with locoregional radiotherapy. Tumour volume regression (>75 %) was observed in 41 % of the patients and complete clinical regression in 30 % of the patients. The 5-year disease-free survival (DFS) rates were 100 %, 82 %, 61 %, 46 % and 52 % for stage I, stage IIA, stage IIB, stage IIIA and stage IIIB patients, respectively. At 5 years, the rate of breast preservation was 94 % with excellent cosmetic results [14]. Meanwhile, Veronesi [15] proved that it was possible to decrease locoregional treatment from radical mastectomy to more conservative approaches such is lumpectomy or segmentectomy without affecting survival.

Since the Jacquillat trial, there has been a substantial evolution in this therapeutic approach, which has been evaluated in a number of clinical studies [16, 17]. The largest study, to date, has been conducted by the National Surgical Adjuvant Breast and Bowel Project (NSABP) [18], a randomised study that involved 1,523 patients in a comparison of the efficacy of an anthracycline-based chemotherapy regimen (doxorubicin plus cyclophosphamide: AC) administered before surgery with that of the same regimen administered in the adjuvant setting. It was shown that the use of induction chemotherapy allowed greater use of breast-conserving surgery (12 %). These results are in agreement with those of other randomised clinical studies, so it may be concluded that the administration of chemotherapy before surgery results in an increased likelihood of breast conservation. Even though no overall survival (OS) benefit is seen for induction chemotherapy compared with adjuvant chemotherapy (HR=0.99; 95 % CI, 0.85–1.16; $P=0.90$), the subset of patients who achieve pathological complete remission (pCR) after induction chemotherapy have significantly higher DFS and OS ($p < 0.001$) [18].

A meta-analysis was conducted by Kong and co-workers [19] in order to determine whether achieving a pathological complete response to induction treatment will predict long-term outcome. Papers were selected from the PubMed database based on defined inclusion and exclusion criteria. Parameters such as number/percentage of patients having pCR and outcome statistics (i.e., overall survival (OS), disease-free survival (DFS), relapse-free survival (RFS)) were collected for 3,776 patients. The summary odds ratio (OR) estimating the association of OS with pCR was 3.44 (95 % CI: 2.45–4.84), with similar findings for DFS (OR = 3.41, 95 % CI: 2.54–4.58) and RFS (OR = 2.45, 95 % CI: 1.59–3.80). This meta-analysis confirmed that pathologic response is a prognostic indicator for RFS, DFS and OS and suggested that patients achieving pCR after induction therapy have favourable outcomes [19].

Biomarkers that might have a predictive value in patients treated with preoperative therapy include the degree of ER expression, grade, histological type and markers of proliferation such as Ki-67 labelling index. The presence of elevated Ki-67 before induction therapy has been found to predict response to chemotherapy LABC. In retrospective studies conducted on a large number of patients, high baseline Ki-67 was found to be an independent factor predictive for pCR by multivariate analyses [20]. Recent results indicate that Ki-67 might represent a valid surrogate of outcome in patients with ER-positive breast cancer treated with induction endocrine therapy [20].

Active studies are in progress to identify agents and biologic markers that could be used to predict treatment response. Recently, DNA microarray analysis and gene expression profiles have been assessed to see if they may be used as predictive markers identifying patients who would benefit from chemotherapy while avoiding toxicities from unnecessary treatment [6].

Patients with inflammatory, locally advanced and operable breast cancer could benefit from a multidisciplinary approach involving chemotherapy, hormonotherapy and monoclonal antibody-based therapy (such as trastuzumab, pertuzumab and bevacizumab). There are potential induction therapeutic options available today for the different subtypes of breast cancer [21, 22] with results indicating that 60–90 % of patients with invasive breast cancer will show clinical responses although only 3–30 % achieve pCR.

Induction anthracycline and/or taxane-based chemotherapy resulted in an increase of 10–30 % in the rate of pCR of unselected patients. The addition of trastuzumab to chemotherapy in patients with HER-2 neu, overexpressed or amplified increases pCR from 30 % to 60 %. The rate of pCR is very low after short-course hormonotherapy at less than 5 %. By contrast, patients with triple receptor-negative (ER-, PR-, HER-2-negative), basal-like (which are 77 % triple negative), HER-2 neu overexpressed, small tumour burden or high-nuclear grade tumours have a higher rate of pCR [6, 23].

Patients who obtain breast and axillary pCR after induction chemotherapy have a better DFS and OS than patients with residual disease (RD). However, several reports have demonstrated that minimal residual disease (RD of less than 1 cm: MRD) is also associated with a good outcome. The pCR rate in patients with invasive lobular carcinoma is low (3 %) compared with invasive ductal carcinoma patients (15 %). More patients with lobular carcinoma are ER positive (92 % vs. 62 %; $p < 0.001$) and are more responsive to endocrine therapy. This difference in pCR rate persists after adjusting for ER status suggesting that lobular carcinoma is an independent predictive factor for pCR [24, 25].

9.1.1 Subgroups of Breast Cancer

Breast cancer is not a single illness but should be considered as a heterogeneous disease with different subtypes of molecular, histopathological and clinical features leading to different prognostic and therapeutic consequences. Gene expression characteristics of breast cancer suggest that it should be classified into five biologically distinct inherent subtypes: luminal A, luminal B, basal-like, normal-like and HER-2 overexpressed [26, 27] (Table 9.1).

Among these subtypes, the basal-like breast cancer is a molecular subtype of breast cancer with a poor prognosis. Follow-up studies of long-term outcome in these patients demonstrate that they can be separated into two clinical groups: those who succumb to their disease within the first 5 years and those expected to show excellent long-term survival. Using data derived from basal-like breast cancer patients, Hallet et al. [28] identified and validated 14-gene signatures in basal breast cancer patients. The ability to distinguish two subgroups of basal breast cancer patients at diagnosis also permits tailoring aggressive therapeutic regimens to those patients with a poor prognosis and conversely avoiding such therapy in low-risk patients. The presence of amplification of the HER2 gene confers sensitivity to the anti-HER2 monoclonal antibodies trastuzumab and pertuzumab and the tyrosine kinase inhibitor lapatinib. Breast cancer molecular types respond differently to preoperative chemotherapy [27, 29].

Rouzier et al. [30] investigated whether the molecular subtype of a tumour affected chemosensitivity. They evaluated the gene expression profile of 82 patients treated with induction paclitaxel followed by 5-fluorouracil, doxorubicin and cyclophosphamide (FAC). The pCR rate was 45 % for basal-like and HER-2 positive subtypes and only 6 % for luminal tumours. Oestrogen receptor-negative tumours were also more sensitive to chemotherapy. The gene profile signature suggested the existence of groups of patients who have a good prognosis despite residual disease after induction chemotherapy [31] (Table 9.2).

Table 9.1 Prognostic factors according to different breast cancer types

Good prognosis unlikely present pCR	Intermediate	Poor prognosis high pCR
Luminal A	Normal-like	Basal-like
Luminal B	–	–
ER+ PR+		ER- PR-
HER2 normal		HER2 overexpressed
Grade I	Grade II	Grade III
Ki67 low		Ki67 high

Table 9.2 Chemosensitivity according to different breast cancer types [30, 31]

More chemosensitive	More chemoresistant
Triple-negative tumour	ER+, PR+
HER2 neu +++	HER2 neu normal
Basal-like	Luminal A, luminal B
Small tumour burden	Low nuclear grade
High nuclear grade	Or
Or	Grade I
Grade III	Lobular carcinoma

Defined by gene expression or immunochemistry

Two tests for the gene profile are currently available: MammaPrint is a microarray-based diagnostic, which evaluates the expression of 70 genes [32]. OncotypeDX2 [33] is a 21-gene quantitative RT-qPCR assay, that predicts the likelihood of a cancer recurrence, the likelihood of benefit from adjuvant chemotherapy and the likelihood of survival in patients with newly diagnosed breast cancer node negative and hormone receptor positive. Intense clinical research is ongoing in order to determine the role of these in guiding induction therapy [34] (Table 9.2).

9.2 Trials Using Drug Sensitivity to Guide Treatment

9.2.1 Chemotherapy

Several clinical trials have attempted to apply information on drug sensitivity to clinical management on the hypothesis that non-cross-resistant chemotherapy agents increase pCR and ultimately improve survival.

Further, the NSABP B-27 [35] trial was designed to determine the impact of adding docetaxel after four cycles of induction AC on clinical and pCR rates and on DFS and OS. In this trial 2,411 women with operable invasive breast cancer were randomly assigned to receive: in arm I, four cycles of induction doxorubicin plus cyclophosphamide followed by surgery; in arm II, four cycles of AC followed by four cycles of induction docetaxel before surgery; and in arm III, AC regimen before surgery and then four cycles of postoperative docetaxel. Higher pCR at the time of local therapy was reached in patients of group II compared to those of groups I and III; however, this had no impact on DFS and OS. Nevertheless, a DFS advantage was observed in patients experiencing clinical partial response having received preoperative docetaxel compared to postoperative administration of this drug (HR 0.71; 95 % CI 0.55–091, $P=0.007$) [35].

Comparable results were observed by the EORTC trial 10902 (European Organization for Research and Treatment of Cancer). In this randomised trial, 698 patients with BC received four cycles of fluorouracil, epirubicin and cyclophosphamide (FEC) administered either pre- ($n=350$) or postoperatively ($n=348$). No difference was observed between the two groups in terms of OS and progression-free survival (PFS) and time to locoregional recurrence (HR 1.16; 95 % CI 0.83–1.63,

$p=0.38$; HR 1.15; 95 % CI 0.89–1.48, $p=0.27$; HR 1.13; 95 % CI 0.70–1.81, $p=0.61$, respectively) [36].

In the German Preoperative Adriamycin and Docetaxel Study (GEPARTRIO) [37], 2,090 patients, with large operable or locally advanced breast cancer, received two cycles of induction docetaxel in combination with doxorubicin and cyclophosphamide (TAC). Patients with 50 % or greater tumour reduction, assessed by ultrasound imaging, were treated with an additional four or six cycles of TAC. Subsequently, the non-responder patients were randomly allocated to receive either four cycles of TAC or four cycles of vinorelbine and capecitabine (NX). Patients who responded after two cycles of TAC have a high chance of achieving pCR. The pCR rates were 24 % in early responders and 6 % in non-responders. There were no statistical differences between six and eight cycles of TAC in responder patients ($p=0.27$) or between TAC and the vinorelbine and capecitabine combination in non-responder patients ($p=0.73$) who were considered as resistant to the initial regimen. An exploratory analysis permitted the authors [38] to observe that DFS after "response-guided" chemotherapy (TAC 8 or TAC-NX) was significantly longer (HR, 0.71; 95 % [CI, 0.60–0.85]; $P=0.003$); nevertheless, TA6 and 8 were not different. Overall survival (HR, 0.79; 95 % [CI, 0.63–0.99]; $P<0.048$) compared to conventional chemotherapy (TAC 6) disease-free survival was longer after "response-guided" chemotherapy in all hormone receptor-positive tumours (luminal A HR=0.55, luminal B [HER2- negative] HR=0.40 and luminal B [HER2-positive] HR=0.56), but not in hormone receptor-negative tumours (HER2 positive [non-luminal] HR=1.01 and triple-negative HR=0.87). Pathological complete response did not predict these survival effects. Pathological complete response predicted an improved DFS in triple-negative (HR=6.67), HER2-positive (non-luminal; HR=5.24) or luminal B (HER2-negative) tumours (HR=3.74). This approach, "response-guided chemotherapy," in the neoadjuvant setting might improve survival in hormone receptor-positive tumours.

In the Aberdeen Study [39], the same category of patients received four induction therapy cycles of cyclophosphamide, vincristine, doxorubicin and prednisone (CVAP). Patients who achieved partial or complete response were allocated to randomly receive four additional cycles of CVAP or four cycles of docetaxel (100 mg/m^2). The addition of sequential docetaxel to CVAP significantly increased response rate (94 % vs. 66 %) and the rate of pCR (34 % vs. 16 %, $p<0.004$) compared with patients receiving CVAP alone. Non-responder patients after four cycles of CVAP received four cycles of docetaxel, and although the clinical response rate was 51 %, the pCR rate was only 2 %. Patients with minimal residual disease (<1 cm, residual cancer burden [RCB]-1) were considered as a good prognosis group and received the same therapy as patients who obtained pCR (RCB-0). By contrast, extensive residual disease was associated with a poor prognosis. The RCB was considered to be an independent prognostic factor in a multivariate model that included age, hormone receptor status, pretreatment, clinical stage, hormonal therapy and pCR.

The role of non-cross-resistant regimens in patients with residual disease after anthracycline-based therapy was evaluated by Valero V et al. (MD Anderson Cancer Center) [40] in two studies. For the first trial [41], 193 patients with locally advanced breast cancer were studied (80 %, stage III). They received three courses of vincristine, doxorubicin, cyclophosphamide and prednisone (VACP) before surgery. Patients with residual disease less than 1 cm received an additional five cycles of VACP and patients with more than 1 cm residual disease were randomly allocated to received five cycles of VACP or five cycles of vinblastine, methotrexate and 5FU-leucovorin (VbMF). Patients who had clinical or pathological CR had improved survival compared with patients with any lesser response. Five-year relapse-free survival (RFS) and OS after VbMF in addition to VACP were 10 % and 18 %, respectively.

In the second study [42], 88 patients were treated with four or six cycles of doxorubicin + docetaxel (AT), 74 obtained adequate response and 72 of them underwent surgery. Pathological complete response, pPR and pMR were observed in 13.9 %, 30.5 % and 55.5 % of patients, respectively. Fourteen patients were considered non-operable after AT and underwent salvage cyclophosphamide, methotrexate and 5-FU combination (CMF) therapy. Five of these patients underwent surgery and one had achieved a pCR. Patients received adjuvant chemotherapy according to the pathological response: if pCR, two more cycles of AT were administered; if pPR, two cycles of AT were given followed by six cycles of CMF; and if pathological minimal response (MR), they received six additional cycles of CMF. The estimated 5-year recurrence-free survival (RFS) rates for patients with pCR, pPR and pMR were 80 %, 77 % and 59 %, respectively, and the estimated 5-year overall survival (OS) rates were 90 %, 91 % and 74 %, respectively. The 5-year OS rates were 82 % for initially operable compared to 21 % for initially inoperable patients ($P \leq 0.001$) [42].

Bevacizumab is a recombinant humanised monoclonal IgG1 antibody that binds to and inhibits the biologic activity of human vascular endothelial growth factor (VEGF) in in vitro and in vivo assay systems. Bevacizumab contains human framework regions and the complementarity-determining regions of a murine antibody that binds to VEGF. Bevacizumab binds VEGF and prevents the interaction of VEGF to its receptors (Flt-1 and KDR) on the surface of endothelial cells. The interaction of VEGF with its receptors leads to endothelial cell proliferation and new blood vessel formation in in vitro models of angiogenesis. Administration of bevacizumab to xenotransplant models of colon cancer in nude mice caused reduction of microvascular growth and inhibition of metastatic disease progression [43].

Bear et al. [44] conducted a trial involving 1,206 HER2-negative pts who were randomly assigned to receive either docetaxel, docetaxel plus capecitabine or docetaxel plus gemcitabine for four cycles, followed by four cycles of doxorubicin plus cyclophosphamide. Patients were randomised to receive or not bevacizumab for the first six cycles of chemotherapy. The addition of bevacizumab significantly increased the pCR rates (28.2 % vs. 34.5 %, $p = 0.02$), with a more marked advantage in terms of pCR in the hormone receptor-positive subcategory of patients (15.1 % without bevacizumab vs. 23.2 % with bevacizumab, $p = 0.007$) with weaker effect in the hormone receptor-negative subgroup (47.1 % vs. 51.5 %, $p = 0.34$). The addition of bevacizumab resulted in increased rates of hypertension, impairment of left ventricular fraction ejection, hand-foot syndrome and mucositis [44].

GeparQuinto, carried out by von Minckwitz et al. [45], included 1,948 patients with HER2-negative BC who were randomly assigned to receive induction therapy with epirubicin and cyclophosphamide followed by docetaxel, with or without concomitant bevacizumab treatment. The addition of bevacizumab leads to a significant increase of pCR rate (odds ratio with addition of bevacizumab, 1.29; 95 % CI 1.02–1.65, $p = 0.04$). In this case, the benefit of bevacizumab treatment on pCR was observed in the hormone receptor-negative subgroup (27.9 % vs. 39.3 %, $p = 0.003$), whereas there was no benefit observed in the hormone receptor-positive patients (7.8 % vs. 7.7 %, $p = 1.00$). In terms of safety profile, a higher incidence of grade 3 or 4 adverse events such as febrile neutropenia, mucositis, hand-foot syndrome, infection and hypertension was observed in the arm containing bevacizumab, with no impact on surgical complications. Subsequent analyses of the GeparQuinto GBG 44 study showed that adding everolimus to paclitaxel in nonresponsive patients to induction epirubicin plus cyclophosphamide regimen, with or without bevacizumab, did not improve the pCR rate in the 403 primary HER2-negative patients [46].

Surgical complications and significant toxicities were associated with bevacizumab combinations, including cardiac infarction, congestive heart failure and pulmonary embolism [47, 48].

9.2.2 Endocrine Induction Therapy

Induction endocrine treatment in postmenopausal, ER-positive, breast cancer patients was limited to patients who were not suitable for chemotherapy and surgery. Earlier phase II studies with tamoxifen that focused primarily on elderly and/or frail patients often unselected for hormone receptor status of the tumour showed response rates ranging from 49 % to 68 % [49]. Conflicting results are reported in the literature on the value of factors predictive of response in the neoadjuvant or induction therapy approach. In the subset of patients with ER-positive tumours, pCR rates range from 2 % to 10 % in patients who express oestrogen receptors (ERs), which suggests that other primary endpoints must be considered within this tumour subset.

Results from two randomised trials on induction endocrine therapy in ER-positive postmenopausal patients support the theory of a relationship between the probability of response and the degree of ER expression [50, 51]. Higher ER levels are significantly related to a greater probability of response in both studies. In addition, a positive significant correlation between the ER level and the degree of Ki-67 suppression after 2 and 12 weeks of endocrine treatment was reported by Dowsett et al. [52]. The level of expression of ER and progesterone (PgR) might be associated with the probability of response to induction chemotherapy. In a retrospective analysis involving 533 patients, no pCR was observed within the cohort of patients considered as highly endocrine responsive (ER and PgR ≥ 50 %), which compares with 3.3 % of those with ER or PgR expressed in 0–49 % of the cells and 17.7 % of those patients hormonal receptor negative ($P < 0.0001$) [53]. On the other hand, even with the higher incidence of pCR, a statistically significantly worse DFS and OS was observed for patients with ER and PgR absent tumours versus patients with tumours expressing high ER and PgR (HR 6.4, 95% CI 3.5–11.6, for DFS; HR 3.6 95% CI 2.4–5.6 for OS). Even though this study conducted by Colleoni et al. [53] shows that response and outcome after induction chemotherapy are correlated with the degree of expression of steroid hormone receptors, more studies on tailored preoperative therapies are necessary [53].

Aromatase inhibitors (AIs) block the conversion of androgens to oestrogens and reduce oestrogen levels in tissue and plasma [54]. Third-generation AIs include the nonsteroidal inhibitors, letrozole and anastrozole, and the steroidal inhibitor, exemestane. The results of large trials conducted in the metastatic and adjuvant setting [52, 55], indicating better outcomes among women given AIs than those given tamoxifen, stimulated the investigation of these agents in the induction setting in postmenopausal women with hormone receptor-positive tumours.

The P024 trial (a randomised, double-blind, multicentre study) compared the efficacy of 4 months of letrozole or tamoxifen as induction therapy for postmenopausal women with ER- and/or PgR-positive stage II or III breast cancer. The patients were not considered as candidates for BCS at baseline and 14 % of them were not eligible for resection. Letrozole increased the clinical response rate (55 % vs. 36 %, $P<0.001$) and the BCS rate (45 % vs. 35 %, $P=0.022$) when compared with tamoxifen [56]. The letrozole arm induced a higher degree of Ki-67 reduction (87 %) compared to [50] the tamoxifen arm 75 % [50].

In the IMPACT study, postmenopausal women with ER-positive, operable breast cancer were randomly assigned to induction tamoxifen, anastrozole or a combination of tamoxifen and anastrozole for 3 months. The response rates were similar for all treatments, 37 % versus 36 % versus 39 % respectively, while patients receiving anastrozole were significantly more likely to undergo breast conservation (46 % vs. 22 %) [51].

In the PROACT trial, anastrozole and tamoxifen yielded a similar response rate. In the subgroup of patients treated with anastrozole who did not receive concurrent chemotherapy, the response rate was statistically similar (36.2 % vs. 26.5 %, $P=0.09$) [57]. Seo et al. conducted a meta-analysis on three studies to show an improved breast conservative surgery rate in patients receiving AI [58].

In another randomised study comparing exemestane to tamoxifen in which 151 postmenopausal patients with ER- and/or PgR-positive breast cancer were included, exemestane significantly increased the clinical response rate (76 % vs. 40 %, $P=0.05$) and the rate of breast conservative surgery (36.8 % vs. 20 %, $P=0.05$) [59].

The ACOSOG Z1031 [60] trial largely confirmed the usefulness of AIs in the induction treatment of ER-positive patients. In this trial, 374 postmenopausal women with clinical stage II or III ER-positive breast cancer were randomly assigned to receive anastrozole, exemestane or letrozole for 16–18 weeks before surgery. The response rates observed were not statistically different. Aromatase inhibitor treatment markedly improved surgical outcomes. Ki67 and preoperative endocrine prognostic index (PEPI) data demonstrated that the three agents tested are biologically equivalent and therefore likely to have similar adjuvant activities.

Luminal A tumours were more likely to have favourable biomarker characteristics after treatment; however, occasional paradoxical increases in Ki67 (12 % of tumours with more than 5 % increase after therapy) suggest treatment-resistant cells that are present in some luminal A tumours that can be detected by posttreatment profiling [60].

The optimal duration of induction endocrine therapy is not determined yet. However, an improved response rate has been reported with induction letrozole when the duration of therapy was prolonged beyond 3 months [61]. According to these observations, several authors recommend prolonging endocrine therapy for a minimum of 4–8 months [49].

Crosstalk between the oestrogen receptor (ER) and the phosphoinositide-3-kinase (PI3K)/Akt/mammalian target of rapamycin (mTOR) pathways is a mechanism of resistance to endocrine therapy, and blockade of both pathways enhances antitumour activity in preclinical models [61, 62]. A new approach to restore endocrine responsiveness in breast cancer might be to use the combination of an AI with a signal transduction inhibitor as a PI3K/mTOR antagonist [63].

Baselga et al. [64] included 270 postmenopausal women with operable ER-positive breast cancer who were randomly assigned to receive 4 months of induction treatment with letrozole (2.5 mg/day) and either everolimus (10 mg/day) or placebo. The primary endpoint was clinical response. Biopsies were obtained at baseline and after 2 weeks of treatment (i.e., day 1) in order to assess PI3K mutation status (PIK3CA) and pharmacodynamic changes of Ki67, phospho-S6, cyclin D1 and progesterone receptor (PgR) by immunohistochemistry. Clinical response rate in the everolimus arm was higher than that with letrozole alone (i.e., placebo; 68.1 % vs. 59.1 %), which was statistically significant ($P = 0.062$). Marked reductions in progesterone receptor and cyclin D1 expression occurred in both treatment arms, and dramatic downregulation of phospho-S6 occurred only in the everolimus arm. An antiproliferative response, as defined by a reduction in Ki67 expression, occurred in 57 % of 91 patients in the everolimus arm and in 30 % of 82 patients in the placebo arm ($P < 0.01$). Everolimus significantly increased letrozole efficacy in the therapy of patients with ER-positive breast cancer.

Limited data are available on induction treatments for premenopausal patients.

Masuda et al. [65] performed the unique double-blind, multicentre, randomised trial, in which 197 premenopausal women with oestrogen receptor (ER)-positive, HER2-negative, operable breast cancer were enrolled. All patients received monthly goserelin plus either anastrozole and tamoxifen-placebo ($n = 98$) or tamoxifen and anastrozole-placebo ($n = 99$) over 24 weeks before surgery. More patients in the anastrozole group achieved complete or partial response compared to the tamoxifen group (anastrozole 70.4 % vs. tamoxifen 50.5 % [$p = 0.004$]).

These studies suggest that induction endocrine therapy with a combination of GnRH analogue and AIs is effective in selected premenopausal patients. But no conclusions can be drawn due to the limited results available. The combination of GnRH analogues and AIs should only currently be given in the context of a clinical trial.

9.2.3 Systemic Induction Therapy for ERb2 Overexpressed Patients

About 20 % of patients with breast cancer will show overexpressed HER2 gene amplification which is associated with an aggressive clinical course of the disease. Trastuzumab, a monoclonal antibody (mAb) targeting HER2, has established activity in both the metastatic and adjuvant settings for these patients. Several single-arm phase II trials in the induction therapy setting have been performed suggesting that the addition of trastuzumab to conventional chemotherapy shows promising antitumour activity, with pCR rates ranging between 12 % and 76 % [66].

Buzdar et al. conducted the first randomised trial of induction therapy with or without trastuzumab. Forty-two patients with HER2-positive disease with operable breast cancer were randomly assigned to either four cycles of paclitaxel followed by four cycles of fluorouracil, epirubicin and cyclophosphamide or to the same chemotherapy with simultaneous weekly trastuzumab for 24 weeks. The primary objective was to demonstrate a 20 % improvement in pCR (assumed 21–41 %) with the addition of trastuzumab to chemotherapy. The planned sample size was 164 patients. The addition of trastuzumab led to a significant increase of pCR rate (pCR 26 % vs. 65.2 %, $p=0.016$), leading to premature closure of the trial ($n=42$). No clinical congestive heart failure was observed. More than 10 % decrease in the cardiac ejection fraction was observed in five and seven patients in the chemotherapy arm and trastuzumab plus chemotherapy arm, respectively. Even though the sample size was small, this pioneer study indicates that adding trastuzumab to chemotherapy significantly increases pCR and stimulated studies in this setting [67].

The NOAH (NeOAdjuvant Herceptin) study conducted by Gianni and Coll [68] involved 235 patients with HER2-positive locally advanced or inflammatory disease. They were randomly assigned to receive doxorubicin/paclitaxel/cyclophosphamide, methotrexate and fluorouracil chemotherapy with or without simultaneous administration of trastuzumab for 30 weeks. This study achieved a significant increase in 3-year event-free survival (EFS) of 71 % with trastuzumab versus 56 % without (HR 0.59, 95 % CI 0.386–0.90, $p=0.013$) as its primary objective and improvement in the secondary endpoint, in terms of an increase in the pCR rate of 38 % versus 19 % ($p=0.001$) [68].

In another study, 120 patients with stage II and III HER2-positive BC, ineligible for breast conservative surgery, were randomly assigned to receive four cycles of epirubicin/cyclophosphamide, followed by four cycles of docetaxel with or without trastuzumab concurrently with the docetaxel induction therapy, resulting in increased pCR rates (26 % with trastuzumab vs. 19 % without) [69].

The Austrian Breast and Colorectal Cancer Study Group randomised 93 patients with HER2-positive BC to receive six cycles of epirubicin-docetaxel or epirubicin-docetaxel-capecitabine induction therapy with or without trastuzumab. The difference between the groups, in terms of pCR, was not statistically significant (pCR 38.6 % vs. 26.5 %, $p=0.212$) [70].

Buzdar and Coll [71] investigated the effect of the timing of trastuzumab administration with anthracycline and taxane induction chemotherapy in a randomised phase III trial (282 patients). Women with operable HER2-positive invasive breast cancer were randomly assigned into two groups. A "sequential group" (140 pts): FEC-75 for four cycles followed by weekly paclitaxel (80 mg/m^2) plus weekly trastuzumab for 12 weeks and a "concurrent treatment" group (142 pts): weekly paclitaxel and trastuzumab for 12 weeks followed by four cycles of FEC-75 and weekly trastuzumab. Surgery, including evaluation of the axilla, was performed within 6 weeks of completion of induction treatment. The pCR rate was the primary endpoint. In the sequential groupw, pCR rate reached 56·5 % compared to 54·2 % in the concurrent group. No treatment-related deaths occurred. The most common severe toxic effects were neutropenia and fatigue. Left ventricular ejection fraction dropped in 0.8 % of patients who received sequential treatment and in 2.9 % patients who received concurrent treatment; by week 24, LVF had dropped in 7·1 % patients and 4·6 % of patients, respectively. Both treatments reached a high response rate but it should be stressed that concurrent administration of trastuzumab with anthracyclines offers no additional benefit and is not warranted [71].

Lapatinib is an epidermal growth factor receptor inhibitor for use in combination with capecitabine for the treatment of advanced or metastatic HER2-positive breast cancer in women who have received prior therapy and also for use in combination with letrozole to treat hormone-positive and HER2-positive advanced breast cancer in postmenopausal women for whom hormonal therapy is indicated. Lapatinib is established as an effective treatment for HER2-positive locally advanced or metastatic breast cancer (MBC), including cancers progressing on prior trastuzumab-based therapy [72].

The GeparQuinto phase III trial led by the German Breast Group studied 620 women with untreated, HER2-positive, primary invasive breast cancer; 162 patients were randomised to receive four cycles of epirubicin/cyclophosphamide followed by docetaxel administered concurrently with either trastuzumab or lapatinib. The primary endpoint, pCR, was achieved in 30.3 % of patients who received trastuzumab plus chemotherapy compared with 22.7 % of patients who received lapatinib plus chemotherapy (odds ratio 0.68 [95 % Cl, 0.47–0.97]; $P<0.04$). Oedema and dyspnoea occurred more frequently in the trastuzumab group, while diarrhoea and skin rash occurred more frequently in the lapatinib group. This face-to-face comparison of trastuzumab and lapatinib showed that pCR rate with chemotherapy and lapatinib was significantly lower than that with chemotherapy and trastuzumab. Therefore, lapatinib should not be used outside of clinical trials as single anti-HER2 treatment in combination with induction chemotherapy [73].

Baselga et al. [74] conducted the NeoALTTO trial in which 455 patients with HER2-positive primary breast cancer were randomly assigned to receive lapatinib plus paclitaxel (154 pts), versus trastuzumab plus paclitaxel (149 pts), versus concomitant lapatinib and trastuzumab plus paclitaxel (152 pts). The results showed that the pCR rate was 51.3 % (95 % Cl, 43.1–59.5) in the combination of lapatinib plus trastuzumab arm compared to 24.7 % (Cl, 18.1–32.3) for the lapatinib alone arm and 29.5 % (Cl 22.4–37 0.5) for the trastuzumab arm. This difference was statistically significant ($P=0.0001$), while the pCR rate difference between the lapatinib and trastuzumab arms was not [74]. An updated analysis performed by Piccart-Gebhart M et al. [75] demonstrated that patients achieving pCR had a better outcome compared with patients not achieving pCR. These studies confirm that the use of HER2-targeted therapy as induction therapy is important for HER2-positive breast cancer and that dual inhibition of HER2 might be a valid approach to induction treatment of HER2-positive breast cancer patients [74].

The National Comprehensive Cancer Network Panel (NCCN) [13] stated their view that regimens recommended in the adjuvant setting are also appropriate to be considered in the preoperative chemotherapy setting. In women with HER2-positive tumours treated with induction chemotherapy, the addition of induction trastuzumab to paclitaxel after FEC chemotherapy was associated with an increase in the pCR rate from 26 % to 65.2 % ($P=0.016$). Thus, the incorporation of trastuzumab into induction chemotherapy regimens appears important in HER2-positive tumours.

Pertuzumab is a recombinant humanised monoclonal antibody that targets the extracellular dimerisation domain (subdomain II) of HER2 and thus blocks ligand-dependent heterodimerisation of HER2 with other HER family members, including EGFR, HER3 and HER4. Pertuzumab inhibits ligand-initiated intracellular signalling through both mitogen-activated protein (MAP) kinase and phosphoinositide 3-kinase (PI3K) signalling pathways, resulting in cell growth arrest and apoptosis. Pertuzumab also mediates antibody-dependent cell-mediated cytotoxicity [76].

When administered together in HER2-positive tumour models and in humans, trastuzumab and pertuzumab provide a greater overall antitumour effect than pertuzumab as a single agent. This approach was developed in metastatic HER2-overexpressed breast cancer leading to significant OS benefit [76] and this fact enhanced use of this concept in adjuvant [77] and induction (neoadjuvant) therapy settings [78].

Two pivotal clinical studies have been performed with pertuzumab, trastuzumab and docetaxel in induction treatment for patients with HER-2 positive with operable (T2-3, N0-1), locally advanced (T2-3, N2 or N3, T4a-c, any N) or inflammatory (T4d, any N0) breast cancer and a primary tumour size >2 cm. The results with this combination in this setting resulted in an accelerated approval by the FDA. This accelerated approval was based on the results of the TRYPHAENA and NEOSPHERE trials. In the first trial, the highest pCR was observed in patients who received pertuzumab, trastuzumab, docetaxel and carboplatin chemotherapy (pCR: 66.2 %). Induction pertuzumab and trastuzumab, given concurrently or sequentially with an anthracycline-based or concurrently with a carboplatin-based chemotherapy regimen, result in a low incidence of LVSD [78].

In the second study, 417 previously untreated women, with HER2-positive breast cancer, were randomly assigned to four groups: group A (107 pts), four induction cycles of trastuzumab plus docetaxel; group B (107 pts), pertuzumab plus trastuzumab plus docetaxel; group C, pertuzumab and trastuzumab; and group D (96 pts), pertuzumab plus docetaxel.

Patients assigned to group B had a significantly improved pCR rate (45·8 % [95 % CI 36·1–55·7]) compared to group A (29·0 % [20·6–38·5]; $p=0.0141$) and to group D (24·0 % [15·8–33·7] and 16·8 % [10·3–25·3]) included in group C. The most common adverse events of grade ≥3 were neutropenia (57 %, 45 %, <1 %, 55 % in groups A, B, C, D, respectively), febrile neutropenia (8 %, 9 %, 0 % and 7 %, in A, B, C and D groups respectively) [77].

9.2.4 Induction Therapy in Patients with Triple-Negative Breast Cancer

Triple-negative (TNBC) tumours have been characterised by several aggressive clinicopathological features including onset at a younger age, higher mean tumour size, higher-grade tumours and, in some cases, a higher rate of node positivity. A histological study of basal-like tumours, of which all were ER/HER2-negative, illustrated marked increases in mitotic count, geographic necrosis, pushing borders of invasion and stromal lymphocytic response. The majority of TNBC carcinomas are ductal in origin; however, several other aggressive phenotypes appear to be over-represented, including metaplastic, atypical or typical medullary and adenoid cystic. It is important to clarify the relationship between TNBC and the basal-like phenotype. Triple negative is a term based on clinical assays for ER, PR and HER2, whereas basal-like is a molecular phenotype that was defined using cDNA microarrays. Although most TNBC do cluster within the basal-like subgroup, these terms are not synonymous and there is up to 30 % discordance between the two groups [79]. The term "basal-like" is used when microarray or more comprehensive immunohistochemical profiling methodology is employed and "triple negative" when the salient studies have relied on clinical assays for definition, this pathology accounts for 15 % of all breast cancer cases. TNBC is highly aggressive, with a high propensity for metastasis and a poor survival rate. Therefore, chemotherapy is the only systemic therapy available [26, 30] because endocrine and molecularly targeted therapies are inappropriate for patients with TNBC.

It is accepted that tumours which lack expression of hormone oestrogen and progesterone receptor and HER2 oncogene will respond well to chemotherapy. Evidence from accumulated induction studies revealed that pCR, defined as no residual disease present in both the breast and axilla, provides a surrogate marker that is predictive for long-term clinical response and survival in TNBC patients [80].

Huober et al. [81] reported a high pCR rate of 39 % in 509 patients with TNBC treated with TAC (docetaxel/doxorubicin/cyclophosphamide) or TAC-NX (docetaxel/doxorubicin/cyclophosphamide-vinorelbine/capecitabine). Di Leo et al. [82] suggested a beneficial outcome of anthracyclines compared with CMF therapy in terms of DFS in 294 patients with TNBC. However, recent studies cast doubt on the role of anthracyclines in early-stage TNBC [80].

An analysis conducted by von Minckwitz et al. concluded that for patients with TNBC in particular, treatment with higher cumulative doses of anthracyclines ($\geq$300 mg/m^2) and taxanes ($\geq$400 mg/m^2) provides higher pCR rates compared to with lower cumulative dose regimens [83].

Recently, the use of platinum agents has received renewed interest in the treatment of TNBC. The CALGB 40603 [84] study was performed in order to determine the impact of adding carboplatin and bevacizumab in the induction therapy. In this study, 443 patients received weekly paclitaxel (80 mg/m2) for 12 weeks followed by doxorubicin 60 mg/m2 and cyclophosphamide 600 mg/m2 once every 2 weeks with GCSF support (dose dense: ddAC) for four cycles. They were randomly assigned to receive weekly paclitaxel with or without concurrent carboplatin AUC 6 once every 3 weeks for four cycles and independently to treatment with or without fortnightly bevacizumab (10 mg/kg) for nine cycles during administration of weekly paclitaxel and the first three cycles of ddAC. Patients were examined every 2–3 weeks; patients experiencing progression during weekly paclitaxel administration were switched to ddAC, whereas progression while receiving ddAC resulted in early surgery. Carboplatin or bevacizumab combined with chemotherapy resulted to an increase of pCR rates. In fact, adding either agent significantly increased the pCR breast rate; 60 % of patients who received carboplatin achieved pCR breast compared with 46 % of those who did not (odds ratio [OR], 1.76; P 0.0018). Patients treated with a bevacizumab-containing regimen had a pCR breast rate of 59 % compared with 48 % of those who were not (OR, 1.58; P 0.0089). Patients assigned to both agents (arm four) had the highest pCR breast rate (67 %), with no significant interaction between their effects ($P=0.52$). A major limitation of this study was that it was not powered to demonstrate any difference on RFS and OS. Even in TNBC, demonstrating that a 13–14 % absolute increase in pCR rates (as seen with the addition of carboplatin) leads to significant improvements in long-term outcomes would require a study with many more patients included in order to answer this question [84].

The addition of induction carboplatin to a regimen of a taxane, an anthracycline and bevacizumab significantly increases, in TNBC patients, the rate of patients achieving a pCR. In the GeparSixto study [85], patients were treated for 18 weeks with weekly paclitaxel (80 mg/m^2) and weekly non-pegylated-liposomal doxorubicin (20 mg/m^2); HER2+ patient group concurrently received trastuzumab every 3 weeks and daily lapatinib. TNBC patients received concurrently bevacizumab (15 mg/kg i.v. q3w). Patients were randomised to receive concurrently weekly carboplatin ($n=295$ pts, AUC 1.5–2) or not ($n=299$). In the carboplatin group, 43·7 % achieved a pCR, compared with 36·9 % without carboplatin (odds ratio 1·33, 95 % CI 0·96–1·85; $p=0.107$). Meanwhile, among patients with triple-negative breast cancer, 53·2 % achieved a pCR with carboplatin, compared with 36·9 %, without ($p=0.005$). For patients with HER2-positive tumours, 32·8 % of patients treated with carboplatin achieved a pCR compared to 36·8 % without ($p=0.581$).

A meta-analysis realised on 11 studies by Xiao-Son Cheng indicated that novel induction schedules in TNBC patients have achieved a significant improvement of pCR rate, particularly among those treated with carboplatin ($p=0.001$)- or bevacizumab ($p=0.003$)-containing regimens. These results could help to design appropriate trials in the adjuvant setting. Moreover, adding carboplatin for TNBC results in an absolute benefit of 13.8 % compared with control arms [86]

Another meta-analysis involving eight studies ($n=1,349$ patients) revealed that the pCR rate in TNBC patients treated with a platinum-based regimen was significantly higher than that in those treated with a non-platinum-based regimen (49.2 % and 64.3 %, respectively). Meanwhile, DFS and OS were not significantly different in TNBC patients treated with a platinum-based regimen and those treated with a non-platinum-based regiment ($P>0.05$). These results suggest that future multicentre randomised controlled trials are required to validate these findings and to determine whether platinum-based chemotherapy particularly can extend the long-term outcomes (RFS, DFS and OS) of TNBC in BRCA 1/2-mutated patients [87].

Other drugs have been tested for TNBC as induction therapy. There are two phase II trials combining cetuximab or panitunumab, which have permitted the identification of biologically defined signatures predicting treatment impact.

Triple-negative breast cancer is a heterogeneous group of tumours for some of which the epithelial growth factor receptor (EGFR) pathway may play an important role. Nabholtz et al. [88] performed a clinical trial in which 60 patients were included and treated with panitumumab combined with FEC100 followed by docetaxel. The pCR rates according to Chevalier and Sataloff classifications were 46.8 % [95 % CI: 32.5–61.1 %] and 55.3 % [95 % CI: 41.1–69.5 %], respectively. This trial concluded that the combination of high EGFR and low cytokeratin 8/18 expression in tumour cells on one hand and high density of CD8+ tumour-infiltrating lymphocytes on the other hand was significantly predictive of pCR. Panitunumab in combination with FEC100 followed by docetaxel appeared to be efficient, with acceptable toxicity, as induction therapy of operable TNBC [88].

The development of poly (adenosine diphosphate [ADP]) ribose polymerase (PARP) inhibitors (PARPi) has progressed significantly and has shown encouraging results in the BRCA1/2 mutation-related cancers particularly in breast and ovarian cancers [89].

Breast cancer patients with BRCA1 mutations also display marked platinum sensitivity; treatment with induction cisplatin in such individuals results in high pathological complete response rates. The majority of breast cancers in BRCA mutation carriers are considered as TNBC. Non-*BRCA*-mutated TNBC appears to harbour a "BRCA*ness*" phenotype due to homologous recombination deficiency (HRD); responses to PARPi in this population are being investigated in a number of phase I and II trials [89].

Several PARPi molecules are under development in this field such as olaparib, veliparib, talazoparib, niraparib and rucaparib, as single or in combination with other targeted agents or chemotherapy. These studies will establish the role of the PARPi in the management of TNBC [90].

A three-arm, double-blinded, placebo-controlled phase III trial of veliparib (ABT-888) in TNBC with carboplatin and paclitaxel after induction chemotherapy (doxorubicin and cyclophosphamide) in early-stage TNBC is currently ongoing.

Mrozek E et al. [91] analysed the rate of pCR achieved by 33 women with HER2-negative (12 TNBC- and 21 HR-positive) breast cancer treated with induction nanoparticle albumin-bound paclitaxel (nab-P), carboplatin and bevacizumab. Six patients achieved pCR (6/33 pts: 18 %). All pCRs were seen in the subgroup of 12 pts with TNBC (50 % pCR). It is interesting observe that in this trial patients were followed by dynamic resonance imaging (DCE-MRI) in order to detect early changes in tumour vascularity and enhance conservative surgery in this setting [91].

9.2.5 Induction Therapy for Inflammatory Breast Cancer (IBC)

Inflammatory breast cancer is an aggressive form of locally advanced breast cancer. Inflammatory breast cancer is usually hormone receptor negative and is more frequently HER2 positive than the usual ductal breast cancers. The gene expression profiling of IBC has demonstrated that all the subtypes of IBC exist, but overexpressed and basal HER2 are relatively more frequent [13, 92].

Multimodality therapy, with systemic induction chemotherapy followed by locoregional therapy, has become the standard approach. However, the optimal chemotherapy regimen, including the sequence of agents and duration of treatment, is undefined because there are no large randomised trials evaluating the ideal systemic treatment. IBC is considered to be a rare disease and conventional anthracycline and taxane-based adjuvant chemotherapy regimens are widely used for induction chemotherapy. Results from a large retrospective study of patients with IBC performed over a 20-year period at the MD Anderson Cancer Center demonstrated that initial treatment with doxorubicin-based chemotherapy followed by local therapy (radiotherapy or mastectomy or both) and further postoperative chemotherapy resulted in a 15-year DFS rate of 28 % [93]. The addition of taxane to an anthracycline-based treatment improved PFS and OS in patients with ER-positive IBC. Kim et al. [94] in a systematic review found evidence for an association between the intensity of preoperative therapy and the probability to achieve a pCR [94]. Patients with axillary lymph node involvement receiving an anthracycline/taxane-based induction therapy have a greater probability of achieving a pCR compared those who received only anthracycline-based therapy; moreover patients who had pCR in the axillary lymph nodes had superior OS and DFS compared with those with residual axillary involvement [95].

All patients with hormone receptor-positive IBC are recommended to receive endocrine therapy sequentially after completing the planned preoperative systemic therapy [13].

For women with HER2-positive disease, the addition of trastuzumab to primary systemic chemotherapy is associated with better response rates. This recommendation was supported by a prospective study that randomised patients with locally advanced breast cancer, including those with IBC, to induction anthracycline-based chemotherapy with or without trastuzumab for 1 year. In this trial, the addition of trastuzumab significantly improved the response rate and event-free survival [68, 96].

The BEVERLY-2 phase II trial assessed the efficacy and safety of combining induction chemotherapy with bevacizumab and trastuzumab for the treatment of HER2-positive inflammatory breast cancer (IBC). All 52 patients accrued received fluorouracil, epirubicin, cyclophosphamide and bevacizumab (cycles 1–4) and docetaxel, trastuzumab and bevacizumab (cycles 5–8) before surgery, followed by trastuzumab and bevacizumab for 30 weeks after surgery. Circulating tumour cell (CTC) and endothelial cell (CEC) counts were assessed at baseline, cycle 5, preoperative, postoperative and 1 year. Encouraging results were obtained with this regimen. In fact, the 3-year DFS rate and OS were 68 % and 90 %, respectively. The centrally reviewed pCR rate was strongly associated with 3-year DFS [80 % and 53 % in patients with/without pCR, respectively $(P=0.03)$]. CTC detection independently predicted 3-year DFS (81 % vs. 43 % for patients with patients with <1 vs. >1 CTC/7.5 ml at baseline; $P=0.001$). Patients with no CTCs detected at baseline and achieving pCR had a high 3-year DFS (95 %). CEC had no prognostic value. The early haematogenous dissemination of cancer cells observed so far should be taken into consideration when evaluating prognosis in IBC [96].

9.2.6 Treatment Evaluation

Patients undergoing systemic induction treatment for breast cancer should have a periodic clinical evaluation during treatment to assess response and ensure that tumour is not progressing. There are no formal rules regarding the ideal assessment strategy during induction treatment. Nevertheless, it makes sense for patients under induction therapy to undergo a clinical examination prior to each cycle of treatment including the affected breast and ipsilateral axilla. In case of induction endocrine therapy, clinical assessments every 4–8 weeks are suitable considering that the response could be expected to take a longer time to be obvious.

Imaging studies (ultrasound or magnetic resonance imaging [MRI]) should only be performed if disease progression is suspected based on the clinical examination. Repeat biopsy of the index tumour during induction treatment is not justified unless it is as part of an assessment foreseen in a clinical trial protocol. Although repeat measurement for biologic factors (such as Ki-67) may identify patients who are unlikely to respond to induction endocrine therapy, validation of such tests is needed before repeat pathological assessment during treatment is incorporated into clinical practice [60]. One systematic review has documented the capacity of breast magnetic resonance imaging (MRI) staging to alter surgical treatment in 7.8–33.3 % of women but no differences in outcome were demonstrated in that analysis. Patients should not be denied the option of breast conservation therapy based upon MRI findings alone in the absence of tissue sampling. In the case of multicentric lesions post chemotherapy MRI, consideration should be given to obtain histological confirmation of these lesions before deciding to proceed with mastectomy [13, 97].

Limited data suggest that fluoro-2-deoxyglucose positron emission tomography (FDG-PET) may have a sensitivity and specificity as high as 80 %, but there are insufficient prospective data to evaluate the ability of FDG-PET to correctly predict response to induction therapy.

The randomised multicentre study AVATAXHER showed the importance of PET scan changes after the first cycle of chemotherapy plus bevacizumab and trastuzumab in early-stage HER2-positive patients. Adding bevacizumab to docetaxel/trastuzumab as induction therapy in patients with low-likelihood pCR tumour predicted by PET-SUV increased the pCR rate from 24.0 % to 42.5 %. PET-SUV by selecting low responding tumours may be a useful tool for optimisation of induction chemotherapy [98]. Therefore, FDG-PET assessment should not be routinely performed outside of clinical trials.

Mghanga FP et al. [99] evaluated the diagnostic performance of fluorine-18 fluorodeoxyglucose positron emission tomography (FDG-PET) in monitoring the response of breast cancers to induction chemotherapy in 15 studies (745 patients). The results of this analysis suggest that FDG-PET has moderately high sensitivity and specificity in early detection of responders from non-responders and can be applied in the evaluation of breast cancer response to induction chemotherapy in patients with breast cancer. Nevertheless, no single diagnostic procedure is capable of accurately assessing the response to induction therapy; the combination of different imaging approaches is recommended [13, 100, 101].

9.2.7 Surgical Treatment

Surgical treatment after induction chemotherapy focuses on the management of the tumour itself and the axillary spread. It is important to consider that one of the purposes of induction chemotherapy is breast conservation with accurate disease staging allowing avoidance of a broad axillary dissection. The development of sentinel node biopsy provides a remarkable advantage for breast conservation after induction chemotherapy.

If the tumour responds to induction therapy, lumpectomy plus axillary lymph node dissection or sentinel lymph node procedure may be considered. If induction therapy results in non-response, progressive disease or lumpectomy are not possible, so mastectomy is considered with axillary staging. If a pre-chemotherapy sentinel lymph node procedure was performed and the sentinel lymph node was pathologically negative, then further axillary lymph node staging is not necessary. If a pre-chemotherapy sentinel lymph node procedure was performed and the sentinel lymph node was positive, then a level I/II axillary lymph node dissection should be performed [13].

In the case of an inoperable tumour that fails to respond or where response is insufficient after several courses of induction therapy, an alternative induction must be taken into consideration followed by local treatment using either radiotherapy or surgery or both.

Surgery should be followed by individualised chemotherapy such as taxanes if the full course of planned chemotherapy was not administered preoperatively, as well as breast and regional lymph node irradiation. The consensus of the NCCN is that there is no role for postoperative chemotherapy if a full course of standard chemotherapy has been completed preoperatively and endocrine therapy in women with ER- and/or PR-positive tumours.

Post-operative radiotherapy in patients who underwent surgery having received previous induction treatment must be decided based on pre-chemotherapy tumour features, irrespective of tumour response to preoperative systemic therapy. It is generally recommended that patients who have axillary nodal metastases receive radiotherapy to the chest wall and regional nodes after mastectomy or to breast and regional nodes after lumpectomy. Conversely, in patients with negative axillary nodes, radiotherapy is not typically recommended after mastectomy and is confined to the breast alone after lumpectomy [13, 102].

9.3 In Summary

Induction or neoadjuvant therapy refers to the systemic treatment of breast cancer preceding surgical therapy.

Such treatment is administered with the aim to downstage the primary tumour, to increase the likelihood of breast conservation and to abolish occult systemic metastases in order to improve survival and eventually to test the tumour's chemosensitivity. Induction therapy is administered with the objective to improve surgical outcomes in patients with breast cancer for whom a primary surgical approach is technically not feasible and for patients with operable breast cancer who desire breast conservation, but for whom either a mastectomy is required or a partial mastectomy would result in a poor cosmetic outcome.

Induction chemotherapy is suitable for patients with HER2-positive or TNBC (ER-negative, PR-negative and HER2-negative) who are most likely to have a good locoregional response to treatment, irrespective of the size of their breast cancer at presentation.

The most frequently recommended regimen for patients undergoing induction chemotherapy is the combination of an anthracycline (doxorubicin or epirubicin) + cyclophosphamide ± 5-FU followed by weekly paclitaxel. For patients who cannot receive anthracycline therapy, docetaxel in combination with cyclophosphamide is a good compromise.

The addition to induction treatment of HER2-directed therapy for patients whose tumours are HER2-positive is strongly advised. Currently, trastuzumab is largely used in this category of patients but recent data are available to suggest that pertuzumab in this setting improves long-term outcomes, including overall survival. The administration of both trastuzumab and pertuzumab increases the pCR rate compared to trastuzumab alone.

Chemotherapy rather than endocrine therapy in the induction therapy setting is usually suggested for patients with hormone receptor-positive, HER2-negative breast cancers. For patients with hormone receptor-positive, HER2-negative breast cancers who are not candidates for chemotherapy, endocrine therapy is reasonable with an aromatase inhibitor in post menopausal patients. For premenopausal women, not enough data is available about the benefits of this approach. The addition of carboplatin in the induction therapy of TNBC strongly increases the rate of pCR in this setting.

Patients receiving systemic induction therapy should be followed by clinical exam at regular intervals during treatment to ensure that disease is not progressing. At the end of treatment, the assessment of tumour response is important to help guide the surgical approach.

Acknowledgment   We recognise Dr Steve Johnson MD, PhD, and Madame Jennifer Tavassoli for their useful expertise and advice.

References

1. GLOBOCAN (IARC). Estimated breast cancer incidence world wide. Section of cancer Surveillance). 2012 globocan.iarc, updated in Mar 2015.

2. Ferlay J, Soerjomataram I, Dikshit R, et al. Cancer incidence and mortality worldwide: sources, methods and major patterns in GLOBOCAN 2012. Int J Cancer. 2015;135(5):359–86.

3. Ferlay J, Soerjomataram I, Ervik M, et al. GLOBOCAN 2012 v1.0, cancer incidence and mortality worldwide: IARC CancerBase No. 11 [internet]. Lyon: International Agency for Research on Cancer; 2013. Available from: http://globocan.iarc.fr, accessed in December 2013.

4. Ferlay J, Steliarova-Foucher E, Lortet-Tieulent J, et al. Cancer incidence and mortality patterns in Europe: estimates for 40 countries in 2012. Eur J Cancer. 2013;49:1374–403.

5. Malvezzi M, Bertuccio P, Levi F, et al. European cancer mortality predictions for the year 2012. Ann Oncol. 2012;23(4):1044–52.

6. Gil-Delgado MA, Delgado FM, Khayat D. In: Aigner KR, Stephens FO, editors. Induction systemic chemotherapy for breast cancer. Berlin: Springer; 2011. p. 127–37.

7. Berry DA, Cronin KA, Plevritis SK, et al. Effect of screening and adjuvant therapy on mortality from breast cancer. N Engl J Med. 2005;353(17):1784.

8. Nissen-Meyer R, Kjellgren K, Malmio K, et al. Surgical adjuvant chemotherapy: results of one short course with cyclophosphamide after mastectomy for breast cancer. Cancer. 1978;41:2088–98.

9. Mansour EG, Gray R, Shatila AH, et al. Efficacy of adjuvant chemotherapy in high-risk node negative breast cancer. N Engl J Med. 1989;320:485–90.

10. Early Breast Cancer Trialists' Collaborative Group. Effects of adjuvant tamoxifen and cytotoxic therapy on mortality in early breast cancer: an overview of 61 randomized trials among 28,896 women. N Engl J Med. 1988;319:1681–92.

11. Early Breast Cancer Trialists' Collaborative Group and. Systemic treatment of early breast cancer by hormonal, cytotoxic, or immune therapy. 133 randomised trials involving 31,000 recurrences and 24,000 deaths among 75,000 women. Lancet. 1992;339:71–85.

12. Hortobagyi GN. Adjuvant systemic therapy for early breast cancer: progress and controversies. Clin Cancer Res. 2001;7:1839–42.

13. National Comprehensive Cancer Network (NCCN). NCCN clinical practice guideline in oncology: breast cancer.V2. 2015: www.nccn.org.

14. Jacquillat C, Weil M, Baillet F, et al. Results of neoadjuvant chemotherapy and radiation therapy in the breast-conserving treatment of 250 patients with all stages of infiltrative breast cancer. Cancer. 1990;66:119–29.

15. Veronesi U, Saccozzi R, del Vecchio M, et al. Comparing radical mastectomy with quadrantectomy, axillary dissection and radiotherapy in patients with small cancers of the breast. N Engl J Med. 1981;305:6–11.

16. Bonadonna G, Valagussa P. The contribution of medicine to the primary treatment of breast cancer. Cancer Res. 1988;48:2314–24.

17. Bonadonna G, Veronesi U, Brambilla C, et al. Primary chemotherapy to avoid mastectomy in tumors with diameters of three centimeters or more. J Natl Cancer Inst. 1990;82:1539–45.

18. Fisher B, Bryant J, Wolmark N, et al. Effect of preoperative chemotherapy on the outcome of women with operable breast cancer. J Clin Oncol. 1998;16:2672–85.

19. Kong X, Moran MS, Zhang N, et al. Meta-analysis confirms achieving pathological complete response after neoadjuvant chemotherapy predicts favourable prognosis for breast cancer patients. Eur J Cancer. 2011;47:2084–90.

20. Colleoni M, Montagna E. Neoadjuvant therapy for ER-positive breast cancers. Ann Oncol. 2012;23(supplement 10):243–8.

21. Harris LN, Kaelin CM, Bellon JR, et al. Preoperative therapy for operable breast cancer. In: Harris JR, Lippman MC, Morrow M, editors. Diseases of the breast. 3rd ed. Philadelphia: Lippincott Williams and Wilkins; 2004. p. 929–43.

22. Buzdar AU. Preoperative chemotherapy treatment of breast cancer- a review. Cancer. 2007;110:2394–407.

23. Gralow JR, Burstein HJ, Wood W, et al. Preoperative therapy in invasive breast cancer: pathologic assessment and systematic therapy issues in operable disease. J Clin Oncol. 2008;26:814819.

24. Cristofanilli M, Gonzales-Angulo A, Sneige N, et al. Invasive lobular carcinoma classic type: response to primary chemotherapy and survival outcomes. J Clin Oncol. 2005;23:41–8.

25. Loibl S, Volz C, Mau C, et al. Response and prognosis after neoadjuvant chemotherapy in 1,051 patients with infiltrating lobular breast carcinoma. Breast Cancer Res Treat. 2014;144:153–1516.

26. Perou CM, Jeffrey SS, van de Rijn M, et al. Distinctive gene expression patterns in human mammary epithelial cells and breast cancer. Proc Natl Acad Sci U S A. 1999;96:9212–7.

27. Liu Z, Zhang XS, Zhang S. Breast tumor subgroups reveal diverse clinical prognostic power. Sci Rep. 2014;4:4002.

28. Hallett RM, Dvorkin-Gheva A, Bane A, et al. A gene signature for predicting outcome in patients with basal-like breast cancer. Sci Rep. 2012;2:227–35.

29. Prat A, Adamo B, Cheang MC, et al. Molecular characterization of basal-like and non-basal-like triple-negative breast cancer. Oncologist. 2013;18:123–33.

30. Rouzier R, Perou CM, Symmans WF, et al. Breast cancer molecular types respond differently to preoperative chemotherapy. Clin Cancer. 2005;11:5678–85.

31. Ignatiadis M, Singhal SK, Desmedt C, et al. Gene modules and response to neoadjuvant chemotherapy in breast cancer subtypes: a pooled analysis. J Clin Oncol. 2012;30:1996–2004.

32. van 't' Veer LJ. Gene expression profiling predicts clinical outcome of breast cancer. Nature. 2002;415:530–6.

33. Paik S, Shak S, Gong T, et al. A multigene assay to predict recurrence of tamoxifen-treated, node-negative breast cancer. N Engl J Med. 2004;351:2817–26.

34. Markopoulos C. Overview of the use of oncotype as additional treatment decision tool in early breast cancer. Expert Rev Anticancer Ther. 2013;2:179–94.

35. Bear HD, Anderson S, Smith RE, et al. Sequential preoperative or postoperative docetaxel added to preoperative doxorubicin plus cyclophosphamide for operable breast cancer: national surgical adjuvant breast and bowel project protocol B-27. J Clin Oncol. 2006;24(13):2019–27.

36. van der Hage JA, van de Velde CJ, Julien JP, et al. Preoperative chemotherapy in primary operable breast cancer: results from the European Organization for Research and Treatment of Cancer trial 10902. J Clin Oncol. 2001;19:4224–37.

37. von Minckwitz G, Kümmel S, Vogel P, et al. Intensified neoadjuvant chemotherapy in early-responding breast cancer: phase III randomized GeparTrio study. J Natl Cancer Inst. 2008;100:552–62.

38. von Minckwitz G, Blohmer JU, Costa DS. Response-guided neoadjuvant chemotherapy for breast cancer. J Clin Oncol. 2013;31(29):3623–30.

39. Heys SD, Hutcheon AW, Sarkar TK, et al. Neoadjuvant docetaxel in breast cancer: 3-year survival results for the Aberdeen trial. Clin Breast Cancer. 2002;3(S2):S69–74.

40. Valero V. The role of systemic treatment for patients with residual disease after neoadjuvant chemotherapy. In: ASCO educational book, American Society of clinical oncology. The role of systemic treatment for patients with residual disease after neoadjuvant chemotherapy. 2009.

41. Thomas E, Holmes FA, Smith TL, et al. The use of alternate, non-cross-resistant adjuvant chemotherapy on the basis of pathologic response to a neoadjuvant doxorubicin-based regimen in women with operable breast cancer: long-term results from a prospective randomized trial. J Clin Oncol. 2004;22(12):2294–302.

42. Alvarez R, Booser D, Cristofanilli M, et al. Phase 2 trial of primary systemic therapy with doxorubicin and docetaxel followed by surgery, radiotherapy, and adjuvant chemotherapy with cyclophosphamide, methotrexate, and 5-fluorouracil based on clinical and pathologic response in patients with stage. Cancer. 2010;116:1210–7.

43. Ellis LM, Hicklin DJ. VEGF-targeted therapy: mechanism of anti-tumor activity. Nat Rev. 2008;8:579–91.

44. Bear HD, Tang G, Rastogi P, et al. Bevacizumab added to neoadjuvant chemotherapy for breast cancer. N Engl J Med. 2012;366(4):310–20.

45. Von Minckwitz G, Eidtmann H, Rezai M, et al. Neoadjuvant chemotherapy and bevacizumab for HER2-negative breast cancer. N Engl J Med. 2012;366(4):299–309.
46. Huober J, Fasching PA, Hanusch C, et al. Neoadjuvant chemotherapy with paclitaxel and everolimus in breast cancer patients with non-responsive tumours to epirubicin/cyclophosphamide (EC) ± bevacizumab – results of the randomised GeparQuinto study (GBG 44). Eur J Cancer. 2013;49(10):2284–93.
47. Gerber B, Loibl S, Eidtmann H, et al. Neoadjuvant bevacizumab and anthracycline-taxane-based chemotherapy in 678 triple-negative primary breast cancers; results from the geparquinto study (GBG 44). Ann Oncol. 2013;24:2978–84.
48. Kansal KJ, Dominici SM, Tolaney S, et al. Neoadjuvant bevacizumab: surgical complications of mastectomy with or without reconstruction. Breast Cancer Res Treat. 2013;141:255–9.
49. Abrial C, Mouret-Reynier M-A, Curé H, et al. Neoadjuvant endocrine therapy in breast cancer. Breast. 2006;15:9–19.
50. Ellis MJ, Coop A, Singh B, et al. Letrozole is more effective neoadjuvant endocrine therapy than tamoxifen for ErbB-1- and/or ErbB-2-positive, estrogen receptor positive primary breast cancer: evidence from a phase III randomized trial. J Clin Oncol. 2001;19:3808–16.
51. Smith IE, Dowsett M, Ebbs SR, et al. Neoadjuvant treatment of postmenopausal breast cancer with anastrozole, tamoxifen, or both in combination: the Immediate Preoperative Anastrozole, Tamoxifen, or Combined with Tamoxifen (IMPACT) multicenter double-blind randomized trial. J Clin Oncol. 2005;23:5108–16.
52. Dowsett M, Smith IE, Ebbs SR, et al. Short-term changes in Ki-67 during neoadjuvant treatment of primary breast cancer with anastrozole or tamoxifen alone or combined correlate with recurrence-free survival. Clin Cancer Res. 2005;11:951s–8.
53. Colleoni M, Bagnardi V, Rotmensz N, et al. Increasing steroid hormone receptors expression defines breast cancer subtypes non responsive to preoperative chemotherapy. Breast Cancer Res Treat. 2009;116:359–69.
54. Mouridsen H, Gershanovich M, Sun Y, et al. Superior efficacy of letrozole versus tamoxifen as first-line therapy for postmenopausal women with advanced breast cancer: results of a phase III study of the International Letrozole Breast Cancer Group. J Clin Oncol. 2001;19:2598–606.
55. Dowsett M, Cuzick J, Ingle J, et al. Meta-analysis of breast cancer outcomes in adjuvant trials of aromatase inhibitors versus tamoxifen. J Clin Oncol. 2010;28:509–18.
56. Eiermann W, Paepke S, Appfelstaedt J, et al. Preoperative treatment of postmenopausal breast cancer patients with letrozole: a randomized double-blind multicenter study. Ann Oncol. 2001;12:1527–32.
57. Cataliotti L, Buzdar AU, Noguchi S, et al. Comparison of anastrozole versus tamoxifen as preoperative therapy in postmenopausal women with hormone receptor-positive breast cancer: the Pre-Operative 'Arimidex' Compared to Tamoxifen (PROACT) trial. Cancer. 2006;106:2095–103.
58. Seo JH, Kim YH, Kim JS, et al. Meta-analysis of pre-operative aromatase inhibitor versus tamoxifen in postmenopausal woman with hormone receptor-positive breast cancer. Cancer Chemother Pharmacol. 2009;63:261–6.
59. Semiglazov V, Kletsel A, Semiglazov V, et al. Exemestane (E) vs tamoxifen (T) as neoadjuvant endocrine therapy for postmenopausal women with ER+ breast cancer (T2N1-2, T3N0-1, T4N0M0). J Clin Oncol. 2005;23:16S (Abstract 530).
60. Ellis ME, Suman VJ, Hoog J, et al. Randomized phase II neoadjuvant comparison between letrozole, anastrozole, and exemestane for postmenopausal women with estrogen receptor-rich stage 2 to 3 breast cancer: clinical and biomarker outcomes and predictive value of the baseline. PAM50-based intrinsic subtype. ACOSOG Z1031: s.n. J Clin Oncol. 2011;29:2342–9.
61. Miller WR. Aromatase inhibitors: prediction of response and nature of resistance. Expert Opin Pharmacother. 2010;11:1873–87.
62. Crowder RJ, Phommaly C, Tao Y, et al. PIK3CA and PIK3CB inhibition produce synthetic lethality when combined with estrogen deprivation in estrogen receptor- positive breast cancer. Cancer Res. 2009;6:3955–62.

63. Aiderus AAB, Dunbier AK. Aromatase inhibition resistance via non-endocrine signalling pathways; a, larionow in resistance to aromatase inhibitors in breast cancer. London: Springer; 2015. p. 169–90.

64. Baselga J, Semiglazov V, van Dam P, et al. Phase II randomized study of neoadjuvant everolimus plus letrozole compared with placebo plus letrozole in patients with estrogen receptor-positive breast cancer. J Clin Oncol. 2009;27:2630–7.

65. Masuda T, Sagara Y, Kinoshita T, et al. Neoadjuvant anastrozole versus tamoxifen in patients receiving goserelin for premenopausal breast cancer (STAGE): a double-blind, randomised phase 3 trial. Lancet Oncol. 2012;13:345–52.

66. Zardavas D, Piccart M. Neoadjuvant therapy for breast cancer. Annu Rev Med. 2015;66:19.1–19.18.

67. Buzdar A, Ibrahim NK, Francis D, et al. Significantly higher pathologic complete remission rate after neoadjuvant therapy with trastuzumab, paclitaxel, and epirubicin chemotherapy: results of a randomized trial in human epidermal growth factor receptor 2–positive operable breast cancer. J Clin Oncol. 2005;16:3676–85.

68. Gianni L, Eiermann W, Semiglazov V, et al. Neoadjuvant chemotherapy with trastuzumab followed by adjuvant trastuzumab versus neoadjuvant chemotherapy alone, in patients with HER2-positive locally advanced breast cancer (the NOAH trial): a randomised controlled superiority trial with a parallel HER2- negative cohort. Lancet. 2010;375:377–84.

69. Pierga J-Y, Delaloge S, Espie' M, et al. A multicenter randomized phase II study of sequential epirubicin/cyclophosphamide followed by docetaxel with or without celecoxib or trastuzumab according to HER2 status, as primary chemotherapy. For localized invasive breast cancer patients. Breast Cancer Res Treat. 2010;122(2):429–37.

70. Steger GG, Greil R, Lang A, et al. Epirubicin and docetaxel with or without capecitabine as neoadjuvant treatment for early breast cancer: final results of a randomized phase III study (ABCSG-24). Ann Oncol. 2014;25(2):366–71.

71. Buzdar AU, Suman VJ, Meric-Bernstam F, et al. Fluorouracil, epirubicin, and cyclophosphamide (FEC-75) followed by paclitaxel plus trastuzumab versus paclitaxel plus trastuzumab followed by FEC- 75 plus trastuzumab as neoadjuvant treatment. For patients with HER2-positive breast cancer (Z1041): a randomised, controlled, phase 3 trial. Lancet Oncol. 2013;14(13):1317–25.

72. Kaufman B, Trudeau M, Awada A, et al. Lapatinib monotherapy in patients with HER2-overexpressing relapsed or refractory inflammatory breast cancer: final results and survival of the expanded HER2+ cohort in EGF103009, a phase II study. Lancet Oncol. 2009;10:581–8.

73. Untch M, Loibl S, Bisochoff J, et al. Lapatinib versus trastuzumab in combination with neoadjuvant anthracycline-taxane-based chemotherapy (GeparQuinto, GBG 44): a randomised phase 3 trial. Lancet Oncol. 2012;13(2):135–44.

74. Baselga J, Brandbury I, Eidtmann H, et al. Lapatinib with trastuzumab for HER2-positive early breast cancer (NeoALTTO): a randomised, open-label, multicentre, phase 3 trial. Lancet. 2012;379(9816):633–40.

75. Piccart-Gebhart M, Holmes A, de Azambuja E, et al. The association between event-free survival and pathological complete response to neoadjuvant lapatinib, trastuzumab or their combination in HER2-positive breast cancer. Survival follow-up analysis of NeoALTTO study (BIG 106). San Antonio Breast Cancer Symposium, S101. 2013.

76. Baselga J, Cortés J, Kim S-B, et al. Pertuzumab plus trastuzumab plus docetaxel for metastatic breast cancer. N Eng Med. 2012;368:109–19.

77. Swain SM, Baselga J, Kim S-B, et al. Pertuzumab, trastuzumab, and docetaxel in HER2-positive metastatic breast cancer. N Engl J Med. 2015;372:724–34.

78. Schneeweiss A, Chia S, Hickish T, et al. Pertuzumab plus trastuzumab in combination with standard neoadjuvant anthracycline containing and anthracycline-free chemotherapy regimens in patients with HER2-positive early breast cancer: a randomized phase II cardiac safety study (TRYPHAENA). Ann Oncol. 2013;24:2278–84.

79. Cleere DW. Triple-negative breast cancer: a clinical update. Community Oncol. 2011;7:203–11.

80. von Minkwitz G, Martin M. Neoadjuvant treatments for triple-negative breast Cancer (TNBC). Ann Oncol. 2012;23 suppl 6:vi35–9.
81. Huober J, von Minckwitz G, Denkert C, et al. Effect of neoadjuvant anthracyclinetaxane-based chemotherapy in different biological breast cancer phenotypes: overall results from the GeparTrio study. Breast Cancer Res Treat. 2010;124:133–40.
82. Di Leo A, Gancberg D, Larsimont D, et al. HER-2 amplification and topoisomerase II alpha gene aberrations as predictive markers in node-positive breast cancer patients randomly treated either with an anthracycline-based therapy or with cyclophosphamide, methotrexate, and 5-fluorouracil. Clin Cancer Res. 2008;8:1107–16.
83. von Minckwitz G, Untch M, Nuesch E, et al. Impact of treatment characteristics on response of different breast cancer phenotypes: pooled analysis of the German neo-adjuvant chemotherapy trials. Breast Cancer Res Treat. 2011;125:145–56.
84. Sikov WM, Berry DA, Perou CM, et al. Impact of the addition of carboplatin and/or bevacizumab to neoadjuvant once-per-week paclitaxel followed by dose-dense doxorubicin and cyclophosphamide on pathologic complete response rates in stage II to III. Triple-negative breast cancer: CALGB 40603 (alliance). J Clin Oncol. 2015;33:13–21.
85. von Minckwitz G, Schneeweiss A, Loibl S, et al. Neoadjuvant carboplatin in patients with triple-negative and HER2-positive early breast cancer (GeparSixto; GBG 66): a randomised phase 2 trial. Lancet Oncol. 2014;15:747–56.
86. Chen X-S, Yuan Y, Garfield DH, et al. Both carboplatin and bevacizumab improve pathological complete remission rate in neoadjuvant treatment of triple negative breast cancer: a meta-analysis. PLoS ONE. 2014;9(9):e108405.
87. Tian M, Zhong Y, Zhou F, et al. Platinum-based therapy for triple-negative breast cancer treatment: a meta-analysis. Mol Clin Oncol. 2015;3:720–4.
88. Nabholtz JM, Abrial C, Mouret-Reynier MA, et al. Multicentric neoadjuvant phase II study of panitumumab combined with an anthracycline/taxane-based chemotherapy in operable triple-negative breast cancer: identification of biologically defined signatures predicting treatment impact. Ann Oncol. 2014;25:1570–7.
89. Benafif S, Hall M. An update on PARP inhibitors for the treatment of cancer. Oncol Targets Ther. 2015;8:519–28.
90. BreastCancerTrials. Breast cancer trials. https://www.breastcancertrials.org/bct_nation/home.seam.
91. Mrózek E, Layman R, Ramaswamy B, et al. Phase II trial of neoadjuvant weekly nanoparticle albumin-bound paclitaxel, carboplatin, and biweekly bevacizumab therapy in women with clinical stage II or III HER2-negative breast cancer. Clin Breast Cancer. 2014;14(4):228–34.
92. Dawood S, Cristofanilli M. What progress have made in managing inflammatory breast cancer? Oncology. 2007;21:673–9.
93. Ueno NT, Buzdar AU, Singletary SE, et al. Combined-modality treatment of inflammatory breast carcinoma: twenty years of experience at M.D. Anderson Cancer Center. Cancer Chemother Pharmacol. 1997;40:321–9.
94. Kim T, Lau J, Erban J. Lack of uniform diagnostic for inflammatory breast cancer limits interpretation of treatment outcomes: systematic review. Clin Breast Cancer. 2006;7:386–95.
95. Hennessy BT, Gonzalez-Angulo AM, Hortobagyi GN, et al. Disease-free and overall survival after pathologic complete disease remission of cytologically proven inflammatory breast carcinoma axillary lymph node metastases after systemic chemotherapy. Cancer. 2006;106:1000–6.
96. Pierga JY, Thierry P, Levy C, et al. Pathological response and circulating tumour cell count identifies treated HER2+inflammatory breast cancer patients with excellent prognosis! BEVERLY 2 survival data. Clin Res. 2015;21:1298–303.
97. Lobbes M, Prevos R, Smidt M. Response monitoring of breast cancer patients receiving neoadjuvant chemotherapy using breast MRI a review of current knowledge. J Cancer Ther Res. 2012;1:34–43.
98. Coudert B, Pierga JY, Mouret-Reynier MA, et al. Use of [18F]-FDG PET to predict response to neoadjuvant trastuzumab and docetaxel in patients with HER2-positive breast cancer, and

addition of bevacizumab to neoadjuvant trastuzumab and docetaxel. In patients with HER2-positive breast cancer, and addition of bevacizumab to neoadjuvant trastuzumab and docetaxel in [18F]-FDG PET-predicted non-responders (AVATAXHER): an open-label, randomised phase 2 trial: s.n. Lancet Oncol. 2014;15:1493–502.

99. Maghanga FP, Lan X, Hassan K, et al. Fluorine-18 fluorodeoxyglucose positron emission tomography–computed tomography in monitoring the response of breast cancer to neoadjuvant chemotherapy: a meta–analysis. Clin Breast Cancer. 2013;13:271–9.

100. Graham LJ, Shupe MP, Schneble EJ, et al. Current approaches and challenges in monitoring treatment responses in breast cancer. J Cancer. 2014;5:58–68.

101. Cheng X, Li Y, Liu B, et al. 18F-FDG PET/CT and PET for evaluation of pathological response to neoadjuvant chemotherapy in breast cancer: a meta-analysis. Acta Radiol. 2012;53:615–27.

102. White J, Mamounas E. Locoregional radiotherapy in patients with breast cancer responding to neoadjuvant chemotherapy: a paradigm for treatment individualization. J Clin Oncol. 2014;32:494–5.

Patients with Locally Advanced Breast Cancer Receiving Intra-arterial Induction Chemotherapy: Report of a Phase II Clinical Study

10

Giammaria Fiorentini, Camillo Aliberti, Paolo Coschiera, Virginia Casadei, Luca Mulazzani, Anna Maria Baldelli, Andrea Mambrini, and David Rossi

10.1 Introduction

Breast cancer is the second leading cause of cancer deaths in women today (after lung cancer) and is the most common cancer among women, excluding nonmelanoma skin cancers. According to the American Cancer Society, about 1.3 million women will be diagnosed with breast cancer annually worldwide and about 465,000 will die from the disease. Locally advanced breast cancer constitutes approximately 15 % of the newly diagnosed breast cancers [1] and up to 75 % of breast cancers in developing countries [1].

The modern treatment approach of breast cancer has changed during the past two decades. Conservative surgery is the first treatment to have been changed. Radical axillary dissection has been replaced by removal of sentinel lymph node in the first attempt. Radiotherapy maintained its presence in combination therapies for destruction of potentially axillary lymph node metastases or for prevention of local

G. Fiorentini, MD (✉)
Oncology Unit, Departments of Oncology-Hematology, Azienda Ospedaliera Ospedali Riuniti Marche Nord, via C.Lombroso 1, Pesaro 61121, Italy
e-mail: g.fiorentini@ospedalesansalvatore.it

C. Aliberti
Department of Radiology, Istituto Oncologico Veneto-IRCCS, Padova, Italy

P. Coschiera • L. Mulazzani
Departments of Radiology, Azienda Ospedaliera Ospedali Riuniti Marche Nord, Pesaro, Italy

V. Casadei • A.M. Baldelli • D. Rossi
Departments of Oncology-Hematology, Azienda Ospedaliera Ospedali Riuniti Marche Nord, Pesaro, Italy

A. Mambrini
Department of Oncology, General Hospital, Carrara, Italy

© Springer-Verlag Berlin Heidelberg 2016
K.R. Aigner, F.O. Stephens (eds.), *Induction Chemotherapy,*
DOI 10.1007/978-3-319-28773-7_10

recurrences. More importance is given to multidisciplinary management of the disease with the combination of adjuvant chemotherapy, endocrine therapy, and new drug directed on biomolecular target as trastuzumab [2–4]. Today many antineoplastic drugs are active and used in induction, adjuvant, and palliative settings [2, 3]. Combination chemotherapy regimens are frequently favored over single agents for the treatment of metastatic breast cancer, in an attempt to achieve superior tumor response rates [4].

Doxorubicin and mitoxantrone are among the most active drugs in treating advanced breast cancer, with single-agent response rates from 35 to 50 % [5, 6]. These drugs have been efficaciously used as IAC [9, 10, 17–24] because of the high response rates of these drugs have been adopted as the basis for several combination chemotherapy regimens. The most commonly administered combinations are fluorouracil, doxorubicin, and cyclophosphamide given intravenously, which yielded responses in 40–70 % of the patients [2, 4]. In Europe doxorubicin has often been replaced by epirubicin and mitoxantrone without loss of effectiveness and with low toxicity. Anthracycline- or mitoxantrone-containing regimens have not prolonged survival in patients with metastatic breast cancer because only 16 % can be rendered free of detectable disease and the median duration of response is short [1–6]. It is not known however whether giving more intensive chemotherapy regimens results in better health outcomes, when both survival and toxicity are considered, and whether better response rates and rates of progression-free survival actually translate to better overall survival [4, 5].

Many patients LABC suffering have large tumors without evidence of distant metastases at presentation. LABC is defined as T3 (tumors larger than 5 cm), T4 (chest wall invasion and/or skin), primary tumor and N2 (with fixed axillary nodes), and N3 (internal mammary) node metastasis [7].

Conventionally, these patients would receive systemic neoadjuvant chemotherapy followed by mastectomy, but it is frequent that some months are lost waiting for surgery. Moreover systemic toxicity remains high with significant risks of cardiotoxicity [3], and the local recurrence rate after surgical therapeutic procedures rates up to 30 % [6].

Regional chemotherapy is a well-known and attractive approach even if it is under evaluated method of treating locally advanced breast cancer [8–15, 26–28].

Lately, IAC is being increasingly used especially in Asia, thus representing an alternative method for the local treatment of breast cancer [17–24]. Regional chemotherapy aims at delivering higher than systemic doses of chemotherapeutic agents to the tumor by first-order targeting, directly perfusing the tumor mass via its arterial supply. Recently some authors developed methods to reduce the arterial flow or developed positioning of implantable infusion ports [19, 29, 30]. For IAC to be effective, the tumor-bearing tissue must be perfused directly by the chosen vessel for infusion. The effectiveness of the method depends on the location and the arterial supply of the tumor. Angiographically guided placement of the catheters into the internal mammary artery (IMA) and the lateral thoracic artery (LTA) should eliminate unwanted perfusion to the arm, shoulder, and neck [8–13]. Alternatively, the subclavian artery may be utilized in cases with inconclusive arteriograms and, although it may be less effective in terms of tumor response, it still offers considerable advantages when compared to systemic chemotherapy [29, 30].

Due to lacking conclusive remarks and to never-ending interest, we carried out a phase II clinical study to assess the efficacy of induction IAC with epirubicin and mitoxantrone in terms of local response, feasibility and safety of IAC, time to surgery, pathological response of the tumor, time to progression, and overall survival.

10.2 Patients and Methods

The study was conducted in compliance with the protocol and the principles laid down in the Declaration of Helsinki, in accordance with the ICH Harmonized Tripartite Guideline for good clinical practice (GCP). Ethical committee approval was obtained before starting the study. Informed consent was obtained from each participant prior to evaluation, screening, and treatment. The study was initiated to apply the criteria for appraisal of the quality of a study. We present a well-reported patient population with high-quality data and quality control and with good clinically significant follow-up without loss of patients.

Eligibility criteria included histologically confirmed carcinoma of the breast, a life expectancy of more than 3 months, WHO performance status <2, measurable disease, adequate bone marrow (absolute neutrophil count >1.500/ml, platelet count >100,000 and hemoglobin >11 g/dL), renal and liver function (total bilirubin and creatinine <1.25 times the upper normal limit), and a normal cardiac function, as demonstrated by ECG and left ventricular ejection fraction (LVEF) measurement. Previous chemotherapy with cyclophosphamide, methotrexate, fluorouracil, or taxanes regimen was accepted, but an interval of 1 month since the end of therapy should have elapsed; prior hormonal therapy or radiotherapy must have been discontinued for at least 4 weeks before protocol entry. No other concomitant anticancer treatment was allowed. All patients gave their informed consent to participate in the trial. The patients' characteristics are listed in Table 10.1.

10.3 Treatment

In all cases, IAC was performed in the angio-suite under aseptic conditions. According to standard Seldinger technique, after the administration of local anesthesia, a 6 F 11 cm long sheath was inserted percutaneously into the femoral artery, and subsequently an arteriogram of the subclavian, internal mammary, and lateral thoracic arteries was obtained initially in all patients. The internal mammary artery (IMA) was catheterized by the use of a 5 F IMA catheter (H1 Cordis, Johnson & Johnson Medical Spa, Milan, Italy) together with a hydrophilic guidewire (Terumo, Japan). When arterial catheterization was technically demanding due to its origin from a tortuous right subclavian artery, the 5 F catheter was exchanged for a 6 F IMA catheter and, alternatively, a 7 F 80–100 cm long sheath was inserted with its tip positioned to the IMA ostium in order to support the catheter-guidewire

Table 10.1 Patient characteristics

No. of patients	72
Age, years median	64
Range	44–75
WHO performances status	
Median	1
Range	0–3
Hormonal receptor status	
Positive	44
Negative or unknown	28
Hercept test	
Positive	12
Negative or unknown	60
Premenopausal	28
Postmenopausal	44
Prior radiotherapy	16
Prior chemotherapy	44
No previous therapy	12
Prior hormonal therapy	40
T3a	20
T3b	28
T4	24

combination during catheterization manipulations. After successful catheterization, the 5 F IMA catheter was exchanged for a hydrophilic 5 F Headhunter (Terumo, Japan), through which embolization was performed at the level of distal IMA and beyond the last branch to the breast with 0.035 platinum coils (Target, USA) 3–4 mm in diameter, when necessary. The embolization was to abolish unwanted perfusion of the anterior abdominal wall, at the same time achieving a higher concentration of chemotherapeutic agent to the distribution of the IMA within the breast. For inner quadrant tumors IMA usually is used, whereas for tumors of the outer quadrants the lateral thoracic artery, the subcapsular trunk, and occasionally the superior thoracic artery are usually used for IAC. Following IMA infusion, tumors involving the outer quadrants of the breast were selectively given chemotherapeutic agents via the lateral thoracic artery, the subscapular trunk, and occasionally the superior thoracic artery, provided there was no skin perfusion from these. If multiple smaller unnamed subclavian and axillary branches were identified, careful selection of one or two of the most suitable among them was adequate for effective lateral-breast perfusion. In the event that we were unable to catheterize one or more of the main arteries supplying the lateral aspect of the breast, only then were the chemotherapeutic agents infused selectively to the subclavian artery. During subclavian infusion, a brachial sphygmomanometer cuff was inflated to 10 mmHg above systolic blood pressure in order to prevent local toxicity to the ipsilateral arm. Prior to IAC, 2 ml of patent blue dye solution with 1 ml of xylocaine, 2 % was injected through the catheter into the internal mammary and lateral thoracic artery in order to confirm the vessels that supply the tumor area. IAC followed, via the appropriate route, using epirubicin 30 mg/mq diluted 1 mg/1 mL over 10 min and mitoxantrone 10 mg/mq diluted in 30 mL of normal saline over 10 min, with cycles repeated every 3 weeks. Antiemetic treatment consisted of an antiserotonin agent plus dexamethasone in a 15-min infusion before starting chemotherapy. Treatment was postponed by a maximum of 2 weeks if a local painful skin reaction appeared, the absolute neutrophil count was less than 1,500, or the platelet count was less than 100,000/μL. The chemotherapeutic agents were administered with the use of an infusion pump during an overall period of about 20 min. Each patient was submitted to three to six cycles.

Pretreatment evaluation included history and physical examination, automated blood cell count, biochemical profile, chest X-ray, liver ultrasound, bone scan, ECG, and resting LVEF determination by echocardiography or multigated radionuclide angiography scan. The blood count and biochemical profile were repeated every 3 weeks. All measurable parameters of disease were re-evaluated every cycle. Cardiac monitoring was performed at baseline and after the conclusion of the program. In case of a LVEF decrease more than 10 % and/or below the lower limits of normal, a repeat measurement in 3 months was required. Otherwise, during follow-up, cardiac toxicity was assessed only in case of clinical signs and symptoms of congestive heart failure (CHF).

Patients were evaluated for response to chemotherapy after every cycle of treatment. Responses were assessed by at least two observers. Tumor response was calculated using either mammography, contrast-enhanced spiral computed tomography (CT), or magnetic resonance imaging (MRI) with quantification of tumor response according to either response evaluation criteria in solid tumors (RECIST).

All adverse events were recorded per standards and terminology set forth by the cancer therapy evaluation program, common terminology criteria for adverse events, version 3.0.

Time to surgery and duration of response were measured from the initiation of treatment. Time to progression and survival were calculated starting from the date of the first IAC cycle to the date of disease progression or the date of death (or last follow-up evaluation), respectively.

The primary objective of this study was to estimate the overall response rate of the IAC regimen, the overall resectability of the breast, and the time to mastectomy. The Simon two-stage phase II design was used to determine the sample size. The regimen would be considered worthy of further testing if at least 20 out of 35 eligible patients had an objective response (60 %), with a significance level of 5 % and a power of 90 %. In the second stage, 37 additional patients would be needed, with an overall sample size of 72 eligible patients. The duration of response, time to progression, and overall survival were assessed using the Kaplan-Meier method for descriptive data, and comparisons were made using the k2 test.

10.4 Results

From October 1997 to March 2006, 109 patients were considered to entry in the study but only 72 out of them presented locally advanced breast cancer without evidence of clinical metastases. Follow-up has been closed in March 2011. Among the patients enrolled, 8 had T4 tumors (>13 cm tumor diameter) and 16 had T4 ulcerated tumors, 5 of which presented with complete disappearance of normal mammary gland tissue, 20 patients presented T3a, and 28 presented T3b tumors. Twenty-nine patients had two sessions of IAC chemotherapy; in 39 patients a third cycle had been administered, while for the remaining 4 patients a fourth session was delivered. No major technical difficulties or procedure-related complications were encountered during those 248 catheterizations. Analysis of the photographic record of the patent blue dye distribution showed that in 18 patients the breast tumor was not exclusively supplied by IMA alone, while in 14 patients the tumor was not adequately supplied by either IMA or LTA. In two patients, the arteriogram of the right subclavian artery showed that the origin of IMA was located just opposite the junction of the subclavian and right vertebral artery. Among 72 patients, we observed 6 (8.3 %) complete responses and 44 (61 %) partial remissions, while 22 patients did not present clear evidence of response (30.5 %) due to local progression (8 cases) or to systemic disease (14 cases). The application of IAC resulted in an overall response rate of 50 patients (70 %), thus making the operative removal of the breast feasible in 50 patients (70 %). No significant differences were seen in response rate according to estrogen receptor status, hercept test positivity, age, previous chemotherapy and response, and disease-free interval. The median number of cycles infused was 2.7 (range 1–4). The median time to response was 3 weeks after the first administration of drugs (range 1–7 weeks) without differences between complete response and partial response. The median time of disease-free survival without systemic progression was 13 months (range 5–34 months) (Fig. 10.1), and in 66 cases the metastatic site was 18 bones, 10 lungs, 14 livers, and 24 multiple, and median survival was 23 months (range. 9–39 months) (Fig. 10.2). Time to mastectomy was short: 9 weeks after completion

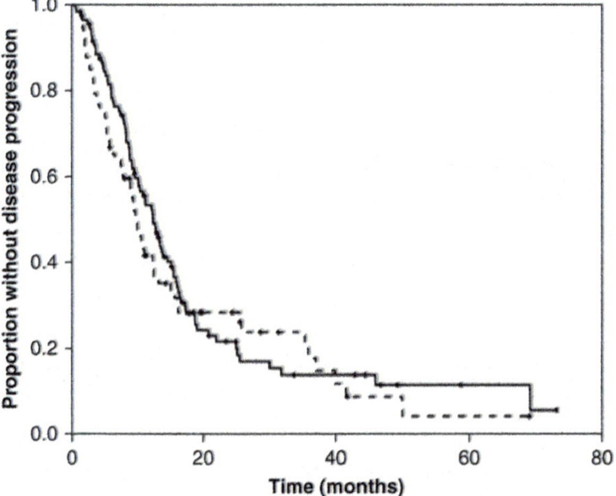

Fig. 10.1 Disease-free survival (T4 *dashed line*, T3a-b continued line)

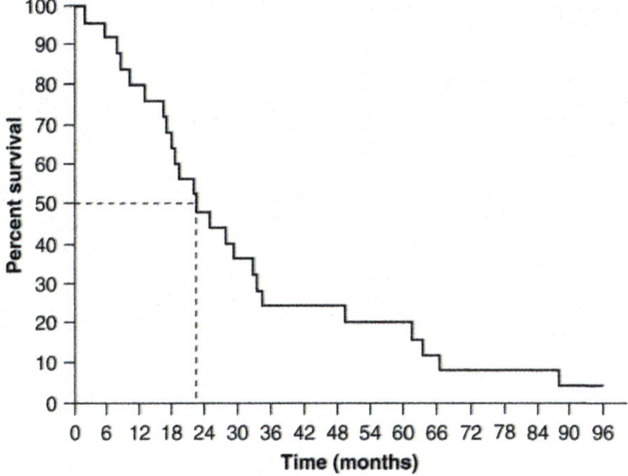

Fig. 10.2 Global survival

Table 10.2 Toxicity observed

Type of toxicity	Grade 1 (% of patients)	Grade 2 (% of patients)	Grade 3 (% of patients)
Thrombocytopenia	12	6	0
Anemia	8	4	0
Mucositis	16	10	0
Nausea/vomiting	12	6	6
Skin chemical burns	20	6	0
Neutropenia	12	6	0
Transient neurotoxicity	20	4	0
Pain in the site of injection	10	0	0
Myalgia	10	0	0
Cardiac toxicity	0	0	0
Hair loss	10	0	0

of IAC (range 3–14). The toxicity data are listed in Table 10.2. No patient required a dose reduction; however treatment was postponed in 20 patients because of delay of local pain or inflammatory skin reactions. Grade 1 nausea and vomiting was encountered in 12 % of the patients, 6 % of patients presented grade 2, and 6 % grade 3, respectively. Mucositis grade 1 and grade 2 was reported in 16 % and ten of patients. Grade 1 and Grade 2 transient peripheral neurotoxicity ipsilateral to the procedure was recorded in 15 (20 %) and 3 (4 %) of patients, respectively. Grade 1 local pain in the site of arterial injection and myalgia was observed in eight patients (10 %). There were no instances of CHF or grade 1–3 cardiotoxicity, even though two patients died of a sudden heart attack 3 years after mastectomy, with pulmonary and liver metastases. In all the specimens of resected tissue, necrosis of tumor (complete 6 cases, partial 32 cases, minimal 12 cases) and fibrosis (extended 33 cases, mild 17 cases) were observed.

10.5 Discussion

Cancer of the breast is considered to be a systemic disease, and therefore regional chemotherapy has been ranked as not justified, treating only the target. The problem arising, however, is that systemic chemotherapy, in case of a bulky primary tumor, can hardly generate adequate drug exposures required for tumor shrinkage. As others have shown, best long-term survival results have been achieved in patients whose primary tumor was completely eradicated, so the first objective in treating breast cancer should be total eradication of the primary cancer. IAC is not an isolated procedure confined exclusively to one well-defined segment of the body like surgery or irradiation. It is both regional and systemic therapy given with its first pass through the area to be treated first, which is the primary tumor in the breast and all its lymphatic drainages. The first pass through the arterial supply causes a concentration-dependent higher tissue uptake of drugs in the area to be treated, but also a systemic drug exposure from the drugs exiting the tumor area through the venous drainage. Anthracycline-containing combinations in locally advanced breast cancer or with systemic disease induce objective response rates in the range of 40–80 %, with median duration of response between 10 and 18 months and median survival between 18 and 24 months [2–6]. Responding patients usually experience short remissions and a low percentage of return to operability and, if this occurs, mastectomy is possible only after prolonged and toxic chemotherapy. Therefore, the need for new combinations and strategies such as induction IAC with active agents has become necessary. This approach appears to be particularly promising with high response rates, quick time to response, and short time to surgical approach [8–26] even in elderly patients [27]. IAC has become an attractive treatment for LABC in an attempt to gain better control of local disease in a short time, permitting removal of an otherwise unresectable tumor and minimizing the adverse effects of systemic chemotherapy [10–26]. Selective infusion of the anticancer drugs into arteries supplying the tumor-bearing tissue prevents chemotherapeutic-agent leakage to surrounding areas, allowing at the same time higher tissue-drug concentration [10–14]. There is growing evidence that selective intra-arterial infusion of chemotherapeutic agents seems more effective in local control when compared to systemic chemotherapy when the same doses are given intravenously. Takatsuka et al. reported a prospective randomized study of neoadjuvant chemotherapy on 73 patients with locally advanced breast cancer. Group A (n26) received no neoadjuvant therapy, group B (n22) received intra-arterial infusions of epirubicin, and group C (n25) received intravenous epirubicin. The regression of the primary tumor was significantly higher in group B than in group C (68.2 vs 36.0 %, $P < 0.05$). The postoperative survival of responders to neoadjuvant therapy was better than that of nonresponders. Side effects were milder in group B than in group C. There was, however, no difference among the three groups in terms of overall and disease-free survivals. Thus, neoadjuvant intra-arterial chemotherapy was effective for achieving loco-regional control of locally advanced breast cancer with a low toxicity, but could not improve survival [18]. Although no patient in our series presented with significant manifestations of systemic toxicity, local side effects in the perfused area were encountered in a significant number of patients, confirming the relatively high reported incidence of those complications [10–26]. Eight out of 72 (10 %,) patients presented with various degree skin chemical burns, a percentage that is absolutely comparable with the results reported by others [8–13]. Apart from the high tissue-drug levels achieved by IAC, one of the most important eliciting factors for local skin complications is the relatively high-infusion pressure under which these drugs are administered. This leads to an accumulation of drugs into the skin through the dilated anastomotic network between intrathoracic IMA, deeply located lateral arteries, and superficial skin vessels [9–13]. Indeed, to facilitate drug penetration into a tumoral mass, the intra-arterial pressure must exceed the interstitial tumor pressure, which is generally higher than that of the surrounded healthy tissue [10, 13, 24]. Although administration of drugs by a constant flow pump causes an initial increase of intra-arterial pressure, it maintains it stable throughout the infusion, thus eliminating further dilatation of skin capillaries and finally leading to a reduction of skin burns. Indeed, in all 20 patients who presented with skin chemical burns in our series, a bolus injection via a hand syringe instead of a constant flow pump was used, allowing fluctuations of intra-arterial pressure. It is generally accepted that the greater the selectivity of infusion, the lower the possibility of systemic side effects and the higher the concentration of drugs at the perfused area. Distal coil embolization of IMA has been described and used to prevent unwanted perfusion in areas other than the breast [8–15]. However, although 26 patients in our series had no distal coil embolization of their IMAs, thus allowing the chemotherapeutic agents to perfuse the upper half of their anterior abdominal wall via the superior epigastric arteries, none of them developed upper abdominal wall skin chemical burns or ulcerations in contrast with other's observations [10–15, 23–25]. Interestingly, when compared with the patients in whom coil embolization took place, there was the same response to the administration of anticancer drugs where tumor shrinkage is concerned. Distal coil embolization results in an increase in IMA intra-luminal pressure during the infusion of drugs solution, potentially producing a backflow toward the subclavian artery stem. Anticancer drugs may thus diffuse at neighboring areas perfused by that artery. This may be the reason for the development of neurological signs in six (16 %) of our patients soon after the administration of drugs. Indeed, in a preoperative arteriogram of one patient, the origin of IMA was found to be just opposite to the subclavian-right vertebral arteries junction. The presence of neurological signs could be explained by the reflux of chemotherapeutic agent solution from distally occluded IMA to the ipsilateral vertebral artery. We recommend a detailed interpretation of the arteriogram in breast cancer patients before coil embolization of distal IMA is employed. The main arteries used for selective infusion of anticancer drugs are IMA and LTA. However, it is well known that the vessels supplying the lateral aspect of the breast differ in anatomy, in contrast with IMA which has a remarkably constant angiographic appearance [8–15]. It is also known that there is a great variability between areas of breast perfused by an artery in different individuals [10–16]. This means that there might be areas in the breast that are hypoperfused or not perfused at all, even if drugs are infused through both the above main supplying arteries. Given the fact that skin perfusion adequately reflects perfusion of the underlying breast tissue, the use of patent blue dye injected through both arteries accurately shows the distribution of the vessels and their contribution to breast cancer-bearing tissue perfusion [9, 22, 24]. In 28 out of the 72 patients enrolled in our study, after injection of patent blue dye, breast tumor was found to be perfused by several arteries except IMA, while 1 patient's tumor was not adequately supplied by either IMA or LTA. In both instances, infusion of anticancer agents solely via IMA would result in treatment failure. Doughty et al. reported 28 patients with locally advanced breast cancer received four doses of regional chemotherapy via angiographically placed percutaneous catheters into the IMA and LTA. Patent blue dye was injected to outline the relative contribution to perfusion of each of these vessels. The IMA was found to perfuse 67 (range 20–95) percent of the breast and the LTA 15 (range 0–35) percent. In one-third of patients, the LTA did not contribute to breast perfusion, and a large area of the lateral aspect of the breast was perfused from a further branch of the subclavian or axillary artery. The blood supply to the breast is extremely variable and must be determined in each patient before delivering regional chemotherapy. We therefore strongly recommend a detailed mapping of the distribution of patent blue dye in the breast of all patients prior to infusion of the chemotherapeutic drugs. According to general practice [8–24], if the lateral aspect of the breast tumor was inadequately perfused via LTA or other main arterial stems, the subclavian artery was used for drug infusion, while a tourniquet was applied to protect the arm from unwanted perfusion. In our study, IAC has been proved to be effective in controlling local disease since six patients (9 %) presented complete tumor response and complete tissue necrosis histologically confirmed. In the Gorich et al. series, 20 % of the patients had no residual tumor identified after IAC [10]. Yet in contrast with our findings, a considerable proportion of patients in that series had tumor remission of less than 50 %. Although Murakami et al. [16] reported a 9 % complete clinical response in patients with primary locally advanced or recurrent breast cancer after IAC, the incidence of positive cancer in the resected margin after toilet mastectomy was reported to be as high as 67 %. Fourteen out of 39 patients (36 %) in the Gorich et al. series developed distant metastases within 18 months from IAC, and 9 died of systemic disease. Furthermore, although local control rates at 5 years after IAC were as high as 90 % in the Murakami et al. series, distant metastases were seen in a great proportion of patients either with primary cancer (44 %) or recurrent tumor (63 %). Since 66 patients in our series presented with metastasis during follow-up – 18 bones, 10 lungs, 14 livers, and 24 multiple – and median survival was 23 months (range. 9–39 months), it is evident that systemic spread of the disease may occur despite adequate local tumor control, as happens after radiotherapy or surgery. Several IAC-related complications have been described, most of which are minor [10–20]. Local dissection of IMA, groin hematoma, arterial thrombosis, and catheter dislodgment has been reported to be the most common of these complications, yet easy to treat percutaneously. Occasionally, the presence of advanced atheroma or arterial tortuosity may result in failure of selective catheterization as reported by McCarter et al. [11] and confirmed by our results. Six patients in our series had no distal coil embolization of their IMA because selective catheterization of the arteries was incomplete due to advanced atheromatosis. Infusion of chemotherapeutic agents via the subclavian artery combined with exclusion of blood flow to the arm by application of a tourniquet is an acceptable alternative. Pacetti et al. reported an interesting study in the elderly evaluating feasibility, toxicity, and local response rates of IAC in patients with LABC over 75 years. Ten patients were treated with the catheter tip placed into the internal mammary artery. In order to evaluate the vessels perfusing the tumor, blue dye solution was infused before drug administration. The patients received fluorouracil 750 mg/m^2, epirubicin 30 mg/m^2, and mitomycin 7 mg/m^2 by bolus infusion. All patients were evaluated for toxicity and response. Twenty-two cycles were administered. The toxicity was mild and did not influence the patients' quality of life. A response rate of 80 % (eight out of ten) was obtained, the median overall survival was 33.5 months, and no patient had local recurrence. They conclude that IAC is an effective and safe treatment for LABC in the elderly. Other authors report an interesting activity in T4 cancer comparable to our data. Chang et al. reported 11 patients with T4 breast cancer received IAC as the first step in multidisciplinary therapy. The IAC agents (epirubicin and mitomycin C) were delivered weekly in the outpatient department by bolus injection through an implantable port-catheter system. A modified technique of port-catheter system implantation was used. The precise localization of the catheter was dually confirmed by angiography and dye test. The effectiveness of the treatment was evaluated by clinical appearance, image study, and microscopic examination. A 91 % response rate was obtained, and the lesions were resectable in < or = 8 weeks. No obvious systemic toxicity resulted from the IAC. They showed that weekly IAC by bolus injection through a port-catheter system for treating locally advanced T4 breast cancer is feasible and efficacious [19]. Toda et al. to evaluate the effects of IAC for LABC examined the grade of histological responses of preoperative IAC on tumors at the time of operation and estimated the patients' prognoses for 19 years [31]. IAC was done preoperatively using timely epochal anticancer drugs on 105 patients with locally advanced (stage IIIa, IIIb) and metastatic (stage IV) breast cancer. The survival rate of the stage IIIb patients who showed a good histological response (grade IIb < or =) to IAC was 68.1 % for 5 years and 62.4 % for 10 years, respectively. This was in contrast to that of the patients classified as stage IIIb who showed a poor histological response (grade IIa > or =) to IAC. On the other hand, there was no significant difference in the survival rates between the stage IIIa and IV patients with good and poor histological responses to IAC. However, the findings showed that a good histological response to IAC reflected a prolonged survival, while the stage IIIb and IV patients acquired a "down clinical staging" by IAC. These results strongly suggest that IAC thus appears to be a useful modality in the multidisciplinary treatment of advanced breast cancer, especially for stage IIIb patients. Kitagawa et al. reported a study on seven patients with LABC (stage IIIb) underwent IAC for one to three times (mean, 1.7) until tumors became resectable. Anticancer drugs were injected into both the IMA and the distal subclavian arteries. There was no major complication related to the procedure. The mean tumor size was significantly decreased from 10.0 ± 3.9 to 5.1 ± 2.5 cm ($P = 0.0086$). Skin and muscle invasions were improved in two patients (28 %) and lymph nodes disappeared in one patient (14 %). In two patients (28 %), downstaging was achieved from stage IIIb to stage IIIa. All tumors turned into resectable, and mastectomy was performed with a mean period of 35 days (range 9–60 days) after IAC. Marked decrease in tumor size allowed one patient to receive breast-conserving surgery. There was no local recurrence in any patient. However, five patients (71 %) experienced distant metastases. The 3-year disease-free and overall survival were 0 % and 71.4 %, respectively. They conclude that IAC for LABC is useful in reducing tumor size and achieving downstaging in a relatively short period, leading to an expanded surgical indication [21]. Shimamoto et al. reported in 2011 a study to evaluate the efficacy and safety of redistributed subclavian arterial infusion chemotherapy (RESAIC). They have focused on the local response, quality of life (QOL), and complications; they also investigated factors that influence the local response of RESAIC. The subjects were patients with LABC whose tumors were resistant to standard systemic chemotherapy (at least more than two regimens), those who were physically unable to tolerate systemic chemotherapy, and patients with locally recurrent breast cancer. The registration period was between April 2006 and May 2009. A total of 24 cases in 22 patients (mean age 59.5 years, range 36–82 years) were entered in the study. The local response rate of RESAIC was 77.3 % (17/22). The QOL score showed improvement on average. There were no serious complications during catheter port implantation, and there was hematological toxicity over grade 3 in 27.3 % (6/22) of patients. A significant difference between responders and nonresponders was seen in patients with a replaced-type tumor (on imaging, diffuse contrast enhancement was seen in whole quadrants) ($P=0.043$), and the patients underwent radiotherapy ($P=0.043$). They conclude that RESAIC is an effective, safe treatment for LABC [23]. Koyama reported a multidisciplinary treatment including intra-arterial infusion chemotherapy as an induction therapy was administered to 55 patients with locally advanced breast cancer. Intra-arterial chemotherapy conducted preoperatively produced marked responses in primary and lymph node lesions with 78 % complete + partial response (CR + PR), subsequently permitting extended radical mastectomy. Histologic examination of resected specimens also revealed that 33 % of the patients had no viable cancer cells remaining in their lesions. Five-year and 10-year survival rates were 57 % and 41 %, respectively, compared with 24 % and 18 %, respectively, for the 17 patients of historic control. Patients showing better local responses to intra-arterial chemotherapy had longer survival time with less frequent local recurrences. Intra-arterial chemotherapy is an effective modality for the treatment of locally advanced breast cancer [22]. Noguchi reported 28 patients with inflammatory breast cancer were treated with combined-modality therapy consisting of (1) IAC through the internal thoracic artery and subclavian artery, (2) surgical ablation, (3) extended radical mastectomy, and (4) adjuvant chemotherapy in that order. The IAC chemotherapy included adriamycin ($n=14$) and mitomycin plus 5-fluorouracil ($n=14$) was used. The response rate of the primary breast lesions to IAC chemotherapy was as high as 83 %, and complete necrosis of the tumor was histologically documented in 43 % of the cases. The median interval from the initiation of IAC to surgery was 7 weeks. Toxicity was acceptable and every patient completed the treatment. The 5- and 10-year disease-free survival rates were 59 % and 53 %, respectively. These results suggest that IAC is a very useful induction therapy for inflammatory breast cancer in terms of excellent local effects and the short time required for therapy before surgery [23]. De Dycker administered IAC with mitoxantrone to 18 patients with primary LABC of inflammatory or ulcerating type. Two patients had a bilateral carcinoma. Eight weeks after regional chemotherapy 18 of 20 tumors had become operable. Regression of tumor size by at least 50 % (checked by mammography) was achieved in seven patients. Axillary lymphadenectomy gave negative results in 6 of 17 patients. Conversion of the receptor status occurred in only 2 of 12 patients. There were only few side effects: alopecia in 20 %, leukopenia 18 %, thrombocytopenia in 7 % of patients. After a follow-up period of up to 28 months, local recurrence was noted in two, distant metastases in three cases. A totally disease-free period was achieved in 14 patients [24]. Bilbao reported 18 eligible patients (median age 50.5 years) with inflammatory breast carcinoma treated with neoadjuvant IAC. The treatment regimen includes cisplatin, adriamycin, mitomycin C, and thiotepa on day 1 and intravenous 5-fluorouracil on days 1 and 2. An objective clinical response rate of 100 % (eight complete and ten partial) has been observed. The median disease-free and overall survivals are 27 months (range 5–85+ months) and 33 months (range 8–85+ months), respectively. With a median follow-up of 21.5 months, 6 (33.3 %) patients remain alive and free of disease and 12 patients have died because of distant metastases. No local recurrences have been observed. IAC is an attractive technique for the treatment of LABC with mild toxicity and high local control rate [25]. We conclude that induction IAC with epirubicin and mitoxantrone seems to be a safe and well-tolerated method in the treatment of LABC, allowing excellent results in terms of quick local responses followed by mastectomy or conservative surgery. IAC can be an important tool, once the technique of application is well done and standardized, allowing tumor shrinkage within a short time and good quality of life. However, the presence of residual tumor in the axillary lymph nodes after IAC is a predictor of local recurrence, and patients with a better clinical response were also less likely to experience local disease recurrence. The size and degree of pathological response did not predict patients most likely to experience recurrence of disease.

References

1. Giordano SH. Update on locally advanced breast cancer. Oncologist. 2003;8(6):521–30.
2. Specht J, Gralow JR. Neoadjuvant chemotherapy for locally advanced breast cancer. Semin Radiat Oncol. 2009;19(4):222–8.
3. Bergh J, Jönsson PE, Glimelius B, Nygren P. A systematic overview of chemotherapy effects in breast cancer. Acta Oncol. 2001;40(2–3):253–81.
4. Carrick S, Parker S, Thornton CE, Ghersi D, Simes J, Wilcken N. Single agent versus combination chemotherapy for metastatic breast cancer. Cochrane Database Syst Rev. 2009;15(2):CD003372.

5. Heidemann E, Stoeger H, Souchon R, Hirschmann WD, Bodenstein H, Oberhoff C, Fischer JT, Schulze M, Clemens M, Andreesen R, Mahlke M, König M, Scharl A, Fehnle K, Kaufmann M. Is first-line single-agent mitoxantrone in the treatment of high-risk metastatic breast cancer patients as effective as combination chemotherapy? No difference in survival but higher quality of life were found in a multicenter randomized trial. Ann Oncol. 2002;13(11):1717–29.

6. Mathew J, Asgeirsson KS, Cheung KL, Chan S, Dahda A, Robertson JF. Neoadjuvant chemotherapy for locally advanced breast cancer: a review of the literature and future directions. Eur J Surg Oncol. 2009;35(2):113–22.

7. Singletary SE, Greene FL, Breast Task Force. Revision of breast cancer staging: the 6th edition of the TNM classification. Semin Surg Oncol. 2003;21(1):53–9.

8. Lewis WG, Walker VA, Ali HH, Sainsbury JR. Intra-arterial chemotherapy in patients with breast cancer: a feasibility study. Br J Cancer. 1995;71(3):605–10.

9. Stephens FO. Intra arterial induction chemotherapy in locally advanced stage III breast cancer. Cancer. 1990;66(4):645–50.

10. Gorich J, Hasan I, Majdali R, et al. Previously treated, locally recurrent breast cancer: treatment with superselective intra arterial chemotherapy. Radiology. 1995;197:199–203.

11. McCarter DHA, Doughty JC, Cooke TG, Mc Ardle CS, Reid AW. Angiographic embolization of the distal internal mammary artery as an adjunct to regional chemotherapy in inoperable breast carcinoma. JVIR. 1995;6:249–51.

12. Doughty JC, Anderson JH, Wilmutt N, Mc Ardle CS. Intra arterial administration of Adriamycin-loaded albumin microspheres for locally advanced breast cancer. Postgrad Med J. 1995;71:47–9.

13. Doughty JC, McCarter DH, Kane E, Reid AW, Cooke TG, McArdle CS. Anatomical basis of intra-arterial chemotherapy for patients with locally advanced breast cancer. Br J Surg. 1996;83(8):1128–30.

14. Cantore M, Fiorentini G, Cavazzini G, Molani L, Morandi C, Caforio M, Caleffi G, Mambrini A, Zamagni D, Smerieri F. Four years experience of primary intra-arterial chemotherapy (PIAC) for locally advanced and recurrent breast cancer. Minerva Chir. 1997;52(9):1077–82.

15. Mc Carter DHA, Doughty JC, Cooke TG, Mc Ardle CS, Reid AW. Selective angiographically delivered regional chemotherapy in patients with locally advanced or recurrent breast cancer: a feasibility study. JVIR. 1998;9:91–6.

16. Murakami M, Kuroda Y, Nishimura S, et al. Intra arterial infusion chemotherapy and radiotherapy with or without surgery for patients with locally advanced or recurrent breast cancer. Am J Clin Oncol. 2001;24(2):185–91.

17. Ichikawa W, Osanai T, Shimizu C, Uetake H, Iida S, Yamashita T, Nishi N, Togo S, Miyanaga T, Nihei Z, Sugihara K. Intra-arterial injection therapy of mitoxantrone for locally advanced breast cancer. Gan To Kagaku Ryoho. 1998;25(9):1333–5.

18. Takatsuka Y, Yayoi E, Kobayashi T, Aikawa T, Kotsuma Y. Neoadjuvant intra-arterial chemotherapy in locally advanced breast cancer: a prospective randomized study. Osaka Breast Cancer Study Group. Jpn J Clin Oncol. 1994;24(1):20–5.

19. Chang HT, Mok KT, Tzeng WS. Induction intraarterial chemotherapy for T4 breast cancer through an implantable port-catheter system. Am J Clin Oncol. 1997;20(5):493–9.

20. Yuyama Y, Yagihashi A, Hirata K, Ohmura T, Suzuki Y, Okamoto J, Yamada T, Okazaki Y, Watanabe Y, Okazaki A, Toda K, Okazaki M, Yajima T, Kameshima H, Araya J, Watanabe N. Neoadjuvant intra-arterial infusion chemotherapy combined with hormonal therapy for locally advanced breast cancer. Oncol Rep. 2000;7(4):797–801.

21. Kitagawa K, Yamakado K, Nakatsuka A, Tanaka N, Matsumura K, Takeda K, Kawarada Y. Preoperative transcatheter arterial infusion chemotherapy for locally advanced breast cancer (stage IIIb) for down-staging and increase of resectability. Eur J Radiol. 2002;43(1):31–6.

22. Koyama H, Nishizawa Y, Wada T, Kabuto T, Shiba E, Iwanaga T, Terasawa T, Wada A. Intra-arterial infusion chemotherapy as an induction therapy in multidisciplinary treatment for locally advanced breast cancer. A long-term follow-up study. Cancer. 1985;56(4):725–9.

23. Noguchi S, Miyauchi K, Nishizawa Y, Koyama H, Terasawa T. Management of inflammatory carcinoma of the breast with combined modality therapy including intraarterial infusion chemotherapy as an induction therapy. Long-term follow-up results of 28 patients. Cancer. 1988;61(8):1483–91.
24. de Dycker RP, Timmermann J, Neumann RL, Wever H, Schindler AE. Arterial regional chemotherapy of advanced breast cancer. Dtsch Med Wochenschr. 1988;113(31–32):1229–33.
25. Bilbao JI, Rebollo J, Longo JM, Mansilla F, Muñoz-Galindo L, Vieitez JM. Neoadjuvant intra-arterial chemotherapy in inflammatory carcinoma of the breast. Br J Radiol. 1992;65(771):248–51.
26. Fiorentini G, Tsetis D, Bernardeschi P, Varveris C, Rossi S, Kalogeraki A, Athanasakis E, Dentico P, Kanellos P, Biancalani M, Almarashdah S, Zacharioudakis G, Saridaki Z, Chalkiadakis G, Xynos E, Zoras O. First-line intra-arterial chemotherapy (IAC) with epirubicin and Mitoxantrone in locally advanced breast cancer. Anticancer Res. 2003;23:4339–46.
27. Pacetti P, Mambrini A, Paolucci R, Sanguinetti F, Palmieri B, Della Seta R, Muttini MP, Fiorentini G, Cantore M. Intra-arterial chemotherapy: a safe treatment for elderly patients with locally advanced breast cancer. In Vivo. 2006;20(6A):761–4.
28. Aigner KR, Gailhofer S, Selak E. Subclavian infusion as induction and adjuvant chemotherapy for breast conserving treatment of primary breast cancer. Cancer Ther. 2008;6:67–72.
29. Shimamoto H, Takizawa K, Ogawa Y, Yoshimatsu M, Yagihashi K, Okazaki H, Kanemaki Y, Nakajima Y, Ohta T, Ogata H, Fukuda M. Clinical efficacy and value of redistributed subclavian arterial infusion chemotherapy for locally advanced breast cancer. Jpn J Radiol. 2011;29(4):236–43.
30. Takizawa K, Shimamoto H, Ogawa Y, Yoshimatsu M, Yagihashi K, Nakajima Y, Kitanosono T. Development of a new subclavian arterial infusion chemotherapy method for locally or recurrent advanced breast cancer using an implanted catheter-port system after redistribution of arterial tumor supply. Cardiovasc Intervent Radiol. 2009;32(5):1059–66.
31. Toda K, Hirata K, Sato T, Okazaki M, Asaishi K, Narimatsu E. Histological evaluation of the effects of intra-arterial chemotherapy for advanced breast cancer: a long-term follow up study with respect to the survival rate. Surg Today. 1998;28(5):509–16.

Regional Chemotherapy for Thoracic Wall Recurrence and Metastasized Breast Cancer

Karl Reinhard Aigner, Stefano Guadagni, and Giuseppe Zavattieri

11.1 Introduction

With breast cancer the treatment strategy has fundamentally changed over the last three decades. While in the past local radical surgical interventions were indicated, such as mastectomy and inclusion of the pectoralis major muscle, the treatment standards have changed increasingly from initially mastectomy alone toward breast-conserving measures. Radical surgical interventions are considered local overtreatment. Similarly, the primary axillary dissection was abandoned in favor of the initial diagnostic removal of the sentinel lymph node. After the breast cancer is potentially capable of metastasizing early and is thus considered a systemic disease, the endeavor in treatment protocols is primarily breast-conserving local tumor excision with removal of the sentinel lymph node rather than invasive procedures. Radiation therapy, however, is an integral part of combination treatments to destroy any microscopic axillary lymph node metastases or prevention of local recurrences on the thoracic wall. The range of indications of anti-hormonal therapy is clearly defined, as is induction and adjuvant chemotherapy. Nevertheless, breast cancer remains a tumor, in which local recurrences or distant metastases may occur at any given time – 2 months or 15 years and more after a guideline-based therapy. The patient's prognosis at the stage of metastasis is bleak in the medium to long term. For this reason quality of life must be assigned special significance under any therapeutic measures. For the treatment of tumor masses that are mainly localized at a defined region such as the thoracic wall, lung, or liver, which mainly or exclusively cause discomfort there or are

K.R. Aigner, MD (✉) G. Zavattieri
Department of Surgical Oncology, Medias Klinikum GmbH & Co KG,
Krankenhausstrasse 3a, Burghausen 84489, Germany
e-mail: info@prof-aigner.de; prof-aigner@medias-klinikum.de

S. Guadagni
Department of General Surgery, University Hospital of L'Aquila, L'Aquila, Italy

© Springer-Verlag Berlin Heidelberg 2016
K.R. Aigner, F.O. Stephens (eds.), *Induction Chemotherapy*,
DOI 10.1007/978-3-319-28773-7_11

life-threatening, regional treatment measures can be used. Their advantage is a faster onset of action with fewer side effects and better quality of life.

11.2 Thoracic Wall Recurrences

11.2.1 Indication

The indication of regional chemotherapy of thoracic wall recurrences depends on the pretreatment. If it has been more than 6–8 months since radiation therapy of the thoracic wall, local hypoperfusion of the area to be treated exists due to radiation fibrosis of the connective tissue. This can be clarified before treatment with intra-arterial blue dye. If the tumor area to be treated does not change color, no form of chemotherapy has any prospect of success, neither regional nor systemic. For regional chemotherapy of thoracic wall recurrences, two procedures may be used, depending on their local proliferation: arterial infusion via the subclavian artery and mammary artery or isolated thoracic perfusion.

11.2.2 Intra-arterial Infusion

11.2.2.1 Subclavian Artery Angiocatheter

Initial treatment is usually carried out by angiography with the Seldinger technique via the femoral artery. For arterial infusion of the thoracic wall including the axilla, the catheter tip is placed in the subclavian artery. If the thoracic wall recurrence is located exclusively in the supply area of the mammary artery, which can be clearly distinguished by the injection of indigo carmine blue in the same (see Fig. 11.3b), treatment can be carried out here. As micrometastasis outside the infusion area of the mammary artery can never ultimately be ruled out, a combination treatment of two arterial infusions via the mammary artery proved of value, followed by two infusions via the subclavian artery after repositioning the catheter tip. The treatment regimens adapted to the situation consist of a dose of 5-fluorouracil, mitomycin C, Adriamycin, and cisplatin. If chemoresistance occurs, a switch can be made to mitoxantrone, gemcitabine, or taxanes. The preferred arterial infusion times are 7–15 min. With arterial infusion of the mammary artery, attention should be paid in diluting the infusion volume of the chemotherapeutic agent sufficiently. Otherwise local damage will occur with infused skin and soft tissue in terms of the "drug streaming."

11.2.2.2 Subclavian Artery Jet Port Catheter

The *subclavian artery Jet Port catheter* consists of a plastic port with a silicone membrane and a polyurethane catheter of 0.6 mm inner and 1.05 mm outer diameter.[1] For fixation in the artery, the tip is olive shaped. The implantation occurs via a transverse incision lateral to the jugulum above the clavicle. After exposure and

---

[1] Jet Port all-round catheter PfM Cologne

lateral displacement of the jugular vein, the carotid artery is identified and the subclavian artery is snared dorsolaterally from it. The catheter tip is inserted end to side into the subclavian artery after the stab incision and fastened with a Prolene purse-string suture at the extravasally situated olive (Fig. 11.1). The fine catheter tip protrudes only 1–2 mm into the vessel lumen. As a thrombosis prophylaxis, the daily administration of aspirin over 2 months is sufficient. Jet Port Allround subclavian artery catheters are not regularly flushed, as this raises the risk of port chamber infection and catheter thrombosis. The advantage of the subclavian artery Jet Port catheter system is that the patient is mobile, in contrast to angiographic therapy.

11.2.3 Case Studies

11.2.3.1 Preoperative Irradiation

A patient with extensive thoracic wall recurrence, especially in the cranial area beyond the infusion zone of the mammary artery, had been treated postoperatively with systemic chemotherapy and local radiation. Six months after the radiotherapy, in response to a rapidly spreading local recurrence, regional chemotherapy was conducted as an infusion via an axillary implanted Jet Port Allround catheter with the catheter tip 1 cm behind the outlet of the subclavian artery. The progressive metastasis under systemic chemotherapy was strongly regressive under the regional arterial infusion. After three cycles there was complete clinical remission (Fig. 11.2).

11.2.3.2 Dose or Concentration-Response Behavior

Dose-response behavior applies to both antibiotic and cytostatic chemotherapy [1]. A clear example is provided by the case of local recurrence in the midline presternally after a mastectomy on the right. The intra-arterial infusion via the right

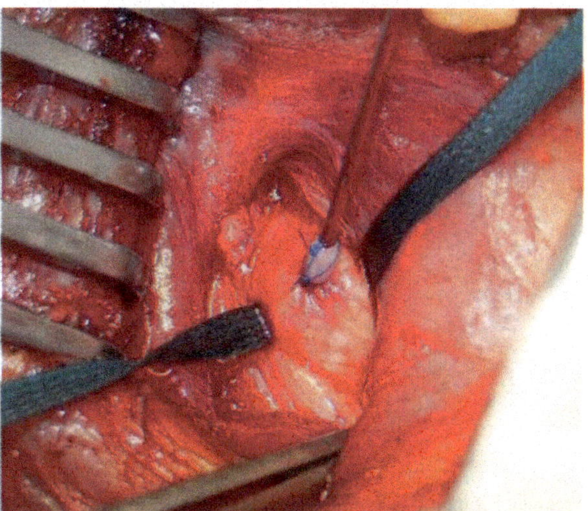

Fig. 11.1 End-to-side implantation of a Jet Port Allround catheter

subclavian artery led to complete remission of the right half of the tumor as a result of the increased flow concentration with the short-term infusion. The short arterial exposure time of 7–15 min with high concentrations of cytostatic agents is enough to create the concentrations of active ingredients required in the tumor tissue. In the venous reflow from the tumor area, the applied drug dose takes effect in the second circulation passage but diluted on both sides via both mammary arteries. The locally too low effective concentration is not sufficient here to cause remission in the left half of the tumor (Fig. 11.3). In this particular case, a complete response of the left tumor section was also induced after therapy via the left subclavian artery in the second cycle of therapy.

11.2.3.3 Recurrence After Lumpectomy

After local excision of a carcinoma measuring 23 mm in diameter between both lower quadrants, a massive recurrence appeared 1 year later, which covered almost half the volume of the right breast (Fig. 11.4a). The patient had refused any adjuvant therapy after the resection. In order to clarify the tumor perfusion, indigo carmine blue dye was injected through a mammary artery catheter inserted femorally using the Seldinger technique. In the process, the mammary artery supply area on the right including the entire

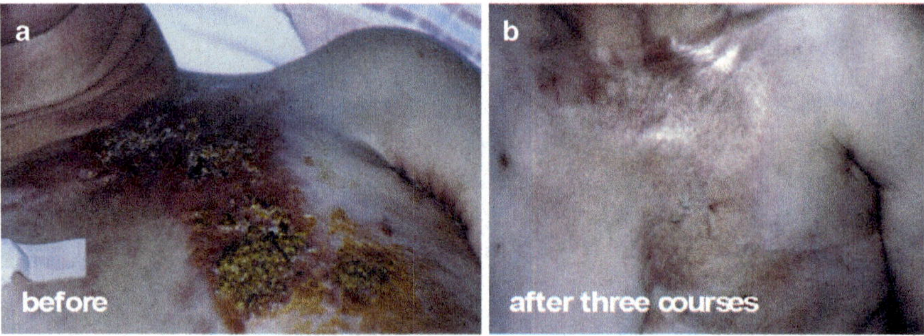

Fig. 11.2 (**a**) Thoracic wall recurrence after radiochemotherapy; (**b**) complete remission after three cycles of subclavian artery infusion with mitomycin C, Adriamycin, and cisplatin

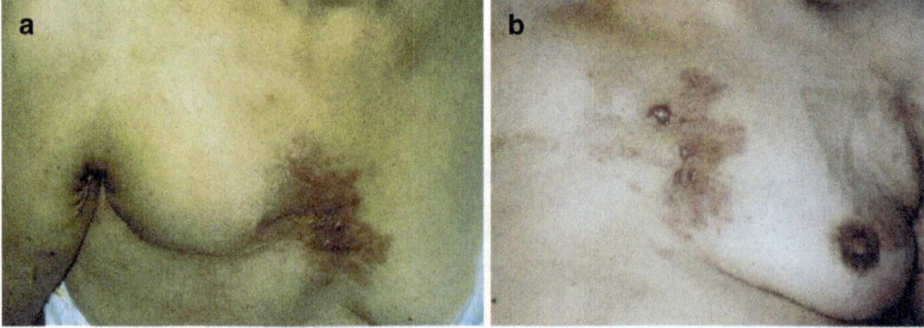

Fig. 11.3 (**a**) Presternal recurrence after mastectomy on the right; (**b**) complete remission of the right half of the tumor after arterial infusion of the right subclavian artery

tumor volume turned deep blue (Fig. 11.4b). The first cycle of intra-arterial therapy began with two infusions via the mammary artery (day 1, mitomycin; day 2, Adriamycin), and after repositioning the catheter tip to proximal just before the mammary artery outlet, it was completed with two short-term infusions of Adriamycin and cisplatin of 15 min each through the subclavian artery. After just the first cycle of therapy shrinkage of the tumor was observed, which had increased further after two cycles (Fig. 11.4c). Due to the positive response to the initial treatment, a Jet Port Allround catheter was implanted in the right subclavian artery for the second cycle. All the subsequent therapy cycles were administered through this. After six cycles there was complete clinical and histological response after excision of the old lumpectomy scar, which had become visible again. The entire infusion area of the subclavian artery showed a reddish brown hyperpigmentation in terms of a mild flow phenomenon (Fig. 11.4d).

11.2.4 Isolated Thoracic Perfusion

The indication for isolated thoracic perfusion is given when the metastasis pattern extends outside the supply area of the subclavian artery and mammary artery. The

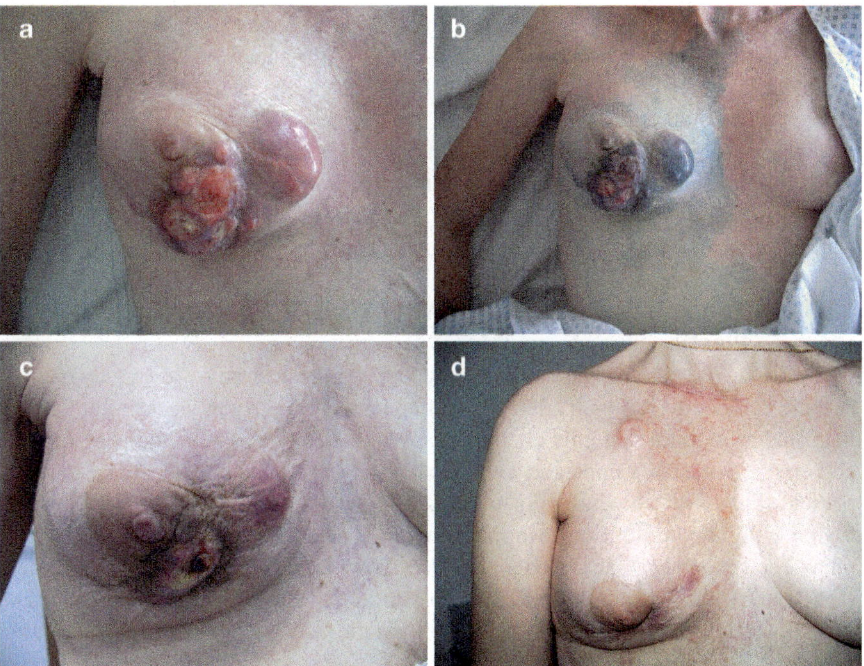

Fig. 11.4 (**a**) Tumor recurrence after lumpectomy; (**b**) indigo carmine blue staining of mammary artery supply area; (**c**) local findings after two therapy cycles; (**d**) clinical and histological complete remission after six cycles (on the anterior thoracic wall, hyperpigmentation is revealed in the arterial infusion area in terms of a mild streaming phenomenon)

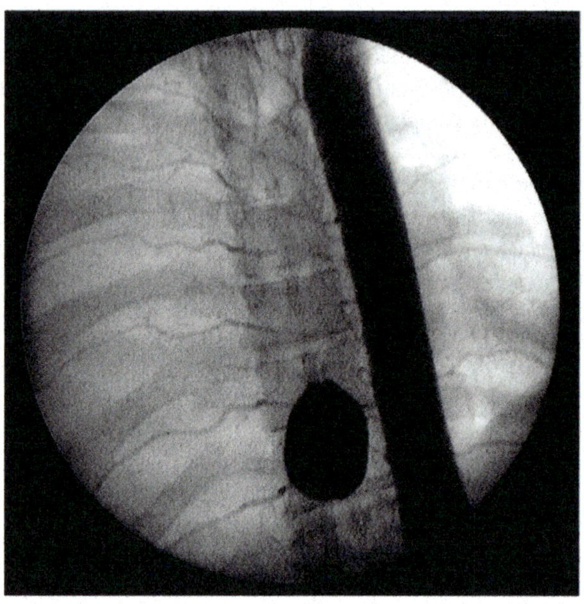

Fig. 11.5 Contrast agent injection through the central channel of the stop-flow balloon catheter after balloon blockage of the aorta. The intercostal arteries are presented with the vena cava balloon filled with contrast agent alongside

isolated thoracic perfusion technique with metastatic breast cancer is identical to the procedure with lung cancer [2]. After blocking the aorta and vena cava with balloon perfusion catheters at the diaphragm level and both upper arms with blood pressure cuffs, the chemotherapy is injected into the thoracic aorta via the central therapy channel of the perfusion catheter as a protracted bolus. This allows for an additional collective arterial infusion of the intercostal arteries, which supply the thoracic wall (Fig. 11.5). The high local exposure to cytostatic agents thereby achieved leads to very rapid remissions in zones not previously irradiated in the vast majority of cases.

11.2.4.1 Thoracic Wall Recurrence After Excision and Pedicle Flap Plastic

In a 40-year-old patient, a local recurrence after a mastectomy was largely excised and the defect covered with a latissimus flap (Fig. 11.6). Three weeks after the surgery under ongoing systemic chemotherapy with Taxol and gemcitabine, skin and soft tissue metastases appeared again on the lateral thoracic wall, adjacent to the pedicle skin soft tissue graft (Fig. 11.6a). After two cycles of isolated thoracic perfusion with chemofiltration using mitomycin C, Adriamycin, and cisplatin, complete remission was achieved 8 weeks after the initial perfusion treatment (Fig. 11.6b). Contralateral axillary lymph node metastases were significantly and palpably reduced within 2 weeks after the first thoracic perfusion. Four weeks after the second isolated perfusion, the control CT scan revealed a hypodense zone in terms of destruction of the metastases (Fig. 11.6c).

11.2.4.2 Major Local Recurrence with Thoracic Invasion

A 38-year-old patient with a gigantic, partly ulcerated tumor of the left breast, which had also infiltrated the left superior lobe of the lung and the pericardium, was

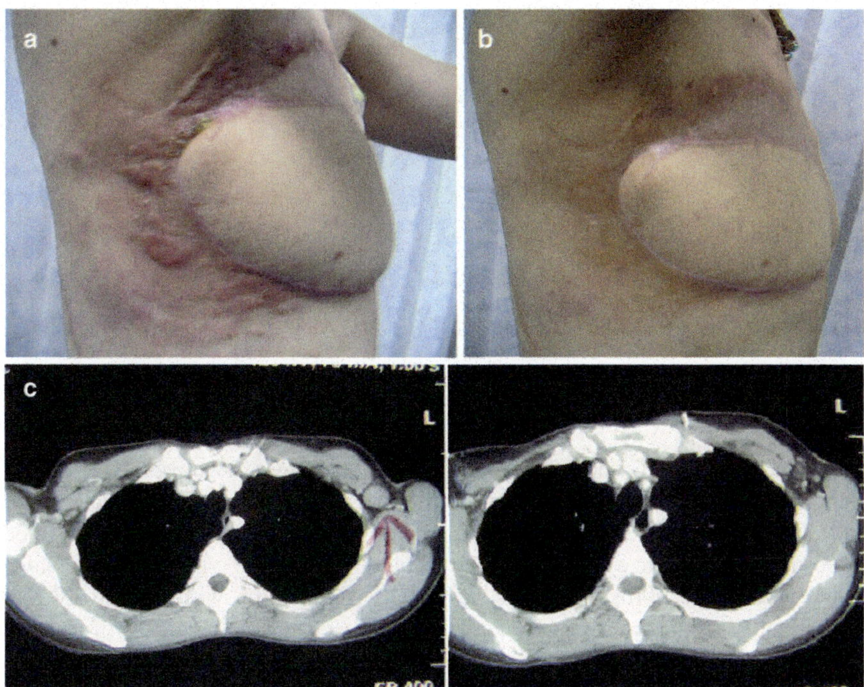

Fig. 11.6 (**a**) Progressive, early local recurrence after latissimus flap and systemic chemotherapy. Site 3 weeks after surgery with still encrusted upper wound edge; (**b**) site 8 weeks later, after two isolated thoracic perfusions; (**c**) CR on axillary lymph node metastases after isolated thoracic perfusion

treated as the only remaining option with isolated thoracic perfusion and chemofiltration. After just the first treatment, there was a clearly visible reduction in the tumor with local necroses. The patient had a high temperature in the first week following treatment every afternoon, which then improved again after the necrotic tissue had drained from the tumor. After the second and third thoracic perfusion at 4-week intervals, there was a continuous reduction in tumor size (Fig. 11.7). The residual tumor on the left axilla was chemoresistant, no longer responded to further perfusion treatment, and was excised locally. In the angiographic indigo carmine blue coloring, this part of the tumor showed hardly any contrast.

11.2.5 Responses and Prognosis

Most thoracic wall recurrences occur in the pre-irradiated area or have already been irradiated. In more than half of cases, there is further metastasis elsewhere, such as in the liver or bones. This is where local therapy is applied with a purely palliative intention, in order to minimize a tumor as quickly as possible, which is bleeding or painful due to nerve or nerve plexus irritation. This often succeeds in non-pre-irradiated findings within two to three isolated perfusions and especially (due

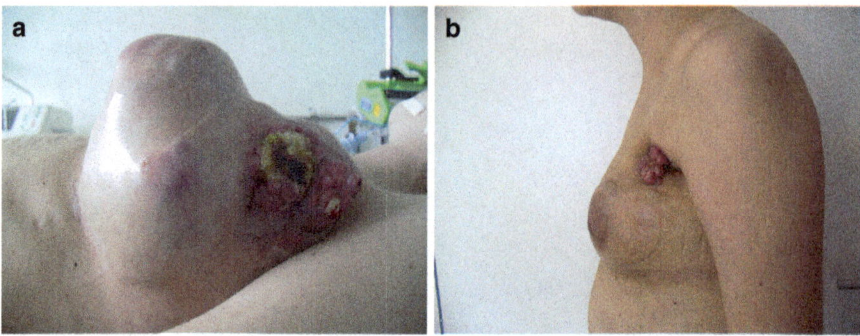

Fig. 11.7 (**a**) Gigantic breast cancer; (**b**) findings after three isolated thoracic perfusions

to the accompanying chemofiltration) without having a negative effect on the patients' quality of life. Large-scale pre-irradiated thoracic wall recurrences, however, also respond hardly or usually not at all to isolated perfusion, with intensified exposure to cytostatic agents due to the local hypoperfusion with radiation-related connective tissue fibrosis. Due to the palliative indication with intensively pre-treated and secondary metastatic patients, the survival time for 25 % of cases is 27 months, the median survival time only 15 months. If complete clinical remission can be achieved without visible and palpable skin and soft tissue infiltration and without regional lymph node metastases, the median period of remission is 11.8 months, after partial remission 6.7 months and after weak response or stable disease 4.4 months [3].

11.3   Toxicity and Side Effects

Hematological toxicity is not very pronounced. The leukocytes rarely fall below 1,000–1,200/m³, just as a clinically relevant thrombocytopenia below 60,000–100,000/µl occurs extremely rarely. The subjective condition is not or hardly impaired by the therapy due to chemofiltration. Less than 5 % of all patients complain about nausea. Due to the 15-min ischemia of the body parts below the diaphragm, a temporary elevation of liver enzymes occurs, but this returns to normal within 8 days. A temporary elevation of creatinine readings will also normally return to the normal range by the time of the second therapy after 4 weeks. In less than 1 % of cases do we observe a mitomycin-induced nephrotoxicity with long-lasting but usually also declining elevation in creatinine. With these patients mitomycin is no longer used.

The only side effect that occurs in 98 % of patients, despite the use of a cold cap during therapy, is alopecia. The stomatitis prophylaxis to prevent oral and mucosal toxicity by local application of an ice bag in the oral cavity, which is inserted right at the start of general anesthesia, prevents this complication entirely. The by far main complication after isolated thoracic perfusion is lymphatic fistula from the femoral cannulization area in the groin. This occurs with femoral access in 30–50 % of cases, while with parailiac access virtually never. Removing the Redon drainage prematurely may result in wound dehiscence and local infections with secondary wound healing. If the drainage is left in with strong lymph secretion for 14 days, there will be a consistent drainage channel, which normally closes up without complications within a few days. The posttreatment time in bed for safe assessment of primary wound healing is 4–5 days.

11.4 Response Criteria

Within the first five postoperative days, if the lesions respond to the therapy, an already measurable reduction in size and central softening of the metastases can be observed. With foci disseminated across the thoracic wall, central liquefaction and greasy deposits are often seen from day 3 to day 5. A decrease in the tumor marker CA 15-3 is observed continuously even after the therapy if the metastases respond. If spontaneous necrosis of a larger area occurs, this is expressed in an increase in the tumor marker by approx. 20 to 100 % and more, from the first and second day following surgery already, followed by a steep decline in the days after that.

11.5 Isolated Thoracic Perfusion with Lung Metastases of Breast Cancer

Lung metastases of breast cancer respond very sensitively to increased exposure to cytostatic agents as with isolated thoracic perfusion. The overall response rate is 71 %, of which 26 % is complete remission and 45 % partial remissions; 25 % of patients survive for 3 years. The median survival time is 20 months and as many as 75 % of patients are still alive after 13 months (Fig. 11.8). The median progression-free survival (PFS) is 14 months. If perfusion therapy is effective, with breast cancer this can normally be verified very quickly using imaging methods. Figure 11.9 shows disseminated lung metastases of breast cancer in both superior lobes of the lung before and 4 weeks after isolated thoracic perfusion. Even very large metastases of this tumor often show very rapid regression behavior. Figure 11.10 shows the complete disappearance of lung metastases after the third cycle of isolated thoracic perfusion (apart from one small residual defect in the left lower field).

11.6 Liver Metastases

Liver metastases occupy a special position in the spectrum of distant metastasis and are the localized metastases that threaten patients' lives most immediately. If they are centrally located in the liver hilum, this may result in a rapid occlusion of

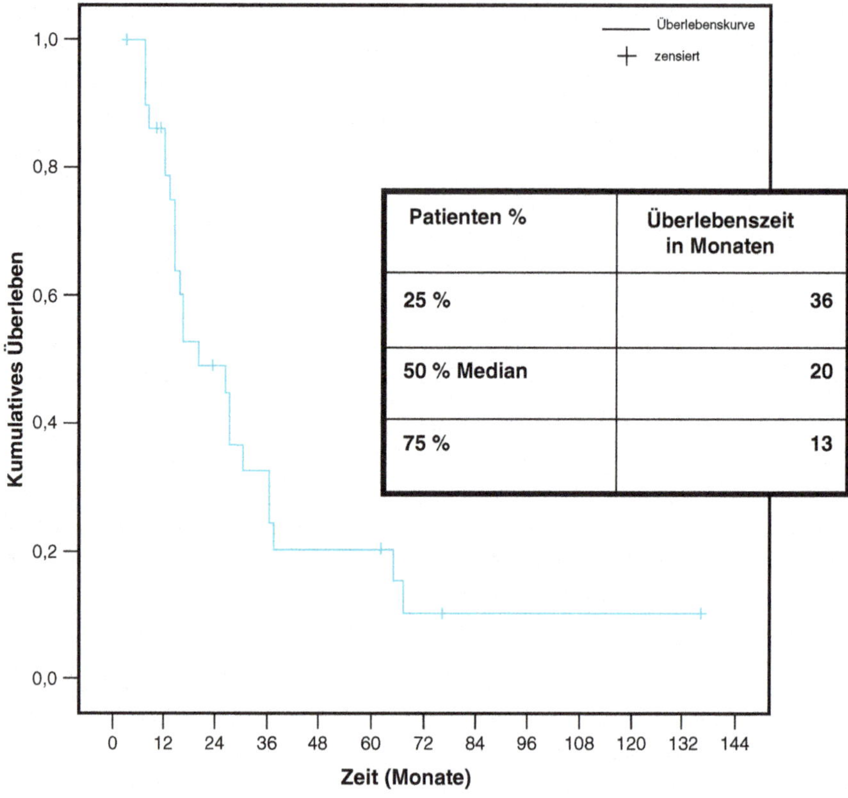

Patienten %	Überlebenszeit in Monaten
25 %	36
50 % Median	20
75 %	13

Fig. 11.8 Kaplan-Meier survival curve after ITP-F with lung metastases of breast cancer

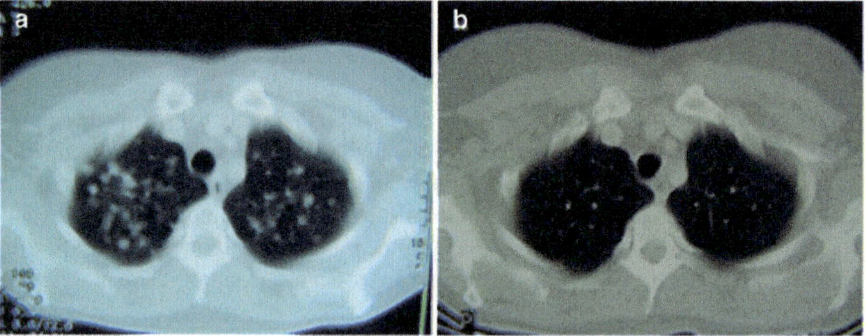

Fig. 11.9 Disseminated lung metastases of breast cancer before (**a**) and 4 weeks after ITP-F (**b**)

the main bile ducts. If they occur multiplied and disseminated, they cause diffuse stenoses and occlusions of small and medium bile ducts, which results in a progressive jaundice that no longer responds to treatment. The short-term prognosis is very poor.

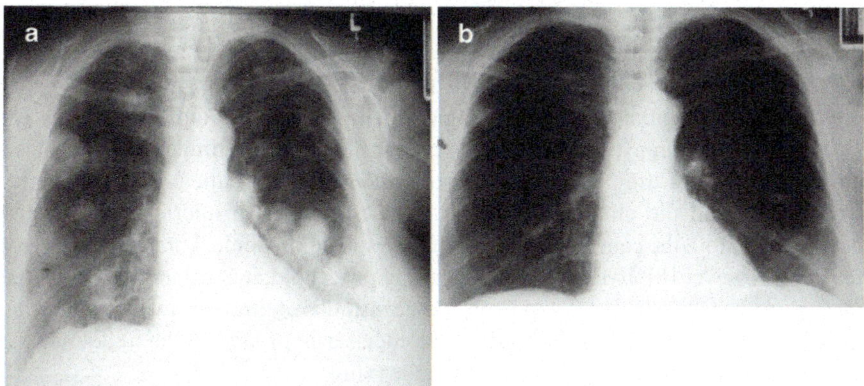

Fig. 11.10 Lung metastases on both sides before (**a**) and after three cycles of isolated thoracic perfusion with chemofiltration (**b**)

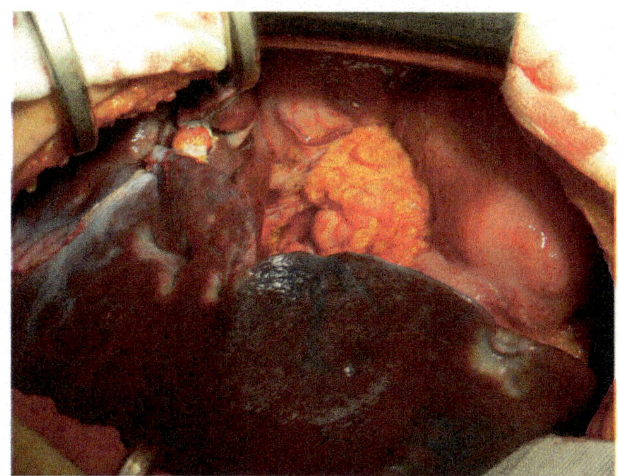

Fig. 11.11 Crater-shaped contractions in regressive liver metastases. Histology: complete remission following regional chemotherapy

After the breast cancer itself shrinks very rapidly in the event of a response to chemotherapy with sufficient exposure in contrast to some other tumor entities, this is an option to prevent the manifestation of bile congestion. The therapy is conducted using an angiographically positioned hepatic artery catheter, which is discussed elsewhere in this book [4, 5]. Alternatively the arterial infusion or chemoembolization can also be carried out via implanted port catheters. The rate of complete remissions is fairly constant at 25 %, as with thoracic wall recurrences or lung metastases. If complete remission is the result under regional chemotherapy with adequate application of cytostatic agents, deep transformed strangulation marks are formed in the connective tissue within two to four treatment cycles, instead of the former metastases in the liver tissue (Fig. 11.11). The median survival time for systemically pretreated patients with non-resectable metastases is 15.3 months and for non-pretreated patients 20.2 months.

11.7 Discussion

As soon as the breast cancer has exceeded the boundaries of the primary tumor site, the disease is potentially systemic. Logically, this means the indication given for systemic chemotherapy, as all the sites where the tumor has ultimately metastasized are unknown. If a drug were available that could be systemically administered, would tackle all the clinically manifest and still unknown micrometastases and destroy them too, the cancer problem would be solved. In clinical practice this is not feasible, however [6]. Even though the therapy takes hold, it does not destroy all the metastases because the local exposure – concentration × time – is insufficient. This is very clearly illustrated in the case of the metastasis located in the middle of the sternum and arterially supplied from two sides (Fig. 11.3).

A consequence of this is that the whole patient cannot be treated with the tumoricidal exposure required, as this would either lead to no longer tolerable side effects or would jeopardize the patient's life; the only alternative solution is to treat the patient "segmentally." In this case it is possible to generate sufficient exposure to cytostatic agents in relation to parts of the body such as the thorax, the liver, or the abdomen in order to achieve a sustainable tumor response in the particular area treated without major systemic side effects for the patient. In a study of 100 patients with breast cancer, it was possible to show that this escalation of the local intra-arterially administered cytostatic concentration leads to higher response rates [7]. This confirmed the statement by E. Frei III and G.P. Canellos, "Dose a critical factor in cancer chemotherapy" [8].

Carrying out randomized studies in the event of a critical involvement of organs or a part of the body is difficult, as most patients have already been pretreated multiple times and are committed to an alternative form of therapy. A randomized trial, which could clarify the issue of "regional or systemic chemotherapy?" is possible with non-pretreated patients, however. With regard to liver metastasis, the advantage of regional chemotherapy is its very rapid response and the high complete remission rate. If metastases that are centrally located or which obstruct the bile ducts are quickly shrunk or eliminated, this will have a life-prolonging effect.

With lung metastases the behavior is similar. If they respond to regional chemotherapy, this occurs almost exclusively within the first two to three cycles. Lung metastases in contrast to liver metastases, however, are not considered as imminently life-threatening so that even here the question of regional or systemic chemotherapy could be clarified with a randomized study.

Extended thoracic wall recurrences, if intensively pretreated, confound any further meaningful therapeutic measures. After frequent systemic chemotherapies, an insurmountable chemoresistance may have occurred, and after more than 6–8 months of previous radiation therapy, even highly concentrated regional chemotherapy is ineffective as a result of the connective tissue radiation fibrosis. On the other hand, extended, heroic surgical interventions can be carried out by including the ribs and/ or the entire sternum or part of it with technically complicated defect coverages [9–11]. This could even be regarded as overtreatment in view of the potentially systemic nature of breast cancer. No guarantee is given that no metastases will appear elsewhere after the intervention, similar to the clinical case in Fig. 11.6a.

The persistent question with thoracic wall recurrence or metastatic breast cancer continues to be, "How should we deal with it?" It is possible to treat the whole patient systemically. With the appropriate and properly dosed therapy regimens, comparable complete response rates of 25 % can certainly be achieved with regional chemotherapy. Xin Yao's study of docetaxel, doxorubicin, and cyclophosphamide [12] included only 20 patients, but as many as five of them had a histologically confirmed complete response. After the breast cancer responds similarly in all manifestations, primary tumor and metastases, also in contrast to some other tumors, such as pancreatic cancer, comparable results should be achievable with the appropriately adjusted systemic chemotherapy.

The argument in favor of regional chemotherapy in this context is the fact established at the beginning that the metastatic patient has limited life expectancy with a very poor prognosis. For this reason precisely every effort should be made in these cases to make her remaining lifetime as agreeable as possible. With high-dose or dose-intensive treatment regimens, high response rates can be achieved, as in the cited study with 25 % complete remissions. The only problem here is the systemic toxicity, for example, with febrile neutropenia in around one-third of cases or even hand-foot syndrome, which is very restrictive to quality of life. The side effects under regional chemotherapy exceed WHO grade 1–2 extremely rarely and patients often hardly notice them. At this stage of the disease, surrogate parameters such as progression-free survival should also play only a subordinate role [13]. The therapeutic result to strive for is progression-free survival with good quality of life.

References

1. Aigner KR, Gailhofer S, Selak E. Subclavian artery infusion as induction and adjuvant chemotherapy for breast conserving treatment of primary breast cancer. Cancer Therapy Vol. 2008;6:67–72.
2. Aigner KR, Selak E. Isolated thoracic perfusion with chemofiltration (ITP-F) for advanced and pre-treated non-small-cell-lung cancer. In: Aigner KR, Stephens FO, editors. Induction chemotherapy. New York: Springer; 2011. p. 321–9.
3. Aigner KR, Müller H, Jansa J, Kalden M. Regional chemotherapy for locally recurrent breast cancer – a phase II study with mitomycin C, fluorouracil/folinic acid. In: Taguchi T, Aigner KR, editors. Mitomycin C in cancer chemotherapy today. Excerpta Medica; Tokyo, Japan. 1991. p. 17–26.
4. Arai Y. Interventional radiological procedures for port-catheter implantation. In: Aigner KR et al. editors. Induction chemotherapy. Berlin: Springer; 2011. p. 221–36.
5. Loberg C. Transarterial treatment of primary and secondary liver tumors. In: Aigner KR et al. editors. Induction chemotherapy – systemic and locoregional. Berlin: Springer; 2011.
6. Aigner KR, Gailhofer S, Selak E, Jansa J. Das metastasierte Mammakarzinom – State of the Art. Pharma Fokus Gynäkologie, 5. Jahrg. 2010.
7. Aigner KR. Regional chemotherapy for breast cancer – the effect of different techniques of drug administration on tumor response. Reg Cancer Treat. 1996;7:127–31.
8. Frei III E, Canellos GP. Dose: a critical factor in cancer chemotherapy. Am J Med. 1980;69:585–94.

9. Gazyakan E, Engel H, Lehnhardt M, Pelzer M. Bilateral double free-flaps for reconstruction of extensive chest wall defect. Ann Thorac Surg. 2012;96:1289–91.
10. Dast S, Berna P, Qassemyar Q, Sinna R. A new option for autologous anterior chest wall reconstruction: the composite thoracodorsal artery perforator flap. Ann Thorac Surg. 2012;93:e67–9.
11. Nierlich P, Funovics P, Dominkus M, Aszmann O, Frey M, Klepetko W. Forequarter amputation combined with chest wall resection: a single-center experience. Ann Thorac Surg. 2011;91:1702–8.
12. Yao X, Hosenpund J, Chitambar CR, Charlson J, Chung Cheng Y. A phase II study of concurrent docetaxel, epirubicin and cyclophosphamide as a neoadjuvant chemotherapy regimen in patients with locally advanced breast cancer. J Cancer. 2012;3:145–51.
13. Aigner KR, Stephens FO. Guidelines and evidence-based medicine – evidence of what? EJCMO. 2012. Published online. http://www.slm-oncology.com/Guidelines_and_Evidence_Based_Medicine_Evidence_of_What_,1,272.html.

Cytoreductive Surgery and "Hyperthermic Intraperitoneal Chemotherapy (HIPEC)"

12

Markus Hirschburger and Winfried Padberg

12.1 Introduction

For a long time malignant tumor manifestation of the peritoneum, peritoneal carcinomatosis (PC) was regarded as terminal. This meant that both medical and surgical palliation treatments came into question which aimed to keep quality of life as long as possible. These methods are known as "best supportive care."

We must differentiate between tumors with primary peritoneal manifestation such as peritoneal mesothelioma and peritoneal carcinomas and secondary tumors of the peritoneum from gynecological and gastrointestinal primaries.

The French EVOCAPE 1 study [1] examined the median survival rate of tumors originating in the gut that were treated with best supportive care. Gastric cancer was found to have a median survival rate of 3 months and colorectal carcinomas of 6 months. By comparison, ovarian cancer can have a median survival time as long as 2 years [2–4]. Assuming that the peritoneal manifestation of a tumor was not a systemic disease but, as the first author Sampson described in 1931 [5], was rather a local progression of tumor mass into the peritoneal cavity, the first aggressive intraperitoneal treatments were developed in the 1980s [6, 7]. The effectivity of aggressive surgery for the treatment of PC was first shown for ovarian cancer in a multimodal therapeutic approach [8]. The proof that aggressive surgical treatment of colorectal metastases of the liver [9] led to a longer survival rate caused a change of perspective in the oncological treatment of this disease and following it the treatment of PC. At the end of the 1980s, the concept of treatment by the combination of the radical reduction of peritoneal tumor mass – cytoreductive surgery – and intraoperative hyperthermic intraperitoneal chemotherapy (HIPEC) was developed [10],

M. Hirschburger (✉) • W. Padberg
Klinik für Allgemein-, Viszeral-, Thorax-, Transplantations- u. Kinderchirurgie,
Universitätsklinikum Gießen, Rudolf-Buchheim-Straße 7, Gießen 35385, Germany
e-mail: markus.hirschburger@klinikum-worms.de;
Winfried.Padberg@chiru.med.uni-giessen.de

© Springer-Verlag Berlin Heidelberg 2016
K.R. Aigner, F.O. Stephens (eds.), *Induction Chemotherapy,*
DOI 10.1007/978-3-319-28773-7_12

mainly through the work of Paul Sugarbaker and team. He was able to show that a considerable improvement of the prognosis could be achieved for a selected group of patients [11–13]. In the 1990s, several phase II studies were published [14–19] showing improved survival rates and in some cases even curative results, in patients treated with cytoreduction and HIPEC. These results were confirmed in the first meta-analysis by Glehen in 2004 [20] with 28 phase II studies including 506 patients with mainly colorectal carcinomas. The median survival rate was 19.2 months. Patients with a macroscopic complete cytoreduction showed a higher survival rate of 32.4 months compared to patients where a total resection was not possible. The latter had a median survival rate of 8.4 months, comparable to patients just receiving best supportive care. The morbidity of 23 % and mortality of 4 % are acceptable considering the very limited treatment alternatives. However, it is shown that this high risk can only be tolerated in patients who undergo total cytoreduction because it is only then that there is a prospect of improved prognosis or even total recovery [13, 20–22]. This means that the operating surgeon's decision carries a huge responsibility but also that the interaction of the perioperative anesthetists and the subsequent ICU treatment plays a major part in the success of the procedure [23, 24].

12.2 Epidemiology and Pathophysiology

The peritoneal manifestation rate of tumors is varied. Whereas primary peritoneal tumors are rare, secondary manifestation of the peritoneum by gynecological or gastrointestinal tumors is common. For example, PC is manifest in 10–15 % of cases with first diagnosis of colon cancer [20, 25, 26]. Of these 10 %, 25 % have isolated PC. With 70,000 first diagnosis of colon cancer annually in Germany [27], this means about 1800 patients. In patients with tumor recurrence, even 10–35 % shows an isolated PC [25, 28].

Further risk factors for PC are mucinous carcinoma, perforated tumors, or iatrogenic tumor perforation. Secondary adhesion of free tumor cells then causes tumor progression. Systemic therapy fails because the limited peritoneal vascularization does not permit adequate therapeutic levels of pharmaceuticals in the peritoneum [28].

12.3 Patient Selection and Preoperative Diagnostics

Selection of suitable patients is extremely important in cytoreductive surgery, and HIPEC as a genuine improvement in prognosis can only be achieved in patients with optimal cytoreduction [29]. The operation is often very prolonged and invasive; therefore, patients should be in a good preoperative condition (ECOG performance status <2). The entity of the tumor and the spread of the tumor both play an important role. Tumor spread is diagnosed by all modern scanning methods. However, it has been shown that the tumor spread found intraoperatively is often not identical to that diagnosed preoperatively [30]. CT diagnostic often underestimates the degree of tumor spread. This is mainly on the small intestine where disseminated spread of small tumor lesions can lead to incomplete cytoreduction. In individual cases, diagnostic laparoscopy can be helpful [29]. However, CT scans are a firm part of preoperative diagnostics because they are needed for excluding further metastases despite their limited use in determining local peritoneal tumor spread. The Peritoneal Surface Malignancy Group has laid down eight clinical and radiological criteria that may increase the probability of total cytoreduction for colorectal tumors and which may be valid for other tumors too [31, 32]:

1. ECOG performance status <2
2. No extraabdominal tumor manifestation
3. No more than three small liver metastases easily resectable
4. No cholestasis
5. No stricture of the ureters
6. No more than one intestinal stenosis
7. No small intestine mesenterium involved
8. No involvement of the hepatic duodenal ligament

12.3.1 Cytoreduction

After successful scanning and decision-making to operate, intraoperative assessment is of greatest importance. First the spread of the PC both in size of the lesions and distribution over the peritoneal surface must be determined. Several indices are available to do this. Paul Sugarbaker's "peritoneal cancer index" (PCI) [13] is the most commonly used internationally (Fig. 12.1). The abdomen is divided in 13 regions. The small intestine alone into four regions shows its considerable importance in the index. The size of the lesions is determined for each region (lesion size = LS). LS-0 signifies that there is no macroscopically identifiable tumor. LS-3 means that the tumor is >5 cm in that region. This way, a maximum score of 39 can be achieved. Different PCI levels for different tumor entities are seen as the limit for viable resection. In the case of colon cancer, it has been shown that resection is possible with a PCI <20, whereas with gastric cancer, the PCI should lie between 10 and 15 [31, 33]. A PCI >20 is no exclusion for viable resection with pseudomyxoma peritonei (PMP). Yet the PCI is only an aid for determining the tumor spread and does not permit a definite assessment about total tumor resectability. Advanced involvement of the small intestine or of anatomically "critical" regions, such as the hepatic duodenal ligament, may make total tumor reduction impossible and lead to a bad prognosis even with a low PCI.

To be able to evaluate the prognosis, it is important to determine the degree of tumor removal. This is measured in the "completeness of cytoreduction score" (CC) ([13], Table 12.1). A CC score of 0 means there is no macroscopic residual tumor at the end of the operation. A CC score of 1 means residual tumor <2.5 mm. Whereas with a score of two, residuals between 2.5 mm and 2.5 cm remain. Finally, a CC score of 3 means residuals >2.5 cm. Several studies [34–37] have confirmed the prognostic relevance of the CC index.

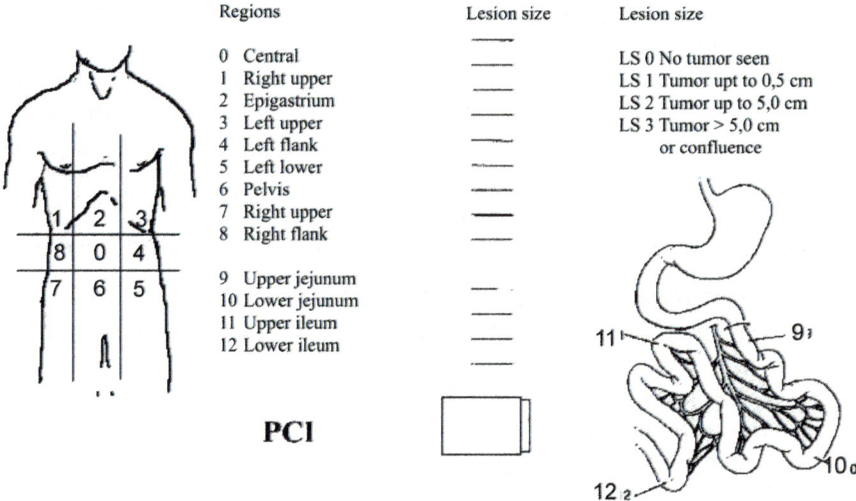

Fig. 12.1 "Peritoneal cancer index" (PCI) defined by Sugarbaker for intraoperative determination of the extense of peritoneal carcinomatosis spread

Table 12.1 Completeness of cytoreduction (CC)

Score	Size of remnant tumor
CC-0	No tumor remnants macroscopically
CC-1	Tumor remnants <0.25 cm
CC-2	Tumor remnants 0.25–2.5 cm
CC-3	Tumor remnants >2.5 cm

To achieve total cytoreduction, the complete affected visceral and parietal peritoneum must be resected. This is relatively easy in the case of the parietal peritoneum of the lateral abdominal wall. It is more difficult in the pelvis and diaphragm as well as the visceral peritoneum of the small intestine stomach and hepatic arch. This often necessitates multivisceral resections and several visceral anastomoses. Sugarbaker described the techniques for the most common visceral and parietal peritoneal resections [11, 38] and grouped these in six operative sections.

He starts with a median laparotomy from the xiphoid to the pubic symphysis to allow complete exploration of both diaphragm and the pelvis. If the greater omentum is affected or an omental cake has formed, the omentum is resected. This is carried out removing the gastroepiploic arch and the gastrica brevis vessels along the greater curvature. Then the peritoneal resection is continued in the left upper abdomen (Fig. 12.2). The peritoneal coating of the diaphragm, the rear wall of the rectus abdominis, the adrenal gland, the fascia of Gerota, parts of the pancreas, and the transverse colon are removed. If there is tumor occurrence in the splenic hilum or the pancreas tail, splenectomy and/or left pancreatic resection may be necessary [39]. In the right abdomen, the procedure is similar (Fig. 12.3), and the dissection is removed "en bloc" along the lateral abdominal wall, the diaphragm, and the Morrison pouch right over to the inferior vena cava. Should the tumor be adherent to the tendinous part of the diaphragm a partial diaphragm resection will be necessary. The resection

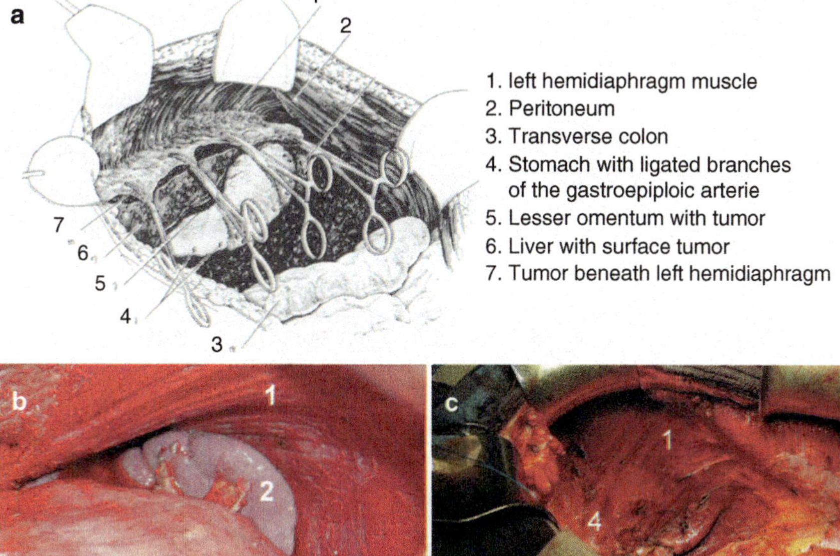

1. left hemidiaphragm muscle
2. Splen
3. Stomach with ligated branches of the
   gastroepiploic arterie

1. left hemidiaphragm muscle
2. Transverse colon
3. Pancreas
4. sutured hemidiaphragm after partial
   resection

Fig. 12.2 (**a**) Peritoneal resection in the upper left abdomen (Sugarbaker), (**b**) intraoperative site after peritoneal resection in the upper left abdomen retaining the spleen, (**c**) intraoperative site after peritoneal resection involving splenectomy and partial resection of the tendinous diaphragm

in the upper abdomen finishes with peritoneal resection of the greater omental pouch along the hepatic duodenal ligament and the superior surface of the pancreas to the celiac trunk and finally the affected parts of the lesser omental pouch.

For the pelvic peritoneal resection (Fig. 12.4), the peritoneum is mobilized along the laparotomy. Caudally, the rectus muscles are identified and the peritoneum swept off the bladder. Laterally, the ureters are identified and followed down to the bladder. In female patients, both round ligaments and ovarian veins are divided. Following this, the mesorectal layer is opened; the rectum is mobilized below the peritoneum and then separated so the complete peritoneal funnel can be removed from the lower pelvis. In female patients, the uterine artery is divided at the crossing point with the ureters, and the uterus and adnexes are removed en bloc with the rest of the lower pelvis.

The effectiveness of the resection is considerably determined by the involvement of the visceral peritoneum despite the systematic method described. An extended cytoreductive resection may often lead to a multivisceral resection with parietal and

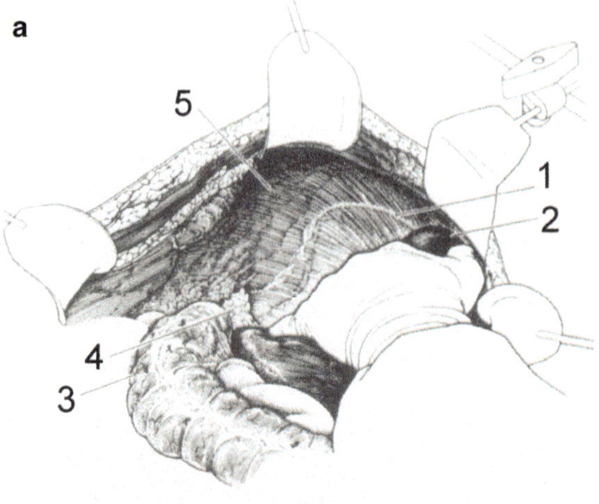

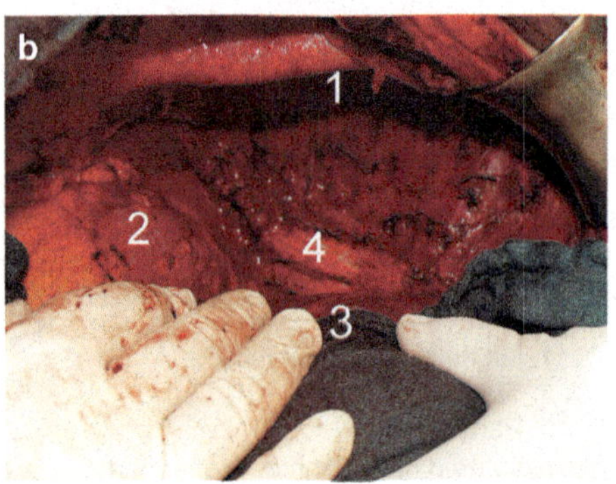

Fig. 12.3 (**a**) Peritoneal resection in the upper right abdomen (Sugarbaker), (**b**) intraoperative site after peritoneal resection

visceral peritoneal resections; resection of the omentum, spleen, parts of the pancreas, lesser sac, and liver capsule; atypical liver resection; cholecystectomy (partial); gastric resection (multiple); small intestine resections; colonic and rectum resection; ovariectomy; hysterectomy; and occasional partial bladder resection. This means that severe reflection about the postoperative quality of life is necessary when determining the extent of the resection.

12.3.2 The Rationale and Technique of Hyperthermic Intraperitoneal Chemotherapy: HIPEC

After termination of the cytoreductive surgery, the hyperthermic intraperitoneal chemotherapy follows. HIPEC is the most commonly applied form of local perioperative chemotherapy. The rationale of intraperitoneal chemotherapy is that this form of application allows high concentrations of chemotherapy locally while the

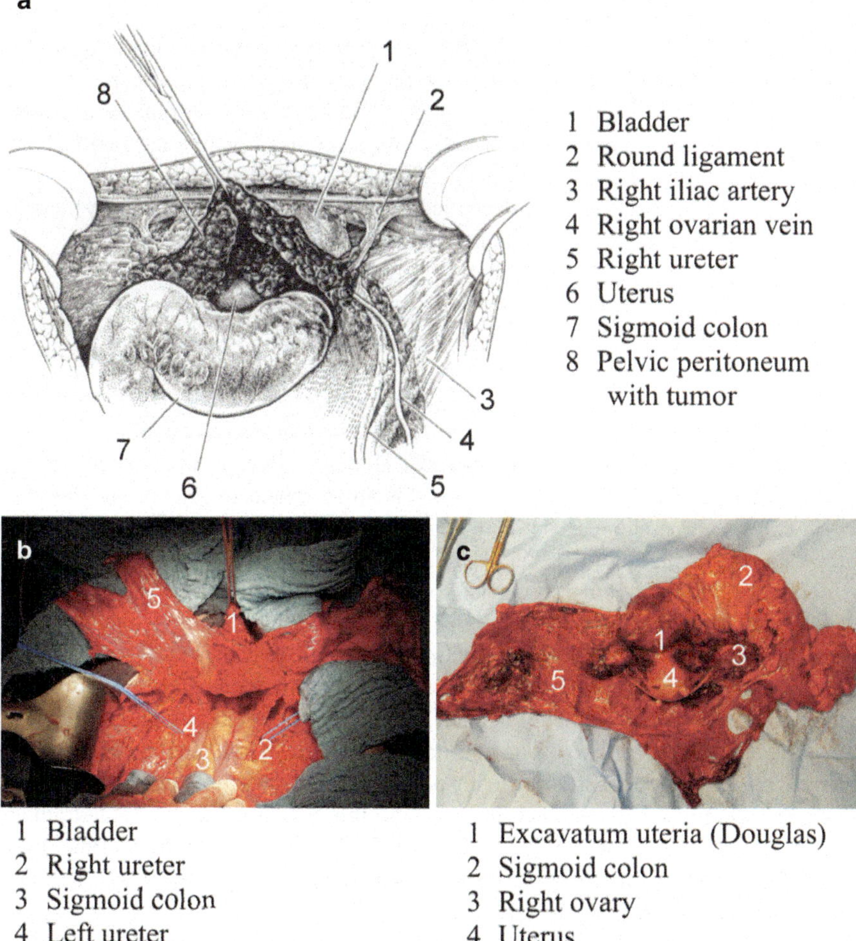

Fig. 12.4 (**a**) Peritoneal resection in the lower pelvis (Sugarbaker), (**b**) intraoperative site with both ureters looped, (**c**) the resection of the lower pelvis with rectum, uterus, both ovaries and parietal peritoneum

systemic concentration levels remain low [40]. This concentration gradient is sustained by the peritoneal plasma barrier (ppb) [41, 42]. Surprisingly even extended peritoneal resection does not change the pharmacokinetics of chemotherapeutics applied intraperitoneally [43]. However, the ppb does lead to diminished chemotherapeutic tissue penetration which limits the effect of intraperitoneal chemotherapy. Estimates of the depth of tissue penetration range from a few cell layers to a depth of 5 mm [44–48]. This is the reason that cytoreductive surgery precedes chemotherapy and the resection is rated as optimal when at most tumor lesions of

<2.5 mm remain (CC 0–1). The hyperthermia has varied effects. First hyperthermia between 41° and 43 °C has a cytotoxic effect, especially on malignant cells [49–51]. Hyperthermia leads to an increase in lysosomes and lysosomal enzymatic activity in malignant cells. Further, hyperthermia in malignant tumors causes a decrease in cell perfusion [52] with resulting acidosis which again increases lysosomal activity and thus accelerates death of malignant cells [50]. Increased membrane permeability and transport mechanisms of malignant cells allow increased intake of pharmaceuticals and so an increase of pharmaceutical activity [47, 51, 53]. However, the synergistic effect of different chemotherapeutics under hyperthermia differs.

12.3.3 HIPEC Procedure

HIPEC is carried out – as mentioned – after the cytoreductive surgery has been completed. However, opinions differ as to whether the reconstruction of the gut should be carried out before or after HIPEC. Theoretically, the concern about recurrence of the carcinoma in the anastomoses is an argument for reconstruction after HIPEC; however, no increased rate of anastomosal recurrences has been found after preceded reconstruction [40]. The drug is given in a standard dose related to body surface area and the volume of carrier solution [54, 55]. Basically, HIPEC may be carried out as an open procedure or with a closed abdomen. The open technique is often referred to as the "coliseum technique" by Sugarbaker [13]. Here, the laparotomy remains open; the skin is fixed continuously on a frame and elevated so that a crater-like opening is formed. Inlet and outlet catheters are brought in through the abdominal wall and get fixed. The optimal temperature is regulated by temperature gauges in inlet and outlet sluices during perfusion. The system is covered with a foil to ensure that theater contamination is at a minimum and below the foil a drainage system is installed. The foil may be opened by the surgeon permitting intraabdominal manipulation to ensure even perfusion of each region by the chemotherapeutics (Fig. 12.5). The perfusion solution is introduced via a heat exchange and perfusion pump at a rate of about 1 l/min (Fig. 12.5). When a temperature between 41 and 43 °C is reached on the inlet and outlet catheters, the chemotherapeutic is added, and perfusion is performed for 30–90 min according to the therapeutic regime. The advantage of the open technique lies in the homogenic distribution, yet there is a greater heat loss, and the theater staff is potentially endangered. In the closed technique, perfusion is commenced after the catheters have been placed and the wound has watertight closure. The advantages of the closed technique are that the target temperature is achieved rapidly and remains stable [56]. Furthermore, the theater staff is less exposed to contamination. The disadvantages lie in a proven inhomogeneous distribution of the chemotherapeutic as well as the risk of local overheating and overloading with chemotherapeutic with the risk of postoperative complications [40].

Over the last years, so-called bidirectional HIPEC methods have become established. Here the intravenous (iv) chemotherapy is applied simultaneously with HIPEC. Elias performed this with 5-FU and folic acid i.v. and oxaliplatin

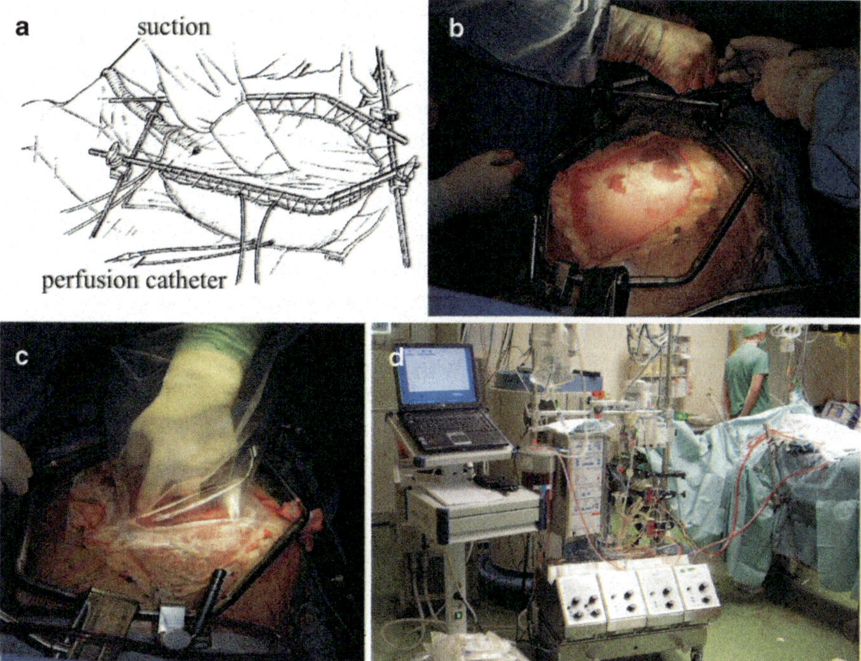

Fig. 12.5 (**a**) Coliseum technique by Sugarbaker. (**b**) Variation of the Coliseum technique as carried out in Giessen. (**c**) Intestinal manipulation during perfusion. (**d**) Heart lung machine for generating the hyperthermia

intraperitoneally [54]. Van der Speeten showed that under these circumstances, it came to an increase in the concentration of 5-FU in the peritoneal cavity [57].

Up till now, there are no standards for the chemotherapeutics used or the time of perfusion. This has led to worldwide different standards of which chemotherapeutic is perfused for how long on which tumor. From all used drugs, mitomycin C is the most commonly used one. The standard drugs of systemic chemotherapy cisplatin, doxorubicin, oxaliplatin, and irinotecan are being applied increasingly especially in cases of bidirectional treatment of colorectal cancer.

For example, in bidirectional HIPEC, leucovorin (20 mg/m^2) and 5-FU (400–450 mg/m^2) are given intravenously over 30 min, 30–60 min before HIPEC with oxaliplatin being carried out.

12.3.4 Aspects of Risks and Safety for Theater Staff

Intraoperative administration of chemotherapeutics does potentially endanger theater staff. Above all, the open coliseum technique involves risks of contamination of the staff and the operating table. When using mitomycin in the coliseum technique, Stuart took urine samples of the theater staff and air samples above and below the foil and checked the theater gloves for permeability for this chemotherapeutic. All the tests for contamination were negative [58]. Similar test with platin-based chemotherapeutics showed low contamination, but significantly higher levels were measured at the HIPEC pump and around the theater table especially when the pump reservoir was filled with the chemotherapeutic with a syringe [59, 60]. Contamination may however be kept at lower levels if certain safety measures are adhered to [40, 61]. Reusable drapes must not be used. Theater staff must be kept to a minimum during and after perfusion. Theater doors must be closed with warnings about HIPEC to keep staff translocation and so air disturbance at a minimum. The theater floor around the table should be covered with absorbent nonreusable cloths. All the staff involved in the process must wear water repellant protective clothing. All potentially contaminated material must be removed in specially labeled stabile containers after HIPEC so that cleaning staff is not endangered. Within the first 48 h after HIPEC, all the patients' body liquids must be regarded as contaminated and treated as such. Low-permeability double gloving is compulsory for every contact with the chemotherapeutic [58]. In cases of continual contact with the chemotherapeutic, the gloves must be changed every 30 min. Air evacuation above the theater table is compulsory. Should contamination still occur, it must be removed with every possible regard to personal safety but without causing an aerosol effect. Theater instruments must be washed several times before clearance. Contamination of theater staff can be kept to a minimum if these methods are adhered to.

12.4 Perioperative Management

The perioperative management during cytoreduction and HIPEC involves different phases, each needing specific individual care [24]. During resection, the large laparotomy, the long operation time, and the enormous wound surface result in considerable fluid loss [62]. Further, hypothermia threatens with negative effects on coagulation, patient neurology, immunology, as well as the metabolic situation [63–65]. Fluid control remains important during perfusion. Patient's hyperthermia during perfusion of up to 40.5 °C increases the metabolic rate requiring more O_2 [66]. Further, a higher pulse rate, lactate levels, and metabolic acidosis [62, 66–69] require adjustments in pulmonary ventilation. This means that one of the aims of the anesthesia is to achieve normothermia but be able to react correctly to changes in body temperature [24]. Next to temperature control, fluid management is as important during intraoperative care of the patient. Maintaining normovolemia has a very important effect on both systemic and regional perfusion, something extremely important especially when performing HIPEC. Hyperthermia causes a drop in the peripheral resistance and so leads to further unwanted fluid distribution. If it comes to a relevant fluid deficit, decreased perfusion of internal organs leading to kidney failure may occur [68]. On the other side, hypervolemia has severe side effects in the future course [70]. Several factors have to be considered to estimate the necessary volume substitution. Fluid need is higher than normal and may reach 12 ml/kg/h, the extensive resection causes severe protein loss through the large wound surface [71], and the blood loss may be high. All factors and also the coagulation situation mean that a balanced substitution with crystalline and colloid solutions as well as fresh plasma and red blood cell concentrates is necessary [24]. Under HIPEC conditions, the perfusion solution and the type of chemotherapeutic must be taken into account. Using oxaliplatin, a 5 % glucose solution is normally used as a carrier causing hyperglycemia and hyponatremia [72, 73]. When cisplatin is administered, its cardiotoxic side effects must be considered [74].

In the first postoperative phase, fluid control is still at the center of our efforts as the enormous wound surface causes considerable fluid and protein loss leading to late volume redistribution [23, 69, 75]. So it can be clearly followed that postoperative respiratory training with continuous positive airway pressure (CPAP) improves the pulmonary situation and convalescence [23]. In the postoperative phase, the peridural thoracic catheter has many advantages. Postoperative ventilation time is reduced as well as the i.v. opioid therapy regime causing bowel movement to commence earlier. A recent publication [76] has shown that there may even be an oncological advantage in using supplementary peridural anesthesia. On the other hand, there are several publications describing higher complication rates of peridural anesthesia under HIPEC [77–79]. A possible alternative pain therapy could be continuous local wound infiltration as carried out in our center in cases of suspected coagulation disorders using a "PainBuster system®" [80].

12.5 Morbidity, Mortality, and Quality of Life (QoL)

Up till now, there is no unitary scheme to document complications after cytoreduction and HIPEC. Postoperative complications may occur through extended resections or through toxic effects caused by HIPEC. These may interact additively. In the joint paper of Milan [81], an expert committee agreed to use the "common terminology criteria for adverse events (CTCAE)" by the National Institutes of Health (NIH) for the documentation of postoperative complications following cytoreduction and HIPEC as the general classification. Here minor complications (grade 0–2) and major complications (grade 3–5) are differentiated by a detailed classification of 28 categories to clearly define morbidity. Increased fluid transfer, bowel atony, anastomosis failure, bleeding, thrombosis, pulmonary embolism, and wound infections are common postoperative complications. Direct complications of the chemotherapeutic are cardio- and hematotoxicity as well as liver and kidney damage. Major complications grade 3 and 4 are described in 30–40 % of the cases with a mortality between 0 % and 8 % [29].

In large centers performing cytoreduction and HIPEC, the morbidity and mortality rate is comparable to that of other multivisceral resections [82].

After cytoreduction and HIPEC, the QoL of the patient is severely limited in the postoperative phase due to the extended operation and the high rate of complications.

However, studies by McQuellon showed that after an initial worsening, patients showed a better QoL 3.6 and 12 months after the operation compared with the preoperative status. Seventy-four percent of the patients had renewed more than half their activities of daily life 1 year postoperatively. An acceptable QoL with little pain can be achieved after 3–6 months. At the time of operation, one third of the patients show signs of depression, and these persist in 24 % of the cases after 1 year of follow-up [83, 84].

An actual meta-analysis by Shan et al. including McQuellon's data shows similar results. If individual aspects of the QoL score are analyzed, patients show a significant improvement in emotional health 3 months after cytoreductive surgery and HIPEC, most easily explained by a newly resolved hope for a new lease of life [85].

The present state of the studies shows that cytoreduction and HIPEC have acceptable results in patients who appreciate the prognostic outcome of their disease and that despite the enormity of the treatment, the postoperative QoL is improved as well as the emotional situation because of the new hope of a longer lease of life.

12.6 Results of Different Tumor Entities

12.6.1 Primary Peritoneal Malignomas

12.6.1.1 Malignant Peritoneal Mesothelioma (MPM)

The malignant mesothelioma is a rare tumor which can develop from the pleura, peritoneum, pericard, or the tunica vaginalis testis [86]. Its rate of occurrence has increased in the past decades due to the widespread exposure to asbestos and will probably reach its maximum in the next 20 years [87]. The diffuse malignant peritoneal mesothelioma (DMPM) represents about 10–30 % of all mesothelioma diseases [88]. The causality of asbestos exposure and DMPM is far less conclusive than in pleura mesothelioma [89, 90]. Histologically, there are three subtypes: epithelial, sarcomatous, and mixed type. The diagnostic classification is not easy as the tumor morphology is very variable, and it is often difficult to differentiate between mesothelioma and benign reactive changes or metastases of an adenocarcinoma [91]. Immunohistology is helpful although there is no typical mesothelioma marker. The tumor can often be defined by its constellation of positive or negative immunoreactivity.

Generally, the disease remains in the abdomen. Autopsies have shown that in 78 % of the cases, patients died of complications of the locoregional tumor growth [92]. It is because of this locoregional tumor progression that treatment with cytoreduction and HIPEC seems a good policy. Without aggressive therapy, the median survival rate lies between 6 and 12 months due to the rapid tumor growth [93]. Under the treatment with cytoreduction and HIPEC, it can be extended and presently lies between 30 and 92 months [94]. An actual meta-analysis showed the 1-, 3-, and 5-year survival rates to be 84 %, 59 %, and 42 %, respectively [95]. Patients with an epithelial mesothelioma have a longer median survival rate [96]. As the disease progresses, the small intestine is involved to a high degree [94]. In a controlled trial, Baratti et al. examined the outcome of patients in whom only affected peritoneum was resected compared with a group in which, regardless of the tumor spread, the entire peritoneum was removed. The median survival time in the subtotally resected group was 29.6 months; in the second, the median survival time had not been reached after a follow-up of 50.3 months. The 5-year survival rate was 40 % in the first group and 63.9 % in the second group. This difference is significant so that the total peritoneal resection is associated with a higher survival rate [97].

Special forms of peritoneal mesothelioma are multicystic peritoneal mesothelioma (MPM) and well-differentiated papillary peritoneal mesothelioma (WDPPM). Both subtypes are rare and show questionable malignant growth behavior. Recurrence is common, and the transformation to malignant mesothelioma is possible. Both forms appear mainly abdominally in fertile females with no case history of asbestos exposure. Different therapeutic approaches have been developed because of the recurrence and transformation rate to malignant tumors, but because of the low number of cases documented, no standards can be advised. Baratti [98] describes cytoreduction and HIPEC in 12 patients with a 5-year survival rate of 90 %. One of the patients suffered transformation to malignant mesothelioma. Considering these results, cytoreduction and HIPEC seem to be a justifiable strategy.

12.6.2 Secondary Peritoneal Malignomas

12.6.2.1 Colorectal Cancer and Appendiceal Cancer

The most common indication for cytoreductive surgery and HIPEC is colorectal cancer with PC. As the appendiceal cancer is included in many studies, it will be included here too. Glehen's meta-analysis [20] from 2004 on 506 patients showed that the median survival time was 32.4 months for patients with macroscopic total tumor removal and HIPEC. In comparison, the median survival time of patients with best supportive care (EVOCAPE 1) was 6 months [1]. Patients without total resection had no benefit. The colorectal cancer was the first tumor entity examined in a randomized controlled trial. This was carried out by Verwaal et al. in the Netherlands examining the effectivity of the combination therapy [21]. The median survival time of the control cohort was 12.6 months compared with 21.6 months in the trial cohort with cytoreductive surgery and HIPEC. Patients with macroscopic total resection showed even better results. The follow-up data on this study after 8 years showed a 5-year survival rate of 45 % on patients with total resection [21]. Several phase II studies showed 5-year survival rates up to 50 % [99, 100]. The results of these studies have made cytoreductive surgery and HIPEC the therapy of choice for the treatment of colorectal cancer with PC in many countries.

In the group of colorectal cancer, it seems that rectal cancer is less respondent to therapy than colon cancer in other regions. Da Silva [101] has shown that the median survival time of patients with rectal cancer was 17 months, whereas that for other colonic regions was 33 months. Furthermore, the histology of the cancer seems to play an important part in the effect of the therapy. The long-term prognosis for signet-ring cell carcinoma is bad despite cytoreductive surgery and HIPEC, and so the indication for this treatment in such cases must be carefully considered [102, 103].

Elias [104] carried out second look operations after 1 year on patients thought to have a high risk of developing PC. These were patients with local PC on the primary operation, ovarian metastases, or a perforated cancer. This collective of 29 patients showed 16 patients (55 %) having PC which was not visible in the CT scan in most cases. Even if there are no long-term results available for this collective as yet, the strategy does seem reasonable for patients at a high risk of developing PC.

12.6.2.2 Pseudomyxoma Peritonei (PMP)

PMP is a rare disease identified by mucinous ascites and peritoneal spreading [105, 106]. During disease progress, large volumes of mucinous ascites are formed causing obstruction and occlusion of the intestine. The disease was first described by Rokitansky in 1842 in a patient with a mucocele of the appendix [107]. For a long time, there was no consensus as to the origin and the pathological classification of PMP. According to pathological examinations, the majority of PMP evolves from low-grade tumors of the appendix [108–110], in rare cases from other organs. These are mainly the ovaries but also the stomach, colon, pancreas, and other intra-abdominal organs [111, 112]. PMPs do not just differ in their origin but also in their growth rate. Ronnett [108] suggested a now popular classification on the results of a retrospective tumor analysis. Three subtypes were described. Low-grade tumors were defined as disseminated peritoneal adenomucinosis (DPAM), high-grade tumors as peritoneal mucinous carcinomatosis (PMCA), and the intermediate type (IG) whose long-term behavior is not different to that of PMCA. Further classifications have been put forward, all of which differentiate between aggressive and less aggressive forms of PMP.

Symptomatic PMP patients often underwent repeated tumor reductive surgery. This led to a short-term improvement in the symptoms but had little influence on the long-term survival rate [105, 106]. Almost all patients had recurrences, and as the number of reoperations increased, the therapy became less effective and the complication rate increased. Histopathologically, it was shown that in some cases, the low aggressive forms transformed to high aggressive forms. Under these conditions, 10-year survival rates between 10 % and 30 % [113, 114] were achieved even though in some cases extremely aggressive treatment with intraperitoneal radiation and chemotherapy was applied.

Many studies showed that therapy with cytoreduction and HIPEC shows improved survival rates when compared to past control groups [116]. With a cohort of 501 patients, Sugarbaker et al. showed that a median survival time of 156 months and a 5- and 10-year survival rate of 72 and 55 % can be achieved [115]. Based on these studies and despite the fact that there were no large randomized studies, the leading HIPEC centers working on the treatment of PMP published a consensus paper in 2008 stating that the combination of cytoreductive surgery and HIPEC is the only scientifically based, promising treatment available [116].

In a study by Chua et al. [117], the data of a multicentric retrospective data bank involving 2298 patients from 16 centers were analyzed. A mortality of 2 % and a complication rate of 24 % were shown for cytoreductive surgery and HIPEC. The median survival time was 196 months with a 10- and 15-year survival rate of 63 and

59 %. Independent factors for a low survival rate were old age, severe postoperative complications, preoperative chemotherapy, and aggressive histological subtype (PMCA).

12.6.2.3 Gastric Cancer

PC is found in 5–20 % of patients with a planned curative gastrectomy [118, 119]. This has a terrible prognosis and a mean survival time of 3 months [1]. Sixty percent of gastric cancer patients die because of PC [120]. Polychemotherapy is the preferred therapy in advanced gastric cancer and is superior to best supportive care [121]. However, several studies have shown that as with other tumor forms, PC does not respond as well as organ metastases to systemic chemotherapy because of the blood peritoneal barrier [122, 125]. The results shown for cytoreductive surgery and HIPEC were not convincing for a long time. The PCI level for gastric cancer which makes a resection an option is lower than for colon cancer [126–128], and a total cytoreduction (CC-0) is a must to improve the prognosis. A meta-analysis and systematic reviews have shown that if these conditions are fulfilled then, an improvement of the prognosis can be achieved by cytoreductive surgery and HIPEC [118, 129, 130]. The median survival time in these studies lays between 7.9 and 15 months and the 5-year survival rate between 6 % and 16 %. Glehen and Yonemura published better results for patients with total cytoreduction (CC-0) with a median survival time between 15.4 and 21.3 months and a 5-year survival rate between 15 % and 29.4 % [131, 132].

The preoperative staging is very important in cases of gastric cancer because of the high incidence of PC. Unfortunately, CT scan is unsuitable to detect the typical tiny PC lesions. It has been shown that spreads of less than 5 mm were only detected with a sensitivity of 11 % [133] and that the PCI determined by CT scan often underestimated the spread [128].

In comparison, laparoscopic staging shows good results with 90 % accuracy. Valle could show in a cohort of 97 patients that the laparoscopic score only varied from the intraoperative score in 2 out of 97 patients [134]. As new neoadjuvant treatments have become available, the initial staging is of tremendous importance, and the staging laparoscopy is therefore the method of choice.

12.6.2.4 Neoadjuvant Strategy for Advanced Gastric Cancer with PC

Various neoadjuvant concepts have been developed to transform an initially nonresectable gastric cancer into a resectable one. Classical neoadjuvant systemic chemotherapy with various drug combinations is able to increase the share of patients in whom a total cytoreduction is possible and thus increase the life expectancy [123, 124, 135]. Realizing that the advantages of local chemotherapy were counterbalanced by the low penetration depth, Yonemura developed a bidirectional neoadjuvant intraperitoneal and systemic chemotherapeutic strategy (NIPS). The results of this method appear favorable. In a group of 79 patients, 65 had positive ascites cytology at first diagnosis. After NIPS, 41 (63 %) of these 65 patients had negative ascites cytology. In half of the patients with PC, it came to a complete remission, and in the rest the rate of total cytoreduction was very high [132, 136, 137]. As a whole, few studies have been performed with favorable results; therefore, the treatment should only be carried out under controlled study conditions.

12.6.2.5 Ovarian Cancer

Ovarian cancer is one of the most common gynecological malignant diseases [138]. Epithelial ovarian cancer represents the most common form with over 70 %. When diagnosed, the disease is usually in an advanced stage with peritoneal involvement [139]. As ovarian cancer is generally chemosensitive, standard therapy is cytoreductive surgery followed by adjuvant systemic chemotherapy with paclitaxel and a platin-based therapeutic [140]. Recurrence is common and chemoresistance develops. The 5-year survival rate for advanced tumor is under 25 % [141]. The degree in which cytoreduction can be carried out in ovarian cancer is highly relevant. A meta-analysis on almost 7000 patients showed that maximal cytoreduction is the most relevant factor for survival [8]. Adjuvant intraperitoneal chemotherapy was tried with success as the initial high chemosensitivity was well known [142]. The logical deduction seems that cytoreductive surgery and HIPEC could be used successfully in the treatment of this tumor form. However, the evidence is unclear and this has several reasons. In many studies, the cohorts of patients are not standardized. In a systematic review [143], Chua et al. show that in the examined cohorts, patients with first diagnosis of ovarian cancer, patients with recurrent cancer, patients who have undergone chemotherapy, patients with chemoresistant tumors, and patients with chemosensitive tumors are grouped together, so making the conclusions of the examinations very questionable. Furthermore, there are different interpretations of the definition of "optimal" cytoreduction [144]. On one hand, extensive multivisceral resection to achieve total cytoreduction (CC-0) leads to high morbidity in the treatment of a chemosensitive tumor, whereas on the other hand, the radicality of the resection is diminished to reduce the morbidity. There are enough arguments to defend either position. Winter et al. [145] showed that in a study with 360 patients, radically resected patients had significantly higher survival rate in an otherwise identical therapeutic regime.

Different points of time can be used to evaluate the effectivity of cytoreductive surgery and HIPEC in ovarian cancer. Primary therapy at first diagnosis of ovarian cancer or secondary therapy at persisting, progressing, or recurrent disease [146]. A French multicenter study [147] has recently been published involving 92 patients who underwent primary therapy with cytoreduction and HIPEC. The median survival time was 35.4 months. Those who had total cytoreduction had a median survival time of 41.5 months.

In the first randomized trial of patients with recurrent ovarian cancer published by Spiliotis, treatment with cytoreductive surgery and systemic chemotherapy was compared to cytoreductive surgery and HIPEC with the same adjuvant systemic chemotherapy. The HIPEC group was found to have a significantly longer survival time of 26.7 months compared to 13.4 months. The 3-year survival rate was 75 % in the HIPEC group but only 18 % in the non-HIPEC group [148]. At the moment, several randomized controlled trials are being carried out to position the value of cytoreductive surgery and HIPEC. The Netherlands Cancer Institute is comparing cytoreductive surgery with HIPEC to cytoreductive surgery alone [149]. The second study from Sidney is comparing the effect of cytoreductive surgery and HIPEC on primary ovarian cancer and on recurrent disease [150]. In a French study [151] (CHIPOR), patients with recurrent ovarian cancer are treated with systemic chemotherapy followed by maximal cytoreductive surgery with and without HIPEC.

After these studies have been completed, we can expect a new evaluation of the combination of cytoreductive surgery and HIPEC in ovarian cancer.

12.7 Summary

The combination of cytoreductive surgery and HIPEC has left the experimental stage for some tumor entities. In large-scale meta-analysis, good results could be achieved for PMP, colorectal cancer, and appendiceal cancer, even in randomized trials. This has lead France and the Netherlands to include this treatment in their guidelines for the treatment of colorectal cancer. Similar results for gastric and ovarian cancer have not yet been achieved although there are signs that under certain conditions, cytoreductive surgery and HIPEC are of use. Still there are many unanswered questions. There are no standardized therapeutic regimes, neither for the choice of chemotherapeutic or for the time of perfusion. The extense of peritoneal resection is not standardized, so in some centers only macroscopically affected peritoneum is resected; in others, a total peritoneal resection is carried out with proven long-term success [95].

The most important factor overall is patient selection because it is only by maximal cytoreduction (CC-0, CC-1) that an improvement of the prognosis may be achieved.

References

1. Sadeghi B, Arvieux C, Glehen O, Beaujard AC, Rivoire M, Bauliuex J, Fontaumard E, Brachet A, Caillot JL, Faure JL, Porcheron J, Peix JL, Francois Y, Vignal J, Gilly FN. Peritoneal carcinomatosis from non-gynecologic malignancies. Cancer. 2000;15:358–63.
2. Hardy JR, Wiltshaw E, Blake PR, Slevin M, Perren TJ, Tan S. Cisplatin and carboplatin in combination for the treatment of stage IV ovarian carcinoma. Ann Oncol. 1991;2:131–6.
3. Curtin JP, Malik R, Venkatramann ES, Barakat RR, Hoskins WJ. Stage IV ovarian cancer: impact of surgical debulking. Gynecol Oncol. 1997;64:9–12.
4. Akahira JI, Yoshikawa H, Shimizu Y, Tsunematsu R, Hirakawa T, Kuramoto H, Kuzuya K, Shiromizu K, Kamura T, Kikuchi Y, Kodama S, Yamamoto K, Sato S. Prognostic factors of stage UV epithelial ovarian cancer: a multicenter retrospective study. Gynecol Oncol. 2001;81:398–403.
5. Sampson JA. Implantation peritoneal carcinomatosis of ovarian origin. Am J Pathol. 1931;7:423–6.
6. Spratt JS, Adcock RA, Muskovin M, Sherrill W, McKeown J. Clinical delivery systems for intraperitoneal hyperthermic chemotherapy. Cancer Res. 1980;40:256–60.
7. Fujimoto S, Shrestha RD, Kokubun M, Kobayashi K, Kiuchi S, Konno C, Takahashi M, Okui K. Pharmacokinetic analysis of mitomycin C for intraperitoneal hyperthermic perfusion in patients with far-advanced or recurrent gastric cancer. Reg Cancer Treat. 1989;2:198–202.

8. Bristow RE, Tomacruz RS, Armstrong DK, Trimble EL, Montz FJ. Survival effect of maximal cytoreductive surgery for advanced ovarian carcinoma during the platinum era: a meta-analysis. J Clin Oncol. 2002;20:1248–59.
9. Sugarbaker PH, Hughes KA. Surgery for colorectal metastasis to liver. In: Wanebo H, editor. Colorectal cancer. St. Louis: Mosby; 1993. p. 405–13.
10. Sugarbaker PH, Cunliffe WJ, Belliveau J, de Brujin EA, Graves T, Mullins RE, Schlag P. Rationale for integrating early postoperative intraperitoneal chemotherapy into the surgical treatment of gastrointestinal cancer. Semin Oncol. 1989;16:83–97.
11. Sugarbaker PH. Peritonectomy procedures. Ann Surg. 1995;221:29–42.
12. Sugarbaker PH. Observations concerning cancer spread within the peritoneal carcinomatosis: principles and management. Boston: Kluwer Academic Publ; 1996. p. 79–100.
13. Sugarbaker PH. Management of peritoneal-surface malignancy: the surgeon's role. Langenbeck's Arch Surg. 1999;384:576–87.
14. Glehen O, Mithieux F, Osinsky D, Beuajard AC, Freyer G, Guertsch P, Francois Y, Peyrat P, Panteix G, Vignal J, Gilly FN. Surgery combined with peritonectomy procedures and intra-peritoneal chemohyperthermia in abdominal cancers with peritoneal carcinomatosis: a phase II study. J Clin Oncol. 2003;21:799–806.
15. Elias D, Blot F, El Otmany A, Antoun S, Lasser P, Boige V, Rougier P, Ducreux M. Curative treatment of peritoneal carcinomatosis arising from colorectal cancer by complete resection and intraperitoneal chemotherapy. Cancer. 2001;92:71–6.
16. Glehen O, Gilly FN, Sugarbaker PH. New perspectives in the management of colorectal cancer: what about peritoneal carcinomatosis? Scand J Surg. 2003;92:178–9.
17. Shen P, Levine EA, Hall J, Case D, Russell G, Fleming R, McQuellon R, Geisinger KR, Loggie BW. Factors predicting survival after intraperitoneal hyperthermic chemotherapy with mitomycin C after cytoreductive surgery for patients with peritoneal carcinomatosis. Arch Surg. 2003;138:26–33.
18. Pestieau SR, Sugarbaker PH. Treatment of primary colon cancer with peritoneal carcinomatosis: comparison of concomitant vs. delayed management. Dis Colon Rectum. 2000;43:1341–6.
19. Witkamp AJ, de Bree E, Kaag MM, Boot H, Beijnen JH, van Slooten GW, van Coevorden F, Zoetmulder FA. Extensive cytoreductive surgery followed by intra-operative hyperthermic intraperitoneal chemotherapy with mitomycin C in patients with peritoneal carcinomatosis of colorectal origin. Eur J Cancer. 2001;37:979–84.
20. Glehen O, Kwiatkowski F, Sugarbaker PH, Elias D, Levine EA, De Simone M, Barone R, Yonemura Y, Cavaliere F, Quenet F, Gutman M, Tentes AA, Lorimier G, Bernard JL, Bereder JM, Porcheron J, Gomez-Portilla A, Shen P, Deraco M, Rat P. Cytoreductive surgery combined with perioperative intraperitoneal chemotherapy for the management of peritoneal carcinomatosis from colorectal cancer: a multi-institutional study. J Clin Oncol. 2004;22:3284–92.
21. Verwaal VJ, van Ruth S, de Bree E, van Sloothen GW, van Tinteren H, Boot H, Zoetmulder FA. Randomized trial of cytoreduction and hyperthermic intraperitoneal chemotherapy versus systemic chemotherapy and palliative surgery in patients with peritoneal carcinomatosis of colorectal cancer. J Clin Oncol. 2003;20:3737–43.
22. Verwaal VJ, Bruin S, Boot H, van Slooten G, van Tinteren H. 8-year follow-up of randomized trial: cytoreduction and hyperthermic intraperitoneal chemotherapy versus systemic chemotherapy in patients with peritoneal carcinomatosis of colorectal origin. Ann Surg Oncol. 2008;15:2426–32.
23. Arakeljan E, Gunningberg L, Larsson J, Norlen K, Mahteme H. Factors influencing early postoperative recovery after cytoreductive surgery and hyperthermic intraperitoneal chemotherapy. Eur J Surg Oncol. 2011;37:897–903.
24. Raspe C, Piso P, Wiesnack C, Bucher M. Anesthetic management in patients undergoing hyperthermic chemotherapy. Curr Opin Anesthesiol. 2012;25:348–55.
25. Dawson LE, Russell AH, Tong D. Adenocarcinoma of the sigmoid colon: sites of initial dissemination and clinical patterns of recurrence following surgery alone. J Surg Oncol. 1983;22:95–9.

26. Chu DZ, Lang NP, Thompson C. Peritoneal carcinomatosis in nongynecologic malignancy: a prospective study of prognostic factors. Cancer. 1989;63:364–7.
27. Glockzin G, Ghali N, Lang SA, Schlitt HJ, Piso P. Results of cytoreductive surgery and hyperthermic intraperitoneal chemotherapy for peritoneal carcinomatosis from colorectal cancer. J Surg Oncol. 2009;100:306–10.
28. Brodsky JT, Cohen AM. Peritoneal seeding following potentially curative resection of colonic carcinoma: implications for adjuvant therapy. Dis Colon Rectum. 1991;34:723–7.
29. Glockzin G, Schlitt HJ, Piso P. Peritoneal carcinomatosis: patients selection, perioperative complications and quality of life related to cytoreductive surgery and hyperthermic intraperitoneal chemotherapy. World J Surg Oncol. 2009;7:5.
30. Esquivel J, Chua TC, Stojadinovic A, Torres Melero J, Levine EA, Gutman M, Howard R, Piso P, Nissan A, Gomez-Portilla A, Gonzalez-Bayon L, Gonzalez-Moreno S, Shen P, Stewart JH, Sugarbaker PH, Barone RM, Hoefer R, Morris DL, Sardi A, Sticca RP. Accuracy and clinical relevance of computed tomography scan interpretation of peritoneal cancer Index in colorectal cancer peritoneal carcinomatosis: a multi-institutional study. J Surg Oncol. 2010;102:565–70.
31. Esquivel J, Elias D, Baratti D, Kusamura S, Deraco M. Consensus statement on the loco regional treatment of colorectal cancer with peritoneal dissemination. J Surg Oncol. 2008;98:263–7.
32. Esquivel J, Sticca R, Sugarbaker P, Levine E, Yan TD, Alexander R, Baratti D, Bartlett D, Barone R, Barrios P, Bieligk S, Bretcha-Boix P, Chang CK, Chu F, Chu Q, Daniel S, de Bree E, Deraco M, Dominguez-Parra L, Elias D, Flynn R, Foster J, Garofalo A, Gilly FN, Glehen O, Gomez-Portilla A, Gonzalez-Bayon L, Gonzalez-Moreno S, Goodman M, Gushchin V, Hanna N, Hartmann J, Harrison L, Hoefer R, Kane J, Kecmanovic D, Kelley S, Kuhn J, Lamont J, Lange J, Li B, Loggie B, Mahteme H, Mann G, Martin R, Misih RA, Moran B, Morris D, Onate-Ocana L, Petrelli N, Philippe G, Pingpank J, Pitroff A, Piso P, Quinones M, Riley L, Rutstein L, Saha S, Alrawi S, Sardi A, Schneebaum S, Shen P, Shibata D, Spellman J, Stojadinovic A, Stewart J, Torres-Melero J, Tuttle T, Verwaal V, Villar J, Wilkinson N, Younan R, Zeh H, Zoetmulder F, Sebbag G. Cytoreductive surgery and hyperthermic intraperitoneal chemotherapy in the management of peritoneal surface malignancies of colonic origin: a consensus statement. Society of surgical Oncology. Ann Surg Oncol. 2007;14(1):128–33.
33. Bozzetti F, Yu W, Baratti D, Kusamura S, Deraco M. Locoregional treatment of peritoneal carcinomatosis from gastric cancer. J Surg Oncol. 2008;98:273–6.
34. Gomez-Portilla A, Sugarbaker PH, Chang D. Second-look surgery after cytoreductive and intraperitoneal chemotherapy for peritoneal carcinomatosis from colorectal cancer: analysis of prognostic features. World J Surg. 1999;23:23–9.
35. Berthet B, Sugarbaker TA, Chang D, Sugarbaker PH. Quantitative methodologies for selection of patients with recurrent abdominopelvic sarcoma for treatment. Eur J Cancer. 1999;3:413–9.
36. Sugarbaker PH. Successful management of microscopic residual disease in large bowel cancer. Cancer Chemother Pharmacol. 1999;42:S15–25.
37. Sugarbaker PH, Schellinx MET, Chang D, Koslowe P, von Meyerfeldt M. Peritoneal carcinomatosis from adenocarcinoma of the colon. World J Surg. 1996;20:585–92.
38. Deraco M, Baratti D, Kusamura S, Laterza B, Balestra MR. Surgical technique of parietal peritonectomy for peritoneal surface malignancies. J Surg Oncol. 2009;100:321–8.
39. Kusamura S, Baratti D, Antonucci A, Younan R, Laterza B, Oliva GD, Gavazzi C, Deraco M. Incidence of postoperative pancreatic fistula and hyperamylasemia after cytoreductive surgery and hyperthermic intraperitoneal chemotherapy. Ann Surg Oncol. 2007;14:3443–52.
40. Gonzalez-Moreno S, Gonzalez-Bayon LA, Ortega-Perez G. Hyperthermic intraperitoneal chemotherapy: rationale and technique. World J Gastrointest Oncol. 2010;2:68–75.
41. Jacquet P, Sugarbaker PH. Peritoneal-plasma barrier. Cancer Treat Res. 1996;82:53–63.
42. Flessner MF. The transport barrier in intraperitoneal therapy. Am J Physiol Renal Physiol. 2005;288:F433–42.

43. De Lima VV, Stuart OA, Mohamed F, Sugarbaker PH. Extent of parietal peritonectomy does not change intraperitoneal chemotherapy pharmacokinetics. Cancer Chemother Pharmacol. 2003;52:108–12.
44. El-Kareh AW, Secomb TW. A theoretical model for intraperitoneal delivery of cisplatin and the effect of hyperthermia on drug penetration distance. Neoplasia. 2004;6:117–27.
45. Los G, Verdegal EM, Mutsaers PH, Mc Vie JG. Penetration of carboplatin and cisplatin into rat peritoneal tumor nodules after intraperitoneal chemotherapy. Cancer Chemother Pharmacol. 1991;28:159–65.
46. Fujimoto S, Takahashi M, Kobayashi K, Nagano K, Kure M, Mutoh T, Ohkubo H. Cytohistologic assessment of antitumor effects of intraperitoneal hyperthermic perfusion with mitomycin C for patients with gastric cancer with peritoneal metastasis. Cancer. 1992;70:2754–60.
47. Panteix G, Guillaumont M, Cherpin L, Cuichard J, Gilly FN, Carry PY, Sayag A, Salle B, Brachet A, Bienvenu J. Study of the pharmacokinetics of mitomycin C in humans during intraperitoneal chemohyperthermia with special mention of the concentration in local tissues. Oncology. 1993;50:366–70.
48. Van de Vaart PJ, Van der Vange N, Zoetmulder FA, van Goethem AR, van Tellingen O, ten Bokkel Huinink WW, Beijnen JH, Bartelink H, Begg AC. Intraperitoneal cisplatin with regional hyperthermia in advanced ovarian cancer: pharmacokinetics and cisplatin-DNA adduct formation in patients and ovarian cancer cell lines. Eur J Cancer. 1998;34:148–54.
49. Cavaliere R, Ciocatto EC, Giovanella BC, Heidelberger C, Johnson RO, Margottini M, Mondovi B, Moricca G, Rossi-Fanelli A. Selective heat sensitivity of cancer cells. Biochemical and clinical studies. Cancer. 1967;20:1351–81.
50. Overgaard J. Effect of hyperthermia on malignant cells in vivo. A review and a hypothesis. Cancer. 1977;39:2637–46.
51. Sticca RP, Dach BW. Rationale for hyperthermia with intraoperative intraperitoneal chemotherapy agents. Surg Oncol Clin N Am. 2003;12:689–701.
52. Dudar TE, Jain RK. Differential response of normal and tumor microcirculation to hyperthermia. Cancer Res. 1984;44:605–12.
53. Benoit L, Duvillard C, Rat P, Chauffert B. The effect of intra-abdominal temperature on the tissue and tumor diffusion of intraperitoneal cisplatin in a model of peritoneal carcinomatosis in rats. Chirurgie. 1999;124:375–9.
54. Elias D, Bonnay M, Puizillou JM, Antoun S, Demirdijan S, El OA, Pignon JP, Drouard-Troalen L, Ouellet JF, Ducreux M. Heated intra-operative intraperitoneal oxaliplatin after complete resection of peritoneal carcinomatosis: pharmacokinetics and tissue distribution. Ann Oncol. 2002;13:267–72.
55. Sugarbaker PH, Mora JT, Carmignani P, Stuart OA, Yoo D. Update on chemotherapeutic agents utilized for perioperative intraperitoneal chemotherapy. Oncologist. 2005;10:112–22.
56. Halkia E, Tsochrinis A, Vassiliadou DT, Pavlakou A, Vaxevanidou A, Datsis A, Efstathiou E, Spiliotis J. Peritoneal carcinomatosis: intraoperative parameters in open (Coliseum) versus closed abdomen HIPEC. Int J Surg Oncol. 2015; Epub 2015 Feb 15.
57. Van der Speeten K, Stuart OA, Sugarbaker PH. Pharmacokinetics and pharmacodynamics of perioperative cancer chemotherapy in peritoneal surface malignancy. Cancer J. 2009;15:216–24.
58. Stuart OA, Stephens AD, Welch L, Sugarbaker PH. Safety monitoring of the coliseum technique for heated intraoperative intraperitoneal chemotherapy with mitomycin C. Ann Surg Oncol. 2002;9:186–91.
59. Schierl R, Novotna J, Piso P, Böhlandt A, Nowak D. Low surface contamination by cis/oxaliplatin during hyperthermic intraperitoneal chemotherapy (HIPEC). Eur J Surg Oncol. 2012;38:88–94.
60. Villa AF, El Balkhi S, Aboura R, Sageot H, Hasni-Pichard H, Pocard M, Elias D, Joly N, Payen D, Blot F, Poupon J, Garnier R. Evaluation of oxaliplatin exposure of healthcare workers during heated intraperitoneal perioperative chemotherapy (HIPEC). Ind Health. 2015;53:28–37.

61. Gonzalez-Bayon L, Gonzalez-Moreno S, Ortega-Perez G. Safety considerations for operating room personnel during hyperthermic intraoperative intraperitoneal chemotherapy perfusion. Eur J Surg Oncol. 2006;32:619–24.

62. Esquivel J, Angulo F, Bland RK, Stephens AD, Sugarbaker PH. Hemodynamic and cardiac function parameters during heated intraoperative intraperitoneal chemotherapy using the open "coliseum technique". Ann Surg Oncol. 2000;7:296–300.

63. Michelson AD, MacGregor H, Barnard MR, Kestin AS, Rohrer MJ, Valeri CR. Reversible inhibition of human platelet activation by hypothermia in vivo and in vitro. Thromb Haemost. 1994;71:633–40.

64. Morris DL, Chambers HF, Morris MG, Sande MA. Hemodynamic characteristics of patients with hypothermia due to occult infection and other causes. Ann Intern Med. 1985;102:153–7.

65. Seekamp A, van Griensven M, Hildebrandt F, Wahlers T, Tscherne H. Adenosine-triphosphate in trauma-related and elective hypothermia. J Trauma. 1999;47:673–83.

66. Kanakoudis F, Petrou A, Michaloudis D, Chortaria G, Konstantinidou A. Anaesthesia for intra-peritoneal perfusion of hyperthermic chemotherapy. Haemodynamic changes, oxygen consumption and delivery. Anaesthesia. 1996;51:1033–6.

67. Shime N, Lee M, Hatanaka T. Cardiovascular changes during continuous hyperthermic peritoneal perfusion. Anesth Analg. 1994;78:938–42.

68. Cafiero T, Di Lorio C, Di Minno RM, Sivolella G, Confuorto G. Non-invasive cardiac monitoring by aortic blood flow determination in patients undergoing hyperthermic intraperitoneal intraoperative chemotherapy. Minerva Anestesiol. 2006;72:207–15.

69. Schmidt C, Creutzenberg M, Piso P, Hobbahn J, Bucher M. Peri-operative anaesthetic management of cytoreductive surgery with hyperthermic intraperitoneal chemotherapy. Anaesthesia. 2008;63:389–95.

70. Raue W, Tsilimparis N, Bloch A, Menenakos C, Hartmann J. Volume therapy and cardiocircular function during hyperthermic intraperitoneal chemotherapy. Eur Surg Res. 2009;43:365–72.

71. Vorgias G, Iavazzo C, Mavromatis J, Leontara J, Katsoulis M, Kalinoglou N, Akrivos T. Determination of the necessary total protein substitution requirements in patients with advanced stage ovarian cancer and ascites, undergoing debulking surgery. Correlation with plasma proteins. Ann Surg Oncol. 2007;14:1919–23.

72. De Somer F, Ceelen W, Delanghe J, De Smet D, Vanackere M, Pattyn P, Mortier E. Severe hyponatremia and hyperlactatemia are associated with intraoperative hyperthermic intraperitoneal chemoperfusion with oxaliplatin. Perit Dial Int. 2008;28:61–6.

73. Raft J, Parisot M, Marchal F, Tala S, Desandes E, Lalot JM, Guillemin F, Longrois D, Meistelman C. Impact of the hyperthermic intraperitoneal chemotherapy on the fluid-electrolytes changes and on the acid-base balance. Ann Fr Anesth Reanim. 2010;29:676–81.

74. Thix CA, Königsrainer I, Kind R, Wied P, Schroeder TH. Ventricular tachycardia during hyperthermic intraperitoneal chemotherapy. Anaesthesia. 2009;64:1134–6.

75. Cooksley TJ, Haji-Michael P. Postoperative critical care management of patients undergoing cytoreductive surgery and heated intraperitoneal chemotherapy (HIPEC). World J Surg Oncol. 2011;9:169.

76. Synder G, Greenberg S. Effect of anaesthetic technique and other perioperative factors on cancer recurrence. Br J Anaesth. 2010;105:106–15.

77. De la Chapelle A, Perus O, Soubielle J, Raucoulles-Aime M, Bernard JL, Bereder JM. High potential for epidural analgesia neuraxial block-associated hypotension in conjunction with heated intraoperative intraperitoneal chemotherapy. Reg Anaesthesiol Pain Med. 2005;30:313–4.

78. Desgranges FP, Steghens A, Rosay H, Méeus P, Stoian A, Daunizeau AL, Pouderoux-Martin S, Piriou V. Epidural analgesia for surgical treatment of peritoneal carcinomatosis: a risky technique ? Ann Fr Anesth Reanim. 2012;31(1):53–9.

79. Desgranges FP, Steghens A, Mithieux F, Rosay H. Potential risks of thoracic epidural analgesia in hyperthermic intraperitoneal chemotherapy. J Surg Oncol. 2010;101:442.

80. Mann V, Mann S, Hecker A, Röhrig R, Müller M, Schwandner T, Hirschburger M, Sprengel A, Weigand MA, Padberg W. Continuous local wound infusion with local anesthetics: for thoracotomy and major abdominal interventions. Chirurg. 2011;82:906–12.

81. Younan R, Kusamura S, Bratti D, Cloutier AS, Deraco M. Morbidity, toxicity and mortality classification systems in the local regional treatment of peritoneal surface malignancy. J Surg Oncol. 2008;98:253–7.

82. Roviello F, Caruso S, Marrelli D, Pedrazzani C, Neri A, De Stefano A, Pinto E. Treatment of peritoneal carcinomatosis with cytoreductive surgery and hyperthermic intraperitoneal chemotherapy: state of the art and future developments. Surg Oncol. 2011;20:e38–54.

83. McQuellon RP, Loggie BW, Fleming RA, Russell GB, Lehmann AB, Rambo TD. Quality of life after intraperitoneal hyperthermic chemotherapy (IPHC) for peritoneal carcinomatosis. Eur J Surg Oncol. 2001;27:65–73.

84. McQuellon RP, Danhauer SC, Russell GB, Shen P, Fenstermaker J, Stewart JH, Levine EA. Monitoring health outcomes following cytoreductive surgery plus intraperitoneal hyperthermic chemotherapy for peritoneal carcinomatosis. Ann Surg Oncol. 2007;14:1105–13.

85. Shan LL, Saxena A, Shan BL, Morris DL. Quality of life after cytoreductive surgery and hyperthermic intraperitoneal chemotherapy for peritoneal carcinomatosis: a systematic review and meta-analysis. Surg Oncol. 2014;23:199–210.

86. Robinson BW, Lake RA. Advances in malignant mesothelioma. N Engl J Med. 2005;353:1591–603.

87. Robinson BW, Musk AW, Lake RA. Malignant mesothelioma. Lancet. 2005;366:397–408.

88. Price B. Analysis of current trends in United States mesothelioma incidence. Am J Epidemiol. 1997;145:211–8.

89. Peterson Jr JT, Greenberg SD, Buffler PA. Non-asbestos-related malignant mesothelioma. A review. Cancer. 1984;54:951–60.

90. Sugarbaker PH, Welch LS, Mohamed F, Glehen O. A review of peritoneal mesothelioma at the Washington Cancer Institute. Surg Oncol Clin N Am. 2003;12:605–21.

91. Husain AN, Colby TV, Ordonez NG, Krausz T, Borczuk A, Cagle PT, Chirieac LR, Churg A, Galateau-Salle F, Gibbs AR, Gown AM, Hammar SP, Litzky LA, Roggli VL, Travis WD, Wick MR. Guidelines for pathologic diagnosis of malignant mesothelioma: a consensus statement from the international mesothelioma interest group. Arch Pathol Lab Med. 2009;133:1317–31.

92. Antmann KH, Blum RH, Greenberger JS, Flowerdew G, Skarin AT, Canellos GP. Multimodality therapy for malignant mesothelioma based on a study of natural history. Am J Med. 1980;68:356–62.

93. Yan TD, Welch L, Black D, Sugarbaker PH. A systematic review on the efficacy of cytoreductive surgery combined with perioperative intraperitoneal chemotherapy for diffuse malignancy peritoneal mesothelioma. Ann Oncol. 2007;18:827–34.

94. Deraco M, Baratti D, Cabras AD, Zaffaroni N, Perrone F, Villa R, Jocolle J, Balestra MA, Kusamura S, Laterza B, Pilotti S. Experience with peritoneal mesothelioma at the Milan National Cancer Institute. World J Gastrointest Oncol. 2010;2:76–84.

95. Helm JH, Miura JT, Glenn JA, Marcus RK, Larrieux G, Jayakrishnan TT, Donahue AE, Gamblin TC, Turaga KK, Johnston FM. Cytoreductive surgery and hyperthermic intraperitoneal chemotherapy for malignant peritoneal mesothelioma: a systemic review and meta-analysis. Ann Surg Oncol. 2015;22:1686–93.

96. Chua TC, Yan TD, Morris DL. Outcomes of cytoreductive surgery and hyperthermic intraperitoneal chemotherapy for peritoneal mesothelioma: the Australian experience. J Surg Oncol. 2009;99:109–13.

97. Baratti D, Kusamura S, Cabras AD, Deraco M. Cytoreductive surgery with selective versus complete parietal peritonectomy followed by hyperthermic intraperitoneal chemotherapy ion patients with diffuse malignant peritoneal mesothelioma: a controlled study. Ann Surg Oncol. 2012;19:1416–24.

98. Baratti D, Kusamura S, Nonaka D, Oliva GD, Laterza B, Deraco M. Multicystic and well-differentiated papillary peritoneal mesothelioma treated by surgical cytoreduction and hyperthermic intra peritoneal chemotherapy (HIPEC). Ann Surg Oncol. 2007;14:1790–7.

99. Elias D, Lefevre JH, Chevalier J, Brouquet A, Marchal F, Classe JM, Ferron GF, Guilloit JM, Meeus P, Goere D, Bonastre J. Complete cytoreductive surgery plus intraperitoneal chemohyperthermia with oxaliplatin for peritoneal carcinomatosis of colorectal origin. J Clin Oncol. 2008;27:681–5.
100. Verwaal VJ, Van Ruth S, Witkamp A, Boot H, van Slooten G, Zoetmulder FA. Long-term survival of peritoneal carcinomatosis of colorectal origin. Ann Surg Oncol. 2005;12(1):65–71.
101. Da Silva GR, Cabanas J, Sugarbaker PH. Limited survival in the treatment of carcinomatosis from rectal cancer. Dis Colon Rectum. 2005;48:2258–63.
102. Pelz JO, Stojadinovic A, Nissan A, Hohenberger W, Esquivel J. Evaluation of a peritoneal surface disease severity score in patients with colon cancer with peritoneal carcinomatosis. J Surg Oncol. 2009;99:9–15.
103. Van Ouheusden TR, Braam HJ, Nienhuijs SW, Wiezer MJ, Van Ramshorst B, Luyer P, De Hingh ICH. Poor outcome after cytoreductive surgery and HIPEC for colorectal peritoneal carcinomatosis with signet ring cell histology. J Surg Oncol. 2015;111:237–42.
104. Elias D, Goerer D, di Pietrantonio D, Boige V, Malka D, Kohneh-Shahri N, Dromain C, Ducreux M. Results of systematic second-look surgery in patients at high risk of developing colorectal peritoneal carcinomatosis. Ann Surg. 2008;247:445–50.
105. Moran BJ, Cecil TD. The etiology, clinical presentation and management of pseudomyxoma peritonei. Surg Oncol Clin N Am. 2003;12:585–603.
106. Sugarbaker PH. New standard of care for appendiceal epithelial neoplasms and pseudomyxoma peritonei syndrome? Lancet Oncol. 2006;7:69–76.
107. Weaver CH. Mucocele of the appendix with pseudomucinous degeneration. Am J Surg. 1937;36:523–6.
108. Ronnett BM, Zahn CM, Kurman RJ, Kass ME, Sugarbaker PH, Shmookler BM. Disseminated peritoneal adenomucinosis and peritoneal mucinous carcinomatosis: a clinicopathologic analysis of 109 cases with emphasis on distinguishing pathologic features, site of origin, prognosis and relationship to "pseudomyxoma peritonei". Am J Surg Pathol. 1995;19:1390–408.
109. Szych C, Staebler A, Connoly DC, Wu R, Cho KR, Ronnett BM. Molecular genetic evidence supporting the clonality and appendiceal origin of pseudomyxoma peritonei in women. Am J Pathol. 1999;154:1849–55.
110. Carr NJ, Emory TS, Sobin LH. Epithelial neoplasms of the appendix and colorectum: an analysis of cell proliferation apoptosis and expression of p53, CD44, bcl-2. Arch Pathol Lab Med. 2002;126:837–41.
111. Kahn MA, Demopoulos RI. Mucinous ovarian tumors with pseudomyxoma peritonei: a clinicopathological study. Int J Gynecol Pathol. 1992;11:15–23.
112. Chejfec G, Rieker WJ, Jablokow VR, Gould VE. Pseudomyxoma peritonei associated with colloid carcinoma of the pancreas. Gastroenterology. 1986;90:202–5.
113. Gough DB, Donohue JH, Schutt AJ, Gonchoroff N, Goellner JR, Wilson TO, Naessens JM, O'Brien PC, van Heerden JA. Pseudomyxoma peritonei. Long-term patient survival with an aggressive regional approach. Am Surg. 1994;219:112–9.
114. Miner TJ, Shia J, Jaques DP, Klimstra DS, Brennan MF, Coit DG. Long-term survival following treatment of pseudomyxoma peritonei: an analysis of surgical therapy. Ann Surg. 2005;241:300–8.
115. Gonzaelz-Moreno S, Sugarbaker PH. Right hemicolectomy does not confer a survival advantage in patients with mucinous carcinoma of the appendix and peritoneal seeding. Br J Surg. 2004;91:304–11.
116. Moran B, Baratti D, Yan TD, Kusamura S, Deraco M. Consensus statement on the locoregional treatment of appendiceal mucinous neoplasms with peritoneal dissemination (pseudomyxoma peritonei). J Surg Oncol. 2008;98:277–82.
117. Chua TC, Moran BJ, Sugarbaker PH, Levine EA, Glehen O, Gilly FN, Baratti D, Deraco M, Elias D, Sardi A, Liauw W, Yan TD, Barrios P, Gomez-Portilla A, de Hingh IH, Ceelen WP, Pelz JO, Piso P, Gonzalez-Moreno S, Van der Speeten K, Morris DL. Early- and long-term

outcome data of patients with pseudomyxoma peritonei from appendiceal origin treated by a strategy of cytoreductive surgery and hyperthermic intraperitoneal chemotherapy. J Clin Oncol. 2012;30:2449–56.

118. Gill RS, Al-Adra DP, Nagendran J, Campbell S, Shi X, Haase E, Schiller D. Treatment of gastric cancer with peritoneal carcinomatosis by cytoreductive surgery and HIPEC: a systematic review of survival, mortality and morbidity. J Surg Oncol. 2011;104:692–8.

119. Ikeguchi M, Oka A, Tsujitani S, Maeta M, Kaibara N. Relationship between area of serosal invasion and intraperitoneal free cancer cells in patients with gastric cancer. Anticancer Res. 1994;14:2131–4.

120. Yonemura Y, Endou Y, Sasaki T, Hirano M, Mizumoto A, Matsuda T, Takao N, Ichinose M, Miura M, Li Y. Surgical treatment for peritoneal carcinomatosis from gastric cancer. Eur J Surg Oncol. 2010;36:1131–8.

121. Roth AD, Fazio N, Stupp R, Falk S, Bernhard J, Saletti P, Köberle D, Borner MM, Rufibach K, Maibach R, Wernli M, Leslie M, Glynne-Jones R, Widmer L, Seymour M, de Braud F, Swiss Group for Clinical Cancer Research. Docetaxel, cisplatin, and fluorouracil; docetaxel and cisplatin; and epirubicin, cisplatin, and fluorouracil as systemic treatment for advanced gastric carcinoma: a randomized phase II trial of the Swiss Group for Clinical Cancer Research. J Clin Oncol. 2007;25:3217–23.

122. Ross P, Nicolson M, Cunningham D, Valle J, Seymour M, Harper P, Price T, Anderson H, Iveson T, Hickish T, Lofts F, Norman A. Prospective randomized trial comparing mitomycin, cisplatin, and protracted venous-infusion fluorouracil (PVI 5-FU) with epirubicin, cisplatin, and PVI 5-FU in advanced esophagogastric cancer. J Clin Oncol. 2002;20:1996–2004.

123. Kochi M, Fujii M, Kanamori N, Kaiga T, Takahashi T, Kobayashi M, Takayama T. Neoadjuvant chemotherapy with S-1 and CDDP in advanced gastric cancer. J Cancer Res Clin Oncol. 2006;132:781–5.

124. Yabusaki Y, Nashimoto A, Tanaka O. Evaluation of TS-1 combined with cisplatin for neoadjuvant chemotherapy in patients with advanced gastric cancer. Jpn J Cancer Chemother. 2003;30:1933–40.

125. Baba H, Yamamoto M, Endo K, Ikeda Y, Toh Y, Kohnoe S, Okamura T. Clinical efficacy of S-1 combined with cisplatin for advanced gastric cancer. Gastric Cancer. 2003;6:45–9.

126. Swellengrebel HA, Zoetmulder FA, Smeenk RM, Antonini N, Verwaal VJ. Quantitative intra-operative assessment of peritoneal carcinomatosis – a comparison of three prognostic tools. Eur J Surg Oncol. 2009;35:1078–84.

127. Yang XJ, Li Y, Yonemura Y. Cytoreductive surgery plus hyperthermic intraperitoneal chemotherapy to treat gastric cancer with ascites and/or peritoneal carcinomatosis: results from a Chinese center. J Surg Oncol. 2010;101:459–64.

128. Yonemura Y, Elnemr A, Endou Y, Hirano M, Mizumoto A, Takao N, Ichinose M, Miura M, Li Y. Multidisciplinary therapy for treatment of patients with peritoneal carcinomatosis from gastric cancer. World J Gastrointest Oncol. 2010;2:85–97.

129. Yan TD, Black D, Sugarbaker PH, Zhu J, Yonemura Y, Petrou G, Morris DL. A systematic review and meta-analysis of the randomized controlled trials on adjuvant intraperitoneal chemotherapy for resectable gastric cancer. Ann Surg Oncol. 2007;14:2702–13.

130. Di Vita M, Capellani A, Piccolo G, Zanghi A, Cavallaro A, Bertola G, Bolognese A, Facchini G, D'Aniello C, Di Francia R, Cardi F, Berretta M. The role of HIPEC in the treatment of peritoneal carcinomatosis from gastric cancer: between lights and shadows. Anti Cancer Drugs. 2015;26:123–38.

131. Glehen O, Gilly FN, Arvieux C, Cotte E, Boutitie F, Mansvelt B, Bereder JM, Lorimier G, Quenet F, Elias D. Peritoneal carcinomatosis from gastric cancer: a multi-institutional study of 159 patients treated by cytoreductive surgery combined with perioperative intraperitoneal chemotherapy. Ann Surg Oncol. 2010;17:2370–7.

132. Yonemura Y, Endou Y, Shinbo M, Sasaki T, Hirano M, Mizumoto A, Matsuda T, Takao N, Ichinose M, Mizuno M, Miura M, Ikeda M, Ikeda S, Nakajima G, Yonemura J, Yuuba T, Masuda S, Kimura H, Matsuki N. Safety and efficacy of bidirectional chemotherapy for treatment of patients with peritoneal dissemination from gastric cancer: selection for cytoreductive surgery. J Surg Oncol. 2009;100:311–6.

133. Koh JL, Yan TD, Glenn D, Morris DL. Evaluation of preoperative computed tomography in estimating peritoneal cancer index in colorectal peritoneal carcinomatosis. Ann Surg Oncol. 2009;16:327–33.
134. Valle M, Garofalo A. Laparoscopic staging of peritoneal surface malignancies. Eur J Surg Oncol. 2006;32:625–7.
135. Yano M, Shiozaki H, Inoue M, Tamura S, Doki Y, Yasuda T, Fujiwara Y, Tsujinaka T, Monden M. Neoadjuvant chemotherapy followed by salvage surgery: effect on survival of patients with primary noncurative gastric cancer. Worl J Surg. 2002;26:1155–9.
136. Yonemura Y, Shinbo M, Hagiwara A. Treatment for potentially curable gastric cancer patients with intraperitoneal free cancer cells. Gastroenterol Surg. 2008;31:802–12.
137. Yonemura Y, Bandou E, Sawa T, Yoshimitsu Y, Endou Y, Sasaki T, Sugarbaker PH. Neoadjuvant treatment of gastric cancer with peritoneal dissemination. Eur J Surg Oncol. 2006;32:661–5.
138. Siegel R, Naishadham R, Jemal A. Cancer statistics, 2012. CA Cancer J Clin. 2012;62:10–29.
139. Goff BA, Mandel L, Muntz HG, Melancon CH. Ovarian carcinoma diagnosis. Cancer. 2000;89:2068–75.
140. McGuire WP, Hoskins WJ, Brady MF, Kucera PR, Partridge EE, Look KY, Clarke-Pearson DL, Davidson M. Cyclophosphamide and cisplatin compared with paclitaxel and cisplatin in patients with stage III and stage IV ovarian cancer. N Engl J Med. 1996;334:1–6.
141. Ozols RF. Treatment goals in ovarian cancer. Int J Gynecol Cancer. 2005;15:3–11.
142. Armstrong DK, Bundy B, Wenzel L, Huang HQ, Baergen R, Lele S, Copeland LJ, Walker JL, Burger RA, Gynecologic Oncology Group. Intraperitoneal cisplatin and paclitaxel in ovarian cancer. N Engl J Med. 2006;354:34–43.
143. Chua TC, Robertson G, Liauw W, Farrell R, Yan TD, Morris DL. Intraoperative hyperthermic intraperitoneal chemotherapy after cytoreductive surgery in ovarian cancer peritoneal carcinomatosis: systematic review of current results. J Cancer Res Clin Oncol. 2009;135:1637–45.
144. Deraco M, Baratti D, Laterza B, Balestra MR, Mingrone E, Macri A, Virzi S, Puccio F, Ravenda PS, Kusamura S. Advanced cytoreduction as surgical standard of care and hyperthermic intraperitoneal chemotherapy as promising treatment in epithelial ovarian cancer. Eur J Surg Oncol. 2011;37:4–9.
145. Winter 3rd WE, Maxwell GL, Tian C, Sundborg MJ, Rose GS, Rose PG, Rubin SC, Muggia F, McGuire WP. Tumor residual after surgical cytoreduction in prediction of clinical outcome in stage IV epithelial ovarian cancer: a Gynecologic Oncology Group Study. J Clin Oncol. 2008;26:83–9.
146. Roviello F, Roviello G, Petrioli R, Marrelli D. Hyperthermic intraperitoneal chemotherapy for the treatment of ovarian cancer: a brief overview of recent results. Crit Rev Oncol Hematol. 2015;11 Epub ahead of print.
147. Bakrin N, Bereder JM, Decullier E, Classe JM, Msika S, Lorimier G, Abboud K, Meeus P, Ferron G, Quenet F, Marchal F, Gouy S, Morice P, Pomel C, Pocard M, Guyon F, Porcheron J, Glehen O, FROGHI (French Oncologic and Gynecologic HIPEC) Group. Peritoneal carcinomatosis treated with cytoreductive surgery and hyperthermic intraperitoneal chemotherapy (HIPEC) for advanced ovarian carcinoma: a French multicenter retrospective cohort study of 566 patients. Eur J Surg Oncol. 2013;39(12):1435–43.
148. Spiliotis J, Halkia E, Lianos E, Kalantzi N, Grivas A, Efsthatiou E, Giassas S. Cytoreductive surgery and HIPEC in recurrent epithelial ovarian cancer: a prospective randomized phase III study. Ann Surg Oncol. 2015;22:1570–5.
149. OVIHIPEC trial; ClinicalTrials.gov identifier:NCT00426257.http://clinicaltrials.gov/ct2/show/NCT00426257.
150. Chua TC, Liauw W, Robertson G, Chia WK, Soo KC, Alobaid A, Al-Mohaimeed K, Morris DL. Towards randomized trials of cytoreductive surgery using peritonectomy and hyperthermic intraperitoneal chemotherapy for ovarian cancer peritoneal carcinomatosis. Gynecol Oncol. 2009;114:137–9.
151. Classe JM, Muller M, Frenel JS, Berton Rigaud D, Ferron G, Jaffré I, Gladieff L. Intraperitoneal chemotherapy in the treatment of advanced ovarian cancer. J Gynecol Obstet Biol Reprod. 2010;39:183–90.

Induction Bidirectional Chemotherapy for Gastric Cancer with Peritoneal Dissemination

13

Y. Yonemura and Paul H. Sugarbaker

13.1 Introduction

Patients with peritoneal seeding from gastric cancer may present themselves to the surgeon without warning that advanced disease exists. Ten to 20 % of patients being explored for potentially curative resection will be found to have peritoneal seeding at the time of abdominal exploration. This occurs most frequently in patients who have the signet ring type of gastric cancer as opposed to intestinal-type pathology. Sometimes, a small amount of fluid on CT scan or on ultrasound may alert the clinician to the presence of peritoneal seeding. On CT, subtle linear densities associated with the fat that constitutes the omentum or small bowel mesentery may suggest peritoneal carcinomatosis (PC). Often, the presence versus absence of PC can only be determined by laparoscopy. When confronted with peritoneal seeding from gastric cancer, the clinician must make a decision regarding the possible risks and benefits of aggressive treatments versus best supportive care. In other diseases where peritoneal surface malignancy is treated, there are reports of a curative approach. The most striking example of this is with appendix cancer and the pseudomyxoma peritonei syndrome [1].

No other treatments for gastric cancer with peritoneal seeding have been shown to be effective. Systemic chemotherapy for patients with peritoneal seeding has been uniformly disappointing. Preusser et al. published a response rate to aggressive chemotherapy of 50 % in patients with advanced gastric cancer, but the response rate was lowest in patients with PC [2]. Ajani et al. treated patients prior to

Y. Yonemura
Peritoneal Surface Malignancy Program, Kasatsu General Hospital,
I-26 Haruki-Motomachi, Kishiwada, Osaka, Japan

P.H. Sugarbaker (✉)
Program in Peritoneal Surface Malignancy, Washington Cancer Institute, Washington Hospital Center, 106 Irving St., N.W, POB 3900, Washington, DC 20010, USA
e-mail: paul.sugarbaker@medstar.net

© Springer-Verlag Berlin Heidelberg 2016
K.R. Aigner, F.O. Stephens (eds.), *Induction Chemotherapy*,
DOI 10.1007/978-3-319-28773-7_13

gastrectomy [3]. At exploration, PC was the most common indication of failure of the intensive chemotherapy regimen. Systemic chemotherapy alone is not an adequate management strategy for primary gastric cancer with PC.

We describe a new induction chemotherapy treatment modality for gastric cancer with peritoneal seeding; it combines intraperitoneal with systemic chemotherapy in an attempt to eradicate disease on visceral peritoneal surfaces and thereby increase the proportion of patients who may receive complete cytoreduction. It is an attempt to eradicate cancer nodules by bidirectional chemotherapy; in this plan, chemotherapy would enter the cancer nodule not only from the systemic circulation but also diffuse into the nodule from a chemotherapy solution in the peritoneal cavity [4]. A prospective phase II study was initiated to demonstrate the efficacy of this treatment in the palliation of patients with gastric cancer and carcinomatosis. The results to date and the toxicities are reviewed in this presentation.

13.1.1 Patients Treated

Patients were enrolled between April 01, 2001, and April 20, 2009. Carcinomatosis was diagnosed by biopsy using laparotomy, laparoscopy, or by the cytologic examination of ascites. The eligibility criteria included: (1) histologically or cytologically proven peritoneal seeding from gastric adenocarcinoma; (2) absence of hematogenous metastasis and remote lymph node metastasis; (3) age 65 years or younger; (4) Eastern Clinical Oncology Group scale of performance status two or less; (5) adequate bone marrow, liver, cardiac, and renal function; and (6) absence of other severe medical conditions or synchronous malignancy.

Informed consent according to the institutional guideline was obtained from all patients.

After the cytological or histological diagnosis of peritoneal dissemination, a peritoneal port system (Bard Port, C.R. Bard Inc., USA) was introduced into the abdominal cavity under local anesthesia, and the tip was placed within the cul-de-sac of Douglas.

13.1.2 Chemotherapy Regimen

For intraperitoneal chemotherapy, 40 mg of Taxotere and 150 mg of carboplatin were introduced over 30 min in 1,000 ml of saline. On the same day, 100 mg/m^2 of methotrexate and 600 mg/m^2 of 5-fluorouracil were infused in 100 ml of saline over 15 min via a peripheral vein. This regimen was repeated in 1 week. Before initiation of the bidirectional chemotherapy, 500 ml of saline was injected into the peritoneal cavity through the port, and fluid was recovered for cytology. Peritoneal wash cytology was performed after the two courses of bidirectional treatment. If the result showed positive cytology, induction chemotherapy was continued for a further two courses. Then, the test was repeated after four courses of treatment and continued again in the cases of positive results for peritoneal wash cytology.

In the patients with negative cytology before the initiation of treatment, endoscopy and CT scan were performed after two courses. If no effect was observed on the tumors, patients additionally received two more courses of therapy. The number of cycles of bidirectional treatments depended on the chemotherapy effect on tumors or the status of peritoneal cytology.

In all studies that address the treatment of carcinomatosis, complete cytoreduction is a requirement for prolonged survival in the management of this condition [5–9]. For this reason, complete or near-complete response of cancer on peritoneal surfaces was the goal of the induction bidirectional chemotherapy.

The peritoneal stage was determined from the Japanese General Rules for Gastric Cancer Study: metastasis to the adjacent peritoneum (P1), a few metastases to distant peritoneal sites (P2), and numerous metastases to the distant peritoneum (P3) [10]. The distributions and sizes of peritoneal metastases were recorded at all laparoscopic or surgical interventions. Effects of induction therapy were evaluated by comparing the size and number of carcinomatosis nodules before and after treatments.

If the peritoneal wash cytology became negative or the tumors showed partial response, laparotomy was done to perform gastrectomy and peritonectomy procedures. Patients showing progressive disease did not undergo laparotomy, and patients with positive cytology even after four or six courses of induction systemic chemotherapy were treated with systemic chemotherapy as definitive treatment.

13.1.3 Surgery for Gastric Cancer with Peritoneal Carcinomatosis

The major objective in performing palliative resection of gastric cancer is the elimination of catastrophic complications caused by the primary malignancy. Also, resection of the gastric cancer greatly reduces the volume of residual cancer. Peritonectomy can be used to further reduce and, in some patients, eliminate all visual evidence of disease. Sugarbaker and Yonemura reported on the use of peritonectomy procedures for carcinomatosis [11, 12]. The peritonectomies that are specific to patients with gastric cancer have been presented [13–15]. These peritonectomy procedures are to maximally cytoreduce the peritoneal surface malignancy and facilitate the total resection of the primary gastric cancer. The epigastric peritonectomy includes any prior midline abdominal scar in continuity with the preperitoneal epigastric fat pad, xiphoid process, and the round and falciform ligaments of the liver (Fig. 13.1). The anterolateral peritonectomy removes the greater omentum with the anterior layer of the peritoneum from the transverse mesocolon, peritoneum of the right paracolic gutter along with the appendix, and the peritoneum in the right subhepatic space. In some patients, the peritoneum covering the left paracolic gutter must be stripped (Fig. 13.2). The subphrenic peritonectomy removes the peritoneal surfaces from the medial half of the right and left hemidiaphragm along with a resection of the left triangular ligament (Fig. 13.3). The omental bursa peritonectomy is initiated with a cholecystectomy. The peritoneal covering of the porta hepatis, the peritoneum covering the anterior and posterior aspects of the

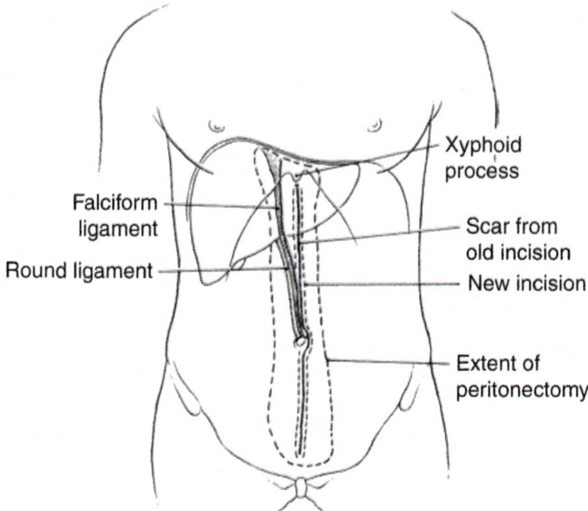

Fig. 13.1 Epigastric peritonectomy

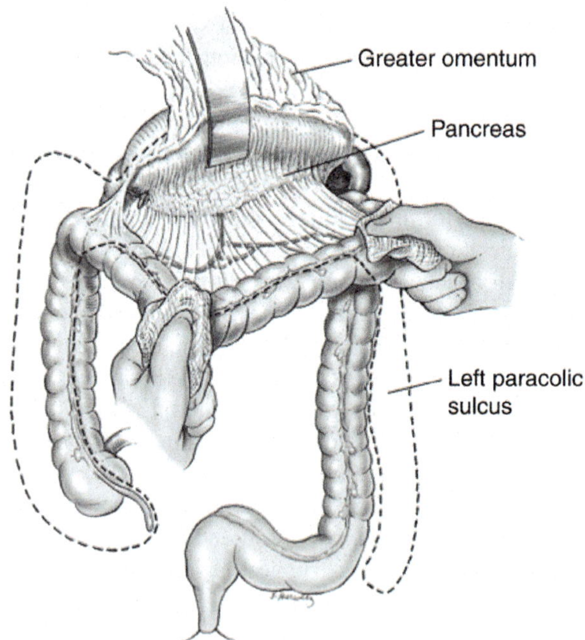

Fig. 13.2 Anterolateral peritonectomy

hepatoduodenal ligament, and the peritoneal floor of the omental bursa including the peritoneum overlying the pancreas are resected (Fig. 13.4). In those patients who have a tumor within the cul-de-sac, a pelvic peritonectomy is indicated.

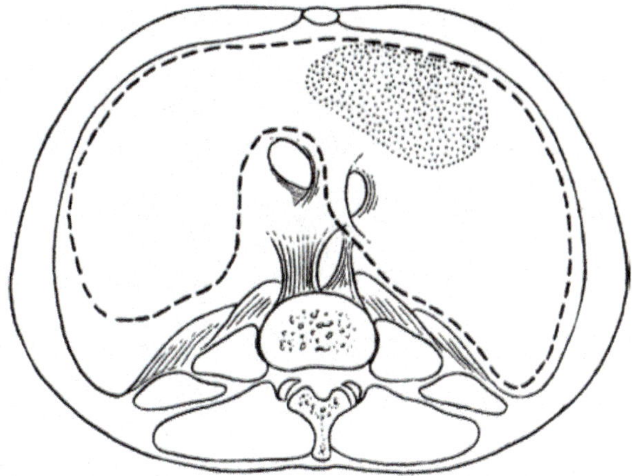

Fig. 13.3 Subphrenic peritonectomy

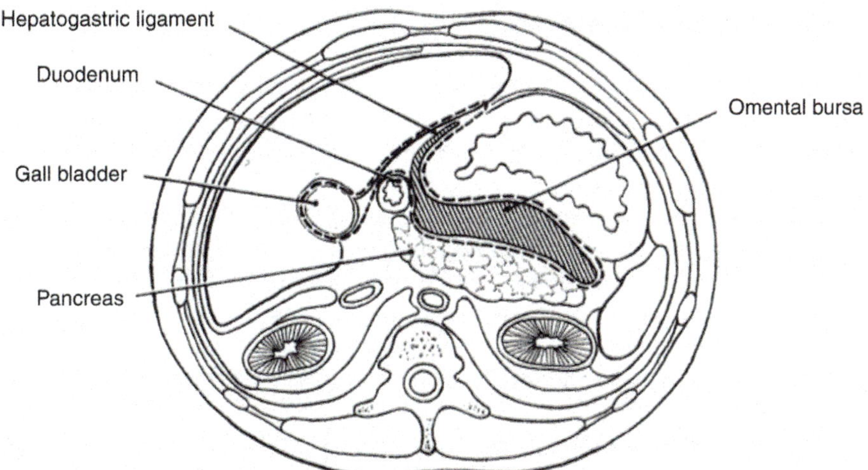

Fig. 13.4 Omental bursa peritonectomy

Electro-evaporative surgery is used to strip the peritoneum from the pouch of Douglas (Fig. 13.5). Occasionally, the pelvic peritonectomy will require removal of the rectosigmoid colon in order to completely remove the tumor from the cul-de-sac. The goal of visceral resections and peritonectomies was the complete removal of all visible cancer.

Complications were prospectively identified and verified by a chart review. All complications related to induction chemotherapy and peritonectomy were recorded.

Outcome data were obtained from medical records and patient interview. Statistical analyses were performed by using SPSS software (SPSS Inc., Chicago, USA). Survival curves are calculated by the Kaplan-Meier method.

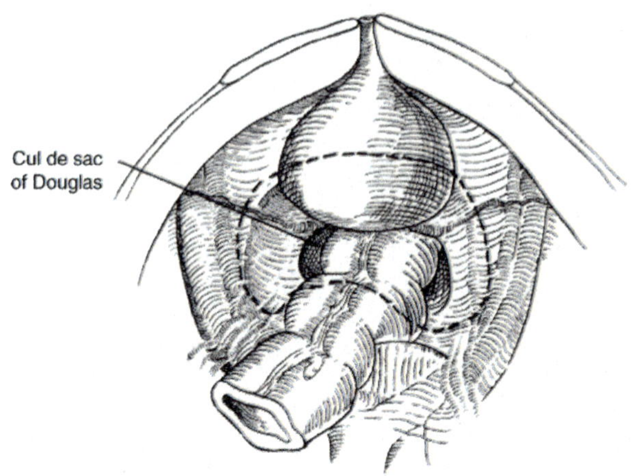

Fig. 13.5 Pelvic peritonectomy

13.2 Results of Treatment

Clinical characteristics of the 133 patients are listed in Table 13.1. The average age was 50.6 years. Fifteen and 118 patients had P2 and P3 dissemination, respectively. Ascites was present in 78 patients. Twenty-eight patients had primary gastric cancer and the remaining 66 patients had recurrent PC.

Prior to induction bidirectional chemotherapy, peritoneal fluid cytology was positive in 85 patients and reverted to negative cytology after treatment in 50. In 68 patients with ascites, all peritoneal fluid disappeared in 33 patients after induction treatment. Seventy-six patients showed partial response (Table 13.2). Following induction treatment, 78 patients had an operative intervention, and the other 45 patients did not undergo surgery due to the progression of disease ($N=33$) and refusal of operation ($N=12$).

Table 13.3 indicates the operation interventions. Total gastrectomy was performed in 54 primary cases, subtotal colectomy in 38, total hysterectomy in combination with bilateral salpingo-oophorectomy in 26, resection of small bowel in 23, and resection of small bowel mesentery in 25. Left and right subdiaphragmatic peritonectomy was performed in 19 and 15 patients, respectively. Pelvic peritonectomy was performed in 31 patients. Fulguration of peritoneal nodules was used as an adjunctive surgical technique in 60 patients. Complete cytoreduction was achieved in 45 (58 %) of 78 patients.

Bone marrow suppression of grade 3 or 4 was recorded in ten patients and diarrhea in four patients, respectively. Bone marrow suppression developed after three courses in three, five courses in three, and six courses in four patients. Port site infection was found in two patients. Renal failure occurred in one patient.

Complications developed in 18 patients (14 %) after cytoreductive surgery with peritonectomy. Pneumonia developed in two patients and renal failure occurred in one patient. There were six instances of anastomotic leakage and two of abdominal

Table 13.1 Patients' characteristics

Age	50.6±13.2 (range 18–81)
Gender	
Male	64
Female	69
Grade of dissemination	
P1	0
P2	15
P3	118
Ascites	
No	65
Yes	68
Peritoneal lavage cytology	
Negative	48
Positive	85
Primary or recurrence	
Primary	67
Recurrence	66
Cycles of NIPS	5.2 (1–20)
Total	133

Table 13.2 Effect of peritoneal dissemination after bidirectional induction chemotherapy

	Surgical exploration	No exploration	Total (%)
No change or progressive disease	19	37	56 (42 %)
Partial response	68	8	76 (57 %)
Complete response	1	0	1 (1 %)

Table 13.3 Operative interventions after bidirectional induction chemotherapy

No operation	45
Complete resection	45
Incomplete resection	33
Operation methods	
Total gastrectomy	54
Colectomy	38
Total hysterectomy/including tubes and ovaries	26
Small bowel resection	23
Resection of mesentery	25
Left subdiaphragmatic peritonectomy	19
Right subdiaphragmatic peritonectomy	15
Pelvic peritonectomy	31
Electrosurgical fulguration	60

abscess. The overall operative mortality rate was 1.5 % (2/133), and the cause of death was multiple organ failure due to sepsis from abdominal abscess.

In all patients with ascites, symptoms from peritoneal fluid resolved. Forty-four patients were alive at the time of analysis. The survival distribution for all patients is shown in Fig. 13.6. Median survival time (MST) of all patients was 13.9 months, with a 1-year survival of 54 %. MST of the 78 patients who had surgical intervention was

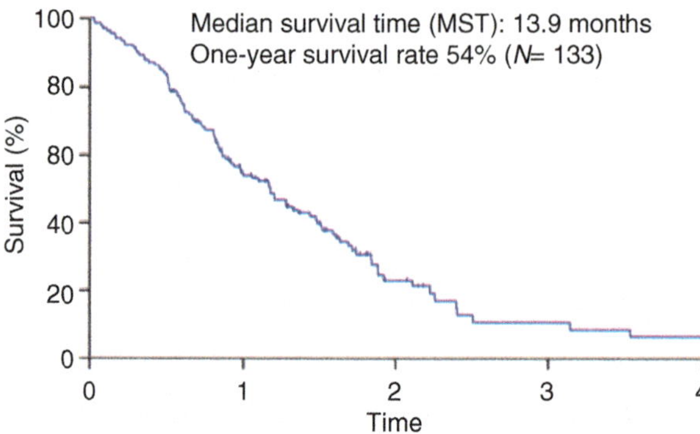

Fig. 13.6 Overall survival of 51 patients with P3 peritoneal dissemination of gastric cancer treated with bidirectional chemotherapy

13.9 months, and that of patients who did not receive the operation was 9.7 months (Fig. 13.2). There was a significant survival difference between the two groups ($P<0.001$, $Z=20.98$). Patients who received a complete resection had a median survival of 20.5 months, and survival of patients who received incomplete cytoreduction was 10.9 months (Fig. 13.7). There was no survival difference between primary and recurrent cases. MST of primary and recurrent cases after cytoreduction was 18.0 and 17.4 months. MST after no operation was 9.6 and 8.2 months, respectively.

13.3 Discussion

13.3.1 Clinical Data Supporting Complete Cytoreduction as the Goal in Management of Gastric Cancer Patients with Peritoneal Seeding

In the surgical treatment of carcinomatosis from appendiceal and colon cancer, complete cytoreduction has been determined to be essential for long-term survival. Culliford et al. reported a 5-year survival of 54 % for complete cytoreduction and 15 % for incomplete cytoreduction [16]. Furthermore, Glehen et al. reported that the median survival rate for colorectal cancer with PC was 32 months for patients with macroscopic complete resection and 8.4 months for patients without macroscopic incomplete cytoreduction [17]. In carcinomatosis from gastric cancer, Yonemura et al. reported that gastric cancer patients receiving complete cytoreduction had a significantly higher survival than did those with residual disease [18]. Although great differences exist in the biological behavior of colon and gastric cancer in both conditions, macroscopic complete cytoreduction may be the most important surgical requirement in the treatment of carcinomatosis to achieve a goal of long-term survival. Unfortunately, complete cytoreduction is not possible in P3 dissemination even with the most aggressive peritonectomy alone. Complete cytoreduction cannot be achieved by surgery alone when small bowel and its mesentery are diffusely involved.

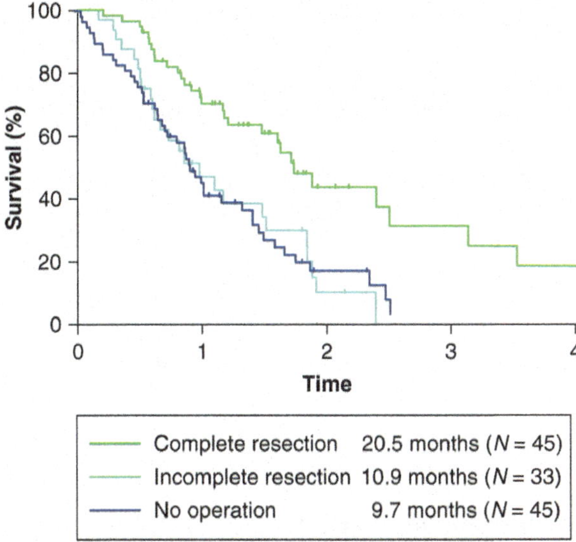

Fig. 13.7 Survival curves of patients in terms of completeness of cytoreduction

In this study, we attempted to eradicate disease from intestinal surfaces using induction bidirectional chemotherapy. This was successfully achieved in approximately half the patients.

13.3.2 Palliative Benefits to All Patients with Cancerous Ascites

In all 78 patients who had ascites, there was a clinical benefit. Symptom control was achieved in 100 % of these patients. These clinical benefits occurred in the group of patients with primary gastric cancer present and also in patients who had a prior gastrectomy.

13.3.3 Rationale for Bidirectional Induction Chemotherapy

Bidirectional induction chemotherapy was developed in order to increase the rate of complete cytoreduction by clearing the peritoneum of cancer nodules. The present study indicates that these treatments can increase the rate of complete cytoreduction as a result of a reduction of distribution and volume of peritoneal cancer nodules.

Furthermore, bidirectional induction chemotherapy was able to eradicate free cancer cells in the peritoneal cavity prior to the operation. Free intraperitoneal cancer cells can be detected in 65 % of patients with peritoneal dissemination [19]. These cells are viable and may be trapped with the peritoneal wound created by the surgical procedure. Accordingly, the free cancer cells should be eradicated before peritonectomy.

In vitro chemosensitivity testing is considered an indicator of clinical chemosensitivity [20]. Tanaka et al. have shown results of such testing in clinically obtained samples from primary gastric cancer, using a collagen gel method [21]. Carboplatin, Taxotere, 5-fluorouracil, cisplatin, and mitomycin C show high chemosensitivity for gastric cancer. From these results, Taxotere, carboplatin, and 5-fluorouracil were selected for induction chemotherapy, and methotrexate was used as a biochemical modulator of 5-fluorouracil [22].

According to Cunliffe, the nutrition for cancer nodules on the peritoneal surface can be derived from the ascites fluid as well as the blood supply [23]. In our management plan, the peritoneal cancer nodule is penetrated bidirectionally, not only through intraperitoneal but also intravenous therapy. Generally, intravenous chemotherapy has little effect on PC [2, 3, 13]. Intraperitoneal chemotherapy alone showed a response rate of less than 30 % [24–26]. The present study showed a response rate of 57 % after combined intravenous and intraperitoneal chemotherapy.

13.3.4 Chemotherapy Agents Selected for Bidirectional Induction Chemotherapy

From the study of the dose-limiting toxicities of intraperitoneal administration of Taxotere, Morgan et al. reported that maximum tolerated dose (MTD) was 125 mg/m^2 and that no grade 3 or 4 toxicities were found after the intraperitoneal administration of a dose lower than 80 mg/m^2 [22]. Furthermore, Fusida et al. reported that there were no hematological toxicities after weekly intraperitoneal administration of 45 mg/m^2 of Taxotere [26]. In the intraperitoneal administration of carboplatin, maximal tolerable dose was determined to be 500, and 300 mg/m^2 of intraperitoneal administration of carboplatin was a safe dose in Japanese patients with ovarian cancer [27, 28]. The doses of 40 mg/m^2 of Taxotere and 150 mg/m^2 of carboplatin which were used in the present study were considered to be safe doses. This combined approach of systemic and intraperitoneal chemotherapy was associated with an absent mortality and a very acceptable morbidity. Also, it was uniformly effective for ascites.

Conclusion

This combination of systemic and locoregional chemotherapy should be considered in patients with carcinomatosis from gastric cancer. It may be even more effective for those patients who have small volumes of disease and symptomatic ascites. Accordingly, the bidirectional chemotherapy may be the preferred strategy for the preoperative chemotherapy of gastric carcinomatosis and should be considered for phase III studies.

References

1. Sugarbaker PH. Epithelial appendiceal neoplasms. Cancer J. 2009;15:225–35.
2. Preusser P, Wilke H, Achterrath W, et al. Phase II study with the combination etoposide, doxorubicin, and cisplatin in advanced measurable gastric cancer. J Clin Oncol. 1989;7(9):1310–7.

3. Ajani JA, Ota DM, Jessup JM, et al. Resectable gastric carcinoma. An evaluation of preoperative and postoperative chemotherapy. Cancer. 1991;68:1501–6.
4. Yonemura Y, Bandou E, Sawa T, Yoshimitsu Y, Endou Y, Sasaki T, et al. Neoadjuvant treatment of gastric cancer with peritoneal dissemination. Eur J Surg Oncol. 2006;32(6):661–5.
5. Yonemura Y, Bandou E, Kinoshita K, Kawamura T, Takahashi S, Endou Y, et al. Effective therapy for peritoneal dissemination in gastric cancer. Surg Oncol Clin N Am. 2003;12:635–48.
6. Yonemura Y, Fujimura T, Fushida S, Takegawa S, Kamata T, Katayama K, et al. Hyperthermochemotherapy combined with cytoreductive surgery for the treatment of gastric cancer with peritoneal dissemination. World J Surg. 1991;15:530–6.
7. Hirose K, Katayama K, Iida A, Yamaguchi A, Nakagawara G, Umeda S, et al. Efficacy of continuous hyperthermic peritoneal perfusion for the prophylaxis and treatment of peritoneal metastasis of advanced gastric cancer. Oncology. 1999;57:106–14.
8. Glehen O, Mithieux F, Osinsky D, Beaujard AC, Freyer G, Guertsch P, et al. Surgery combined with peritonectomy procedures and intraperitoneal chemohyperthermia in abdominal cancers with peritoneal carcinomatosis: a phase II study. J Clin Oncol. 2003;21:799–806.
9. Sugarbaker PH. Results of treatment of 385 patients with peritoneal surface spread of appendiceal malignancy. Ann Surg Oncol. 1999;6(8):727–31.
10. Japanese Research Society for Gastric Cancer. The general rules for gastric cancer study. 1st ed. Tokyo: Kanehara Shuppan; 1995.
11. Sugarbaker PH. Peritonectomy procedures. Ann Surg. 1995;21:29–42.
12. Yonemura Y, Fujimura T, Fushida S, Fujita H, Bando E, Taniguchi K, et al. Peritonectomy as a treatment modality for patients with peritoneal dissemination from gastric cancer. In: Nakashima T, Yamaguchi T, editors. Multimodality therapy for gastric cancer. Tokyo: Springer; 1999. p. 71–80.
13. Sugarbaker PH, Yu W, Yonemura Y. Gastrectomy, peritonectomy and perioperative intraperitoneal chemotherapy: the evolution of treatment strategies for advanced gastric cancer. Semin Surg Oncol. 2003;21:233–48.
14. Yonemura Y, Fujimura T, Fushida S, et al. Techniques of peritonectomy for advanced and recurrent gastric cancer with peritoneal dissemination. In: Siewert JR, Roder JD, editors. 2nd international gastric cancer congress. Bologna: Monduzzi; 1997. p. 1365–9.
15. Yonemura Y, Fujimura T, Fushida S, et al. A new surgical approach (peritonectomy) for the treatment of peritoneal dissemination. Hepatogastroenterology. 1999;46:601–9.
16. Culliford AT, Brooks AD, Sharma S, Saltz LB, Schwartz GK, O'Reilly EM, et al. Surgical debulking and intraperitoneal chemotherapy for established peritoneal metastases from colon and appendix cancer. Ann Surg Oncol. 2001;8:787–95.
17. Glehen O, Kwiatkowski F, Sugarbaker PH, et al. Cytoreductive surgery combined with perioperative intraperitoneal chemotherapy for the management of peritoneal carcinomatosis from colorectal cancer: a multi-institutional study. J Clin Oncol. 2004;22:3284–92.
18. Yonemura Y, de Aretxabala X, Fujimura T, Fushida S, Katayama K, Bandou E, et al. Intraoperative chemo-hyperthermic peritoneal perfusion as an adjuvant to gastric cancer: final results of a randomized controlled study. Hepatogastroenterology. 2001;48:1776–82.
19. Bandou E, Yonemura Y, Takeshita Y, Taniguchi K, Yasui T, Yoshimitsu Y, et al. Intraoperative lavage for cytological examination in 1,297 patients with gastric carcinoma. Am J Surg. 1999;178:256–62.
20. Kubota T, Sasano N, Abe O, Nakao I, Kawamura E, Saito T, et al. Potential of the histoculture drug-response assay to contribute to cancer patient survival. Clin Cancer Res. 1995;1:1537–43.
21. Tanaka M, Obata T, Sasaki T. Evaluation of antitumor effects of docetaxel (Taxotere®) on human gastric cancers in vitro and in vivo. Eur J Cancer. 1996;32:226–30.
22. Newman EM, Lu Y, Kashani-Sabet M, Kesavan V, Scanlon KJ. Mechanisms of cross-resistance to methotrexate and 5-fluorouracil in an A2780 human ovarian carcinoma cell subline resistant to cisplatin. Biochem Pharmacol. 1988;37:443–7.
23. Cunliffe WJ. The rationale for early postoperative intraperitoneal chemotherapy for gastric cancer. In: Sugarbaker P, editor. Management of gastric cancer. Boston: Kluwer; 1991. p. 143–57.

24. Fujimoto S, Takahashi M, Kobayashi K, Kure M, Mutou T, Masaoka H, et al. Relation between clinical and histologic outcome of intraperitoneal hyperthermic perfusion for patients with gastric cancer and peritoneal metastasis. Oncology. 1993;50:338–43.
25. Morgan RJ, Doroshow JH, Synold T, Lim D, Shibata S, Margolin K, et al. Phase I trial of intraperitoneal docetaxel in the treatment of advanced malignancies primarily confined to the peritoneal cavity: dose-limiting toxicity and pharmacology. Clin Cancer Res. 2003;9:5896–901.
26. Fusida S, Furui N, Kinami S, Ninomiya I, Fujimura T, Nishimura G, et al. Pharmacologic study of intraperitoneal docetaxel in gastric cancer patients with peritoneal dissemination. Jpn J Cancer Chemother. 2002;29:1759–63.
27. Malmstrom H, Larsson D, Simonsen E. Phase I study of intraperitoneal carboplatin as adjuvant therapy in early ovarian cancer. Gynecol Oncol. 1990;39:289–94.
28. Ohno M, Hirokawa M, Hando T. Pharmacokinetics of carboplatin after intraperitoneal administration and clinical effect in ovarian cancer. Jpn J Cancer Chemother. 1992;19:2355–61.

Esophageal Cancer

14

Tetsuo Taguchi

14.1 Arterial Infusion Chemotherapy as Induction Treatment for Advanced Esophageal Cancer

Treatment of esophageal cancer has been mainly surgical, combined with various other modalities such as radiotherapy, chemotherapy, immunotherapy, and hyperthermia [1]. Because of its anatomical complexities, arterial infusion chemotherapy in esophageal cancer has not been as commonly investigated as that in cancers of other organs.

At present, there is no optimal indication confirmed for arterial infusion for esophageal cancer. Ishida et al. [1, 2] determine candidates for this therapy by integrating various test results obtained at the time of hospitalization and select those who have thoracic esophageal cancer with suspected infiltration into the other organs and who have angiographically confirmed vessels supplying the cancerous lesion. This decision, however, depends on the site of the lesion and the patient's general condition. They performed this therapy as one of preoperative treatment, but the majority of patients already have advanced disease with malnutrition and impaired reserve of various organs.

The objectives of the arterial infusion therapy are to administer an anticancer drug directly into the artery or arteries supplying the cancerous tissue, thus enhancing its antitumor effect by achieving higher concentrations of the drug in the tissue, to minimize systemic side effects of the anticancer drug, and to lower the dose of both the drug and irradiation when this therapy is employed concomitantly.

This therapy is based on the following concepts: (1) local therapy used with surgery should not adversely affect the outcome of the surgery and should promote reduction and localization of the local tumor mass so that more patients can have

T. Taguchi
Department of Oncologic Surgery, Research Institute for Microbial Disease,
Osaka University, Japan Society for Cancer Chemotherapy, Osaka, Japan
e-mail: len03736@nifty.com

© Springer-Verlag Berlin Heidelberg 2016
K.R. Aigner, F.O. Stephens (eds.), *Induction Chemotherapy,*
DOI 10.1007/978-3-319-28773-7_14

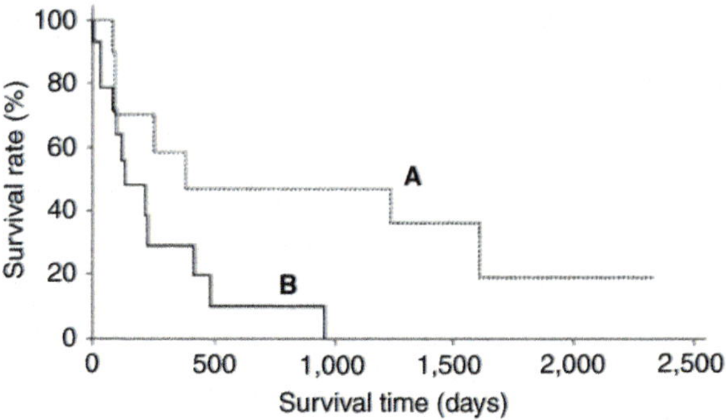

Fig. 14.1 (**a**) Preoperative irradiation with CDDP arterial infusion [2]. (**b**) Preoperative irradiation only log-rank test: $p = 0.069$ excluded hospital death cases

operations and (2) therapy should take into account distant metastasis and it should minimize adverse effects on the patient's general condition and keep them well enough to tolerate systemic treatment for subclinical or apparent distant metastasis both before and after surgery.

Practice of arterial infusion chemotherapy: Arterial infusion chemotherapy is conducted with esophageal angiography. A catheter is introduced by the Seldinger technique. It should be confirmed under radiographic examination that the tip of the catheter is inserted into the thoracic artery and then the tip should be guided along the arterial wall until it finds the opening of the target artery. The drug can be administered either by continuous infusion or by bolus infusion. The drug administered is CDDP (50–100 mg, in 50 ml of saline is infused at a rate of 3 ml/min using a catheter). Radiotherapy was conducted concomitantly. After having received 75 mg of CDDP intra-arterially and 30 Gy of radiation therapy, they elicited long-term results of arterial infusion therapy for esophageal cancer. Figure 14.1 shows the survival curves of preoperatively irradiated patients with or without CDDP arterial infusion, treated between 1984 and 1987 in their clinic. All these patients had very advanced disease and were not scheduled for complete resection at the time of admission. The 1- and 3-year survival rates were 28 % and 0 %, respectively, in patients treated without arterial infusion, compared with 57 % and 45 % in those treated with arterial infusion. The difference between the two groups was not statistically significant ($p = 0.069$ log-rank test), but these results suggest that arterial infusion therapy with concomitant irradiation may be useful for improving survival rates in very advanced esophageal cancer patients.

14.2 Induction (Neoadjuvant) Chemoradiation Therapy for the Treatment of Esophageal Cancer

An esophagectomy with three-field lymph node dissection is the standard therapy for advanced esophageal cancer in Japan. However, the results of esophagectomies are still unsatisfactory in comparison to results of surgical treatment for gastric cancer or colon cancer. Recently, definitive chemoradiation therapy (CRT) has shown progress as a treatment modality for resectable esophageal cancer, with data indicating the potential efficacy of combination therapy with chemoradiation and an esophagectomy. So preoperative chemoradiation for resectable cancer is becoming a standard therapy in Europe and North America. Recently, Matsubara [3] reported overview focuses on induction (neoadjuvant) chemoradiation for resectable esophageal cancer. Table 14.1 shows randomized trials that have been conducted for induction CRT plus surgery versus surgery alone.

In 1992, Nygaard et al. [4] reported the first randomized control trial of induction (preoperative) chemoradiotherapy for esophageal cancer, and they found that preoperative radiotherapy and chemotherapy prolonged survival. However, since then, many phase III trials comparing chemoradiation followed by surgery and surgery alone have not shown a benefit for preoperative chemoradiation. Only Walsh et al. [5] reported the efficacy of preoperative chemoradiation in improving survival, but this randomized control trial was problematic because the survival data in the group treated with surgery alone were insufficient to compare with the surgical procedures, that were not standardized.

After that, Visser et al. [6] in 2003, Malthaner et al. [7] in 2004, and Burmeister et al. [8] in 2005 reviewed adjuvant and induction (preoperative, neoadjuvant) therapy for esophageal cancer. They concluded that preoperative chemoradiation could not be regarded as standard of care and should not be used outside a clinical trial.

However, in 2007, Gebski et al. [9] reported that the result obtained from meta-analysis concerning induction (neoadjuvant) chemoradiotherapy for resectable esophageal cancer that is a significant survival benefit was evident with this finding indicating the results of management decisions to use evidence-based treatment for esophageal cancer. Their analysis was based on eight published randomized control trials and two unpublished randomized control trials. The pooled results of these ten

Table 14.1 Randomized trials of neoadjuvant chemoradiation therapy (CRT) plus surgery versus surgery alone [3]

Author	Surgery alone (*n*)	CRT + surgery (*n*)	Pathology	Radiation dose (Gy)	Chemotherapy	Surgical approach
Apinop et al.	34	35	SCC	40	CDD/5-FU	T/A
Bosset et al.	139	143	SCC	37	CDDP	T/A
Le Prise et al.	42	39	SCC	20	CDD/5-FU	Unknown
NyGaard et al.	41	41	SCC	35	CDDP/Bleo	T/A
Lee et al.	51	50	SCC	45.6	CDDP/5-FU	T/A
Urba et al.	50	50	SCC/Ademo	45	CDDP/5-FU/VBL	Th
Burmeister et al.	128	128	Ademo	35	CDDP/5-FU	T/A
Tepper et al.	26	30	Ademo	50.4	CDDP/5-FU	T/A
Walsh et al.	55	58	Ademo	40	CDDP/5-FU	T/A, Th

SCC squamous cell carcinoma, *Ademo* adenocarcinoma, *CDDP* cisplatin, *5-FU* 5-flurouracil, *T/A* transthoracic and abdominal approach, *Th* transhiatal approach, *n* number of patients

randomized control trials showed a relative reduction in mortality for patients receiving induction chemoradiotherapy (HR), 0.81[95 % CI, 0.70–0.93]; ($p = 0.002$). But Gebski et al. [9] reported that the benefit of the induction (neoadjuvant) treatment was lost by increased risk of death after surgery.

In 2008, Tepper et al. [10] reported a favorable result for induction (neoadjuvant) chemoradiation followed by surgery. However, this trial was closed due to poor accrual. The major limitation of this trial was the small sample size. Therefore, there are still no supportive data for induction chemoradiation followed by surgery in comparison to surgery alone in a well-designed large-scale randomized control trial.

14.2.1 Chemotherapeutic Agents Commonly Trialed

5-FU and cisplatin were the agents most commonly used in most of the trials. Several trials have reported that there was evidence of a dose–response relationship between increasing the protocol-prescribed radiotherapy dose, the 5-FU dose, the cisplatin dose, and pCR. Of note, epirubicin, 5-FU, and cisplatin are widely used in Europe, as well as in North America and Japan. Cunningham's group [11] reported that capecitabine and oxaliplatin were as effective as 5-FU and cisplatin. These new drug combinations containing docetaxel, paclitaxel, and/or other molecular target agents may improve the survival benefit of preoperative chemoradiation for resectable esophageal cancer.

In 2008, JCOG [12] reported promising data by the Japanese group. Patients with locally advanced SCC (squamous cell carcinoma) of the esophagus were randomly allocated to surgery followed by chemotherapy or to induction chemotherapy with surgery. The pre- and post-chemotherapy regimens used the same protocol, with cisplatin and 5-FU. The JCOG reported that preoperative chemotherapy improved overall survival. So, new randomized control trials must be conducted using induction chemotherapy as a standard arm instead of surgery alone.

So far, only one study has compared chemoradiation to chemotherapy alone before an esophageal resection in 2008 by Luu et al. [13]. This study was not a prospective randomized trial but a retrospective examination. A total of 122 cases were collected. Surgical complications did not differ between the two groups. The median survival was 20.7 months in the chemotherapy group and 17.2 months in the chemoradiation group ($p = 0.14$). The 1-, 3-, and 5-year survivals in the induction chemotherapy group did not differ significantly from the survivals in the preoperative chemoradiation group. However, the induction chemotherapy group had a significantly longer median disease-free survival, of 15.8 months, in comparison to that of 13.7 months for the preoperative chemoradiation group ($p = 0.02$). The chemoradiation resulted in a significantly higher rate of complete pCRs in comparison to chemotherapy alone. However, the chemoradiation group did not show improved survival. In addition, preoperative chemoradiation leads to a delay in surgery. Luu et al. concluded that induction (preoperative) chemotherapy might be the preferred preoperative modality to expedite the ability to perform a resection and improve the survival of patients with locally advanced esophageal cancer.

Matsubara [3] concluded by intensive reviews that a well-designed large-scale randomized control trial (RCT) is needed to determine the utility of induction chemoradiation.

14.3 Summary

The practice of arterial infusion chemotherapy: Arterial infusion chemotherapy conducted with esophageal angiography using CDDP (50–100 mg, in 50 ml of saline is infused at a rate of 3 ml/min using a catheter) with radiotherapy conducted concomitantly has elicited the most encouraging long-term results in treating esophageal cancer (Fig. 14.1).

A three-way study is needed to compare results using preoperative induction chemotherapy alone (using intra-arterial and systemic administration of the chemotherapy), with results using preoperative (induction) chemoradiation.

References

1. Taguchi T, Nakamura H, editors. Arterial infusion chemotherapy. Tokyo: Japanese Journal of Cancer and Chemotherapy Publishers Inc; 1994. ISBN 0385-0684.
2. Ishida K, Murakami K. Protocol of therapy for esophageal cancer. Rinsho Geka (JPN). 1987;42:741–9.
3. Matsubara H. Neoadjuvant chemoradiation therapy for the treatment of esophageal carcinoma. Int J Clin Oncol. 2008;13(6):474–8. ISSN 1341-9625.
4. Nygaard K, Hagen S, Hansen HS, et al. Preoperative radiotherapy prolongs survival in operable esophageal carcinoma; a randomized, multicenter study of pre-operative radiotherapy and chemotherapy. The second Scandinavian trial in esophageal cancer. World J Surg. 1992;16(6):1104–9. Discussion 1110.
5. Walsh TN, Noonan N, Hollywood D, et al. A comparison of multimodal therapy and surgery for esophageal adenocarcinoma. N Engl J Med. 1996;335:462–7.
6. Visser BC, Venook AP, Patti MG. Adjuvant and neoadjuvant therapy for esophageal cancer; a critical reappraisal. Surg Oncol. 2003;12:1–7.
7. Malthaner RA, Wong RK, Rumble RB, et al. Neoadjuvant or adjuvant therapy for respectable esophageal cancer; a systemic review and meta-analysis. BMC Med. 2004;2:35.
8. Burmeister BH, Smithers BM, Gebski V, et al. Surgery alone versus chemoradiotherapy followed by surgery for resectable cancer of the esophagus; a randomized controlled phase III trial. Lancet Oncol. 2005;6(9):659–68.
9. Gebski V, Burmeister B, Smithers BM, et al. Chemoradiotherapy or chemotherapy in oesophageal carcinoma; a meta-analysis. Lancet Oncol. 2007;8:226–34.
10. Tepper J, Krasna MJ, Niedzwiecki D, et al. Phase III trial of trimodality therapy with cisplatin, fluorouracil, radiotherapy and surgery compared with surgery alone for esophageal cancer: CALGB 9781. J Clin Oncol. 2008;26:1086–92.
11. Cunningham D, Starling N, Rao S, et al. Capecitabine and oxaliplatin for advanced esophageal gastric cancer. N Engl J Med. 2008;358:36–46.
12. Igaki H, Kato H, Ando N, et al. A randomized trial of postoperative adjuvant chemotherapy with cisplatin and 5-fluorouracil versus neoadjuvant chemotherapy for clinical stage II/III squamous cell carcinoma of the thoracic esophagus (JCOG 9907). J Clin Oncol. 2008;26(suppl):4510.
13. Luu TD, Gaur P, Force SD, et al. Neoadjuvant chemoradiation versus chemotherapy for patients undergoing esophagectomy for esophageal cancer. Ann Thorac Surg. 2008;85(4):1217–23.

Gastric Cancer

15

Tetsuo Taguchi

15.1 Arterial Infusion Chemotherapy as Primary Treatment for Advanced Gastric Cancer

Arterial infusion chemotherapy is a promising route of administration [1]. This therapy is improving with modified drug/dose regimens, including development of multiple drug therapy, and improved dosing methods. In Japan, arterial infusion therapy was first introduced around 1963 by Shiraha et al. [2].

Arterial infusion therapy using 5-FU (5-fluorouracil) + MMC (mitomycin C) as induction for advanced gastric cancer was examined in clinical studies around the 1970s by Yoshikawa et al. [3], Taguchi et al. [4], Nakano et al. [5], Fujita et al. [6], and Awane et al. [7]. They reported the clinical results showing 20–30 % higher response rate could be achieved when chemotherapy was given by intra-arterial infusion rather than systemically.

Indications for consideration of arterial chemotherapy:

1. Patients with inoperable, advanced gastric cancer and patients with multiple metastatic lesions in the liver.
2. The second group who might be considered for likely benefit are patients with infiltration to adjacent organs other than the liver or severe metastases in the third or more distal lymph nodes.
3. The third group who might benefit are patients with peritoneal dissemination. Even if ascites is present, arterial infusion therapy may bestow some benefit. The targets of the therapy are metastases or infiltrated subdiaphragmatic abdominal organs.

T. Taguchi
Department of Oncologic Surgery, Research Institute for Microbial Disease,
Osaka University, Japan Society for Cancer Chemotherapy, Osaka, Japan
e-mail: len03736@nifty.com

© Springer-Verlag Berlin Heidelberg 2016
K.R. Aigner, F.O. Stephens (eds.), *Induction Chemotherapy*,
DOI 10.1007/978-3-319-28773-7_15

Patients with metastases in the brain, lung, bone, or in Virchow's node are excluded.

If metastatic lesions are localized in the liver, an indwelling catheter is inserted into the common hepatic artery. If not, the tip of the catheter should be generally located proximally to the bifurcation of the celiac artery.

Dosing regimens of drugs: There is no established dosing regimen for any drugs. Taguchi et al. [8] initiated using 5-FU and MMC in the 1960s. 5-FU at 250 mg/day and urokinase at 6,000 units/day are given every day by intra-arterial infusion (over 1 h daily). A total dose of at least 10 g of 5-FU should be given. Together with this therapy, intermittent dose of 6–20 mg of MMC (6 mg for weekly injection, 10 mg biweekly; and 20 mg once every 4 weeks) should be given. They concluded that 6 mg weekly is an appropriate dosage.

Response of nonresectable gastric cancer to sub-selective aortic infusion chemotherapy is shown in Tables 15.1 and 15.2 and Fig. 15.1. Response of recurrent gastric cancer to arterial infusion chemotherapy is shown in Fig. 15.2. Response of measurable lesions to arterial infusions, which failed, is shown in Table 15.3. Response in gastric cancer patients with measurable lesions, which failed to show tumor response, is shown in Table 15.4. Improvement in subjective symptoms without improvement in measurable lesions is rare.

Table 15.1 Classification according to chemotherapeutic regimen [1]

Group	No. of cases	Chemotherapeutic regimen
Intensive i.a. chemotherapy	40	5-FU at 250 mg (daily), total dose $\geq$5 g with MMC, ACNU, or ACNU or CQ + ADM bolus i.a.
Incomplete i.a. chemotherapy	16	MMC, ACNU, or CQ + ADM bolus i.a. with or without 5-FU at 250 mg (daily), total dose $\leq$5 g
Non-intra-arterial chemotherapy	47	MMC, 5-FU ADM or ACM bolus i.v., MFC i.v., 5-FUd.s. or FT p.o. or suppo., BMR, etc.

5-FU 5-fluorouracil, *MMC* mitomycin C, *ACNU* nimustine hydrochloride, *CQ* carbazilquinone, *ADM* adriamycin, *ACM* aclacinomycin, *MFC* MMC+5-FU+cytosine arabinoside, *5-FUd.s.* 5-FU dry syrup, *FT* tegafur, *BMR* biological response modifier, *i.a.* intra-arterial, *i.v.* intravenous, *p.o.* per os, *suppo.* suppository

Table 15.2 Response in nonresectable gastric cancer patients by chemotherapy [1]

Group	No. of cases	Survival time (days) median, 50 %		Cases of response $\geq$1-A[a]	$\geq$1 year survival cases
A: intensive i.a. chemotherapy	40	253[b]	189	11	8[b]
B: incomplete i.a. chemotherapy	16	150	134	0	0
C: non-intra-arterial chemotherapy	47	135	131	0	0

Source: Research Institute for Microbial Diseases, Osaka University, January 1978 to December 1981
[a]Criteria by Karnofsky
[b]A:C; $P<0.01$

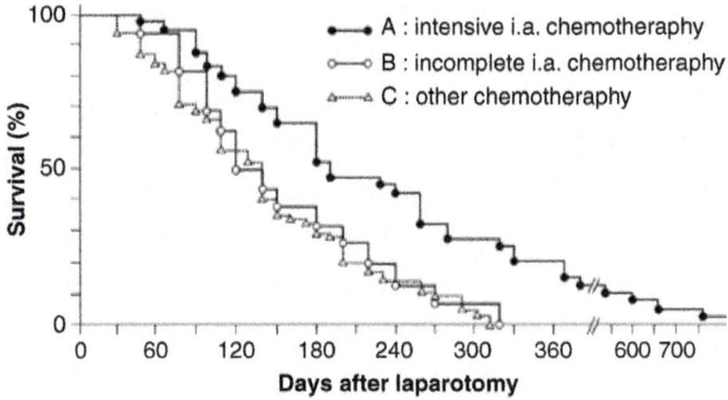

Fig. 15.1 Survival of nonresectable advanced gastric cancer (Calculated according to the method of Kaplan-Meier) [1]

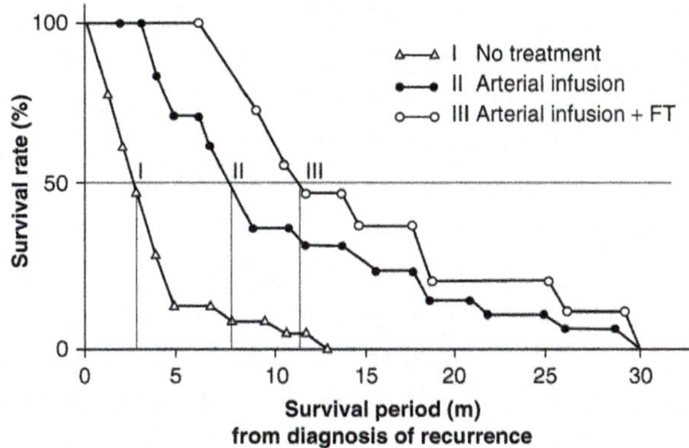

Fig. 15.2 Survival curve of recurrent gastric cancer [1]

Table 15.3 Response of measurable lesions to arterial infusion chemotherapy [1]

Gastric cancer	No. of cases	Response of tumor		
		No.	<50 %	≥50 %
Nonresectable	15	10 (66.7 %)	1 (6.7 %)	4 (26.7 %)
Recurrence	26	14 (53.8 %)	4 (15.4 %)	8 (30.8 %)

Response of patients with gastric cancer which is not measurable to arterial infusion chemotherapy is shown in Table 15.5. Tumor response to each drug given by intra-arterial infusion is shown in Table 15.6 together with the number of patients who survived for at least 1 year. Arterial infusion chemotherapy and adverse reactions to each anticancer drug given by intra-arterial infusion are shown in Table 15.7.

Hypertensive arterial chemotherapy combined with angiotensin II for advanced or recurrent gastric cancer using MMC+5-FU has been reported in several studies [1, 7, 9]. The theoretical purpose of arterial infusion chemotherapy used together with injection of angiotensin II is to increase the delivery of anticancer drugs to the target tumor tissues by increasing blood flow in the tumor tissues.

Table 15.4 Response of gastric cancer patients with measurable lesions, who failed to show tumor response [1]

Mode of response	Nonresectable (10)	Recurrent (14)
None	8	11
Increased appetite	1	1
Relief of pain	0	0
Disappearance of ascites	1	1
Improved ileus	0	1

Table 15.5 Response to arterial infusion chemotherapy of patients with gastric cancer which is not measurable [1]

Mode of response	Nonresectable (27)	Recurrent (8)
None	8	3
Increased appetite	1	0
Relief of pain	5	1
Improved dysphasia	3	0
Disappearance of ascites	1	0
Improvement in general condition	1	2
Relief of jaundice	0	2
Radiological and endoscopic effects	8	0

Table 15.6 Tumor response to each drug given by intra-arterial infusion and more than 1 year survival cases (nonresectable and recurrent gastric cancer) [1]

Mode of administration		Drugs	No. of cases	Tumor response	Effects[a] MR	PR	≥1 year survivors
Bolus (26)		MMC	9	1	1		
		ADR	5				
		MMC+5-FU	10	2	1	1	1
		Others	2	1	1		
5-FU daily, others bolus		MMC	4				
	(19) 5-FU, 5 g	ADR+CQ	8	5	4	1	
		ACNU	2				
		ACM	5				
		MMC	9	2	1	1	2
	(23) 5-FU, 5–10 g	ADR+CQ	5	2	1	1	
		ACNU	7	2	1	1	1
		ACM	2	1	1		
		MMC	10	4	1	3	3
	(44) 5-FU, 10 g	ADR+CQ	6	3	1	2	3
		ACNU	24	10	1	9	9
		ACM	4	3	3	2	
Total			112	36	14	22	21

[a]Criteria by Japan Society for Cancer Therapy

They utilized sub-selective aortic infusion chemotherapy in cases where tumor was confined to the abdominal cavity. But when the tumor was in the liver only, hepatic arterial infusion chemotherapy was used. Regarding the method of

Table 15.7 Adverse reactions to each anticancer drug given by intra-arterial infusion (nonresectable and recurrent gastric cancer) [1]

Mode of administration		Drugs	No. of cases	Adverse reactions[a]									
				0	1	2	3	4	5	6	7	8	9
Bolus (26)		MMC	9	8							1		
		ADR	5	3	2								
		MMC+5-FU	10	5	3		1	1					
		Others	2	1				1					
5-FU daily, others bolus	(19) 5-FU, 5 g	MMC	4	2	1	1		2	1			1	
		ADR+CQ	8	1	4				1	4	1		
		ACNU	2		1			1				1	
		ACM	5	3							2		
	(23) 5-FU, 5–10 g	MMC	9	1	5		1		3		2		
		ADR+CQ	5	2	1		3			1	1		
		ACNU	7		1				1		4		1
		ACM	2								2		
	(44) 5-FU, 10 g	MMC	10	5	5	1	1				1		
		ADR+CQ	6	2	4		2	2	1	2	1		
		ACNU	24	9	8	7	7	2	4		6	2	3
		ACM	4	1					1		1		
Total			112	43	35	9	9	9	12	7	43	4	4

[a]0 no, 1 leucopenia, 2 thrombopenia, 3 GOT↑, GPT↑, 4 albuminuria, 5 dermatitis and pigmentation, 6 alopecia, 7 disorders of alimental tract, 8 infection, 9 others

administration of hypertensive drugs, they did not inject angiotensin II intra-arterially, but it was injected intravenously. After the raised blood pressure was stabilized, MMC was given by intra-arterial infusion over 5–10 min.

Their results were very interesting in that the concurrent use of angiotensin II potentiated response of gastric cancer of a well-differentiated type which was hypervascular, much more than any other types. Signet ring cell carcinoma failed to respond to this therapy.

The randomized study showed increased response if angiotensin II was also used, but this increased response did not prolong life expectancy. The reason for this is unknown but should be clarified in further studies.

In 1989, Nakajima et al. [10] have attempted to treat patients with advanced unresectable gastric cancer with a four-drug regimen of combination chemotherapy as induction chemotherapy delivered systemically and regionally, followed by radical gastrectomy.

Patients and methods: From 1989 to 1995, 30 of 42 patients with incurable gastric cancer (stage IV, M1 disease) were entered into a combined modality treatment trial with intensive chemotherapy 5-FU, leucovorin, etoposide, and cisplatin (FLEP regimen) and surgery (Table 15.8).

Entry criteria were as follows: (a) histologically proved adenocarcinoma of the stomach, with no history of previous treatment; (b) patient's age <75 years, performance status ≤3, and normal liver, renal, and bone marrow functions; (c) unresectable disease due to wide local extension, with intra- or extra-abdominal metastasis;

Table 15.8 Characteristics of patients receiving FLEP therapy [10]

Characteristics	No. of cases
Sex	
Male	18
Female	12
Age (year)	
Average	53 ± 16.2
$\leq$39	4
40–59	13
$\geq$60	13
Unresectable lesions	
One intra-abdominal	
H_3 (H)	1
$N_3 + {}^4$(N)	10
Two intra-abdominal	
$N_4\,H_3$ (H)	5
$N_4\,P_1$ (N)	1
$N_4\,P_3$ (P)	1
$T_4\,P_3$ (P)	3
Three intra-abdominal	
$N_4\,P_2\,H_2$ (N)	1
$T_4\,N_3\,H_1$ (N)	1
$T_4\,N_3\,H_3$ (H)	1
$T_4\,N_4\,H_1$ (N)	1
$T_4\,N_4\,P_2$ (N)	1
$T_4\,N_4\,P_2$ (P)	1
Intra- and extra-abdominal	
$N_4\,H_3\,M$ (M)	1
$T_4\,P_3\,M$ (M)	1
$S_3\,N_4\,M$ (M)	1
Total	30

H, liver metastasis; H1, solitary lesion in one lobe; H2, a few lesions in both lobes; H3, numerous lesions in both lobes; N3, lymph node metastasis to station 3 (retropancreatic, hepatoduodenal ligament, around superior mesenteric vessels); N4, para-aortic node metastasis; P1, a few disseminated lesions around the stomach; P2, a few disseminated foci on the diaphragm or on the mesenterium below the transverse colon; P3, numerous lesions throughout the abdominal cavity; T4, primary lesion filtrating adjacent organ(s) or tissues; M, extra-abdominal hematogenous metastasis to the lung, bone, or brain. For instance, N_4H_2 indicates that the patient had simultaneous metastasis to the para-aortic nodes and to both lobes of the liver. Letters in parenthesis indicate the type of dominant metastasis

(d) provision of informed consent; and (e) patients available for regular follow-up after surgery.

The chemotherapy regimen consisted of systemic delivery of 370 mg/m^2 of 5-FU and 30 mg of leucovorin given intravenously on days 1–5, followed by 70 mg/m^2 of cisplatin and 70 mg/m^2 of etoposide given intra-arterially via an aortic catheter on days 6 and 20. Both drugs were dissolved separately in 200 ml of physiologic saline and infused over 1 h for each drug using an infusion pump.

In most patients, the tip of catheter was placed in the aorta at the level of the ninth thoracic vertebra, a few centimeters above the origin of the celiac artery, and the other end was connected to a subcutaneous implantable vascular access device. The catheter was inserted into the aorta via a branch of the deep femoral artery or via the thoracoabdominal artery. Each treatment cycle was repeated twice every 5 weeks before surgery.

Results: Two courses of chemotherapy were given to 27 of 30 patients with incurable disease; in the remaining 3 patients, treatment was stopped due to toxicity or disease progression. The major adverse effects were GI disturbances, including nausea and vomiting (44 %), mucositis (20 %) of the GI tract, and bone marrow suppression (4 %) (Table 15.9).

Three patients developed combined renal and bone marrow dysfunction, with a fatal outcome in one patient who had extensive multiple liver metastasis.

Local response to chemotherapy was evaluated by the main type of cancer extension, based on the average of scores for each tumor site (Table 15.10). Partial response (PR) was observed in 15 of 30 patients (50 %). Eight patients (28.9 %) showed no change (NC), and seven (21.1 %) showed PD. The highest response rate in terms of dominant type was observed in the node involvement (N) category: 13 of 15 patients showed PR, and 9 of these 13 had curative gastrectomy (radical dissection or RD surgery). Even in patients with distant lymph node metastasis associated with other types of metastasis who failed to achieve PR, nodal metastasis responded well: 20 of 27 lesions (74.1 %) metastatic to para-aortic nodes showed a good response, including two CRs, confirmed by the histologic examination of the resected specimens. Supraclavicular node swelling in two patients completely disappeared macroscopically. Primary lesions responded to chemotherapy in 13 of 30

Table 15.9 Toxicities (≧WHO grade 3) [10]

Bone marrow	
Leukocytopenia	12 (40.0 %)
Thrombocytopenia	3 (8.0 %)
Gastrointestinal	
Nausea, vomiting	12 (44.0 %)
Stomatitis, diarrhea	5 (20.0 %)
Renal failure	3 (12.0 %)

Table 15.10 Local response to chemotherapy according to dominant type of cancer extension [10]

Dominant type	PR	NC+PD	Total	RR (%)
H	2	5	7	13.3
N	13	2	15	86.7
P	0	5	5	0
M		3	3	0
Total	15	15	30	50.0

cases (43.3 %). In cases of either liver metastasis or peritoneal dissemination, response rates were low, and overall evaluation showed no responder in the hepatic (H), peritoneal (P), and widespread metastatic (M) categories.

In addition to nine curative gastrectomies, 6 out of 15 patients with PR, 3 out of 8 with NC, and 1 out of 7 with PD underwent palliative gastrectomy (Table 15.11). The resectability rate was 63 % (19 of 30), and a curative resection was performed in 47 % (9 of 19). Radical "curative" gastrectomy was combined in most cases with resection of involved adjacent organs and extensive dissection of para-aortic lymph nodes. However, intra-and postoperative complications were observed more often in cases of palliative surgery than in curatively resected cases.

Postoperative survival curves are shown in Fig. 15.3. The median survival time was 6.5 months for all cases, 12.7 months for responders, and 4.7 months for non-responders. The survival rate of patients with "curative" gastrectomy has not yet fallen to the 50 % level (55.6 % at 5 years), whereas patients who underwent palliative surgery or no surgery did not survive more than 13 or 11 months, respectively.

During the past 50 years, many reports attest to the clinical benefit of regional chemotherapy for advanced gastric cancer.

Stephens et al. [11] and Aigner et al. [12] also reported the possible advantage of celiac axis infusion chemotherapy for advanced gastric cancer. Scintigraphy with technetium showed a difference in the drug distribution between regional and

Table 15.11 Local response and surgical treatment [10]

	R0	R1	No surgery	Total
PR	9 (60.0)	6 (40.0)	0	15
NC		3 (37.5)	5 (62.5)	8
PD		1 (14.3)	6 (85.7)	7
Total	9 (30.0)	10 (33.3)	11 (36.7)	30

R0 radical surgery, *R1* palliative surgery

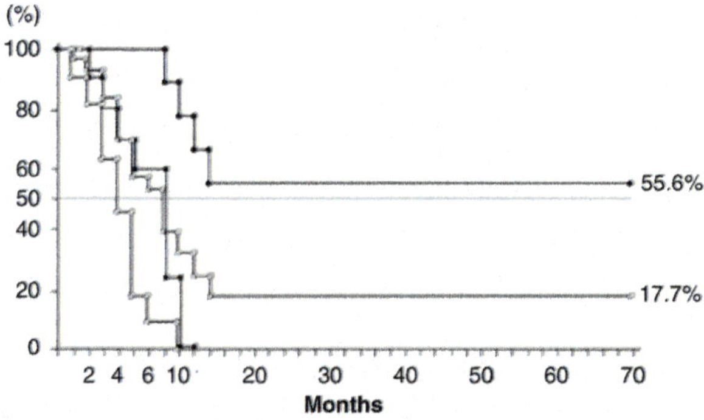

Fig. 15.3 Survival curves according to treatments [10], - all cases treated ($n=30$, MST=6.5); ●-● responders treated with chemotherapy and curative surgery, not reaching MST ($n=9$, 5-year survival rate 55.6 %); ■-■ responders and nonresponders treated with chemotherapy and non-curative surgery ($n=10$, MST=6.5); ○-○ nonresponders treated with chemotherapy ($n=11$, MST=4.7)

system delivery: approximately half of the drug given via an aortic catheter distributed to organs and structures did not exactly reflect the drug concentration at the cellular level, although it may roughly correlate with the local amount of drug on first exposure. Nakajima et al. [10] used a combination chemotherapy of regional (CDDP and etoposide given into the aorta) and systemic delivery (5-FU and leucovorin) for the control of both local and disseminated disease in the intra-and extra-abdominal regions.

The overall response rate (50 %) of their regimen (FLEP) is encouraging in recent trials with response rates ranging from 30 to 50 %. The highest response was observed in the metastatic distant lymph nodes and in primary lesions, whereas peritoneal dissemination and extra-abdominal lesions did not respond to FLEP. Total evaluation by dominant type indicates that patients with locally advanced disease with extended lymphatic spread seem to be the best candidates for the FLEP regimen.

Long-term survival was observed exclusively among the nine patients who showed sufficient local response to allow radical surgery. These patients were initially judged as having unresectable disease because of wide local extension and widespread lymphatic metastasis along the celiac axis and abdominal aorta. The outcome of PR patients with curative surgery was very good, but that of PR patients who underwent palliative gastrectomy was as poor as that of nonresponders.

These above results indicate that although temporary local reduction by chemotherapy or surgery is insufficient to completely eradicate the cancer as a result of the effects of both modalities, there is enhanced long-term survival.

However, results of this pilot study suggest that with combination modality therapy, sufficient tumor reduction is induced to enable a subsequent radical gastrectomy in one third of patients with initially unresectable gastric cancer, especially those with extensive lymphatic spread.

Clinical results from many trials of arterial infusion chemotherapy alone for advanced gastric cancer as induction chemotherapy have shown that a 20–30 % higher response rate can be achieved. However, the benefit of prolonged survival rates and improved quality of life is not consistently realized. These techniques did not gain enthusiastic support and have not been used as frontline therapy in gastric cancer.

However, arterial infusion chemotherapy is still only a part of the multidisciplinary therapy for gastric cancer.

15.2 Systemic Chemotherapy as Primary Treatment for Advanced Gastric Cancer

The development of effective therapy for advanced gastric cancer is still slow, and no globally acceptable standard regimen has yet been established.

For unresectable or recurrent gastric cancer, several phase III trials have demonstrated that a 5-FU-based regimen provides a survival benefit for these patients over best supportive care only [13–15]. Although quite a few randomized trials [16–22], using anthracycline, MMC, 5-FU, MTX, and cisplatin, were carried out before the early 1990s, none of the chemotherapy regimens showed a survival benefit over 5-FU alone, and no worldwide consensus about a standard regimen has been agreed.

Both CF (cisplatin + 5-FU) and ECF (epirubicin + cisplatin + 5-FU) have been considered as reference regimens to date, but the median survival time (MST) of the regimens does not exceed 7–10 months [23].

Recently, several active agents have been used systemically in treating gastric cancer therapy, the taxanes, irinotecan (CPT-11), oxaliplatin, S-1, and capecitabine, and more recently, biological agents such as cetuximab and bevacizumab have been used [24].

Current studies have thus focused on "new-generation agents," and much effort has been directed toward the development of the best regimen in various treatment settings. A series of these trials have provided several regimens that could become a standard treatment: the regimens include docetaxel + cisplatin + 5-FU (DCF) and cisplatin + S-1 for advanced and metastatic cancer, and S-1 monotherapy in the adjuvant setting.

These trials have achieved prolonged survival as compared with results in such trials in the 1990s [24].

In Japan, two recent trials, the Japan Clinical Oncology Group (JCOG) 9912 trial (in which the S-1 arm showed best survival) [25] and the SPIRITS trial (in which the S-1 + cisplatin arm showed best survival times) [26] revealed superior results than seen in the previous JCOG trial 9205 [27]. Considering these results, S-1 + cisplatin would be a most reasonable standard regimen for advanced gastric cancer. However, there still remain questions to be elucidated in the near future: whether S-1 plus cisplatin is superior to the most commonly used regimen worldwide – 5-FU plus cisplatin – and whether cisplatin is the best partner for S-1. These issues will be studied in ongoing trials, such as the FLAGS (5-FU + cisplatin vs. S-1 + cisplatin), TOP002 (S-1 vs. S-1 + irinotecan), and JACCROGC-03 (S-1 vs. S-1 + docetaxel) trials [24–26, 28–32].

Since the development of S-1, there are an increasing number of case reports of the unresectable gastric cancer responding to clinical or pathological complete response or partial response treated with S-1/CDDP, S-1/irinotecan, and S-1/docetaxel regimen as induction (preoperative, primary, or neoadjuvant) chemotherapy in Japan [33–36].

These results suggest that sufficient tumor reduction is induced by S-1-based regimen to enable a subsequent radical gastrectomy in 10–20 % of patients with initially unresectable gastric cancer, especially those with extensive lymphatic spread.

Now, a prospective randomized trial is necessary to confirm the clinical benefit of this systemic induction chemotherapy for advanced gastric cancer (JCOG0501 study ongoing).

References

1. Taguchi T, Nakamura H, editors. Arterial infusion chemotherapy. Tokyo: Japanese Journal Cancer and Chemother Publishers; 1994. ISBN 0385-0684.

2. Shiraha Y, et al. Intraarterial infusion of anti-cancer drugs for malignant tumors. Diagn Ther (Shindan Chiryou). 1964;53:43.
3. Yoshikawa K. Chemotherapy for gastric cancer evaluation of clinical response followed by intraaortic infusion treatment. Jpn J Cancer Clin. 1973;19:776–8.
4. Taguchi T, et al. Arterial infusion chemotherapy for advanced gastrointestinal cancer. Gastroenterol Surg (Shoukaki-Geka). 1979;2:1081–8.
5. Nakano Y, et al. Effect of intra-aortic chemotherapy on advanced gastric cancer and colorectal cancers. Jpn J Cancer Chemother. 1978;5:321–7.
6. Fujita F, et al. Chemotherapy for the patients with non-resectable gastric cancer of Bormann type IV. Jpn J Cancer Chemother. 1977;4:1315–22.
7. Awane Y, Katayanagi T, Kitamura M, et al. Local intra-arterial therapy with adriamycin and 5-FU in progressive cancer. Jpn J Cancer Chemother. 1981;8:1593–9.
8. Taguchi T, et al. Intra-arterial chemotherapy for advanced gastrointestinal cancer. Jpn J Gastroenterol Surg (Shoukaki-Geka). 1974;2:1081–8.
9. Kitamura M, Awane Y, Katayanagi T, et al. An evaluation of complications associated with continued intra-arterial therapy with carcinostatic drugs. Jpn J Cancer Chemother. 1980;7:1432–8.
10. Nakajima T, et al. Combined intensive chemotherapy and radical surgery for incurable gastric cancer. Ann Surg Oncol. 1997;4(3):203–8.
11. Stephens FO, Adams BG, Grea P. Intra-arterial chemotherapy given preoperatively in the management of carcinoma of the stomach. Surg Gynecol Obstet. 1986;162:370–4.
12. Aigner KR, Benthin F, Müller H. Celiac axis infusion (CA1) chemotherapy for advanced gastric cancer. In: Sugarbaker PH, editor. Management of gastric cancer. Boston: Kluwer Academic; 1991. p. 357–62.
13. Murad AM, Santiago FF, Petroianu A, et al. Modified therapy with 5-fluorouracil, doxorubicin and methotrexate in advanced gastric cancer. Cancer. 1993;72:37–41.
14. Glinetius B, Huffmann K, Hoglund U, et al. Initial or delayed chemotherapy with best supportive. Ann Oncol. 1994;5:189–90.
15. Pyrhonen S, Kuitumen T, Nyandoto P, et al. Randomized comparison of fluorouracil, epidoxorubicin and methotrexate (FEMTX) plus best supportive care alone in patients with non-resectable gastric cancer. Br J Cancer. 1995;71:587–91.
16. Cullinan SA, Moertel CG, Fleming TR, et al. A comparison of three chemotherapeutic regimens in the treatment of advanced pancreatic and gastric carcinoma, Fluorouracil versus fluorouracil and doxorubicin versus fluorouracil, doxorubicin and mitomycin. JAMA. 1985;253(14):2061–7.
17. Wils JA, Klein HO, Wagener DJ, et al. Sequential high-dose methotrexate and fluorouracil combined with doxorubicin: a step ahead in the treatment of gastric cancer: a trial of European Organization for Research and Treatment of Gastrointestinal Tract Co-operative Group. J Clin Oncol. 1991;9:827–31.
18. Kelsen D, Atiqu OT, Saltz L, et al. FAMTX versus etoposide, doxorubicin and cisplatin: a randomized trial in gastric cancer. J Clin Oncol. 1992;10:541–8.
19. Kim NK, Park YS, Heo DS, et al. A phase III randomized study of 5-fluorouracil and cisplatin versus 5-fluorouracil, doxorubicin and mitomycin C versus 5-fluorouracil alone in the treatment of advanced gastric cancer. Cancer. 1993;71:3813–8.
20. Culliman SA, Moertel CG, Wieand HS, et al. Controlled evaluation of three drug combination regimen versus fluorouracil alone in the therapy of advanced gastric cancer. J Clin Oncol. 1994;12:412–6.
21. Cocconi G, Bella M, Zironi S, et al. Fluorouracil, doxorubicin and mitomycin combination versus PELF chemotherapy in advanced gastric cancer: a prospective randomized trial of the Italian Oncology Group for Clinical Research. J Clin Oncol. 1994;12(12):2687–93.
22. Webb A, Cunningham D, Scarffe JH, et al. Randomized trial comparing epirubicin, cisplatin and fluorouracil versus fluorouracil, doxorubicin and methotrexate in advanced esophagogastric cancer. J Clin Oncol. 1997;15:261–7.

23. Van Cutsem E, Moiseyenko VM, Tjulandin S, et al. Phase III study of docetaxel and cisplatin plus fluorouracil compared with cisplatin and fluorouracil as first line therapy for advanced gastric cancer: a report of the V325 Study Group. J Clin Oncol. 2006;24:4991–7.
24. Ohtsu A, Fuse N, Yoshino T, et al. Future perspectives of chemotherapy for advanced gastric cancer. Gastric Cancer. 2009;12:60–6.
25. Boku N, Yamamoto S, Shirao K, et al. Randomized phase III study of 5-FU alone versus combination of irinotecan and cisplatin (CP) versus S-1 alone in advanced gastric cancer (JCOG 9912). J Clin Oncol. 2007;25:LBA 4513.
26. Koizumi W, Narahara H, Hara T, et al. S-1 plus cisplatin versus S-1 alone for first line treatment of advanced gastric cancer (SPIRITS trial): a phase III trial. Lancet Oncol. 2008;9:215–21.
27. Ohtsu A, Shimada Y, Shirao K, et al. Randomized phase III trial of fluorouracil alone versus fluorouracil plus cisplatin versus uracil and tegaful plus mitomycin in patients with unresectable advanced gastric cancer: the Japan Clinical Oncology Group Study, (JCOG 9205). J Clin Oncol. 2003;21:54–9.
28. Imamura H, Iiishi H, Tsuburaya A, et al. Randomized phase III study of irinotecan plus S-1 (IRIS) versus S-1 alone as first-line treatment for advanced gastric cancer (GC0301/TOP002). Gastrointestinal cancers symposium, Orlando; 2008, abstract 5.
29. Jin M, Lu H, Li J, et al. Randomized three-armed phase III study of S-1 monotherapy versus S-1/CDDP versus 5-FU/CDDP in patients with advanced gastric cancer SC-101 study. J Clin Oncol. 2008;26:221s (abstract 4533).
30. Boku N. JCOG trials of systemic chemotherapy for unresectable or recurrent gastric cancer. Gastric Cancer. 2009;12:43–9.
31. Takiuchi H. Combination therapy with S-1 and irinotecan (CPT-11) for advanced or recurrent gastric cancer. Gastric Cancer. 2009;12:55–9.
32. Koizumi W. Clinical development of S-1 plus cisplatin therapy as first-line treatment for advanced gastric cancer. Gastric Cancer. 2009;12:10–54.
33. Mori S, Kishimoto H, Tauchi K, et al. Histological complete response in advanced gastric cancer after 2 weeks of S-1 administration as neoadjuvant chemotherapy. Gastric Cancer. 2006;9(2):136–9.
34. Matono D, Horiuchi H, Kishimoto Y, et al. A case of advanced gastric cancer with giant lymph node metastasis responding to S-1/CDDP neoadjuvant chemotherapy. Jpn J Cancer Chemother. 2008;35(9):1573–5.
35. Takasu N, Nomura T, Fukumoto T, et al. Advanced gastric cancer showing complete response to neoadjuvant chemotherapy with CPT-11 and S-1 – a case report. Jpn J Cancer Chemother. 2009;36(1):111–3.
36. Masumura K, Ninomiya M, Nishizaki M, et al. A case of long survival in Stage IV gastric carcinoma responding to combination treatment with paclitaxel and 5-FU followed by surgical resection. Jpn J Cancer Chemother. 2008;35(10):1745–8.

Systemic and Regional Chemotherapy for Advanced and Metastasized Pancreatic Cancer

16

Karl Reinhard Aigner, Sabine Gailhofer, and Gur Ben-Ari

16.1 Introduction

Pancreatic cancer remains a challenge in cancer therapy. The 5-year survival rate does not exceed 5 % because of late symptoms, and there are nearly as many cancer deaths as patients diagnosed each year, reflecting the poor prognosis associated with pancreatic cancer. At the time of diagnosis, only 10–15 % of the patients have still limited disease and are amenable to surgical resection. Systemic chemotherapy in non-resectable tumors has been of modest benefit, and most have been associated with significant toxicity.

In the last two decades, numerous well-designed randomized phase III studies have been performed in order to elucidate the optimal treatment strategy for advanced or metastasized pancreatic cancer. Although they appeared to offer much hope in treating this disease, the outcome has been very limited. Induction chemotherapy for locally advanced or metastasized tumors is the predominant indication in most diagnosed pancreatic cancers. Since, at diagnosis, life expectancy was about 2–4 months, Burris' study with gemcitabine as first-line therapy for advanced pancreatic cancer showing a significant survival advantage of 2 months was a substantial step forward [1]. Gemcitabine also improved clinical benefit response (CBR), and until now its efficiency has not been surpassed by any other single-agent therapy. However, since in multiple trials, single-agent gemcitabine did not exceed overall survival figures of approximately 6 months, new strategies were warranted.

K.R. Aigner, MD (✉) • S. Gailhofer
Department of Surgical Oncology, Medias Klinikum GmbH & Co KG,
Krankenhausstrasse 3a, Burghausen 84489, Germany
e-mail: info@prof-aigner.de

G. Ben-Ari
Department of Surgical Oncology (Emeritus), Sheba Medical Center Ramat-Gan, Tel-Aviv University, Medical School, Tel-Aviv, Israel

© Springer-Verlag Berlin Heidelberg 2016
K.R. Aigner, F.O. Stephens (eds.), *Induction Chemotherapy*,
DOI 10.1007/978-3-319-28773-7_16

It was quite understandable that in view of the lack of success of other mono-therapies, combination therapies were administered, hopefully to improve overall survival. A trial of gemcitabine combined with capecitabine versus gemcitabine alone [2, 3] resulted in a median overall survival of 7.4 months compared with 6 months for gemcitabine alone and an absolute improvement in 1-year survival of 7 % (26 % versus 19 %). Two further trials comparing gemcitabine alone or in combination with capecitabine failed to reveal any substantial differences in efficacy between the two groups [4, 5].

Combination therapies, such as gemcitabine with 5-FU [6], cisplatin [7], irinotecan [8], oxaliplatin [9, 10], siplatin and 5-FU [11] or ISIS-2503 [12], have failed to show improvement. Because of the negative results of randomized phase II studies of gemcitabine at a fixed dose rate or in combination with cisplatin, docetaxel, or irinotecan in patients with metastatic pancreatic cancer, none of these approaches was recommended for routine use [13]. Other phase III studies have been completely negative without any suggestion of increased efficacy such as comparing 5-FU with 5-FU plus cisplatin [14], gemcitabine alone, or with cisplatin [15], 5-FU alone or with mitomycin [16], as well as the combination of gemcitabine with exatecan [17], pemetrexed [18], or the targeted agents tipifarnib [19] or marimastat [20]. Also the addition of targeted agents like bevacizumab and erlotinib to gemcitabine [21] failed to demonstrate an advantage over gemcitabine alone; likewise, the addition of bevacizumab versus placebo could not translate into an improvement in overall survival. Other antiangiogenetic agents, too, have been recently communicated to be ineffective in this setting.

In a phase III study published by Moore et al. [22], the combination of gemcitabine with the tyrosine kinase inhibitor erlotinib showed a statistically significant difference in overall survival compared with gemcitabine alone. This was the first time any drug added to gemcitabine resulted in an improvement of overall survival. In this study including 569 patients totally with locally advanced pancreatic cancer, the survival advantage was 6.24 versus 5.91 months. The 1-year survival was more notable, amounting to 23 % versus 17 %. Analysis conducted to define the population of patients that could benefit most from this therapy revealed that the side effect "skin rash" was an indicator for response. It was also stated that females do not benefit from erlotinib compared to males.

Although the gemcitabine/erlotinib combination therapy reveals a distinct advantage in a selected group of patients, it can be stated that combination therapies have been globally disappointing. Pancreatic cancer, in general, has a propensity of being chemoresistant, and dose-intense systemic chemotherapies did not overcome this resistance.

In numerous recent studies, importance was given to surrogate end points like improvement of objective response rates, decline of the tumor marker CA 19-9, or progression-free survival (PFS) which, however, turned out to have no meaningful impact on overall survival. In addition, it has been noted in most trials that patients with reduced performance status and poor prognosis do not benefit from chemotherapy for advanced disease. Reviewing the achievements in terms of survival and quality of life from therapy of pancreatic cancer, the results are poor, at high cost, financially as well as in terms of adverse effects. It has been suggested that the burden from treatment-related adverse effects should not be added to those already suffering with the disease [11]. Survival benefits of statistically significant, 2 months at the most, at the cost of side effects or unacceptable toxicity demand the development of innovative strategies with better options in the treatment of pancreatic cancer.

16.2 Approaching the Target

Studies conducted so far were based on the evaluation of the effect of various drug combinations on survival. After all it seems reasonable to shift away from studies based on trial-and-error testing [23]. Targeted agents, active theoretically and in xenograft models, might play a paramount role in the future when there is better understanding of the complex interactions of signaling pathways and their possible blockade.

In many tumor models, the increase of local drug exposure actually is an important parameter to improve clinical results [24].

As distinct from other tumors, pancreatic cancer has a characteristic that explains the reason of poor responsiveness of primary tumors as opposed to metastases. There is a high degree of fibrotic encasement in primary tumors with very restricted vasculature [25–29]. Intraoperatively primary pancreatic carcinomas appear almost avascular, whereas liver metastases of the same tumor show an excellent blood supply when patent blue is injected through the hepatic artery for staining (Fig. 16.1). In contrast, normal pancreatic tissue reveals much better staining than the primary tumor itself when patent blue is injected intra-arterially. Better response and reduction of liver metastases were reported in some intra-arterial studies [30–33]. This phenomenon was taken into account in a study mentioned previously [13], where patients who had only locally advanced disease were excluded in order to avoid confounding evaluation of response.

16.3 Intra-arterial Chemotherapy

Studies with intra-arterial chemotherapy are heterogenous and encompass the administration of various drugs in a variety of dosages and times of application [30–33]. So far, there is no uniform standard and know-how about which application is the best. However, despite the great variety throughout all studies, survival time is generally superior and toxicity lower as compared with data from systemic chemotherapy. There are two randomized phase III trials comparing systemic versus regional chemotherapy. One study comparing intravenous application versus celiac axis infusion of the three-drug combination (mitomycin, mitoxantrone, and cisplatin) was terminated early because of the obvious discrepancy in survival in favor of intra-arterial chemotherapy and markedly increased toxicity in the systemic arm [34]. The Italian SITILO prospective randomized phase III study was

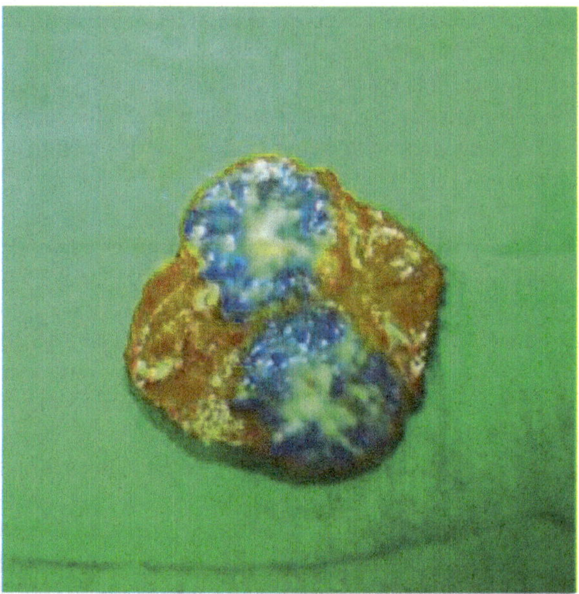

Fig. 16.1 Intra-arterial blue staining of liver metastases from pancreatic cancer. The metastases have more uptake of methylene blue than the surrounding liver parenchyma

conducted with a systemic arm of standard gemcitabine and a locoregional arm with 5-fluorouracil, leucovorin, epirubicin, and carboplatin. A third arm with 5-fluorouracil and leucovorin alone given systemically was soon abandoned, and the study continued with the systemic and locoregional arm [25]. This phase III study is of great interest, because the median overall survival of 5.85 months confirms the results of previous trials with gemcitabine, and on the other hand reveals a significant advantage in median overall survival of 7.9 months in the locoregional arm, where 12 months and 18 months survival are 35 % and 15 %, respectively. Of interest in this study is that there is more systemic toxicity in the intra-arterial arm, because of a different, non-gemcitabine containing intra-arterial drug combination, and a substantial spill of drugs in the venous drainage after the first pass through the arterial access.

16.4   Induction Chemotherapy

Induction chemotherapy for locally advanced disease is suggested to downstage the primary tumor and to achieve resectability, regardless of accompanying liver or local lymph node metastases. A tumor in the head of the pancreas itself is more life-threatening than locoregional or distant metastases.

In a meta-analysis of 111 studies and 4400 patients with primarily non-resectable or borderline resectable pancreatic cancer treated with preoperative induction radio- or chemotherapy, an estimated 33.2 % resectability rate after systemic induction chemotherapy was reported [35]. A comparatively similar rate was achieved with intra-arterial microembolization with degradable starch microspheres in a phase II study on 265 cases [31]. Eighty patients had survived 1 year or more. Out of these 80 patients with favorable results from regional chemotherapy, 39 % became resectable. This translates into a 12 % resectability rate in the entire group of patients. Surgical procedures in long-term survivors are listed in Table 16.1. There were 15/80 (19 %) Whipple resections, 12/80 (15 %) corpus/tail resections, and 4/80 (5 %) enucleations of necrotic tissues (Fig. 16.2). While resections were performed after downsizing of the primary tumor, enucleations had to be considered excavation of complete necrosis of the tumorous lesions, the symptoms of which were undulating fever, lethargy, lowering and unstable blood pressure, and high pulse rate, such as in tumor lysis syndrome. In the overall group of 265 advanced stage and partially pretreated patients, a 9-month median survival was noted. One-year and 18-month survival was 30 % and 25 %, respectively. The paradox responsiveness of liver metastases versus primary tumors is also reflected in the causes of death. More or less every second patient (48 %) died from tumor progression at the primary site, and only 8 % died from liver metastases, 7 % from peritoneal dissemination, and 4 % from lung metastases.

Table 16.1 Surgical procedures

	Patients	Percentage
Tumor resections	31/80	39
Whipple resection	15/80	19
Corpus/tail resection	12/80	15
Drainage of necrosis	4/80	5

Surgical procedures in long-term survivors of more than 1 year ($n=80$)

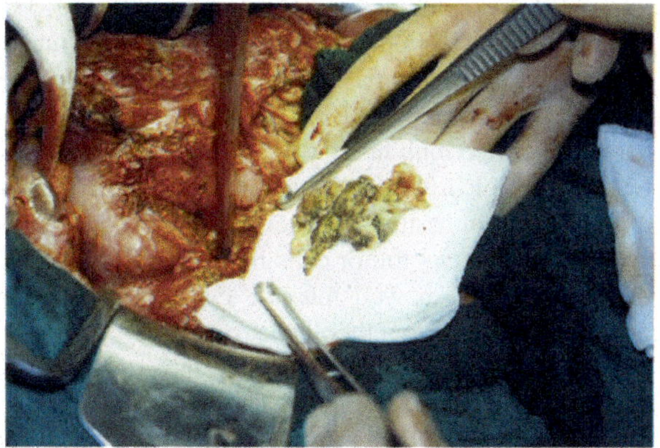

Fig. 16.2 Excavation and drainage of necrotic tumor tissue from the head of the pancreas after regional chemotherapy with DSM microembolization

16.5 Discussion

During the last two decades, achievements in terms of overall survival in the treatment of pancreatic cancer were not done in leaps but were worked out in little steps only. The greatest little step forward was the introduction of gemcitabine in systemic chemotherapy for advanced and metastasized pancreatic cancer [1]. This was a landmark study, the results of which – an improvement of median overall survival from some 4–6 months – could be confirmed by a series of subsequent studies from other previously mentioned groups and were not surpassed so far in overall survival by any other combination therapy. This includes conventional chemotherapeutic drugs as well as newer targeted agents. Studies conducted so far were based on the evaluation of the effect of various drug combinations on survival, in the form of trial-and-error testing, without considering potential advantages of modified handling of drugs such as manipulation of parameters like exposure and drug concentration at the target site.

Dose-dependent tumor toxicity of chemotherapeutics has been a well-known principle [36–39]. The dose–response behavior is steep [40]. In clinical practice with systemic chemotherapy, however, required drug exposures in solid tumors are limited by escalating toxicity. Therefore, the concentration component of the time x concentration product may be managed using techniques such as regional chemotherapy, the rationale behind which is to provide a means for delivering a much higher dose and concentration of the drug directly to the tumor than can be achieved by systemic administration.

When C. T. Klopp in 1950 first injected nitrogen mustard into an artery, the local effect appeared to him like "chemotherapeutic irradiation" [41]. This was the very beginning. During the years and decades since then, pitfalls with regional chemotherapy, in general, were associated with lack of experience in terms of know-how, techniques, and pharmaceutical and pharmacokinetic principles.

Therapy of pancreatic cancer in particular seemed to be an unsurmountable challenge. In recent years, progress has been made with regard to the local effect of intra-arterial chemotherapy on liver metastases [30–33]. This is most evidently due to the better blood supply as compared with the primary tumors in the pancreas that are encased in fibrotic tissue. This phenomenon was demonstrated impressively in second look operations 12 months after regional chemotherapy. Liver metastases, parapancreatic lymph node metastases, and the primary tumor itself showed a different histologic response behavior. Whereas in liver metastases, histologically, no more vital tumor tissue was observed, lymph node metastases showed central necrosis with some intact tumor cells in the periphery, and the biopsy from the primary tumor, however, showed massive cytoplasmatic edema and marked tumor cell degeneration, but altogether the least response [30]. This paradox response between primary tumor and metastases reveals the crucial weak point in the therapy of pancreatic cancer. Since a complete response in the primary can hardly be achieved, and most resections are R1 resections, the most frequent cause of death is relapse and tumor progression at the primary site [31]. Systemic chemotherapy, in what combination so ever, cannot provide the necessary drug exposure that is required. This may be the reason why all combination therapies eventually failed.

Regional chemotherapy, however, provides an advantage in response rates in single studies with consistently elevated median overall survival times of 8–10 months with lower side effects, which should not be imposed on patients with poor life expectancy who suffer already enough from their disease. The prospective randomized phase III study from the Italian SITILO group clearly revealed the superiority of regional chemotherapy [25].

There is still a lot of potential of possible and necessary improvement, especially in the management of the resistant primary tumors. The problem is not solved by far yet. However, ongoing studies with microembolization and isolation techniques show a tendency toward improvement of the response behavior at the primary site (to be published).

Effective therapy of the primary tumor is particularly important in induction chemotherapy for borderline or non-resectable tumors [35]. Actually, there are no phase III trials available that clarify the effect of systemic or intra-arterial induction chemotherapy on resectability. Who judges and decides resectability? Decisions may be individually different. Well-designed and reproducible parameters defining "resectability" are mandatory to decide which tumors are resectable and which are not. It largely depends on the experience and technical skills of the surgeon. Therefore, such a study can hardly be performed as a multicenter study unless the local therapeutic approach is so efficient that it really generates measurable downsizing or tumor necrosis and therefore resectability. Systemic chemotherapy is most unlikely to do so at present. Regional chemotherapy holds this potential but still requires much improvement in order to overcome chemoresistance at the primary tumor site. Therefore, actually, progress is made in little steps and not yet by leaps.

References

1. Burris III HA, Moore MJ, Andersen J, et al. Improvements in survival and clinical benefit with gemcitabine as first-line therapy for patients with advanced pancreas cancer: a randomized trial. J Clin Oncol. 1997;15:2403–13.
2. Cunningham D, Chau I, Stocken D, et al. Phase III randomised comparison of gemcitabine (GEM) with gemcitabine plus capecitabine (GEM-CAP) in patients with advanced pancreatic cancer. Eur J Cancer Suppl. 2005;3(2):12.
3. Cunningham D, Chau I, Stocken D, et al. Phase III randomised comparison of gemcitabine (GEM) versus gemcitabine plus capecitabine (GEM-CAP) in patients with advanced pancreatic cancer. J Clin Oncol. 2009;27:5513–8.
4. Scheithauer W, Schull B, Ulrich-Pur H, et al. Biweekly high-dose gemcitabine alone or in combination with capecitabine in patients with metastatic pancreatic adenocarcinoma: a randomized phase II trial. Ann Oncol. 2003;14:97–104.
5. Herrmann R, Bodoky G, Ruhstaller T, et al. Gemcitabine plus capecitabine compared with gemcitabine alone in advanced pancreatic cancer: a randomized, multicenter, phase III trial of the Swiss Group for Clinical Cancer Research and the Central European Cooperative Oncology Group. J Clin Oncol. 2007;25:2212–7.

6. Berlin JD, Catalano P, Thomas JP, et al. Phase III study of gemcitabine in combination with fluorouracil versus gemcitabine alone in patients with advanced pancreatic carcinoma: Eastern Cooperative Oncology Group Trial E2297. J Clin Oncol. 2002;20:3270–5.

7. Heinemann V, Quietzsch D, Gieseler F, et al. A phase III trial comparing gemcitabine plus cisplatin vs. gemcitabine alone in advanced pancreatic carcinoma. Proc Am Soc Clin Oncol. 2003;22:250.

8. Rocha Lima CM, Green MR, Rotche R, et al. Irinotecan plus gemcitabine results in no survival advantage compared with gemcitabine monotherapy in patients with locally advanced or metastatic pancreatic cancer despite increased tumor response rate. J Clin Oncol. 2004;22:3776–83.

9. Louvet C, Labianca R, Hammel P, et al. Gemcitabine in combination with oxaliplatin compared with gemcitabine alone in locally advanced or metastatic pancreatic cancer: results of a GERCOR and GISCAD phase III trial. J Clin Oncol. 2005;23:3509–16.

10. Poplin E, Feng Y, Berlin J, et al. Phase III, randomized study of gemcitabine and oxaliplatin versus gemcitabine (fixed-dose rate infusion) compared with gemcitabine (30-minute infusion) in patients with pancreatic carcinoma E6201: a trial of the Eastern Cooperative Oncology Group. J Clin Oncol. 2009;27:3778–85.

11. El-Rayes BF, Zalupski MM, Shields AF, et al. Phase II study gemcitabine, cisplatin, and infusional fluorouracil in advanced pancreatic cancer. J Clin Oncol. 2003;21:2920–5.

12. Alberts SR, Schroeder M, Erlichman C, et al. Gemcitabine and ISIS-2503 for patients with locally advanced or metastatic pancreatic adenocarcinoma: a North Central Cancer Treatment Group phase II trial. J Clin Oncol. 2004;22:4944–50.

13. Kulke Matthew H, Tempero Margaret A, Niedzwiecki D, et al. Randomized phase II study of gemcitabine administered at a fixed dose rate or in combination with cisplatin, docetaxel, or irinotecan in patients with metastatic pancreatic cancer: CALGB 89904. J Clin Oncol. 2009;27:5506–12.

14. Ducreux M, Rougier P, Pignon JP, et al. A randomised trial comparing 5-FU with 5-FU plus cisplatin in advanced pancreatic carcinoma. Ann Oncol. 2002;13:1185–91.

15. Colucci G, Giuliani F, Gebbia V, et al. Gemcitabine alone or with cisplatin for the treatment of patients with locally advanced and/or metastatic pancreatic carcinoma: a prospective, randomized phase III study of the Gruppo Oncologia dell'Italia Meridionale. Cancer. 2002;94:902–10.

16. Maisey N, Chau I, Cunningham D, et al. Multicenter randomized phase III trial of protracted venous infusion of 5-fluorouracil with PVI 5-FU plus mitomycin in inoperable pancreatic cancer. J Clin Oncol. 2002;20:3130–6.

17. Abou-Alfa GK, Letourneau R, Harker G, et al. Randomized phase III study of exatecan and gemcitabine compared with gemcitabine compared with gemcitabine alone in untreated advanced pancreatic cancer. J Clin Oncol. 2006;24:4441–7.

18. Oettle H, Richards D, Ramanathan RK, et al. A phase III trial of pemetrexed plus gemcitabine versus gemcitabine in patients with unresectable or metastatic pancreatic cancer. Ann Oncol. 2005;16:1639–45.

19. Van Cutsem E, van de Velde H, Karasek P, et al. Phase III trial of gemcitabine plus tipifarnib compared with gemcitabine plus placebo in advanced pancreatic cancer. J Clin Oncol. 2004;22:1430–8.

20. Bramhall SR, Schulz J, Nemunaitis J, et al. A double-blind placebo-controlled, randomised study comparing gemcitabine and marimastat with gemcitabine and placebo as first line therapy in patients with advanced pancreatic cancer. Br J Cancer. 2002;87:161–7.

21. Van Cutsem E, Vervenne W, Bennouna J, et al. Phase III trial of bevacizumab in combination with gemcitabine and erlotinib in patients with metastatic pancreatic cancer. J Clin Oncol. 2009;27:2231–7.

22. Moore MJ, Goldstein D, Hamm J, et al. Erlotinib plus gemcitabine compared with gemcitabine alone in patients with advanced pancreatic cancer: a phase III trial of the National Cancer Institute of Canada clinical trials group. J Clin Oncol. 2007;25(15):1960–6.

23. Chua YJ, Zalcberg JR. Pancreatic cancer – is the wall crumbling? Ann Oncol. 2008;19(7):1224–30.
24. Stephens FO. Why use regional chemotherapy? Principles and pharmacokinetics. Reg Cancer Treat. 1988;1:4–10.
25. Cantore M, Fiorentini G, Luppi G, et al. Randomised trial of gemcitabine versus flec regimen given intra-arterially for patients with unresectable pancreatic cancer. J Exp Clin Cancer Res. 2003;22:4.
26. Miller DW, Fontain M, Kolar C, et al. The expression of multidrug resistance-associated protein (MRP) in pancreatic adenocarcinoma cell lines. Cancer Lett. 1996;107:301–6.
27. Verovski VN, Van den Berge DL, Delvaeye MM, et al. Low-level doxorubicin resistance in P-glycoprotein-negative human pancreatic tumor PSN1/ADR cells implicates a brefeldin A-sensitive mechanism of drug extrusion. Br J Cancer. 1996;73:596–602.
28. Kartner N, Riorden JR, Ling V. Cell surface P-glycoprotein associated with multidrug resistance in mammalian cell lines. Science. 1983;221:1285–8.
29. Goldstein LJ, Galski H, Fojo A, et al. Expression of the multidrug resistance gene product P-glycoprotein in human cancer. J Natl Cancer Inst. 1989;81:116.
30. Aigner KR, Müller H, Basserman R. Intra-arterial chemotherapy with MMC, CDDP and 5-FU for nonresectable pancreatic cancer – a phase II study. Reg Cancer Treat. 1990;3:1–6.
31. Aigner KR, Gailhofer S. Celiac axis infusion and microembolization for advanced stage III/IV pancreatic cancer – a phase II study on 265 cases. Anticancer Res. 2005;25:4407–12.
32. Ishikawa O, Ohigashi H, Imaoka S, et al. Regional chemotherapy to prevent hepatic metastasis after resection of pancreatic cancer. Hepatogastroenterology. 1997;44(18):1541–6.
33. Beger HG, Gansauge F, Buchler MW, et al. Intraarterial adjuvant chemotherapy after pancreaticoduodenectomy for pancreatic cancer: significant reduction in occurrence of liver metastasis. World J Surg. 1999;23(9):946–9.
34. Aigner KR, Gailhofer S, Kopp S. Regional versus systemic chemotherapy for advanced pancreatic cancer: a randomized study. Hepatogastroenterology. 1998;45:1125–9.
35. Gillen S, Schuster T, Meyer Zum Buschenfelde C, Friess H, et al. Preoperative/neoadjuvant therapy in pancreatic cancer: a systematic review and meta-analysis of response and resection percentages. PLoS Med. 2010;7:e1000267.
36. Collins JM. Pharmacologic rationale for regional drug delivery. J Clin Oncol. 1984;2:498–504.
37. Stephens FO, Harker GJS, Dickinson RTJ, Roberts BA. Preoperative basal chemotherapy in the management of cancer of the stomach: a preliminary report. Aust N Z J Surg. 1979;49:331.
38. Stephens FO, Crea P, Harker GJS, Roberts BA, Hambly CK. Intra-arterial chemotherapy as basal treatment in advanced and fungating primary breast cancer. Lancet. 1980;2:435.
39. Stephens FO. Clinical experience in the use of intra-arterial infusion chemotherapy in the treatment of cancers in the head and neck, the extremities, the breast and the stomach. In: Schwemmle K, Aigner KR, editors. Vascular perfusion in cancer therapy, Recent Results in Cancer Research, vol. 86. Berlin: Springer; 1983. p. 122.
40. Frei E, Canellos III GP. Dose: a critical factor in cancer chemotherapy. Am J Med. 1980;69:585–94.
41. Klopp CT, Alford TC, Bateman J, Berry GN, Winship T. Fractionated intra-arterial cancer chemotherapy with methyl bis-amine hydrochloride; a preliminary report. Ann Surg. 1950;132:811–32.

Interventional Radiological Procedures for Port-Catheter Implantation

17

Yasuaki Arai

17.1 Hepatic Arterial Infusion Chemotherapy

17.1.1 Introduction

Hepatic arterial infusion is now one of the most widely used techniques in regional chemotherapy. Especially, in the treatment of liver metastases from colorectal cancer, it had been recognized as the most powerful treatment before the establishment of recent standard systemic chemotherapy combined with irinotecan or oxaliplatin. However, most of the randomized trials comparing hepatic arterial infusion chemotherapy to systemic chemotherapy have failed to reveal the advantage on survival prolongation [1–12], and the powerful systemic chemotherapies such as FOLFOX and FOLFIRI have been established as the standard for systemic chemotherapy. As a result, at the present time, the role of hepatic arterial infusion chemotherapy has been minimized and used under very limited conditions. The most important issue of hepatic arterial infusion chemotherapy is that the implantation of a port-catheter system is needed to initiate this treatment. Before the development of interventional radiological procedures, the implantation of port-catheter systems was done by a surgical procedure using laparotomy. This caused various complications including a reduction of patients' performance status. Thus, it was recognized that surgical procedures for port-catheter implantation might give negative influence on the results of randomized trials. At present time, the minimally invasive procedure for port-catheter implantation has been well established using techniques of interventional radiology [13–15]. Therefore, had this procedure been employed in the randomized trials, there might have been different outcomes.

Y. Arai
Division of Diagnostic Radiology, National Cancer Center,
5-1-1, tshukiji, Chuo-ku, Tokyo 104-0045, Japan
e-mail: arai-y3111@mvh.biglobe.ne.jp

© Springer-Verlag Berlin Heidelberg 2016
K.R. Aigner, F.O. Stephens (eds.), *Induction Chemotherapy*,
DOI 10.1007/978-3-319-28773-7_17

In such fields as colorectal cancer systemic chemotherapy has been well established, and it became no longer necessary to use the old techniques of hepatic arterial infusion chemotherapy as standard. However, with such established standard systemic chemotherapy, cancer is not cured in the vast majority of patients. Thus, many opportunities to use hepatic arterial infusion chemotherapy with its greater impact chemotherapy are now available for study. Especially, by using minimally invasive interventional procedures, the combination of hepatic arterial infusion chemotherapy combined with systemic chemotherapy may show better clinical outcomes compared with those by systemic chemotherapy alone [16, 17]. Also, in the treatment of hepatocellular carcinoma that is increasing the world over, this technique may be employed for another treatment option replacing chemoembolization [18].

17.1.2 Concept

Arterial infusion chemotherapy achieves significantly higher antitumor activity with limited systemic toxicity. It means that the administrated drug is distributed only to the whole liver but not to extrahepatic organs. Port-catheter implantation with interventional radiological techniques is aimed at achieving three distinct processes of [1] arterial redistribution, [2] easy access with percutaneous catheter placement, and [3] evaluation and management of drug distribution, and after all three processes are completed, the "optimal drug distribution" can be achieved.

17.1.3 Techniques

17.1.3.1 Arterial Redistribution (Fig. 17.1)

The purposes of arterial redistribution are to convert multiple hepatic arteries if present into a single vascular supply and to occlude arteries arising from the hepatic arterial region and supplying extrahepatic organs.

Conversion of Multiple Hepatic Arteries into a Single Vascular Supply

To convert multiple hepatic arteries into a single vascular supply, all hepatic arteries, except the one to be used for drug administration, must be embolized by coils and/or glue such as n-butyl-2-cyano-acrylate (NBCA) mixed with Lipiodol. The replaced right hepatic artery (rep. RHA), the accessory right hepatic artery (acc. RHA) that arises from the superior mesenteric artery (SMA) or the common hepatic artery (CHA), and the replaced left hepatic artery (rep. LHA) are the common target arteries of this procedure. Because of the existence of intrahepatic arterial communications between hepatic arteries, the vascular territory where the feeding artery has been embolized can receive arterial blood supply from the remaining nonoccluded hepatic artery through these communications. By this mechanism, the liver that had been supplied with multiple hepatic arteries can be changed to receive arterial blood supply from the one remaining artery, and then, the liver can be completely perfused by a single indwelling catheter. However, the incidence of hepatic

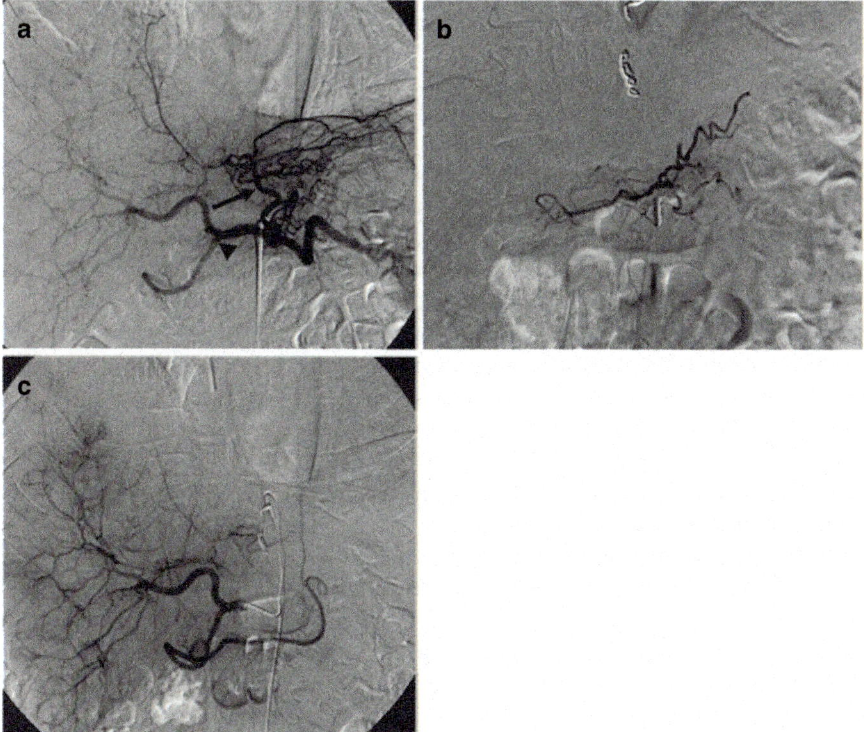

Fig. 17.1 (**a**) The replaced left hepatic artery is originating from the left gastric artery (*black arrow*), and the right gastric artery is originating from the proximal portion of the gastroduodenal artery (*black arrow head*). (**b**) A microcatheter is inserted into the right gastric artery to embolize this artery by a microcoil. (**c**) The common hepatic angiogram (*DSA*) after the embolization of the replaced left hepatic artery and the right gastric artery shows the left lobe of the liver receives blood supply from the common hepatic artery and disappearance of blood supply into the right gastric artery via the gastroduodenal artery

arterial occlusion is high if the indwelling catheter was placed into the replaced hepatic artery; therefore, in a case with the proper hepatic artery and the replaced hepatic artery, the replaced hepatic artery should be embolized to leave the proper hepatic artery as the only patent and functioning hepatic artery.

Occlusion of Arteries Arising from the Hepatic Artery and Supplying Extrahepatic Organs

To prevent toxic events caused by infusion of chemotherapeutic agents into the extrahepatic organs such as the stomach, duodenum, or pancreas, branch arteries arising from the artery to be used for infusion and supplying extrahepatic organs must be embolized. The gastroduodenal artery (GDA), the right gastric artery (RGA), the accessory left gastric artery (acc. LGA), the superior duodenal artery (SDA), the posterior superior pancreaticoduodenal artery (PSPDA), and the dorsal pancreatic artery (DPA) should be considered as the target arteries of this procedure.

To embolize a small artery such as the RGA, the use of microcatheter system and microcoils is efficient and is an easier procedure. In cases with difficulties in inserting even a microcatheter into such small arteries, the glue used carefully will be effective instead of microcoils.

17.1.3.2 Percutaneous Catheter Placement

The most important advantage of the percutaneous placement of an indwelling catheter is its limited invasiveness compared to the surgical method underwent general anesthesia and laparotomy. To prevent complications associated with an indwelling catheter, such as hepatic arterial occlusion, catheter dislocation, and catheter kinking, there are three important points. The first is employing the "tip-fixation method." The cause of hepatic arterial occlusion is usually the mechanical stimulation of catheter tip against the vascular endothelium by patients' movement and breathing. The "tip-fixation method" is inserting an indwelling catheter having a side hole not into the hepatic artery but commonly into the GDA adjusting the position of side hole to CHA and then fixing the distal tip of the indwelling catheter with the GDA using coils. Thus, this method can reduce the mechanical stimulation of catheter tip against the hepatic artery. The second is to keep enough length of an indwelling catheter in the aorta. By keeping enough length of an indwelling catheter, the stretching tension to the indwelling catheter by patient's movement can be avoided, and then, it leads to the reduction of risk of catheter dislocation. The third is to avoid routes with a wide range of motion (e.g., shoulder or hip joint) in the region where an indwelling catheter is traversing. From this point of view, a route via the subclavian artery or the inferior epigastric artery is more suitable to avoid catheter kinking than that via the femoral artery. However, if the "tip-fixation method" and keeping enough length of an indwelling catheter in the aorta are employed, the risk of catheter dislocation and kinking is limited also in the access via the femoral artery. By applying these techniques, the incidence of complications associated with an indwelling catheter can be remarkably decreased.

Access to the Subclavian Artery

The left subclavian artery is commonly used to avoid complications to the intracranial circulation. The traditional approach is to make a surgical cutdown, which makes a 3 cm skin incision 2 cm below the left clavicle on the anterior chest wall under the local anesthesia, insert an indwelling catheter via a branch of the subclavian artery, and fix the catheter by ligation of the branch over the catheter.

The direct puncture of the left subclavian artery is also possible under sonographic or fluoroscopic guidance; however, in case of fluoroscopic guidance, insertion of guide wire into the subclavian artery via a separate access is necessary to make a target of puncture. The direct puncture access is simple and easier than surgical cutdown; however, the incompleteness of fixation caused by lack of ligation with a branch sometimes leads to complications such as bleeding, catheter dislocation, and, rarely, intracranial thrombosis.

Access to the Inferior Epigastric Artery

A "retrograde guide wire guiding method" is useful for interventional radiologists to access to the inferior epigastric artery. In this method, a guidewire is inserted into the inferior epigastric artery by the conventional angiographic manner via the femoral artery, and then the inferior epigastric artery is exposed by a cutdown procedure under fluoroscopic localization of the guidewire. Pulling out the guidewire through the inferior epigastric artery, the angiographic catheter can be easily inserted into the abdominal aorta through the inferior epigastric artery using an over the guidewire technique. After the placement of the indwelling catheter at the adequate position, the catheter is fixed with the inferior epigastric artery by ligation of over the artery.

Access to the Femoral Artery
Access to the femoral artery for the indwelling catheter placement is essentially the same as that for the conventional angiography.

Insertion of the Indwelling Catheter
There are two types of indwelling catheter. One is Anthron PU catheter (B. Braun Medical S.A.S Chasseneuil, France, manufactured by Toray Industries. Inc., Chiba, Japan), and another is W-spiral catheter (Piolax Medical Device, Inc., Kanagawa, Japan). There are many types of catheters; however, and commonly a tapered-type catheter (5 Fr in outer diameter and tapered to 2.7 Fr at 20 cm from the tip) is used. The indwelling catheter must have a side hole to flow out anticancer agents. If using a catheter without a side hole, a side hole must be opened by scissors-cut manipulation (or using the side-hole opener set in the catheter kit of W-spiral catheter). The tip portion of the indwelling catheter must be cut to an adequate length for subsequent tip fixation. Based on the angiography images via the celiac and the superior mesenteric arteries, the artery most suitable for fixation of the tip indwelling catheter will be chosen. The prepared side-holed catheter is inserted by using the catheter exchange method with a 0.018 in. or smaller guidewire (if a non-tapered indwelling catheter is employed, 0.035 in. guidewire can be used). Commonly, the occlusion of an end hole of indwelling catheter is not necessary if a tapered indwelling catheter is used. However, if a non-tapered 5 Fr indwelling catheter is used, the end hole of the indwelling catheter must be occluded by a microcoil inserted into the distal portion to the side hole of the indwelling catheter inserted via a microcatheter placed coaxially. In addition, if using the left subclavian arterial approach, a 5 Fr curved long introducer should be used to prevent kinking.

Tip Fixation
The GDA is the most commonly used for fixation of the tip of the indwelling catheter. However, also other arteries such as the SA, the LGA, the acc. LGA can be used for the tip fixation, if needed. When using the GDA, an indwelling side-holed catheter is inserted into the GDA with the side hole placed within the CHA. Then, the GDA is embolized with coils and if necessary with NBCA-Lipiodol mixture. If a second catheter can be inserted via the other access, coils and NBCA-Lipiodol mixture can be administered through the second catheter (Fig. 17.2). If this process is performed without the use of a second catheter, the indwelling catheter with a side hole in the 5 Fr portion is first inserted into the GDA, and then, a microcatheter

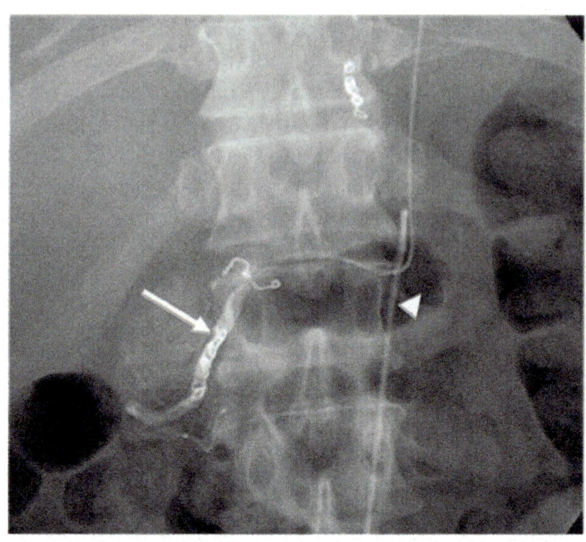

Fig. 17.2 The tip of the indwelling catheter is fixed with the gastroduodenal artery with microcoils and NBCA-Lipiodol mixture (*white arrow*) administered through a microcatheter via the second catheter (*white arrow*)

is coaxially inserted into the GDA through the indwelling catheter and passed through the side hole (Fig. 17.3). After the fixation of the tip, the indwelling catheter should form a loop in the aorta to prevent a direct transmission of patient's movement to the distal portion inserted into the CHA (Fig. 17.4).

Occlusion of the End Hole of the Indwelling Catheter

The end hole of the indwelling catheter is naturally occluded with thrombus between a side hole and the end hole, if a tapered-type indwelling catheter is employed. However, if a non-tapered 5 Fr catheter is used, the end hole of the indwelling catheter should be occluded using a microcoil inserted through a coaxial microcatheter.

Connection with a Port System

The proximal end of the indwelling catheter is connected to the implantable port system. Keeping a natural course of the catheter is very important to prevent troubles such as catheter kinking and breakage. It is also important to have a distance from the joints with wide range of motion (e.g., hip joint, shoulder joint). A Huber-point needle must be used to puncture a silicone septum of the port. After administration of chemotherapeutic agents, enough volume of saline to wash the inner lumen of the catheter and port system must be flushed, and 2 mL (2,000 U) of heparin must be injected into the system at least every 2 weeks to prevent thrombosis of the catheter.

17.1.3.3 Evaluation and Management of Drug Distribution

During long-term hepatic arterial infusion chemotherapy, drug distribution via the indwelling catheter and port system sometimes changes, because of the development of collateral and/or parasitic blood supply to the liver. To achieve good therapeutic results, the "optimal drug distribution" must be maintained.

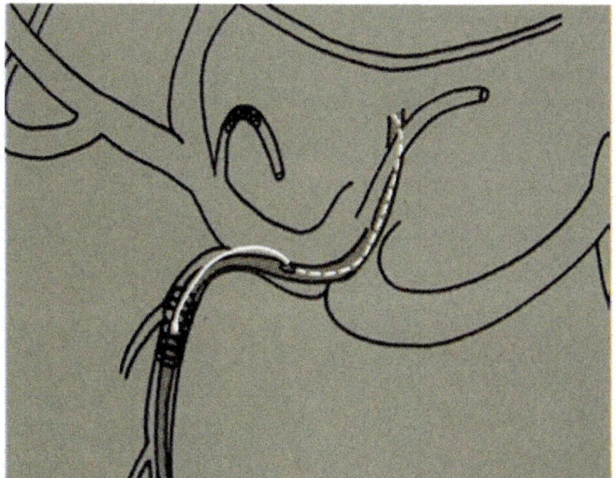

Fig. 17.3 A microcatheter can be inserted into the gastroduodenal artery through the indwelling catheter coaxially and passed through the side hole

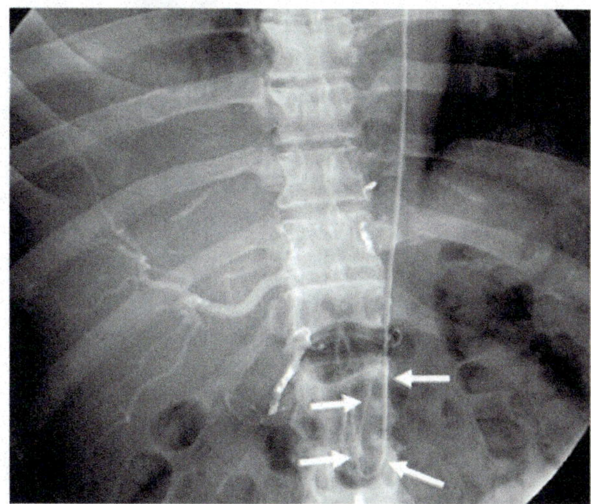

Fig. 17.4 The tapered part of the indwelling catheter forms a loop in the aorta (*white arrows*) to prevent a direct transmission of patient's movement to the distal portion inserted into the common hepatic artery

Evaluation of Drug Distribution (Fig. 17.5)

In the drug distribution evaluation, a computed tomography during angiography (CTA) via the indwelling catheter-port system is needed, as two-dimensional imaging, such as digital subtraction angiography (DSA) via the indwelling catheter-port system, is insufficient. The volume and rate of contrast medium to be used are determined by the scanning time and pitch of the CT scanner. Commonly, 10–20 mL volume of 30–50 % diluted contrast medium is injected via the indwelling catheter-port system at the rate of 0.5–1.5 mL/s. The "optimal drug distribution" in hepatic arterial infusion chemotherapy, defined by CTA, should show contrast enhancement of the entire liver without enhancement of extrahepatic organs. Furthermore, to prevent drug-related complications, it is mandatory to make a thorough evaluation looking for contrast enhancement within the stomach wall, duodenum, or pancreas.

Fig. 17.5 (**a**) DAS image via the indwelling catheter-port system is insufficient to evaluate the details of drug distribution. (**b**) CTA images via the indwelling catheter-port system show the details of drug distribution clearly

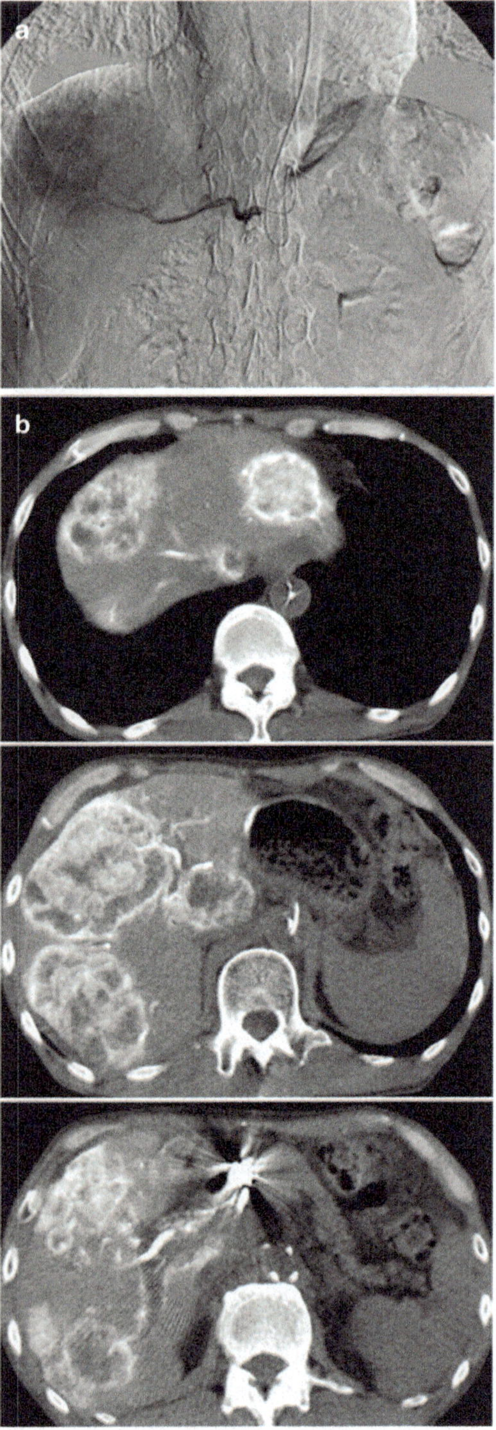

Drug distribution surveillance should be performed at least every 3 months to detect any catheter dislodgement or at any time with unusual clinical symptoms such as abdominal pain, nausea, or fever during and/or after infusion chemotherapy. If there is an area without contrast enhancement in the liver, the presence of parasitic or collateral blood supply in this area should be strongly suspected. In such cases, selective angiography must be performed not only to reveal arteries supplying blood into this area but also to revise the drug distribution. Selective angiography, to become mandatory to look for parasitic or collateral blood supply to the liver, includes CA, the SMA, the inferior phrenic artery, the right renal artery, the right adrenal artery, and, if necessary, the internal mammary artery.

Contrast medium should be injected at the same infusion rate as that for the given chemotherapeutic agent because the distribution of contrast medium should accurately simulate the distribution of chemotherapeutic agent. However, performing CTA at less than 1 mL/min infusion rate such as the continuous infusion of 5-fluorouracil (5-FU) or 5-fluorodeoxyuridine (FUDR) is impossible. In such slow infusion rate, MRI with contrast medium injected via the indwelling catheter system may show more accurate distribution of chemotherapeutic agents than CTA [19].

Management of Drug Distribution (Fig. 17.6)
If a parasitic or collateral artery supplies blood to a part of the liver, embolization of this artery must be performed to revise the drug distribution. However, such parasitic or collateral arteries often have multiple communications with other vessels. Also, proximal embolization with coils may not be enough to stop its blood supply to the liver. Therefore, for the embolization of such parasitic or collateral artery, a complete embolization cast using a NBCA-Lipiodol mixture (diluted six to ten times by Lipiodol) should be performed. If the successful embolization of the artery is performed and if there is no artery supplying blood to the liver (with the exception of the hepatic artery where drug is infused via the system), the improved drug distribution will be seen on CTA.

In cases of extrahepatic organ enhancement on CTA via the indwelling catheter system, the branch artery supplying blood to the extrahepatic organ should be detected by conventional angiography and embolized. For this embolization, it is usually sufficient to occlude the proximal portion of the artery using microcoil. Yet when the artery is too small to insert a microcoil, embolization may be performed using NBCA-Lipiodol (diluted two to three times by Lipiodol).

17.1.4 Therapeutic Results

For hepatic arterial infusion chemotherapy, percutaneous image-guided catheter placement is a technically safe and a viable alternative to traditional methods of hepatic artery access. There have been many reports of percutaneous hepatic arterial catheter placement with techniques of interventional radiology. The technical success rate of catheter placement and 1-year functioning rate that the indwelling

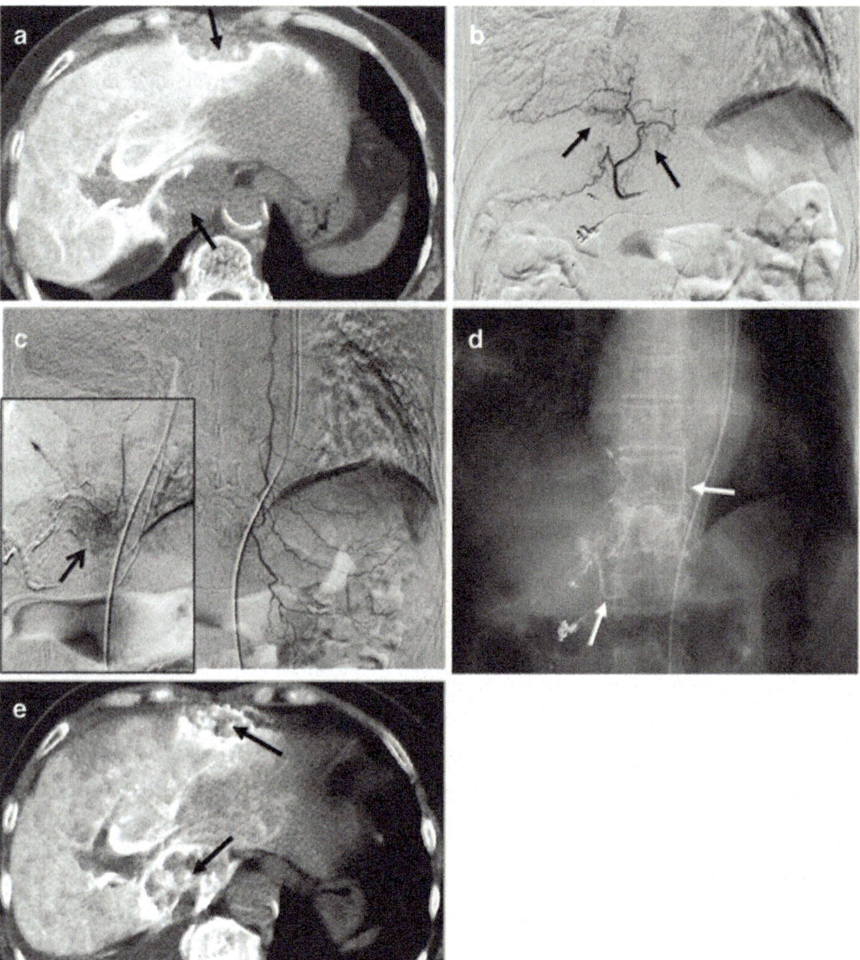

Fig. 17.6 (**a**) CTA via the indwelling catheter-port system shows the intrahepatic areas without contrast enhancement (*black arrows*). (**b**) DSA image of the right inferior phrenic artery shows fine tumor staining in the liver. (**c**) A super selective DSA image of the branch of the left internal mammary artery shows tumor staining in the liver. (**d**) Parasitic arteries supplying blood to the liver are embolized with NBCA-Lipiodol mixture (*white arrows*). (**e**) CTA via the indwelling catheter-port system after the embolization of parasitic arteries shows the significant better drug distribution compared to that before the embolization (**a**). Non-enhanced areas before the embolization are enhanced in this study (*black arrows*)

catheter ports can be used were approximately 97 %, 99 %, and 78–81 %, respectively [20–22]. However, to ensure the high likelihood of tumor-only delivery of chemotherapy, a complete knowledge of hepatic arterial anatomy, potential blood flow complications, and infusion device management is needed.

The response rate and median survival of HAIC using an interventional procedure:

Colorectal cancer (there are two studies):

1. $N=32$, response rate$=78$ %, median survival$=25.8$ months [23]
2. $N=30$, response rate$=83$ %, median survival$=26.0$ months [24]

Gastric cancer (there are two studies):

1. $N=40$, response rate$=72$ %, median survival$=15.0$ months [25]
2. $N=83$, response rate$=56$ %, median survival$=10.5$ months [26]

17.2 Arterial Infusion Chemotherapy for Locally Advanced Breast Cancer

17.2.1 Introduction

There are many kinds of treatment modalities for breast cancer, and the key treatment to prolong survival of patients with advanced stages is systemic chemotherapy. However, the good control of primary lesion is also important to achieve better quality of life for patients with locally advanced primary lesions. Intra-arterial infusion chemotherapy has been tried to manage such locally advanced breast cancer by using a conventional angiography technique or surgical/interventional catheter placement and has shown the proper efficacy. However, this treatment modality had clear limitations, because the locally advanced breast cancers can receive arterial blood supply from various arteries, such as the internal and external thoracic arteries, the intercostal arteries, and the other small braches originating from the subclavian artery. Consequently the standard procedures of the arterial redistribution and catheter placement to obtain the "optimal drug distribution" in the repeated administration of chemotherapeutic agents for the locally advanced breast cancer had not been established.

However, also in this filed, using the techniques and knowledge that has been obtained in the process of establishing the procedures for hepatic arterial infusion chemotherapy, new interventional radiological procedures have been developed [27].

17.2.2 Concept

To simplify the arterial blood supply to the breast tumor, the internal thoracic artery is embolized using NBCA-Lipiodol mixture in this new technique. With this arterial redistribution, the breast tumor receives arterial blood supply via the braches originating from the part of the subclavian artery distal to the origin of the vertebral artery. As a result, most of the infused anticancer agents at the point distal to the origin of the vertebral artery can be infused into the breast region under the stop flow of the brachial artery using the compression by a sphygmomanometer cuff.

17.2.3 Techniques (Fig. 17.7)

17.2.3.1 Arterial Redistribution

The brachial artery is punctured at the level of the elbow joint, and a 4 Fr sheath is inserted. After obtaining the selective angiograms of the subclavian artery and the internal thoracic artery, a 4 Fr hook-shaped catheter is inserted into the internal thoracic artery. A microcatheter is inserted into the internal thoracic artery coaxially into the internal thoracic artery and advanced to approximately 3 cm distal to the tip of the parent catheter, and then NBCA-Lipiodol mixture (diluted around eight times) is injected. The important objective of this procedure is to embolize the peripheral braches of the internal thoracic artery without the over flow of NBCA-Lipiodol mixture into the subclavian artery. Thus, the tips of the parent catheter and microcatheter should be inserted into the deeper portion of the internal thoracic artery, if needed. Additionally, embolization using microcoils in the proximal portion on the internal thoracic artery can be used to occlude proximal portion of the internal thoracic artery safely. After the embolization of the internal thoracic artery, a DSA of the subclavian artery is performed to evaluate the results of arterial redistribution.

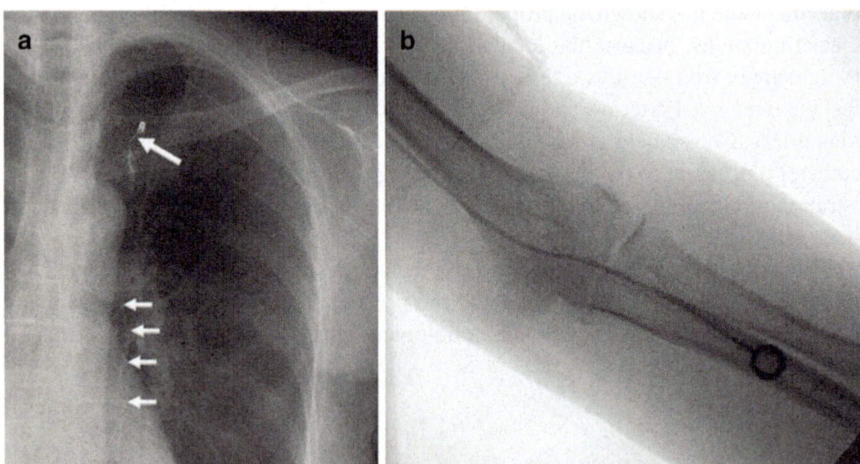

Fig. 17.7 (**a**) The left internal thoracic artery is embolized with NBCA-Lipiodol mixture (*small white arrows*) and microcoils (*big white arrow*). (**b**) The indwelling catheter is connected to a port, and a port is implanted at the subcutaneous pouch in the forearm

17.2.3.2 Indwelling Catheter and Port Placement

After the arterial redistribution, an angiographic catheter is exchanged to a long tapered 5 Fr Anthron PU catheter with tapering to 3.3 Fr in the distal part as an indwelling catheter. The length of tapered part of the indwelling catheter is shortened to match the 5 Fr part adjusting the puncture site. The tip of the indwelling catheter is positioned just distal to the internal thoracic artery. After the placement of the indwelling catheter, the 5 Fr part coming out from the brachial artery is cut, remaining approximately 5 cm, and connected to the implantable port pulling through the subcutaneous tunnel. Finally the port is implanted at the subcutaneous pouch in the forearm.

17.2.3.3 Evaluation of the Drug Distribution

Drug distribution is observed with CTA using the same manner as that for hepatic arterial infusion (Fig. 17.8).

17.2.4 Therapeutic Results (Fig. 17.9)

The therapeutic result using this new technique is still limited. Takizawa et al. reported that 4 CRs and 5 PRs were obtained in 11 patients mainly by the infusion of epirubicin without major toxic events [27].

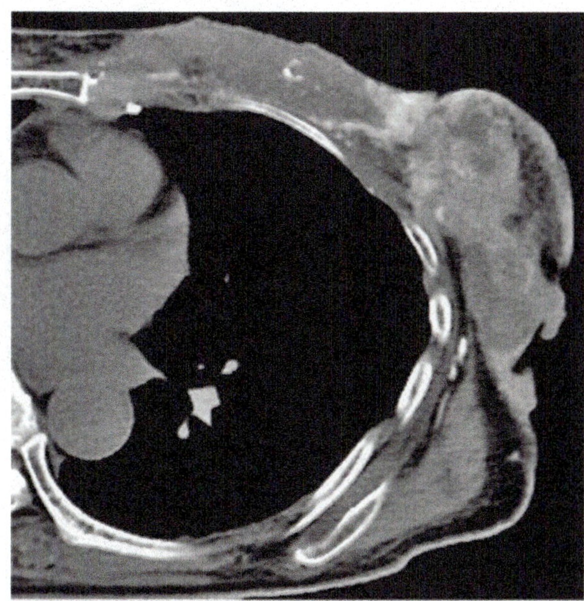

Fig. 17.8 CTA via the indwelling catheter-port system. The median side of the breast tumor is not enhanced because of tumor necrosis, and the lateral side of tumor is well enhanced

Fig. 17.9 The huge tumor of left chest wall (**a**) became significantly smaller in size (**b**) after 2 months by arterial infusion chemotherapy via the implanted catheter-port system

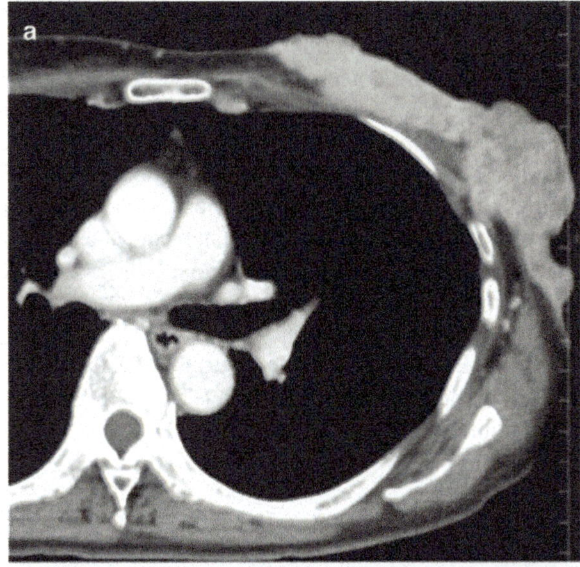

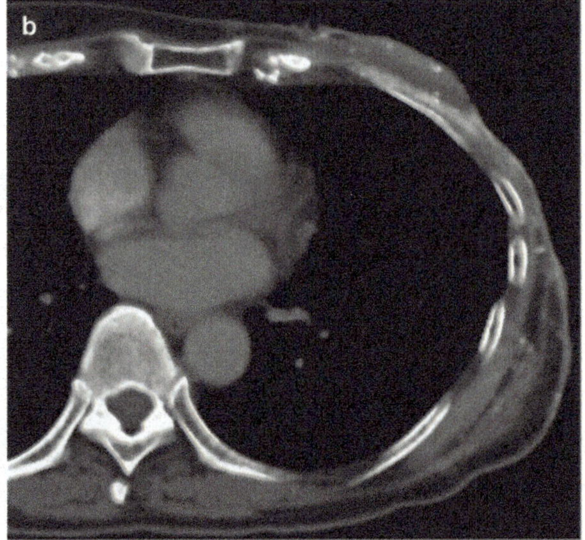

References

1. Kemeny MM, Goldberg DA, Browning S, Metter GE, et al. Experience with continuous regional chemotherapy and hepatic resection as treatment of hepatic metastases from colorectal primaries. A prospective randomized study. Cancer. 1985;55:1265–70.
2. Chang AE, Schneider PD, Sugarbaker PH, et al. A prospective randomized trial of regional versus systemic continuous 5-fluorodeoxyuridine chemotherapy in the treatment of colorectal liver metastases. Ann Surg. 1987;206:685–93.

3. Kemeny N, Daly J, Reichman B, Geller N, et al. Intrahepatic or systemic infusion of fluorodeoxyuridine in patients with liver metastases from colorectal carcinoma. A randomized trial. Ann Intern Med. 1987;107:459–65.
4. Hohn DC, Stagg RJ, Friedman MA, Hannigan Jr JF, et al. A randomized trial of continuous intravenous versus hepatic intraarterial floxuridine in patients with colorectal cancer metastatic to the liver: the northern California Oncology Group trial. J Clin Oncol. 1989;7:1646–54.
5. Martin JK, O'Connell MJ, Wieand HS, Fitzgibbons Jr RJ, et al. Intra-arterial floxuridine vs. systemic fluorouracil for hepatic metastases from colorectal cancer. A randomized trial. Arch Surg. 1990;125:1022–7.
6. Rougier P, Laplanche A, Huguier M, Hay JM, et al. Hepatic arterial infusion of floxuridine in patients with liver metastases from colorectal carcinoma: long-term results of a prospective randomized trial. J Clin Oncol. 1992;10:1112–8.
7. Allen-Mersh TG, Earlam S, Fordy C, et al. Quality of life and survival with continuous hepatic artery floxuridine infusion for colorectal liver metastases. Lancet. 1994;344:1255–60.
8. Lorenz M, Muller HH. Randomized, multicenter trial of fluorouracil plus leucovorin administered either via hepatic arterial or intravenous infusion versus fluorodeoxyuridine administered via hepatic arterial infusion in patients with nonresectable liver metastases from colorectal carcinoma. J Clin Oncol. 2000;18:243–54.
9. Allen-Mersh TG, Glover C, Fordy C, et al. Randomized trial of regional plus systemic fluorinated pyrimidine compared with systemic fluorinated pyrimidine in treatment of colorectal liver metastases. Eur J Surg Oncol. 2000;26:468–73.
10. Kerr DJ, McArdle CS, Ledermann J, et al. Intrahepatic arterial versus intravenous fluorouracil and folinic acid for colorectal cancer liver metastases: a multicentre randomised trial. Lancet. 2003;361:368–73.
11. Begos DG, Ballantyne GH. Regional chemotherapy for colorectal liver metastases: thirty years without patient benefit. J Surg Oncol. 1994;56:139–44.
12. Meta-analysis Group of Cancer. Reappraisal of hepatic arterial infusion in the treatment of nonresectable liver metastases from colorectal cancer. J Natl Cancer Inst. 1996;88:252–8.
13. Arai Y, Inaba Y, Takeuchi Y. Interventional techniques for hepatic arterial infusion chemotherapy. In: Castaneda-Zuniga WR, editor. Interventional radiology. Baltimore: Williams and Wilkins; 1997. p. 192–205.
14. Arai Y, Takeuchi Y, Inaba Y, et al. Percutaneous catheter placement for hepatic arterial infusion chemotherapy. Tech Vasc Interv Radiol. 2007;10:30–7.
15. Ganeshan A, Upponi S, Hon LQ, et al. Hepatic arterial infusion of chemotherapy: the role of diagnostic and interventional radiology. Ann Oncol. 2008;19:847–51.
16. Kemeny N, Jarnagin W, Paty P, et al. Phase I trial of systemic oxaliplatin combination chemotherapy with hepatic arterial infusion in patients with unresectable liver metastases from colorectal cancer. J Clin Oncol. 2005;23:4888–96.
17. Ducreux M, Ychou M, Laplanche A, et al. Hepatic arterial oxaliplatin infusion plus intravenous chemotherapy in colorectal cancer with inoperable hepatic metastases: a trial of the gastrointestinal group of the Federation Nationale des Centres de Lutte Contre le Cancer. J Clin Oncol. 2005;23:4881–7.
18. Obi S, Yoshida H, Toune R, et al. Combination therapy of intraarterial 5-fluorouracil and systemic interferon-alpha for advanced hepatocellular carcinoma with portal venous invasion. Cancer. 2006;106:1990–7.
19. Seki H, Ozaki T, Takaki S, et al. Using slow-infusion MR arteriography and an implantable port system to assess drug distribution at hepatic arterial infusion chemotherapy. AJR Am J Roentgenol. 2003;180:681–6.
20. Seki H, Kimura M, Yoshimura N, et al. Hepatic arterial infusion chemotherapy using percutaneous catheter placement with an implantable port: assessment of factors affecting patency of the hepatic artery. Clin Radiol. 1999;54:221–7.
21. Yamagami T, Iida S, Kato T, et al. Using n-butyl cyanoacrylate and the fixed-catheter-tip technique in percutaneous implantation of a port-catheter system in patients undergoing repeated hepatic arterial chemotherapy. AJR Am J Roentgenol. 2002;179:1611–7.

22. Tanaka T, Arai Y, Inaba Y, et al. Radiologic placement of side-hole catheter with tip fixation for hepatic arterial infusion chemotherapy. J Vasc Interv Radiol. 2003;14:63–8.
23. Arai Y, Inaba Y, Takeuchi Y, et al. Intermittent hepatic arterial infusion of high-dose 5FU on a weekly schedule for liver metastases from colorectal cancer. Cancer Chemother Pharmacol. 1997;40:526–30.
24. Arai Y, Inaba Y, Matsueda K, et al. Weekly 5 hour hepatic arterial infusion of high dose 5-FU for unresectable liver metastases from colorectal cancer in patients without extra-hepatic lesions. Proc ASCO. 1998;17:285a.
25. Arai Y, Sone Y, Tohyama N, et al. Hepatic arterial infusion for unresectable liver metastases from gastric cancer. Proc ASCO. 1992;11:176.
26. Kumada T, Arai Y, Itoh K, et al. Phase II study of combined administration of 5-fluorouracil, epirubicin and mitomycin-C by hepatic artery infusion in patients with liver metastases of gastric cancer. Oncology. 1999;57:216–23.
27. Takizawa K, Shimamoto H, Ogawa Y, et al. Development of a new subclavian arterial infusion chemotherapy method for locally or recurrent advanced breast cancer using an implanted catheter-port system after redistribution of arterial tumor supply. Cardiovasc Intervent Radiol. 2009;32:1059–66.

Induction Chemotherapy for Hepatocellular Carcinoma

18

Takumi Fukumoto and Yonson Ku

Abbreviations

DBE	Drug-eluting beads
HBV	Hepatitis B virus
HCC	Hepatocellular carcinoma
HCV	Hepatitis C virus
MDR1	Multidrug resistance protein 1
MRP	Multidrug resistance protein
PIHP	Percutaneous isolated hepatic perfusion
RFA	Radiofrequency ablation
SHARP	Sorafenib Hepatocellular Carcinoma Assessment Randomized Protocol
TACE	Transcatheter arterial chemoembolization
VEGF	Vascular endothelial growth factor

18.1 Introduction

Hepatocellular carcinoma (HCC) is the fifth most common cancer worldwide and the fourth leading cause of cancer-related death [1]. The incidence of HCC varies by geographic location, and the majority of cases occur in developing countries, especially in Asia and Africa because of the high prevalence of endemic hepatitis B virus (HBV) infection. In contrast, there are an increasing number of HCC cases in the Western countries including North America [2], Europe [3], and Japan, because of the sequel of hepatitis C virus (HCV) infection and alcoholic cirrhosis. There is

T. Fukumoto, MD, PhD (✉) • Y. Ku, MD
Division of Hepato-Biliary-Pancreatic Surgery, Department of Surgery, Kobe University
Graduate School of Medicine, 7-5-1 Kusunoki-cho, Chuo-ku, Kobe 650-0017, Japan
e-mail: fukumoto@med.kobe-u.ac.jp

© Springer-Verlag Berlin Heidelberg 2016
K.R. Aigner, F.O. Stephens (eds.), *Induction Chemotherapy,*
DOI 10.1007/978-3-319-28773-7_18

a steady increase in the incidence of HCC, because of an increasing prevalence of nonalcoholic steatohepatitis as a result of obesity and metabolic syndrome [4].

Surgical resection gives the best chance of longer survival for patients with HCC in well-selected candidates. Local ablative therapies including percutaneous ethanol injection therapy and radiofrequency ablation (RFA) have also been established as a curative treatment for HCC but usually restricted to HCC <3 cm in diameter. However, delayed diagnosis and/or advanced underlying liver cirrhosis has excluded the majority of patients from this type of curative interventions [5]. In addition, after even curative treatment for HCC with these measures, intra- or extra-hepatic recurrence occurs frequently, the rate being as high as 50 % at 2 years [6, 7]. Therefore, there is an urgent need to develop an effective treatment for patients with advanced HCC. In this review, we concisely discuss the role of systemic and locoregional chemotherapies in the treatment of patients with advanced HCC.

18.2 Systemic Chemotherapy for HCC

18.2.1 Cytotoxic Chemotherapy

HCC is a relatively chemoresistant tumor, and HCC cells have intrinsic or acquired drug resistance mediated via enhanced cellular drug efflux of several cytotoxic agents. This phenomenon is associated with increase in a drug transporter family, the adenosine triphosphate-binding cassette proteins that include multidrug resistance protein 1 (MDR1), multidrug resistance protein (MRP), and p-glycoprotein (P-gp). Overexpression of MDR1 accompanied by a decrease in doxorubicin accumulation levels has been reported in HCC cell line [8]. The knockdown of H19 gene suppressed the MDR1/P-glycoprotein expression and increased the cellular doxorubicin accumulation level [8].

Chemotherapeutic agents require p53 to induce apoptosis; tumors with a disruption in p53 pathway are thus resistant to chemotherapy. Mutation of p53 may contribute to HCC drug resistance in HCC cell lines [9]. In fact, HCC in advanced stages acquired the drug resistance and showed the downregulation or inactivation of proapoptotic molecules such as p53, Bax, or Bid and overactivation of antiapoptotic signals [10]. In addition, topoisomerase II alpha encodes an enzyme that is the target for anticancer chemotherapeutic agents such as etoposide and doxorubicin and is associated with drug resistance [11], and its expression is associated with an aggressive tumor phenotype [12]. Lastly, recent evidence suggests that these drug resistances are associated with hypoxia and angiogenesis of HCC [13].

Doxorubicin is a member of the anthracycline ring antibiotics with a broad spectrum of antitumor activity and the most widely used cytotoxic agent, as a single agent or in combination with other drugs [14, 15]. It was shown to produce a response rate of about 10–15 %, but with no survival benefit [16]. Significant grade 3 or above hematological and gastrointestinal toxicities were encountered in patients treated with doxorubicin [17].

Other chemotherapeutic agents such as epirubicin [18], cisplatin [19–21], 5-fluorouracil [22], etoposide [23], mitoxantrone [24], fludarabine, and their combinations have failed to demonstrate meaningful activity [19, 22–25]. The newer chemotherapeutic agents, such as gemcitabine [26–28] and irinotecan [29], have also shown disappointing results.

Nolatrexed, a novel thymidylate synthase inhibitor, was compared with doxorubicin in phase III randomized controlled study. But it failed to show survival benefit. Patients treated with nolatrexed had more treatment-related toxicities and withdrawal [17].

Combination chemotherapy seemed to improve the response rate, but with no impact on survival. In a phase II study, 5-fluorouracil plus leucovorin showed a response rate of 28 % [30]; 5-fluorouracil plus doxorubicin, 13 % [31]; and epirubicin plus etoposide [32], 39 %. Perhaps the most interesting combination of chemotherapy is the interferon-based regimen. The combination of cisplatin, interferon-a-2b, doxorubicin, and fluorouracil (PIAF) was formerly spotlighted. In the phase II study, Leung et al. showed, on average, a 26 % partial response, with four patients achieving a complete pathological response [33]. However, in the phase III study, although this combination had achieved seemingly higher response rates than other combinations, there was no survival advantage compared with supportive care alone and there were considerable toxicities [34]. Recently, phase II studies using a combination of newer agents including gemcitabine, capecitabine, and/or oxaliplatin demonstrated good tumor control rate [35, 36]. However, like the PIAF study [34], these good results need to be further validated in phase III randomized controlled study before they come to be recognized as a standard treatment for HCC.

Taken together, there is no convincing evidence that cytotoxic agents improve overall survival (OS) in advanced HCC patients [37, 38] (Table 18.1). Currently, only HCC patients in whom the standard treatments are contraindicated are considered to be candidates for cytotoxic chemotherapy. Thus, to improve the outcome for patients with advanced HCC, development and validation of alternative cytotoxic agents are clearly needed.

18.2.2 Hormonal Therapy

The gender differences noted in HCC incidence rates have promoted many investigators to examine tumor profiles for hormonal factors and embark on clinical trials of various hormonal modalities. Estrogen is an important target of hormonal therapy for HCC because it is involved in stimulating hepatocyte proliferation in vitro and may promote liver tumor growth in vivo. The antiestrogen compound tamoxifen has been shown to reduce the level of estrogen receptors in the liver [48]. Based on these observations, Barbare et al. conducted a randomized phase III study about tamoxifen in patients with advanced HCC but failed to show survival benefit [49]. Chow et al. also reported tamoxifen did not prolong survival in patients with inoperable HCC [50]. Antiandrogen therapies have also failed to improve survival in

Table 18.1 Pivotal clinical trials of cytotoxic chemotherapy in advanced HCC

Year	Study	Regimen	Sample size	Response rate (%) (months)	Median survival
Single-agent chemotherapy					
1983	Melia [39]	Doxorubicin vs. VP-16	35	28 vs.18	NR
1984	Chlebowski [40]	Doxorubicin	52	11	4.2
1985	Colombo [41]	Doxorubicin	66	24.5	8.0
1988	Lai [42]	Doxorubicin vs. placebo	106	3.3	10.6 vs. 7.5
1999	Mok [43]	Nolatrexed vs. doxorubicin	54	0	4.9 vs. 3.7
2000	Halm [44]	Pegylated liposomal doxorubicin	16	0	4.7
2001	Pohl [18]	Epirubicin	52	9	13.7
2007	Gish [17]	Nolatrexed vs. doxorubicin	54	0	4.9 vs.3.7
1986	Ravry [20]	Cisplatin	42	2.3	NR
1987	Falkson [21]	Cisplatin vs. mitoxantrone	74	17 vs.8	3.3 vs. 3.3
1997	Wall [45]	Topotecan	36	13.9	8.0
2001	O'Reilly [29]	Irinotecan	17	7	8.2
2000	Yang [26]	Gemcitabine	28	17.8	18.7
2002	Fuchs [27]	Gemcitabine	30	0	6.9
2003	Guan [28]	Gemcitabine	48	2.1	3.2
Multi-agent chemotherapy					
1984	Ravry [46]	Doxorubicin + bleomycin	60	16	
1990	Al-Idrissi [47]	5-FU+adriamycin+mitomycin C	40	44	
2004	Lee [15]	Doxorubicin + cisplatin	37	18.9	7.3
2005	Yeo [34]	PIAF vs. adriamycin	188	21 vs. 10.5	8.6 vs. 6.8

PIAF cisplatin, interferon, doxorubicin, and 5-fluorouracil, *NR* not reported

randomized studies in patients with advanced HCC [51, 52]. In spite of many trials, the overall results have been disappointing and survival has remained poor. Nonetheless, such approaches are attractive because the agents used in hormonal therapy are in general less toxic.

18.2.3 Somatostatin Therapy

Somatostatin possesses antimitotic activity against a variety of non-endocrine tumors and HCC cells have somatostatin receptors [53]. Therefore, the somatostatin analog octreotide and the long-acting form lanreotide were used in treating HCC. An early randomized study conducted by Kouroumalis et al. showed survival benefits in employing subcutaneous octreotide in the treatment of advanced HCC patients [54]. Nevertheless, the large placebo-controlled double-blind study conducted by

Becker et al. did not show any survival benefit in using long-acting octreotide in the treatment of patients with advanced HCC [55].

18.2.4 Thalidomide Therapy

Thalidomide was originally developed in the 1960s as a sedative [56] and recently reevaluated as an anticancer drug. It was used in treating advanced HCC patients, mainly due to its anti-angiogenic property. Several phase II studies have examined the efficacy of thalidomide either as a single agent or in combination with epirubicin or interferon and have shown limited treatment activity in patients with HCC [57–59].

18.2.5 Interferon Therapy

Interferon is usually used in the treatment of viral hepatitis and has also been tested in HCC. It has multiple therapeutic mechanisms, including direct antiviral effect, immunomodulatory effect, and direct and indirect antiproliferative effects. Early studies using a high dose of interferon had shown encouraging results with a 30 % response rate and improved overall survival rate. However, there were significant treatment-related toxicities in patients who received high-dose interferon [60]. On the other hand, studies using a lower dosage of interferon have not shown significant beneficial effect [61].

18.2.6 Molecularly Targeted Therapy

Sorafenib is an oral multi-kinase inhibitor that blocks tumor cell proliferation by targeting the intracellular signaling pathway at the level of Raf-1 and B-Raf serine-threonine kinases and exerts an anti-angiogenic effect by targeting the vascular endothelial growth factor receptor-1, 2, and 3 and platelet-derived growth factor receptor-beta tyrosine kinases [62]. Recently, two clinical successful studies, SHARP (Sorafenib Hepatocellular Carcinoma Assessment Randomized Protocol) [62] and Asia-Pacific trial [63], of sorafenib represent a significant advance in the treatment of advanced HCC patients without a curative chance. They have ushered in the era of molecular targeted agents in the treatment of advanced HCC; however, they have some limitations. First, the SHARP trial only included the patients with Child-Pugh Class A cirrhosis. There is no evidence for the efficacy and safety of sorafenib to patients with Child-Pugh Class B and C. Second, the results of both trials show many diverse responses in a subset of HCC patients. There are no reliable clinical parameters which may predict the response to sorafenib. Third, the survival benefit by sorafenib in patients with advanced HCC is only 3 months. On the other hand, the medication cost of sorafenib is approximately >$5,000 per patient per month. There are currently no data available regarding the cost effectiveness of sorafenib in the management of advanced HCC patients. Fourth, the modest improvement of survival benefit in the SHARP trial is still unsatisfactory for HCC patients with a poor prognosis. Fifth, there are no data available about the efficacy of sorafenib in combination with other chemotherapeutic agents and/or treatment modalities to further improvement in survival benefit. In this regard, the phase III study of sorafenib in patients in Japan and Korea with advanced HCC treated after TACE has failed to show any survival benefits. To answer the above limitations, the STORM trial (Sorafenib as Adjuvant Treatment in the Prevention of Recurrence of Hepatocellular Carcinoma) and SPACE trial (Sorafenib or Placebo in Combination with Transarterial Chemoembolization for Intermediate-Stage HCC) were performed but could not provide enough survival benefits.

Sunitinib is a multitargeted tyrosine kinase inhibitor with anti-angiogenic properties. A phase II trial in patients with unresectable HCC was conducted showing a median progression-free survival of 3.9 months and overall survival of 9.8 months [64]. However, the phase III trial comparing sunitinib with sorafenib in patients with advanced HCC was withdrawn because of serious adverse events and failed attempt to demonstrate noninferior efficacy [65]. Consequently, the development of sunitinib for HCC is canceled.

Brivanib is unique dual inhibitor of the fibroblast growth factor (FGF) and vascular endothelial growth factor (VEGF) signaling pathways. In phase II trial, brivanib has demonstrated promising antitumor activity and acceptable tolerability as first-line therapy or as second-line therapy in patients who had failed prior to sorafenib [66]. The incidence of hand-foot syndrome was only 8 %. However, the phase III brivanib study in patients at risk (BRISK) of HCC was disappointing. The BRISK-PS (brivanib-post sorafenib) trial that evaluated brivanib vs. placebo in patients who progressed or were intolerant to sorafenib also failed to meet the primary end point of improving OS (9.4 months vs. 8.2 months, brivanib vs. placebo) [67]. The BRISK-FL study compared the efficacy and safety of brivanib with sorafenib in patients with advanced HCC who had not received systemic therapy before. This research also failed to show improving OS (9.5 months vs. 9.9 months, brivanib vs. sorafenib) [68].

Linifanib is a multitargeted tyrosine kinase inhibitor that inhibits multiple members of the VEGFR and PDGFR families. In the interim phase II trial in patients with advanced HCC, linifanib showed a median time to progression of 3.7 months [69]. However, a phase III trial to evaluate the efficacy and tolerability of linifanib as first-line therapy vs. sorafenib failed to meet its primary end point, showing a similar OS (9.1 months vs. 9.8 months, linifanib vs. sorafenib) [70].

Orantinib is a tyrosine kinase inhibitor of platelet-derived growth factor receptor (PDGFR), FGFR, and VEGFR. This drug has revealed promising preliminary efficacy in a phase I/II trial (2.1 months TTP and 13.1 months OS) [71]. However, an interim analysis of an international multicenter phase III trial of combining TACE with either orantinib or placebo failed to meet its primary end point. Subsequently, this phase III trial was canceled.

Ramucirumab is a monoclonal antibody that selectively inhibits human VEGFR-2. A preliminary phase II clinical trial for advanced HCC has shown encouraging anticancer effect (4.0 months PFS and 12.0 months OS) [72]. However, a large, second-line, randomized phase III trial with ramucirumab or placebo in sorafenib pretreated patients with advanced-stage HCC (REACH) has shown disappointing results (OS: 9.2 months vs. 7.6 months, ramucirumab vs. placebo).

Erlotinib is an oral tyrosine kinase inhibitor, which acts on the epidermal growth factor receptor (EGFR). Erlotinib monotherapy demonstrated the safety but showed only modest efficacy in advanced HCC [73]. A phase III trial that combined sorafenib with erlotinib for HCC patients (SEARCH trial) failed to exhibit survival benefit (OS: 9.5 months vs. 8.5 months, sorafenib vs. sorafenib and erlotinib).

Bevacizumab, an anti-VEGF monoclonal antibody, was the first angiogenesis inhibitor to be approved as an antineoplastic agent. It also showed only modest effect as a single agent in patients with advanced HCC. Therefore, it has been combined with cytotoxic drugs (gemcitabine, oxaliplatin, and capecitabine) or erlotinib [74] in several phase II trials. The result of one randomized phase II trial with sorafenib vs. bevacizumab and erlotinib was presented in ASCO-GI2015. It did not show any survival benefit (OS: 8.6 months vs. 8.6 months, sorafenib vs. bevacizumab and erlotinib).

18.3 Locoregional Chemotherapy

18.3.1 Transcatheter Arterial Chemoembolization (TACE)

The rationale for locoregional chemotherapy is to intensify dose delivery of cytotoxic chemotherapeutic agents with a steep dose-response curve at a cancer-bearing organ, while minimizing systemic exposure to these agents. TACE is the most widely used locoregional chemotherapy for unresectable HCC in palliative intent. It is not usually indicated as first-line treatment, because the treatment results of TACE were worse than that of liver resection or percutaneous ablation [75]. TACE is based on the principle of arterial obstruction which can induce ischemic tumor necrosis and arterial injection chemotherapy. Embolic particles (usually iodized oil) containing the cytotoxic agent (cisplatin, doxorubicin, or mitomycin C) are selectively injected into the feeding artery of the tumor in the liver through the catheter. TACE achieves objective responses in 15–61 % of patients [76–82] and appeared to prevent significant tumor progression compared with conservative or inactive treatments [76, 77]. However, early randomized controlled trials have failed to show survival benefits of TACE, and, until recently, the use of TACE was controversial in HCC patients. In 2002, two sophisticated randomized controlled trials showed the survival benefits of TACE compared to the conservative treatment [78, 82]. In addition, meta-analysis including these randomized controlled trials also confirmed an overall survival benefit for TACE in comparison to the control group [83, 84]. However, the role of cytotoxic drugs in TACE is still obscure because meta-analysis of TACE vs. TAE alone demonstrated no survival difference [85].

A new strategy to improve the treatment effect of TACE is the use of intra-arterial drug delivery system, namely, drug-eluting beads (DEB) [86]. DEB consist of PVA beads and doxorubicin allowing delivery of large amounts of drugs to tumors for a prolonged time. The pharmacokinetic profiles of injected doxorubicin were significantly better in TACE using DEB than in conventional TACE, and

1-year and 2-year survival rate after TACE using DEB was 93 % and 89 %, respectively [86]. There are currently four randomized controlled trials [87–90] between DEB TACE and conventional TACE; however, a clear superiority of DEB TACE over conventional TACE is still lacking.

Another important agent for hepatic arterial embolization is yttrium-90. Yttrium-90 radioembolization has shown clinical effectiveness in intermediate and advanced HCC, with a favorable safety profile. Yttrium-90-loaded glass or resin microspheres are infused via hepatic arterial catheters. These spheres preferentially travel to tumor vessels where they block the main source of blood flow to the tumor and deliver dosed radiation to the tumor. Initial data in patients with advanced HCC [91, 92] show similar effectiveness to TACE (OS: 12.8–16.4 months). The main limitation of this treatment is the lack of phase III randomized studies comparing with standard modalities. Currently, randomized trials between yttrium-90-radioembolization vs. sorafenib, or a sequence of yttrium-90-radioembolization and sorafenib vs. sorafenib alone, are ongoing.

18.3.2 Percutaneous Isolated Hepatic Perfusion (PIHP)

As an ultimate locoregional chemotherapy of the liver, we [93–96] and other research groups [97–99] have independently developed PIHP. PIHP is a novel and simple hepatic venous isolation system that enables administration of cytotoxic agents at a dose of up to ten times the maximally tolerated dose, while reducing exposure of the entire body to the major side effects of the agents (Fig. 18.1). Major cytotoxic agents including doxorubicin [93, 97], MMC [94], cisplatin [95, 96], and melphalan [100] can be effectively eliminated by the PIHP system when administered via the hepatic artery.

Several groups have reported the results of phase I and II clinical trials of PIHP for the treatment of HCC. In 1998, we first reported the long-term results of PIHP in 28 patients with multiple advanced HCC of more than five tumor foci with doxorubicin-based regimen [101]. The response rate was approximately 63 %, and the median duration of response was 10 months. The overall survival rates were 67.5 % and 39.7 % at 1 and 5 years, respectively. Until December 31, 2009, we have treated 136 HCC patients with PIHP and obtained a similar response rate of 60 %, and the 1-year and 5-year survival rates of stage IV-A patients were 80.6 % and 20.3 %, respectively (unpublished data). Curley et al. used the similar system of PIHP for the treatment of 11 patients with unresectable HCC [102]. The patients underwent a total of 17 treatments with doxorubicin at doses of 60–120 mg/m [2]. In this phase I trial, seven out of the ten assessable patients had partial response, and two out of these seven patients had a marked tumor volume reduction. Currently, phase II and III trials for HCC with several chemotherapeutic agents are taking place in the United States as a multicenter study.

The use of PIHP in combination with reductive surgery for previously unresectable HCC has been reported by us [103]. This dual treatment strategy has several oncologic advantages: (i) a large HCC frequently accompanies arterial collaterals from adjacent organs, which may reduce the effect of transarterial chemotherapy,

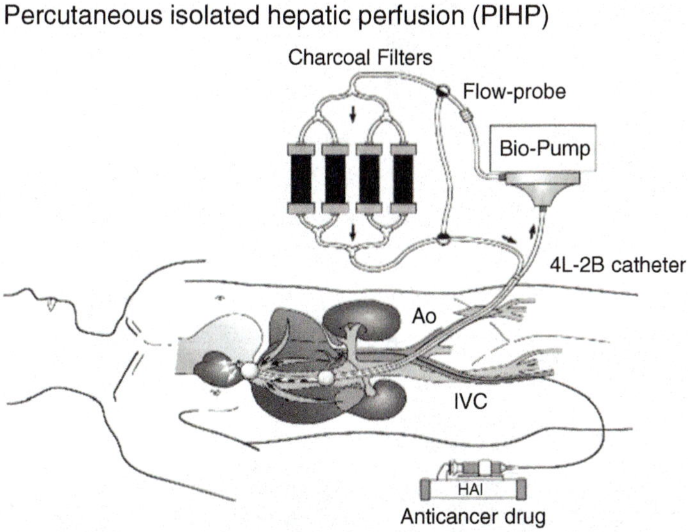

Fig. 18.1 Single catheter technique of PIHP. A 4 lumen −2 balloon catheter was introduced into the retrohepatic inferior vena cava via the femoral vein, and isolated hepatic vein blood was directed to the extracorporeal pump-filter unit. During PIHP, chemotherapeutic agents are administered into the hepatic artery. *Arrows* indicate direction of blood flow. *Ao* aorta, *IVC* inferior vena cava, *HAI* hepatic arterial infusion

and these arterial collaterals could be eliminated at the time of first-line surgical resection; (ii) reductive hepatectomy reduces the vascular bed of the liver, which is theoretically beneficial to increasing the relative dose rate to the residual tumors (Fig. 18.2). An impressively increased response rate achieved by PIHP in this setting (88 %) supports the validity of the dual treatment for patients with advanced HCC [103, 104].

18.4 Combination Treatment

The combination of molecular target agent and locoregional chemotherapy or cytotoxic systemic chemotherapy may act synergistically to generate additive therapeutic effects.

A high incidence of recurrence is a major clinical limitation of TACE. As a result, the combination of TACE with molecular target agent has emerged to improve the efficacy of TACE. A clinical phase II trial of sorafenib with DEB TACE in patients with advanced HCC showed considerable efficacy with 58 % objective response [105]. A retrospective large multicenter study [105] (8.5 months TTP and 12 months OS) and a propensity score matching study [106] (OS: 7.5 months vs. 5.1 months, sorafenib and TACE vs. TACE alone) showed antitumor effects of sorafenib plus TACE for advanced HCC.

Based on the encouraging data from sorafenib plus doxorubicin in HCC [107], a phase III randomized study of sorafenib plus doxorubicin vs. sorafenib alone is

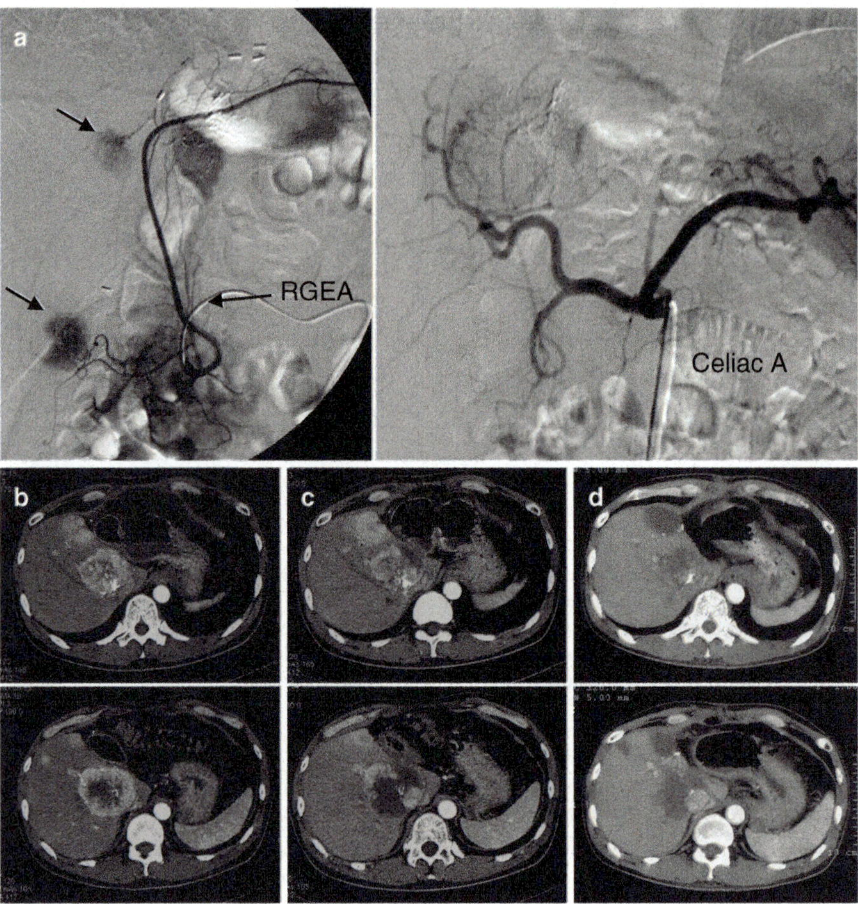

Fig. 18.2 Abdominal angiography and CT scan of a 36-year-old man with multiple recurrent HCC after left lobectomy. He sequentially underwent first PIHP, reductive partial hepatectomy with elimination of arterial collaterals, and second PIHP (each PIHP with 100 mg/m^2 doxorubicin and 30 mg/m^2 MMC). (**a**) Pretreatment angiography demonstrated that two large recurrent tumors were fed by both the right hepatic artery and right gastroepiploic artery. (**b**) CT scan before treatment also demonstrated two massive-type tumors in the right lobe. (**c**) CT scan after first PIHP. No distinct antitumor effects were observed at the perfusion area of the right gastroepiploic artery in the recurrent tumors. (**d**) CT scan 1 month after partial hepatectomy with elimination of arterial collaterals plus second PIHP confirmed almost complete necrosis of the residual tumors. *RGEA* right gastroepiploic artery

underway in patients with advanced HCC. Studies combining sorafenib plus gemcitabine/oxaliplatin, modified FOLFOX, or capecitabine/oxaliplatin are also ongoing.

Conclusions

During the last decade, many molecular targeted agents have been researched in clinical studies. However, as a single agent, all of them except for sorafenib have had disappointing results in the treatment for advanced-stage

HCC. Therefore, many studies combining sorafenib with other molecular target agents, locoregional chemotherapy, or cytotoxic systemic chemotherapy are underway. A substantial improvement in the outcomes of advanced HCC is expected with the advent of new therapeutic approaches as represented by PIHP or new agents which may target alternative crucial pathways or molecules in HCC cells.

References

1. Parkin DM, Bray F, Ferlay J, et al. Global cancer statistics, 2002. CA Cancer J Clin. 2005;55:74–108.
2. El-Serag HB, Mason AC. Rising incidence of hepatocellular carcinoma in the United States. N Engl J Med. 1999;340:745–50.
3. Bosetti C, Levi F, Boffetta P, et al. Trends in mortality from hepatocellular carcinoma in Europe, 1980–2004. Hepatology. 2008;48:137–45.
4. Caldwell SH, Crespo DM, Kang HS, et al. Obesity and hepatocellular carcinoma. Gastroenterology. 2004;127:S97–103.
5. Fan ST, Lo CM, Liu CL, et al. Hepatectomy for hepatocellular carcinoma: toward zero hospital deaths. Ann Surg. 1999;229:322–30.
6. Nagasue N, Kohno H, Chang YC, et al. Liver resection for hepatocellular carcinoma. Results of 229 consecutive patients during 11 years. Ann Surg. 1993;217:375–84.
7. Tanaka H, Kubo S, Tsukamoto T, et al. Recurrence rate and transplantability after liver resection in patients with hepatocellular carcinoma who initially met transplantation criteria. Transplant Proc. 2005;37:1254–6.
8. Tsang WP, Kwok TT. Riboregulator H19 induction of MDR1-associated drug resistance in human hepatocellular carcinoma cells. Oncogene. 2007;26:4877–81.
9. Chan KT, Lung ML. Mutant p53 expression enhances drug resistance in a hepatocellular carcinoma cell line. Cancer Chemother Pharmacol. 2004;53:519–26.
10. Fabregat I, Roncero C, Fernandez M. Survival and apoptosis: a dysregulated balance in liver cancer. Liver Int. 2007;27:155–62.
11. Okada Y, Tosaka A, Nimura Y, et al. Atypical multidrug resistance may be associated with catalytically active mutants of human DNA topoisomerase II alpha. Gene. 2001;272:141–8.
12. Watanuki A, Ohwada S, Fukusato T, et al. Prognostic significance of DNA topoisomerase IIalpha expression in human hepatocellular carcinoma. Anticancer Res. 2002;22:1113–9.
13. Zhu H, Chen XP, Luo SF, et al. Involvement of hypoxia-inducible factor-1-alpha in multidrug resistance induced by hypoxia in HepG2 cells. J Exp Clin Cancer Res. 2005;24:565–74.
14. Hong RL, Tseng YL. A phase II and pharmacokinetic study of pegylated liposomal doxorubicin in patients with advanced hepatocellular carcinoma. Cancer Chemother Pharmacol. 2003;51:433–8.
15. Lee J, Park JO, Kim WS, et al. Phase II study of doxorubicin and cisplatin in patients with metastatic hepatocellular carcinoma. Cancer Chemother Pharmacol. 2004;54:385–90.
16. Lai EC, Choi TK, Cheng CH, et al. Doxorubicin for unresectable hepatocellular carcinoma. A prospective study on the addition of verapamil. Cancer. 1990;66:1685–7.
17. Gish RG, Porta C, Lazar L, et al. Phase III randomized controlled trial comparing the survival of patients with unresectable hepatocellular carcinoma treated with nolatrexed or doxorubicin. J Clin Oncol. 2007;25:3069–75.
18. Pohl J, Zuna I, Stremmel W, et al. Systemic chemotherapy with epirubicin for treatment of advanced or multifocal hepatocellular carcinoma. Chemotherapy. 2001;47:359–65.
19. Okada S, Okazaki N, Nose H, et al. A phase 2 study of cisplatin in patients with hepatocellular carcinoma. Oncology. 1993;50:22–6.
20. Ravry MJ, Omura GA, Bartolucci AA, et al. Phase II evaluation of cisplatin in advanced hepatocellular carcinoma and cholangiocarcinoma: a Southeastern Cancer Study Group Trial. Cancer Treat Rep. 1986;70:311–2.

21. Falkson G, Ryan LM, Johnson LA, et al. A random phase II study of mitoxantrone and cisplatin in patients with hepatocellular carcinoma. An ECOG study. Cancer. 1987;60:2141–5.
22. Stuart K, Tessitore J, Huberman M. 5-Fluorouracil and alpha-interferon in hepatocellular carcinoma. Am J Clin Oncol. 1996;19:136–9.
23. Shiu W, Mok SD, Leung N, et al. Phase 2 study of high dose etoposide (VP16-213) in hepatocellular carcinoma. Jpn J Clin Oncol. 1987;17:113–5.
24. Davis RB, Van Echo DA, Leone LA, et al. Phase II trial of mitoxantrone in advanced primary liver cancer: a Cancer and Leukemia Group B Study. Cancer Treat Rep. 1986;70:1125–6.
25. Zhu AX. Systemic therapy of advanced hepatocellular carcinoma: how hopeful should we be? Oncologist. 2006;11:790–800.
26. Yang TS, Lin YC, Chen JS, et al. Phase II study of gemcitabine in patients with advanced hepatocellular carcinoma. Cancer. 2000;89:750–6.
27. Fuchs CS, Clark JW, Ryan DP, et al. A phase II trial of gemcitabine in patients with advanced hepatocellular carcinoma. Cancer. 2002;94:3186–91.
28. Guan Z, Wang Y, Maoleekoonpairoj S, et al. Prospective randomised phase II study of gemcitabine at standard or fixed dose rate schedule in unresectable hepatocellular carcinoma. Br J Cancer. 2003;89:1865–9.
29. O'Reilly EM, Stuart KE, Sanz-Altamira PM, et al. A phase II study of irinotecan in patients with advanced hepatocellular carcinoma. Cancer. 2001;91:101–5.
30. Porta C, Moroni M, Nastasi G, et al. 5-Fluorouracil and d, l-leucovorin calcium are active to treat unresectable hepatocellular carcinoma patients: preliminary results of a phase II study. Oncology. 1995;52:487–91.
31. Baker LH, Saiki JH, Jones SE, et al. Adriamycin and 5-fluorouracil in the treatment of advanced hepatoma: a Southwest Oncology Group study. Cancer Treat Rep. 1977;61:1595–7.
32. Bobbio-Pallavicini E, Porta C, Moroni M, et al. Epirubicin and etoposide combination chemotherapy to treat hepatocellular carcinoma patients: a phase II study. Eur J Cancer. 1997;33:1784–8.
33. Leung TW, Patt YZ, Lau WY, et al. Complete pathological remission is possible with systemic combination chemotherapy for inoperable hepatocellular carcinoma. Clin Cancer Res. 1999;5:1676–81.
34. Yeo W, Mok TS, Zee B, et al. A randomized phase III study of doxorubicin versus cisplatin/interferon alpha-2b/doxorubicin/fluorouracil (PIAF) combination chemotherapy for unresectable hepatocellular carcinoma. J Natl Cancer Inst. 2005;97:1532–8.
35. Louafi S, Boige V, Ducreux M, et al. Gemcitabine plus oxaliplatin (GEMOX) in patients with advanced hepatocellular carcinoma (HCC): results of a phase II study. Cancer. 2007;109:1384–90.
36. Boige V, Raoul JL, Pignon JP, et al. Multicentre phase II trial of capecitabine plus oxaliplatin (XELOX) in patients with advanced hepatocellular carcinoma: FFCD 03-03 trial. Br J Cancer. 2007;97:862–7.
37. Johnson PJ. Hepatocellular carcinoma: is current therapy really altering outcome? Gut. 2002;51:459–62.
38. Palmer DH, Hussain SA, Johnson PJ. Systemic therapies for hepatocellular carcinoma. Expert Opin Investig Drugs. 2004;13:1555–68.
39. Melia WM, Johnson PJ, Williams R. Induction of remission in hepatocellular carcinoma. A comparison of VP 16 with adriamycin. Cancer. 1983;51:206–10.
40. Chlebowski RT, Brzechwa-Adjukiewicz A, Cowden A, et al. Doxorubicin (75 mg/m2) for hepatocellular carcinoma: clinical and pharmacokinetic results. Cancer Treat Rep. 1984;68:487–91.
41. Colombo M, Tommasini MA, Del Ninno E, et al. Hepatocellular carcinoma in Italy: report of a clinical trial with intravenous doxorubicin. Liver. 1985;5:336–41.
42. Lai CL, Wu PC, Chan GC, et al. Doxorubicin versus no antitumor therapy in inoperable hepatocellular carcinoma. A prospective randomized trial. Cancer. 1988;62:479–83.

43. Mok TS, Leung TW, Lee SD, et al. A multi-centre randomized phase II study of nolatrexed versus doxorubicin in treatment of Chinese patients with advanced hepatocellular carcinoma. Cancer Chemother Pharmacol. 1999;44:307–11.
44. Halm U, Etzrodt G, Schiefke I, et al. A phase II study of pegylated liposomal doxorubicin for treatment of advanced hepatocellular carcinoma. Ann Oncol. 2000;11:113–4.
45. Wall JG, Benedetti JK, O'Rourke MA, et al. Phase II trial to topotecan in hepatocellular carcinoma: a Southwest Oncology Group study. Invest New Drugs. 1997;15:257–60.
46. Ravry MJ, Omura GA, Bartolucci AA. Phase II evaluation of doxorubicin plus bleomycin in hepatocellular carcinoma: a Southeastern Cancer Study Group trial. Cancer Treat Rep. 1984;68:1517–8.
47. al-Idrissi HY. Combined 5-fluorouracil, adriamycin and mitomycin C in the management of adenocarcinoma metastasizing to the liver from an unknown primary site. J Int Med Res. 1990;18:425–9.
48. Jiang SY, Shyu RY, Yeh MY, et al. Tamoxifen inhibits hepatoma cell growth through an estrogen receptor independent mechanism. J Hepatol. 1995;23:712–9.
49. Barbare JC, Bouche O, Bonnetain F, et al. Randomized controlled trial of tamoxifen in advanced hepatocellular carcinoma. J Clin Oncol. 2005;23:4338–46.
50. Chow PK, Tai BC, Tan CK, et al. High-dose tamoxifen in the treatment of inoperable hepatocellular carcinoma: a multicenter randomized controlled trial. Hepatology. 2002;36:1221–6.
51. Manesis EK, Giannoulis G, Zoumboulis P, et al. Treatment of hepatocellular carcinoma with combined suppression and inhibition of sex hormones: a randomized, controlled trial. Hepatology. 1995;21:1535–42.
52. Grimaldi C, Bleiberg H, Gay F, et al. Evaluation of antiandrogen therapy in unresectable hepatocellular carcinoma: results of a European Organization for Research and Treatment of Cancer multicentric double-blind trial. J Clin Oncol. 1998;16:411–7.
53. Verhoef C, van Dekken H, Hofland LJ, et al. Somatostatin receptor in human hepatocellular carcinomas: biological, patient and tumor characteristics. Dig Surg. 2008;25:21–6.
54. Kouroumalis E, Skordilis P, Thermos K, et al. Treatment of hepatocellular carcinoma with octreotide: a randomised controlled study. Gut. 1998;42:442–7.
55. Becker G, Allgaier HP, Olschewski M, et al. Long-acting octreotide versus placebo for treatment of advanced HCC: a randomized controlled double-blind study. Hepatology. 2007;45:9–15.
56. Somers GF. Pharmacological properties of thalidomide (alpha-phthalimido glutarimide), a new sedative hypnotic drug. Br J Pharmacol Chemother. 1960;15:111–6.
57. Lin AY, Brophy N, Fisher GA, et al. Phase II study of thalidomide in patients with unresectable hepatocellular carcinoma. Cancer. 2005;103:119–25.
58. Patt YZ, Hassan MM, Lozano RD, et al. Thalidomide in the treatment of patients with hepatocellular carcinoma: a phase II trial. Cancer. 2005;103:749–55.
59. Zhu AX, Fuchs CS, Clark JW, et al. A phase II study of epirubicin and thalidomide in unresectable or metastatic hepatocellular carcinoma. Oncologist. 2005;10:392–8.
60. Lai CL, Lau JY, Wu PC, et al. Recombinant interferon-alpha in inoperable hepatocellular carcinoma: a randomized controlled trial. Hepatology. 1993;17:389–94.
61. Llovet JM, Sala M, Castells L, et al. Randomized controlled trial of interferon treatment for advanced hepatocellular carcinoma. Hepatology. 2000;31:54–8.
62. Wilhelm SM, Carter C, Tang L, et al. BAY 43-9006 exhibits broad spectrum oral antitumor activity and targets the RAF/MEK/ERK pathway and receptor tyrosine kinases involved in tumor progression and angiogenesis. Cancer Res. 2004;64:7099–109.
63. Cheng AL, Kang YK, Chen Z, et al. Efficacy and safety of sorafenib in patients in the Asia-Pacific region with advanced hepatocellular carcinoma: a phase III randomised, double-blind, placebo-controlled trial. Lancet Oncol. 2009;10:25–34.
64. Zhu AX, Sahani DV, Duda DG, et al. Efficacy, safety, and potential biomarkers of sunitinib monotherapy in advanced hepatocellular carcinoma: a phase II study. J Clin Oncol. 2009;27:3027–35.

65. Cheng AL, Kang YK, Lin DY, et al. Sunitinib versus sorafenib in advanced hepatocellular cancer: results of a randomized phase III trial. J Clin Oncol. 2013;31:4067–75.
66. Raoul JL FR, Kang YK, et al. Phase 2 study of first- and second-line treatment with brivanib in patients with hepatocellular carcinoma. ILCA Third Annual Conference, Milan, 4–6 Sept 2009, abstr O-030. 2009.
67. Llovet JM, Decaens T, Raoul JL, et al. Brivanib in patients with advanced hepatocellular carcinoma who were intolerant to sorafenib or for whom sorafenib failed: results from the randomized phase III BRISK-PS study. J Clin Oncol. 2013;31:3509–16.
68. Johnson PJ, Qin S, Park JW, et al. Brivanib versus sorafenib as first-line therapy in patients with unresectable, advanced hepatocellular carcinoma: results from the randomized phase III BRISK-FL study. J Clin Oncol. 2013;31:3517–24.
69. Toh H, Chen P, Carr BI, Knox JJ, Gill S, Steinberg J, Carlson DM, Qian J, Qin Q, Yong W. A phase II study of ABT-869 in hepatocellular carcinoma (HCC): interim analysis [abstract]. J Clin Oncol. 2009;27(15s):A4581.
70. Cainap C, Qin S, Huang WT, et al. Linifanib versus Sorafenib in patients with advanced hepatocellular carcinoma: results of a randomized phase III trial. J Clin Oncol. 2015;33:172–9.
71. Inaba Y, Kanai F, Aramaki T, et al. A randomised phase II study of TSU-68 in patients with hepatocellular carcinoma treated by transarterial chemoembolisation. Eur J Cancer. 2013;49:2832–40.
72. Zhu AX, Finn RS, Mulcahy M, et al. A phase II and biomarker study of ramucirumab, a human monoclonal antibody targeting the VEGF receptor-2, as first-line monotherapy in patients with advanced hepatocellular cancer. Clin Cancer Res. 2013;19:6614–23.
73. Thomas MB, Chadha R, Glover K, et al. Phase 2 study of erlotinib in patients with unresectable hepatocellular carcinoma. Cancer. 2007;110:1059–67.
74. Thomas MB, Morris JS, Chadha R, et al. Phase II trial of the combination of bevacizumab and erlotinib in patients who have advanced hepatocellular carcinoma. J Clin Oncol. 2009;27:843–50.
75. Arii S, Yamaoka Y, Futagawa S, et al. Results of surgical and nonsurgical treatment for small-sized hepatocellular carcinomas: a retrospective and nationwide survey in Japan. The Liver Cancer Study Group of Japan. Hepatology. 2000;32:1224–9.
76. Bruix J, Llovet JM, Castells A, et al. Transarterial embolization versus symptomatic treatment in patients with advanced hepatocellular carcinoma: results of a randomized, controlled trial in a single institution. Hepatology. 1998;27:1578–83.
77. A comparison of lipiodol chemoembolization and conservative treatment for unresectable hepatocellular carcinoma. Groupe d'Etude et de Traitement du Carcinome Hepatocellulaire. N Engl J Med. 1995;332:1256–61.
78. Llovet JM, Real MI, Montana X, et al. Arterial embolisation or chemoembolisation versus symptomatic treatment in patients with unresectable hepatocellular carcinoma: a randomised controlled trial. Lancet. 2002;359:1734–9.
79. Lin DY, Liaw YF, Lee TY, et al. Hepatic arterial embolization in patients with unresectable hepatocellular carcinoma – a randomized controlled trial. Gastroenterology. 1988;94:453–6.
80. Pelletier G, Roche A, Ink O, et al. A randomized trial of hepatic arterial chemoembolization in patients with unresectable hepatocellular carcinoma. J Hepatol. 1990;11:181–4.
81. Pelletier G, Ducreux M, Gay F, et al. Treatment of unresectable hepatocellular carcinoma with lipiodol chemoembolization: a multicenter randomized trial. Groupe CHC. J Hepatol. 1998;29:129–34.
82. Lo CM, Ngan H, Tso WK, et al. Randomized controlled trial of transarterial lipiodol chemoembolization for unresectable hepatocellular carcinoma. Hepatology. 2002;35:1164–71.
83. Camma C, Schepis F, Orlando A, et al. Transarterial chemoembolization for unresectable hepatocellular carcinoma: meta-analysis of randomized controlled trials. Radiology. 2002;224:47–54.
84. Llovet JM, Bruix J. Systematic review of randomized trials for unresectable hepatocellular carcinoma: chemoembolization improves survival. Hepatology. 2003;37:429–42.

85. Marelli L, Stigliano R, Triantos C, et al. Transarterial therapy for hepatocellular carcinoma: which technique is more effective? A systematic review of cohort and randomized studies. Cardiovasc Intervent Radiol. 2007;30:6–25.

86. Varela M, Real MI, Burrel M, et al. Chemoembolization of hepatocellular carcinoma with drug eluting beads: efficacy and doxorubicin pharmacokinetics. J Hepatol. 2007;46:474–81.

87. Sacco S, Pistoia F, Degan D, et al. Conventional vascular risk factors: their role in the association between migraine and cardiovascular diseases. Cephalalgia. 2015;35:146–64.

88. van Malenstein H, Maleux G, Vandecaveye V, et al. A randomized phase II study of drug-eluting beads versus transarterial chemoembolization for unresectable hepatocellular carcinoma. Onkologie. 2011;34:368–76.

89. Lammer J, Malagari K, Vogl T, et al. Prospective randomized study of doxorubicin-eluting-bead embolization in the treatment of hepatocellular carcinoma: results of the PRECISION V study. Cardiovasc Intervent Radiol. 2010;33:41–52.

90. Golfieri R, Giampalma E, Renzulli M, et al. Randomised controlled trial of doxorubicin-eluting beads vs conventional chemoembolisation for hepatocellular carcinoma. Br J Cancer. 2014;111:255–64.

91. Hilgard P, Hamami M, Fouly AE, et al. Radioembolization with yttrium-90 glass microspheres in hepatocellular carcinoma: European experience on safety and long-term survival. Hepatology. 2010;52:1741–9.

92. Sangro B, Carpanese L, Cianni R, et al. Survival after yttrium-90 resin microsphere radioembolization of hepatocellular carcinoma across Barcelona clinic liver cancer stages: a European evaluation. Hepatology. 2011;54:868–78.

93. Ku Y, Saitoh M, Nishiyama H, et al. Extracorporeal adriamycin-removal following hepatic artery infusion: use of direct hemoperfusion combined with veno-venous bypass. Nippon Geka Gakkai Zasshi. 1989;90:1758–64.

94. Ku Y, Saitoh M, Nishiyama H, et al. Extracorporeal removal of anticancer drugs in hepatic artery infusion: the effect of direct hemoperfusion combined with venovenous bypass. Surgery. 1990;107:273–81.

95. Maekawa Y, Ku Y, Saitoh Y. Extracorporeal cisplatin removal using direct hemoperfusion under hepatic venous isolation for hepatic arterial chemotherapy: an experimental study on pharmacokinetics. Surg Today. 1993;23:58–62.

96. Kusunoki N, Ku Y, Tominaga M, et al. Effect of sodium thiosulfate on cisplatin removal with complete hepatic venous isolation and extracorporeal charcoal hemoperfusion: a pharmacokinetic evaluation. Ann Surg Oncol. 2001;8:449–57.

97. Curley SA, Byrd DR, Newman RA, et al. Hepatic arterial infusion chemotherapy with complete hepatic venous isolation and extracorporeal chemofiltration: a feasibility study of a novel system. Anticancer Drugs. 1991;2:175–83.

98. Beheshti MV, Denny Jr DF, Glickman MG, et al. Percutaneous isolated liver perfusion for treatment of hepatic malignancy: preliminary report. J Vasc Interv Radiol. 1992;3:453–8.

99. August DA, Verma N, Vaerten MA, et al. Pharmacokinetic evaluation of percutaneous hepatic venous isolation for administration of regional chemotherapy. Surg Oncol. 1995;4:205–16.

100. Pingpank JF, Libutti SK, Chang R, et al. Phase I study of hepatic arterial melphalan infusion and hepatic venous hemofiltration using percutaneously placed catheters in patients with unresectable hepatic malignancies. J Clin Oncol. 2005;23:3465–74.

101. Ku Y, Iwasaki T, Fukumoto T, et al. Induction of long-term remission in advanced hepatocellular carcinoma with percutaneous isolated liver chemoperfusion. Ann Surg. 1998;227:519–26.

102. Curley SA, Newman RA, Dougherty TB, et al. Complete hepatic venous isolation and extracorporeal chemofiltration as treatment for human hepatocellular carcinoma: a phase I study. Ann Surg Oncol. 1994;1:389–99.

103. Ku Y, Iwasaki T, Tominaga M, et al. Reductive surgery plus percutaneous isolated hepatic perfusion for multiple advanced hepatocellular carcinoma. Ann Surg. 2004;239:53–60.

104. Fukumoto T, Tominaga M, Kido M, et al. Long-term outcomes and prognostic factors with reductive hepatectomy and sequential percutaneous isolated hepatic perfusion for multiple bilobar hepatocellular carcinoma. Ann Surg Oncol. 2014;21:971–8.
105. Pawlik TM, Reyes DK, Cosgrove D, et al. Phase II trial of sorafenib combined with concurrent transarterial chemoembolization with drug-eluting beads for hepatocellular carcinoma. J Clin Oncol. 2011;29:3960–7.
106. Bai W, Wang YJ, Zhao Y, et al. Sorafenib in combination with transarterial chemoembolization improves the survival of patients with unresectable hepatocellular carcinoma: a propensity score matching study. J Dig Dis. 2013;14:181–90.
107. Abou-Alfa GK, Johnson P, Knox JJ, et al. Doxorubicin plus sorafenib vs doxorubicin alone in patients with advanced hepatocellular carcinoma: a randomized trial. JAMA. 2010;304:2154–60.

Transarterial Treatment of Primary and Secondary Liver Tumors

Christina Loberg

The number of neoplasms increases over the years. Systemic and surgical treatment improves and more patients witness the occurrence of metastases. Therefore, metastases endanger organ function and are the limiting prognostic factor. Metastases are a common cause of death in cancer. With regard to colorectal cancer (CRC), about two-thirds of patients with CRC will die of liver metastases. Tumor control and decrease in tumor load in metastatic disease are normally achieved with systemic treatment. Regional treatment via transarterial approach is a well-established technique in the treatment of primary and secondary liver tumors in a palliative setting. Short hospitalization, effective tumor treatment, and less side effects are the main advantages in comparison to systemic or surgical treatment. Transarterial local therapy results in a higher response rate than systemic chemotherapy.

The aim of local tumor therapy is targeted treatment of metastases in organs of vital importance in addition to surgical and systemic therapy to avid tumor spread. Locoregional therapy can also be used to downstage disease in patients with initially unresectable liver metastases or in combination with systemic regimens.

Organ function is preserved with the benefit or extended survival with good life quality, less side effects, and short time of hospitalization. Therefore, interdisciplinary collaboration in oncology is essential.

Image-guided tumor therapies can be performed with CT, MRI, ultrasound, PET/CT, and fluoroscopy. Regional treatments contain embolization, chemoembolization (TACE), hepatic arterial infusion chemotherapy (HAIC), radioembolization (SIRT), and portal vein embolization.

C. Loberg
Department of Diagnostic and Interventional Radiology, University Hospital RWTH Aachen, Pauwelsstrasse 30, Aachen 52074, Germany
e-mail: cloberg@ukaachen.de

© Springer-Verlag Berlin Heidelberg 2016
K.R. Aigner, F.O. Stephens (eds.), *Induction Chemotherapy,*
DOI 10.1007/978-3-319-28773-7_19

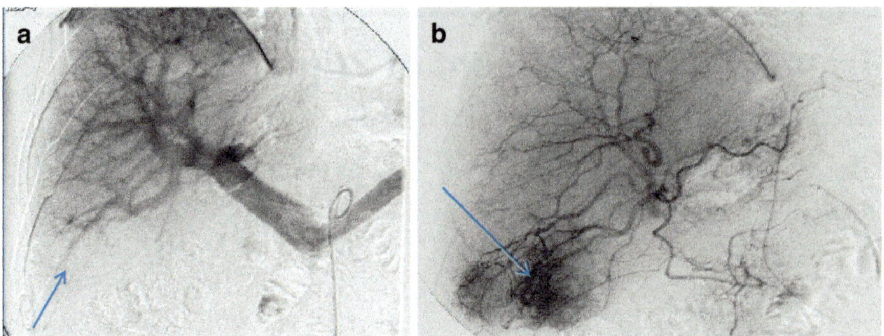

Fig. 19.1 (**a**) Normal liver less than 20 % of arterial supply. (**b**) Metastases, 100 % of arterial supply

19.1 Concept of Transarterial Therapy

Primary and secondary liver tumors receive their blood supply almost exclusively from the artery (100 %) in contrast to normal healthy liver tissue which is supplied by the portal vein (less than 20 % of arterial perfusion) (Fig. 19.1).

19.2 Patient Selection

All patients undergo diligent preinterventional preparation. Current CT and MRI examination of the liver is essential for planning interventional approach. Patients may be considered for locoregional therapy with TACE or 90Y radioembolization if they have liver-only or liver-dominant metastatic disease, and the level of hepatic parenchyma involvement does not exceed 60 %. Liver-dominant metastatic disease is defined as 80 % or more of the overall total body metastatic tumor burden located in the liver. Contraindications for transcatheter procedures originate in severe allergic reaction on iodine contrast media, PLT less than 60,000/ml, PTT >30 s, and INR less than 0.85.

All patients undergo extended informing about adverse events and complication, especially risk of liver failure, abscess, and RILD (radiation-induced liver disease) in case of SIRT.

In cases of hepatocellular carcinoma, Lipiodol or drug-eluting beads are used as embolic agents in combination with or without doxorubicin or alcohol. Superselective approach is essential depending on the underlying cause of liver disease. Different kinds of metastases require different compositions of anticancer agents. In case of cholangiocellular carcinoma (CCC), breast cancer, or metastases of malignant melanoma, triple TACE with combination of cisplatin, mitomycin C, and doxorubicin is used.

19.3   Transarterial Chemoembolization

Indications: patients with unresectable or non-ablatable liver-dominant metastases or patients who cannot undergo surgery because of comorbidity are potential candidates for TACE and SIRT. TACE is applied in cases of colorectal liver metastases, breast cancer, malignant melanoma, uveal melanoma, and NET. Patients undergoing TACE should not have vascular tumor invasion and adequate liver function. Life expectancy should be longer than 3 months and have a sufficient liver reserve. TACE is performed every 4 weeks for three times and can be repeated if follow-up examinations show tumor growth.

Laboratory findings including AST, ALT, tumor marker, and bilirubin are needed. Bilirubin level higher than 2 mg/dl with more than 50 % liver involvement is an independent predictor for patients who are not candidates for potentially curative treatment.

Two-thirds of patients develop postembolization syndrome with nausea, fatigue, and elevated liver enzymes. Complications as liver abscess are less common; tumor rupture is equally rare. Bile duct injury has been reported in 11.3 % of patients being treated; gastrointestinal ischemia due to nontarget embolization occurred in less than 1 % of cases.

Overall survival rates of 62 % (1 year) and 28 % (2 years) in cases of CRC are shown. In cases of NET rates of partial and complete response range between 68 % and 100 % (Fig. 19.2).

19.4   Hepatic Artery Infusion Therapy

The aim is to increase drug concentrations in tumor tissue to achieve higher response rates. The effectiveness of intra-arterial drug delivery is proportional to the first-pass effect of the drug by the liver and inversely proportional to body clearance.

HAIC is repeated every 2 weeks, and a permanent access via a subcutaneous port system linked to an intra-arterial catheter to the hepatic artery is needed. In cases of additional liver arteries, flow remodeling is needed because HAIC needs a single hepatic artery.

Randomized studies showed response rates of 90 % with a disease control rate of 100 % and a progression-free survival of 20 months, combining oxaliplatin with systemic 5-FU and cetuximab as first-line treatment. Disease was downstaged in 48 % of patients for resection and/or radiofrequency ablation (Fig. 19.3).

19.5   Selective Internal Radiotherapy

Normal liver tissue has a low radiation tolerance of approximately 30 Gy when compared with the doses required for effective tumor treatment. Yittrium-90 is a pure beta emitter with a median range in soft tissue between 2.5 and 11 mm, an

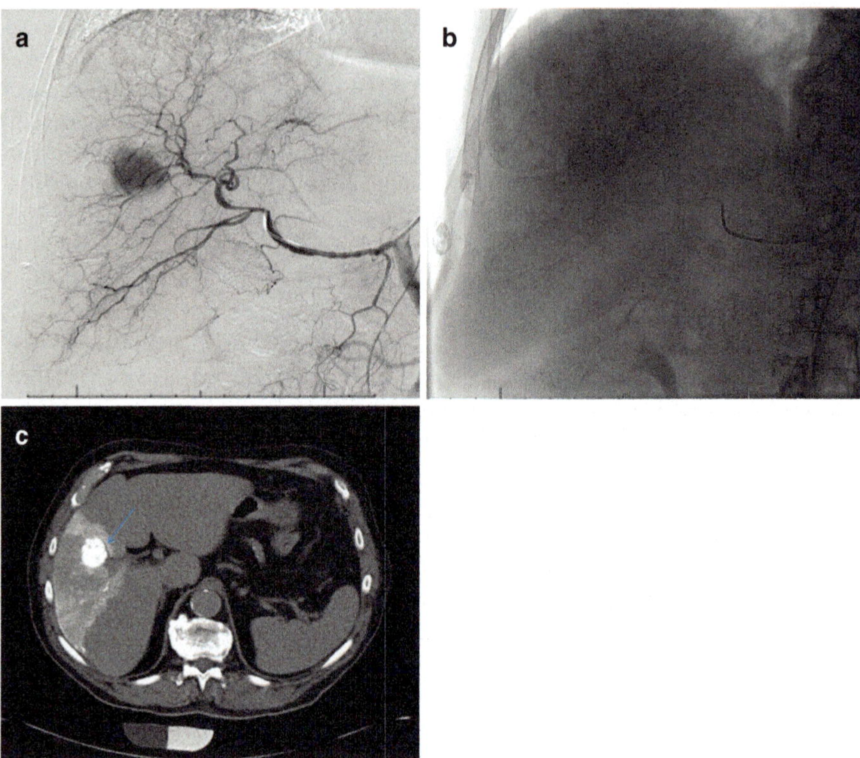

Fig. 19.2 (**a**) Patient with hepatocellular carcinoma in case of liver cirrhosis caused by hepatitis B. (**b**) TACE in case of HCC: *1* Lipiodol or drug-eluting beads, *2* alcohol or doxorubicin, and *3* superselective approach depending of the cause of liver disease. (**c**) CT after TACE using Lipiodol: accumulation of Lipiodol in HCC

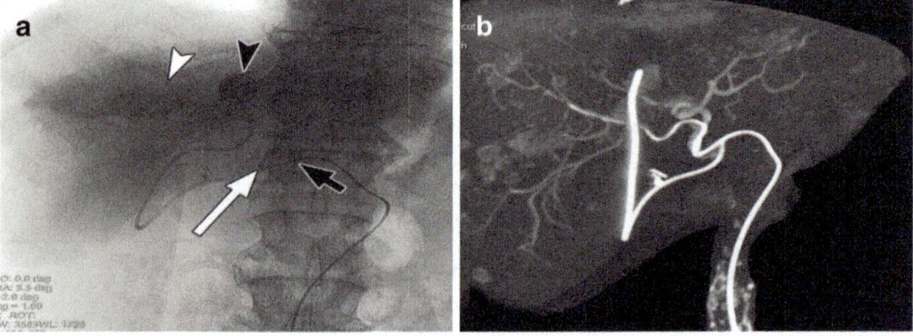

Fig. 19.3 (**a**) Percutaneous implanted catheter, tip in distal branch of the right hepatic artery. (**b**) Injection through femoral port with numerous tumor blushes related to metastases

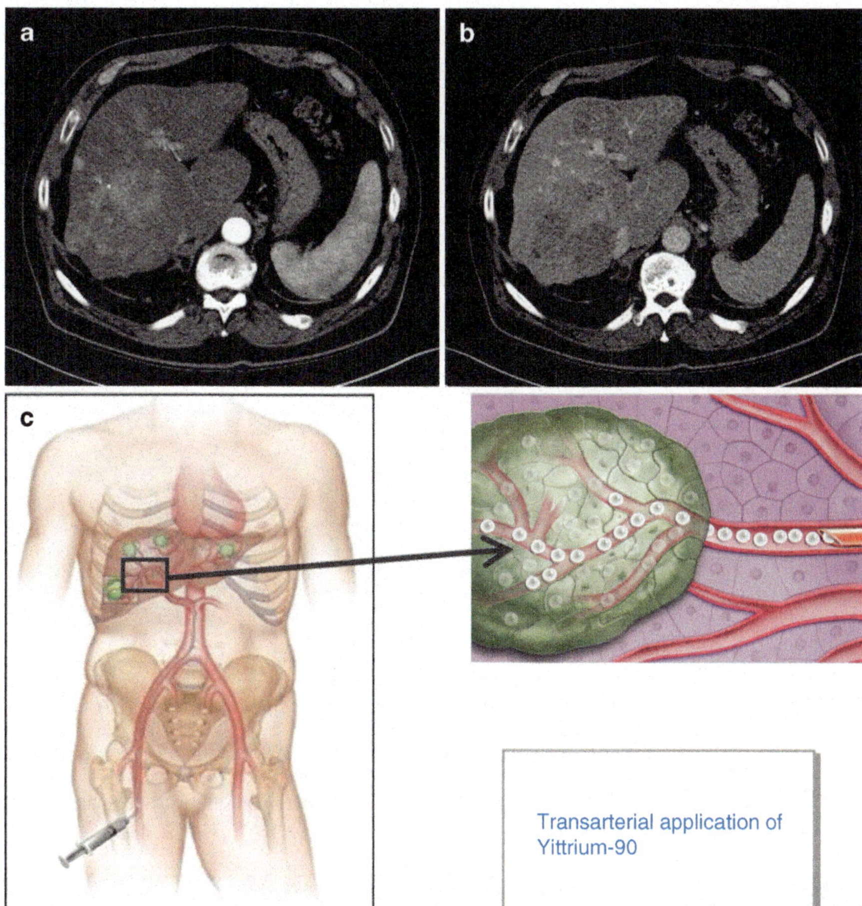

Fig. 19.4 (**a**) Patient with multilocular hepatocellular carcinoma. *1* Chronic hepatitis B. *2* Liver cirrhosis. *3* Radiotherapy (**b**)

average energy of 0.9367 MeV, and a half-life of 64.2 h. Local tumor dose reaches up to 1,000 Gy. At the moment two types of radioactive microspheres are available, resin or glass, specific activity per particle is different. SIRT is performed in cooperation with the Department of Nuclear Medicine. Preinterventional treatment is nearly the same in comparison to TACE, but gastroduodenal artery, right gastric artery, and falciform, cystic, and peripancreatic arterial branches have to be embolized. A lung scan after a single application of TC 99 with 200–400 MBq is performed to identify arteriovenous shunting.

Less than 20 % of patients develop radio-induced liver disease with symptoms as nausea, fatigue, and liver failure. Radiation dose can be reduced in cases of reduced liver function and SIRT can be performed segmentally (Figs. 19.4, 19.5, and 19.6).

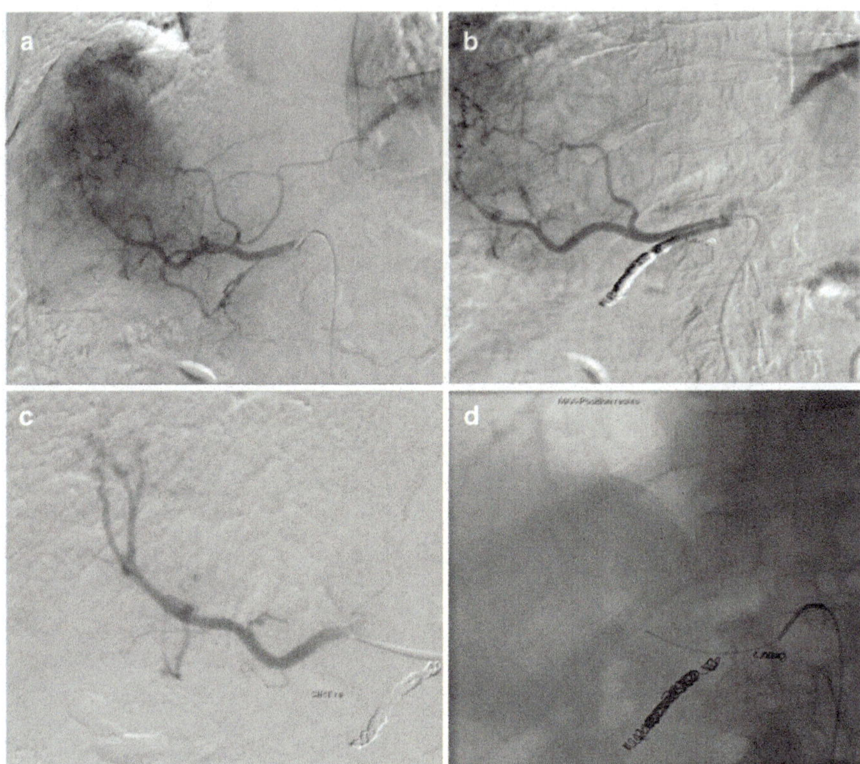

Fig. 19.5 (**a**) Diagnostic angiography. (**b**) Protective coil embolization gastroduodenal artery. (**c**) Test injection of 99-technetium (**d**) SIRT

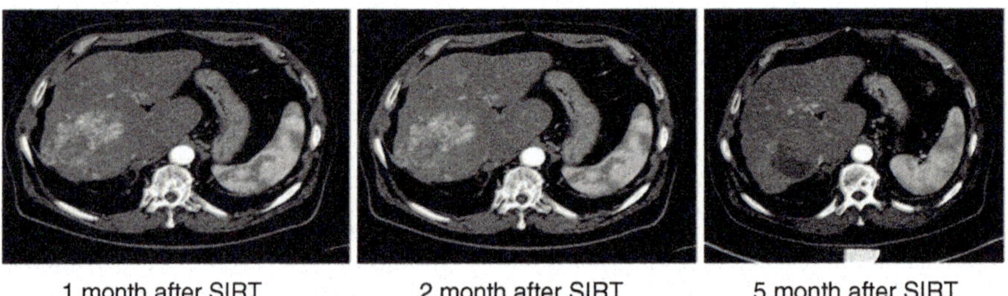

Fig. 19.6 Follow-up after SIRT in case of multifocal hepatocellular carcinoma. One month after SIRT, 2 months after SIRT, and 5 months after SIRT

19.6   Periprocedural Management

Periprocedural medication is extremely important to reduce incidence and severity of adverse events associated with TACE or SIRT. Abdominal pain and dizziness are the most frequent side effects. Several protocols have been used to achieve pain control, including intravenous administration of analgesic agents, steroids in cases with large tumor burden, and intra-arterial injection of lidocaine. In patients with biliodigestive anastomoses, preinterventional administration of antibiotics is recommended to avoid hepatic abscess. In patients with carcinoid tumors, octreotide is recommended to prevent carcinoid crisis.

Diagnostic angiography of celiac and mesenteric arteries is mandatory to identify anatomic variants and to assess tumor vascularization. Arteriovenous fistula and collateral vessels with hepatopetal flow need to be embolized priorly. A selective approach for positioning the microcatheter system is essential.

19.6.1 Embolizing Agents

Most commonly chemotherapeutic and embolizing agents are cisplatin, doxorubicin, and mitomycin C in combination with or without Lipiodol which has a poor embolizing effect. Additional embolic substances as microspheres and gelatin sponges have permanent or temporary effects and are recommended. Irinotecan in combination with drug-eluting beads (DEB) has been recently introduced in cases of HCC and CRC. Injection must be very slow and an injection rate of 1 ml/min is recommended. Maintaining forward flow into the liver is essential during the whole procedure, especially in case of SIRT to avoid radionecrosis of different organs.

19.6.2 Embolization End Point

The aim is delivering the whole dose of anticancer treatment into the liver. If near stasis or vasospasm is observed during the injection, it should be stopped.

19.7   Postinterventional Management

MRI and CT examination is performed in case of SIRT 4–8 weeks after SIRT up to 2 years, in case of TACE intervals range from 1 day after procedure up to 4 weeks, 3 and 6 months according to clinical presentation and progress of tumor marker.

19.8   Conclusion

Transarterial locoregional therapy is an excellent tool in the treatment and control of metastatic disease. It can markedly improve patients' survival and quality of life in a palliative setting.

Further Readings

 1. International Agency for Research on Cancer. World Health Organization. GLOBOCAN 2008: Estimated cancer incidence, mortality, prevalence and disability-adjusted life years worldwide in 2008. Available at http://globocan.iarc.fr/.
 2. Brown RE, Bower MR, Martin RC. Hepatic resection for colorectal liver metastases. Surg Clin N Am. 2010;90:839–52.

3. Martin RC, Salem R, Adam R, Dixon E. Locoregional surgical and interventional therapies for advanced colorectal liver metastasis: consensus statement. HPB (Oxford). 2013;15:131–3.

4. Mahnken AH, Pereira PL, de Baere T. Interventional oncologic approaches to liver metastases. Radiology. 2013;266:407–30.

5. Zannon C, Grosso M, Clara R, et al. Combined regional and systemic chemotherapy by a mini-invasive approach for the treatment of colorectal liver metastases. Am J Clin Oncol. 2001;24(4):354–9.

6. Inaba Y, Arni Y, Matsueda K, Takeuchi Y, Aramaki T. Right gastric artery embolization to prevent acute gastric mucosal lesions in patients undergoing repeat hepatic arterial infusion chemotherapy. J Vasc Interv Radiol. 2001;12(8):957–63.

7. Kemeny NE, Niedzwicki D, Hollis DR, et al. Hepatic arterial infusion versus systemic therapy for hepatic metastases from colorectal cancer. A randomized trial of efficacy, quality of life and molecular markers. J Clin Oncol. 2006;24(9):1395–403.

8. Fiorentini G, Rossi S, Dentico P, et al. Irinotecan hepatic arterial infusion chemotherapy for hepatic metastases from colorectal cancer: a phase II clinical study. Tumori. 2003;89(4):382–4.

9. Geschwind JF, Kaushik S, Ramsey DE, Choti MA, Fishman EK, Koheiter H. Influence of a new prophylactic antibiotic therapy on the incidence of liver abscesses after chemoembolization treatment of liver tumors. J Vasc Interv Radiol. 2002;13(11):1163–6.

10. Lewandowski RJ, Thurson KG, Goin JE, et al. Microsphere (Tera-Sphere) treatment for unresectable colorectal cancer metastases of the liver: response to treatment at targeted doses of 135 – 150 Gy as measured by 18F-FDG-PET and computed tomography imaging. J Vasc Interv Radiol. 2005;16(12):1641–51.

11. Martin RC, Robbins K, Tomalty D, et al. Transarterial chemoembolization (TACE) using Irinotecan-loaded beads for the treatment of unresectable metastases to the liver in patients with colorectal cancer: an interim report. Word J Surg Oncol. 2009;7:80.

12. Vogl TJ, Mack MG, Balzer JO, et al. Liver metastases: neoadjuvant downsizing with transarterial chemoembolization before laser induced thermotherapy. Radiology. 2003;229(2):457–64.

13. Vogl TJ, Naguib NN, Nour-Eldin NE, et al. Repeated chemoembolization followed by laser-induced thermotherapy for liver metastases of breast cancer. AJR Am J Roentgenol. 2011;196(1):W66–72.

14. Vogl TJ, Gruber T, Balzer JO, Eichler K, Hammerstingl R, Zangos S. Repeated transarterial chemoembolization in the treatment of liver metastases of colorectal cancer: a prospective study. Radiology. 2009;250(1):281–9.

15. Martinelli DJ, Wadler S, Baka CW, et al. Utility of chemoembolization as second-line treatment in patients with advanced or recurrent colorectal carcinoma. Cancer. 1994;74(6):1706–12.

16. Albert M, Kiefer MV, Sun W, et al. Chemoembolization of colorectal liver metastases with cisplatin, doxorubicin and mitomycin C, ethiodol and polyvinyl alcohol. Cancer. 2011;117(2):343–52.

17. Poggi G, Pozzi E, Riccardi A, et al. Complications of image guides transcatheter hepatic chemoembolization of primary and secondary tumors of the liver. Anticancer Res. 2010;30(12):5159–64.

18. Riaz A, Lewandowski RJ, Kuklik I, et al. Complications following radioembolization with Yttrium-90 microspheres: a comprehensive literature review. J Vasc Interv Radiol. 2009;20(9):1121–30.

19. Sangro B, Gil-Alzugaray B, Rodriguez J, et al. Liver disease induced by radioembolization of liver tumors: description and possible risk factors. Cancer. 2008;112(7):1538–46.

Pelvic Perfusion for Rectal Cancer

Stefano Guadagni, Karl Reinhard Aigner,
Giammaria Fiorentini, Maurizio Cantore, Marco Clementi,
Alessandro Chiominto, and Giuseppe Zavattieri

20.1 Introduction

Induction chemotherapy is the chemotherapy able to induce changes that make follow-up surgery and/or radiotherapy more likely to be successful. Pelvic perfusion can be used as induction chemotherapy for the treatment of rectal cancer, mainly in case of local recurrence but also in particular patients with advanced primary cancer. This is an innovative approach because pelvic perfusion was normally used as terminal link of a chain in a multimodular treatment. The use of pelvic perfusion with hemofiltration at the beginning of a therapy sequence is mainly suggested by the side effects of systemic chemotherapy and radiotherapy.

20.2 Local Recurrence of Rectal Cancer

The incidence rate of local pelvic recurrence after standard "curative" surgery for rectal cancer varies widely according to the definition employed, accuracy of diagnosis, completeness of follow-up, and whether and how often postmortem examinations were performed [1–5]. In control groups included in prospective randomized

S. Guadagni, MD (✉) • M. Cantore, MD • M. Clementi, MD
A. Chiominto, MD
Department of General Surgery, University Hospital of L'Aquila, L'Aquila, Italy
e-mail: stefanoguadagni@interfree.it

K.R. Aigner, MD • G. Zavattieri
Department of Surgical Oncology, Medias Klinikum GmbH & Co KG,
Krankenhausstrasse 3a, Burghausen 84489, Germany

G. Fiorentini, MD
Azienda Ospedaliera Marche Nord, Ospedale San Salvatore, Pesaro, Italy

© Springer-Verlag Berlin Heidelberg 2016
K.R. Aigner, F.O. Stephens (eds.), *Induction Chemotherapy*,
DOI 10.1007/978-3-319-28773-7_20

trials or in epidemiological studies, the 5-year local recurrence rates vary from 20 % to 35 % [6–13].

The treatment of local recurrence remains a challenge since, without surgical intervention, the reported survival rate of patients with local recurrence of rectal cancer is less than 4 % at 5 years, and the median life expectancy is 7 months [6]. Although 50 % of recurrences are associated with disseminated disease [14], most patients die of local and/or regional progression of disease rather than systemic metastases [15]. Extensive resection (abdominal sacral resection with or without pelvic exenteration) gives the best chance of survival [16–18]. Operative mortality varies from 0 % to 10 %, the 5-year survival rate varies from 20 % to 30 %, and the median life expectancy varies from 39 to 44 months [16–18]. Results from such radical surgery seem to be optimized by applying multimodality approaches, including external beam radiotherapy, sensitizing chemotherapy, and intraoperative radiation therapy [19–21]. The actuarial 2-year overall survival is approximately 50 %, and the actuarial 5-year disease-free survival is approximately 35 % [19–21]. However, if the resected recurrent cancer does not have margins free on histopathologic examination, the actuarial 2-year survival rate is significantly lower (approximately 35 %). Unfortunately, extensive surgery is not feasible in almost two-thirds of patients with recurrent rectal cancer [22]. In general, the demonstration of pelvic side wall involvement, growth into the sciatic notch, involvement of the first and/or second sacral vertebra, and/or encasement of the bladder or iliac vessels contraindicates surgery [19].

Although occasional cases of complete remission have been reported [23], radiotherapy alone or in conjunction with chemotherapy provides palliative benefit and extension of mean or median survival, but long-term survival (>2 years) is rare [24–27]. Studies using radiotherapy alone have reported a median survival time of 17.9 months in a group of patients able to receive a dose of 50–60 Gy [28]; on the other hand, after a mean dose of 30 Gy, a median survival time of 14 months has been observed in chemotherapy- and radiotherapy-naive patients [29], whereas a median survival time of 12 months has been reported for palliative reirradiation [30].

20.3 Pelvic Perfusion

For patients with unresectable recurrent rectal cancer, neither intravenous systemic chemotherapy nor intra-arterial chemotherapy achieves desirable results in terms of pain control and tumor response [31–38]. To improve clinical response, several methods of regional chemotherapy delivery have been suggested. One of these methods is pelvic perfusion. In 1958, Creech et al. [39] proposed the technique of isolated perfusion in which the blood supply of a body region was isolated: the aorta and the vena cava are occluded with vessel clamps and perfused by means of cannulae with thigh tourniquet application to reduce collateral circulation. Actually, the perfused compartment was not fully isolated. Pharmacokinetic evaluations of 5-fluorouracil (5-FU) in patients with pelvic recurrence of colorectal cancer [40] showed that isolation perfusion was advantageous compared with intra-arterial or intravenous administration. This technique is still in use [41].

Isolated perfusion incorporating laparotomic aortic and caval cannulation was modified by the use of femoral cannulation [42–47]. In 1960, Watkins et al. [48] described a technique using balloon catheters to achieve blockage of the aorta and inferior vena cava. In 1963, Lawrence et al. [49] reported a technique using balloon occlusion catheters and a large abdominal external tourniquet. In a 1987 study of hyperthermic pelvic infusion with 5-FU, Wile and Smolin [45] reported the occlusion of the great vessels by means of balloon catheters and femoral cannulation in 11 of 27 patients with refractory pelvic cancer. In 1993, a similar technique was reported by Turk et al. [50] in six patients with recurrent unresectable rectal cancer who underwent perfusion with 5-FU, cisplatin, and mitomycin C (MMC). In 1996, Wanebo et al. [57] published the results of normothermic pelvic perfusion with the same regimen in 14 patients with unresectable and 5 with resectable recurrent rectal cancer. In 1994, Aigner and Kaevel [52] presented the results of pelvic perfusion with MMC and melphalan in 41 patients with recurrent unresectable rectal cancer. Both occlusion of the great vessels and perfusion were done with only two catheters, which were surgically introduced through the femoral vessels. The 2-year survival rate in the group of patients pretreated with radiotherapy and/or chemotherapy was 35 %. A similar technique using percutaneous catheters was later performed by Thompson et al. [53] in seven patients with recurrent rectal cancer who underwent perfusion with MMC and 5-FU or cisplatin.

Microenviromental alterations, including tissue hypoxia and low cellular pH, occur during isolated pelvic perfusion. MMC is ten times more toxic to tumor cells in hypoxic conditions [54, 55]. The pharmacokinetics of MMC in peripheral and inferior vena cava blood was studied by our group [56] in four patients with unresectable recurrent rectal cancer under different types of major vessel occlusion. For the type of pelvic perfusion corresponding to the method used by Aigner and Kaevel [52], the area under the plasma concentration-time curve (AUC) ratio for inferior caval vein blood vs systemic circulation was 11.7:1.

20.4 Hypoxic Pelvic Perfusion (Stop-Flow) Technique

20.4.1 Positioning of Catheters

There are two methods. In the first, which is obligatory when associated lymphadenectomy is indicated, the femoral artery and vein have to be exposed through a short longitudinal incision in the groin. After systemic heparinization (150 U/kg), a three-lumen balloon 12-French catheter (PfM, Cologne, Germany) has to be introduced into the inferior vena cava via the saphenous vein and a second one into the aorta via the femoral artery; these were positioned under fluoroscopic control below the renal vessels and above the aortic and venous bifurcation using a guidewire. In the second, which is useful when the procedure has to be repeated several times, a percutaneous puncture of the femoral vessels has to be performed. The tools used in the procedure are mainly based on two 11-French introducers with hemostatic valve and dilatator. Moreover, two double-lumen 7-French balloon catheters are necessary (PfM, Cologne, Germany). Both blood circulation and perfusion will take place in the space between introducer wall and catheter, a space that corresponds to a long-hollow cylinder at the top of which the blood flows in and out through a ring surface.

20.4.2 Occlusion of Circulation

Both balloons were filled with isotonic sodium chloride solution, containing the radiopaque dye diatrizoate, and blocked. For isolation of the pelvis, two large-cuff orthopedic tourniquets, placed around each of the upper thighs just below the lower level of the femoral triangle, were inflated just before starting the perfusion.

20.4.3 Drug Perfusion

The infusion channels of the arterial and venous stop-flow catheters were connected to a hypoxic perfusion set on a roller pump (RAND, Medolla, Italy). The set was primed with an isotonic sodium chloride solution containing heparin (10,000 U/L). Once flow was established (approx 200 mL/min), drug therapy was started. The drug, diluted in 250 mL of isotonic sodium chloride solution also containing 16 mg

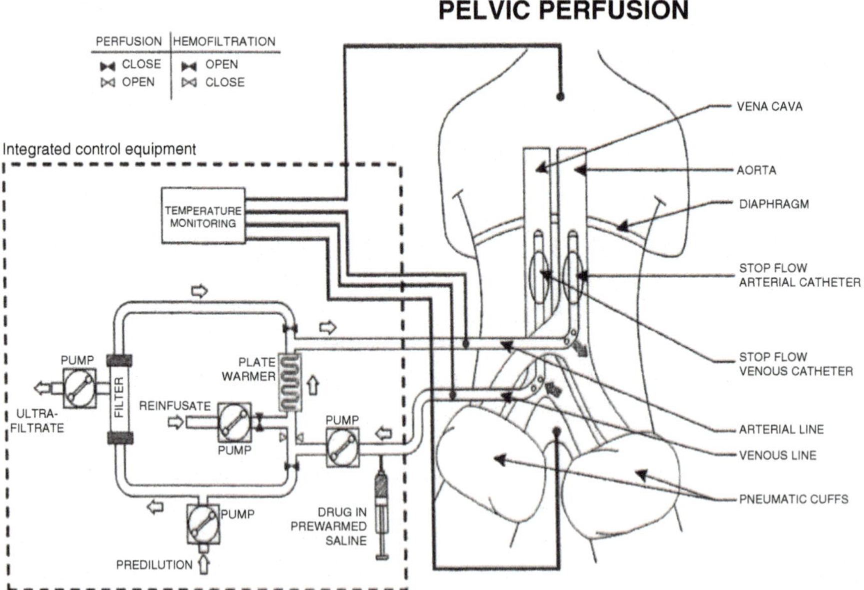

Fig. 20.1 Scheme of hypoxic pelvic perfusion and extracorporeal circuit incorporating both a hemofiltration system and a heater-cooler unit

of dexamethasone sodium phosphate, was administered over 3 min. The extracorporeal circuit (Fig. 20.1) also included both a hemofiltration system and a heater-cooler unit. The hypoxic perfusion circuit was maintained over 20 min (mean 22 ± 4 min). The temperature of the perfusate was 38.5 °C.

20.4.4 Reestablishment of Normal Circulation

After perfusion, both catheter balloons and pneumatic cuffs were deflated and the circulation restored. The extracorporeal circuit also was used in the hemofiltration section for 80 ± 20 min. A polyamide hemofilter with a surface area of 2.1 m^2 was used. Thereafter, the catheters were withdrawn and the vessels repaired. Using the percutaneous approach, hemostasis was done by compression for approximately 30 min.

20.5 Advantages and Limitations of Pelvic Perfusion

For patients with unresectable recurrent rectal cancer, particularly when the surgeon is unable to accomplish a gross total surgical resection of the recurrent cancer, preoperative external irradiation plus continuous infusion chemotherapy, intraoperative irradiation, maximal surgical resection, and systemic chemotherapy are currently being studied in clinical trials [19–21, 57]. When comorbid conditions contraindicate extensive palliative surgery, when intraoperative irradiation is not available, or when external irradiation is not practical, hypoxic pelvic perfusion has been an effective alternative [53].

The relative advantage of intra-arterial over intravenous chemotherapy (R_D) is proportional to the increase of drug concentration in the target organ or compartment (R_T) and to the reduction of drug concentration in the systemic circulation (R_S), as can be seen in the following equation:

$$R_D = \left[\left(R_T / R_S\right)\right] = 1 + \left[Cl_T / Q\left(1 - E\right)\right]$$

where Cl_T represents the overall amount of blood detoxified in the whole body per minute (drug clearance in the whole body), Q represents the blood flow in the artery in which the drug is infused, and E represents the amount of drug cleared by or held by the organ or compartment in which the drug has been infused [58]. The relative advantage of intra-arterial over intravenous chemotherapy (R_D) can be increased by reducing Q and increasing Cl_T and E. Hypoxic perfusion with the balloon occlusion technique can be an effective method for reducing Q. Hemofiltration of venous blood from the infused organ or compartment can increase Cl_T.

Hypoxic pelvic perfusion has potential therapeutic advantages over intra-arterial infusion of chemotherapy, as recently demonstrated by a pilot study in which an approximately tenfold superior MMC pelvic-systemic exposure ratio was measured for hypoxic pelvic perfusion in comparison with intra-aortic infusion in patients with unresectable locally recurrent rectal cancer [56]. After intravenous push injection of

20 mg/m^2 of MMC, Door [59] reported that the peripheral C_{max} was 6.0 μg/mL with an AUC of 73.3 μg/mL × minutes. In our experience [60], after intra-aortic administration of 25 mg/m^2 of MMC during the hypoxic pelvic perfusion, the mean C_{max} in the pelvic compartment was 54.8 μg/mL, the mean peripheral C_{max} was 25 μg/mL, and the mean peripheral AUC was 50.2 μg/mL × minutes.

The efficiency of the simplified balloon occlusion technique used in our experience [60] to perform hypoxic pelvic perfusion has been demonstrated by the good mean pelvic-systemic MMC-AUC ratio (13.3:1) measured in our series of 11 treatments, this being higher than both the value of 9.0:1 reported by Wanebo et al. [51] and the value of 4.4:1 reported by Turk et al. [50]. The high variability in the range of MMC-AUC ratio values (4.3:1–25.7:1), which is attributable in our opinion to the variability of conditions in different individuals (i.e., anastomotic venous leak from the pelvic circulation to the systemic circulation), explains why both the type of tumor response and the extent of toxic effects in this kind of patient are not accurately predictable.

20.5.1 Choice of Drug

Several different chemotherapeutic regimens have been used in pelvic perfusion, often as part of a single study. In the treatments performed for recurrent rectal cancer, the agents more frequently used have been 5-FU [45, 50, 51] and cisplatin [45, 50, 51] in monochemotherapy or in polychemotherapy. Less frequently and often in small series, the use of nitrogen mustard [42, 43, 49], cyclophosphamide [49], 2-deoxy-5-fluorouridine [49], melphalan [52], and mitoxantrone [41] has been reported. The real value of pelvic perfusion in terms of tumor response is consequently difficult to ascertain. After a pilot study on hypoxic pelvic perfusion [56], we planned a phase II trial based on the use of single-agent MMC, which has been shown to be increasingly cytotoxic in a hypoxic environment [53, 54]. Although 5-FU has been considered more effective than MMC against adenocarcinoma of the rectum, also when administered by pelvic perfusion [50], 5-FU was not selected for this study mainly because most patients had disease progression after systemic chemotherapy with this agent.

In our selected series of patients, one course of hypoxic pelvic perfusion with 25 mg/m^2 of MMC resulted in an overall response rate of 36.3 %. These results are comparable to those reported by Turk et al. [50], which were approx 30 % using 5-FU (3,000 mg/m^2), cisplatin (25–75 mg/m^2), and MMC (10 mg/m^2). Aigner and Keavel [52] reported an overall response rate of 32 % in a series of 41 patients treated with MMC (12.5 mg/m^2) and melphalan (12.5 mg/m^2). Wile and Smolin [45] reported an overall response rate of 40 % in 17 patients treated with 5-FU (750–1,500 mg/m^2) by hyperthermic perfusion.

Based on these data, the response rate does not seem to be significantly higher in patients treated with polychemotherapy than in those receiving monochemotherapy. Further studies are necessary to evaluate other drugs that are active in hypoxic conditions (i.e., doxorubicin, tirapazamine), the role of hyperthermia and oxygenation with prolonged isolated perfusion [45], or the use of agents modulating multiple drug resistance [50].

Strocchi et al. [61] reported an overall response rate of 30 % in a series of ten patients with unresectable pelvic recurrence from colorectal cancer, treated with a combination of MMC (20 mg/m^2) plus doxorubicin (75 mg/m^2; eight patients) or epirubicin (75 mg/m^2; two patients) infused into the isolated pelvic compartment. Pain remission was observed in eight out of ten patients.

In 2014, Murata et al. [62] reported an overall response rate of 31 % in a series of 23 patients with unresectable pelvic recurrence or inoperable rectal cancer, treated with cisplatin (from 170 to 200 mg/m^2); the overall mean survival period was 24 months.

Recently, a new rationale has been adopted to the choice of drugs. The improvements in genetic research fields are at the basis of the possibility to administer a tailoring chemotherapy. In particular it is feasible to isolate the cancer cells of a patient from his peripheral blood and to genetically analyze these cells using molecular biology techniques (microarray, PCR, RT-PCR, Southern and Northern blot, etc.) and to investigate on genes that are necessary for the expansion and the survival of the tumor while at the same time they consist targets of the chemotherapeutic compounds. Likewise the mechanisms by which the cancer cells resist the chemotherapeutic drugs (MDR1 protein, LRP protein, glutathione transferase, gene amplification, etc.) may be investigated. In parallel the mechanisms of neovascularization and infiltration of the tumor, which are considered necessary for the ability of the tumor to perform metastasis, may be localized. In this manner, a patient with unresectable recurrent rectal cancer could receive chemotherapeutic agents based

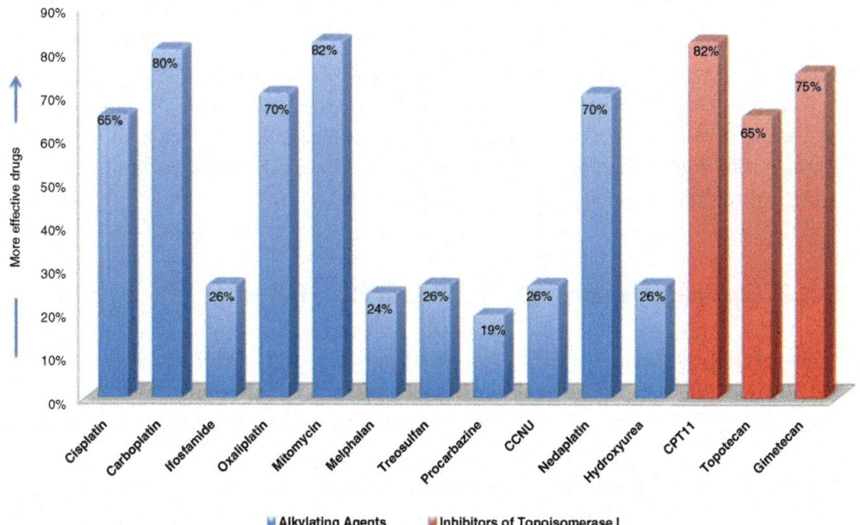

Fig. 20.2 Chemosensitivity test (part 1) in a patient with recurrent rectal cancer. Two drugs only (mitomycin and CPT11) are determining the necrosis of more than 80 % of tumor cells

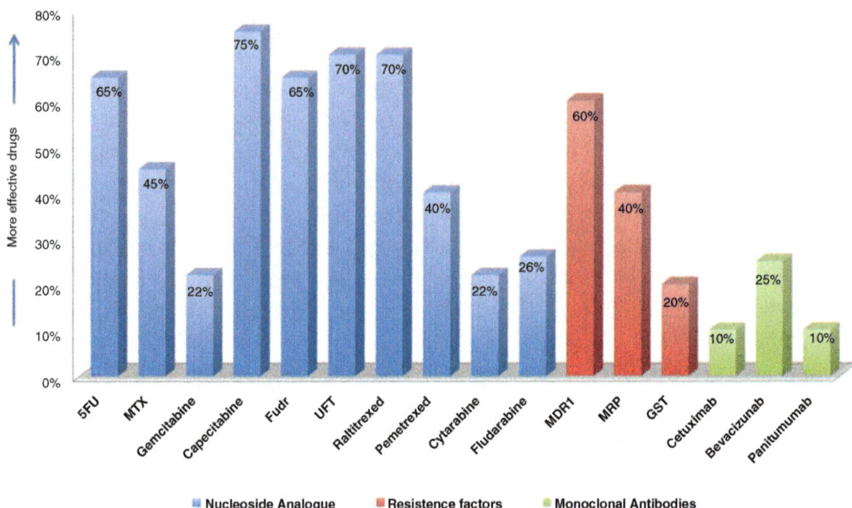

Fig. 20.3 Chemosensitivity test (part 2) in the same patient with recurrent rectal cancer. The specific tumor appears to have resisting populations because of the MDR1 overexpression. Bevacizumab could be considered as inhibitor of neoangiogenesis based on overexpression of tumor-related genes

on sensitivity of his neoplastic cells. Figures 20.2 and 20.3 show the in vitro neoplastic cell necrosis in several cultures when different chemotherapeutic drugs are inserted in the culture medium.

This rationale for the choice of drugs implies that each patient of a homogeneous group of subjects with recurrent rectal cancer could receive a different chemotherapeutic regimen. In a pilot study on 25 patients with unresectable recurrent rectal cancer, hypoxic pelvic perfusion of drugs selected based on chemosensitivity tests (RGCC, Filotas, Greece) provided 13 % of partial responses, 38 % of minor responses, 39 % of stable disease, and 10 % of progressive disease, with an overall response rate higher than 50 %. These results are better than those obtainable with traditional regimens suggesting further trials.

20.5.2 Comparative Response and Survival Rates

When pelvic perfusion has been performed in patients refractory to systemic chemotherapy and/or reirradiation, the response rate of pain relief is greater than 45 %. This result, together with the local control of tumor growth (6 months of median time to disease progression), promotes an improved quality of life. Tumor responses and survival rates are at least comparable to those observed with the other second-line therapies employed in FU-refractory metastatic colorectal cancer such as irinotecan or oxaliplatin [63–65], whereas systemic toxicities are significantly lower [66]. The median survival time (12.2 months) registered after one course of hypoxic

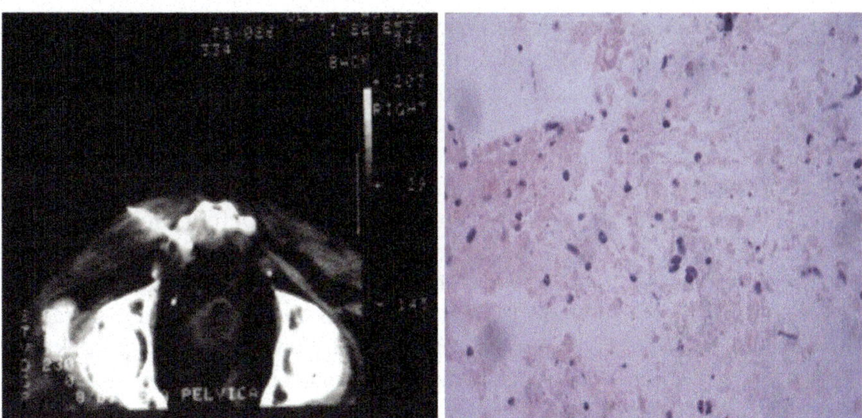

Fig. 20.4 Computed tomography-assisted biopsy of a mass infiltrating the sacrum. Histopathology demonstrated the presence of extensive necrosis and residual adenocarcinoma

pelvic perfusion is comparable to that obtained by irradiation or reirradiation in non-pretreated patients [29, 30]. Considering the vascular damage following radiotherapy, a different sequence in the multimodular treatment of unresectable recurrent rectal cancer could be more useful.

In our experience, when pelvic perfusion has been performed as induction chemotherapy in patients with unresectable recurrent rectal cancer, the tumor response rate is higher than 60 %. Figure 20.4 shows an example of response in a white male aged 82 years. The patient received a regimen of MMC (15 mg/m^2), 5-FU (1,000 mg/m^2), and cisplatin (100 mg/m^2).

20.5.3 Limitations

Since its first description, despite several innovations and significant response rates [39], regional pelvic perfusion has not seen widespread use, first owing to its inherent complexity and second owing to serious adverse effects from local and systemic toxicities. In 1963, Lawrence et al. [49] reported a 70 % occurrence of local toxic effects (30 % of them major) after pelvic perfusion with MMC at a dose of 1 mg/kg. With a dose of 25 mg/m^2 and regional administration of dexamethasone sodium phosphate, no local toxic effects were registered in our series. To reduce systemic exposure, low pressure and flow in the extracorporeal circuit with the aim of reducing leakage [51] as well as hemofiltration [67] were adopted in our experience. It has been reported that chemofiltration reduces immediate cytotoxic effects and postpones cumulative toxic effects in patients treated with abdominal stop-flow infusion [68]. Bioavailability of MMC in the peripheral venous blood can be reduced using safe hemofiltration for 60 min [56], and at the end of the procedure, approx 10 % of the total MMC dose administered can be detected in urine and ultrafiltrate [60]. In 2014, Murata et al. [62], adopted hemodialysis with the same purpose.

20.6 Pelvic Perfusion in Advanced Primary Rectal Cancer

Although postoperative systemic chemotherapy and radiotherapy for patients with stage II and III rectal cancer remain an acceptable option, preoperative chemoradiation is now the preferred treatment modality [69]. Benefits of preoperative chemoradiation include tumor regression, downstaging and improvement in resectability, and a higher rate of sphincter preservation and local control [69]. However, preoperative radiation therapy is associated with increased acute and late complications compared to surgery alone [70, 71]. The interval time before surgery is another topic of discussion. In several Europe institutions, preoperative radiotherapy is delivered in 1 week (25 Gy in five daily fractions), followed by surgery 1 week later. At the contrary in the United States, the long-course chemoradiation approach is preferred (50.4 Gy in 28 daily fractions with 5-FU and folinic acid) according to less severe late effects (i.e., bowel dysfunction) in comparison to high radiation doses per fraction. In 2014, Fung-Kee-Fung [72] has published an exhaustive review; in particular, it has been reported that postoperative complications differed according to the timing of surgery relative to the start date of radiotherapy, being significantly lower in patients who underwent surgery less than 11 days after the start of radiotherapy. Moreover, it has to be considered that in several countries, mostly in those undeveloped concerning health care, approximately 30 % of patients do not accept preoperative chemoradiation or cannot receive it for several reasons or interrupt it. In these particular cases, pelvic perfusion can be used as *induction chemotherapy* 20 days before surgery for rectal cancer. Figure 20.5 shows a computed tomography of a T_3 rectal cancer performed immediately before pelvic perfusion in a 52-year-old patient.

Twenty days after hypoxic pelvic perfusion, the patient was submitted to anterior resection of the rectum. Figure 20.6 shows the resected specimen in which it is evident an extensive fibrosis of the mesorectum, infiltrating the muscular layer, with residual cancer in three foci.

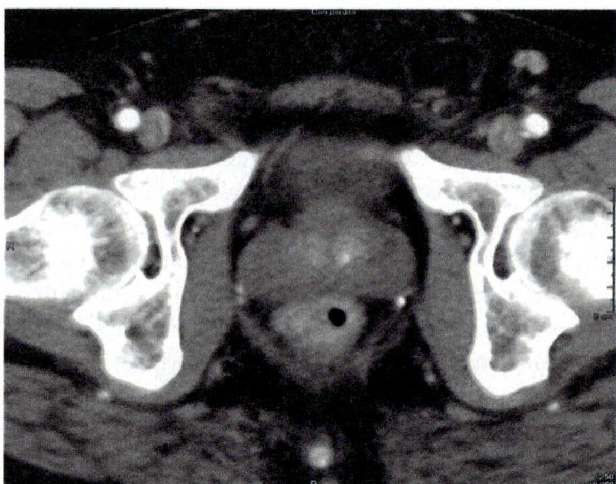

Fig. 20.5 Computed tomography of a T_3 rectal cancer

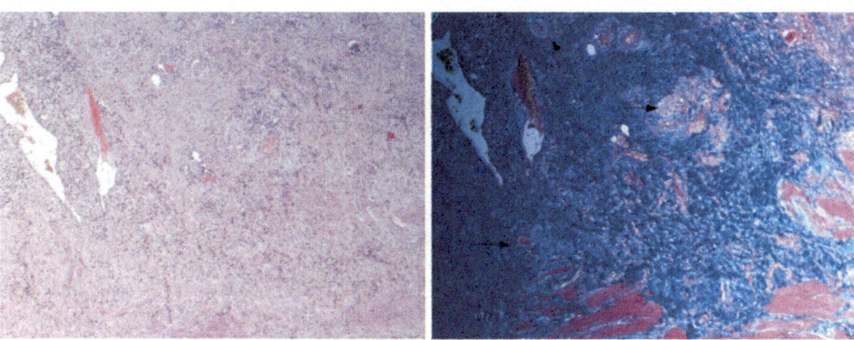

Fig. 20.6 Extensive fibrosis of the mesorectum, more evident in trichromic stain (*right* side). Three foci of residual cancer are indicated by *arrows*

Postoperative chemoradiation was also used in this patient. Further studies are necessary to establish whether hypoxic pelvic perfusion before surgery allows a less difficult dissection in comparison to preoperative chemoradiation and if a lower incidence of specific complications (i.e., wound infection) can be observed. A pilot study in a small number of patients demonstrated that the interval time between perfusion and resection may be always of 15–20 days with no specific complications, and preliminary results showed a comparable response ratio with preoperative chemoradiation. In conclusion, our experience demonstrated that clinical trials are recommendable to evaluate if hypoxic pelvic perfusion can be an alternative for those patients in which, for several reasons, preoperative chemoradiation has not been administered.

Acknowledgments All the authors contributed equally to the realization of this work.

References

1. Quirke P, Durdey P, Dixon MF, Williams NS. Local recurrence of rectal adenocarcinoma due to inadequate surgical resection. Histopathological study of lateral tumor spread and surgical excision. Lancet. 1986;2:996–9.
2. Wiig JN, Wolff PA, Tveit KM, Giercksky KE. Location of pelvic recurrence after curative low anterior resection for rectal cancer. Eur J Surg Oncol. 1999;25:590–4.
3. Bufalari A, Boselli C, Giustozzi G, Moggi L. Locally advanced rectal cancer: multivariate analysis of outcome risk factors. J Surg Oncol. 2000;74:2–10.
4. Holm T, Cedermark B, Rutqvist LE. Local recurrence of rectal adenocarcinoma after "curative" surgery with and without preoperative radiotherapy. Br J Surg. 1994;81:452–5.
5. Marsh PJ, James RD, Schofield PF. Definition of local recurrence after surgery for rectal carcinoma. Br J Surg. 1995;82:465–8.
6. Sagar PM, Pemberton JH. Surgical management of locally recurrent rectal cancer. Br J Surg. 1996;83:293–304.
7. Luna-Perez P, Trejo-Valdivia B, Labastida S, Garcia-Alvarado S, Rodriguez DF, Delgado S. Prognostic factors in patients with locally advanced rectal adenocarcinoma treated with preoperative radiotherapy and surgery. World J Surg. 1999;23:1069–4.

8. Medical Research Council Rectal Cancer Working Party. Randomised trial of surgery alone versus radiotherapy followed by surgery for potentially operable locally advanced rectal cancer. Lancet. 1996;348:1605–10.

9. Marsh PJ, James RD, Schofield PF. Adjuvant preoperative radiotherapy for locally advanced rectal carcinoma. Results of a prospective, randomised trial. Dis Colon Rectum. 1994;37:1205–14.

10. Swedish Rectal Cancer Trial. Improved survival with preoperative radiotherapy in resectable rectal cancer. N Engl J Med. 1997;336:980–7.

11. Heald RJ, Husband EM, Ryall RD. The mesorectum in rectal cancer surgery – the clue to pelvic recurrence? Br J Surg. 1982;69:613–6.

12. Bokey EL, Ojerskog B, Chapuis PH, Dent OF, Newland RC, Sinclair G. Local recurrence after curative excision of the rectum for cancer without adjuvant therapy: role of total anatomical dissection. Br J Surg. 1999;86:1164–70.

13. Merchant NB, Guillem JG, Paty PB, et al. T3N0 rectal cancer: results following sharp mesorectal excision and no adjuvant therapy. J Gastrointest Surg. 1999;3:642–7.

14. Huguier M, Houry S. Treatment of local recurrence of rectal cancer. Am J Surg. 1998;175:288–92.

15. Pilipshen SJ, Heilweil M, Quan SHQ, Sternberg SS, Enker WE. Patterns of pelvic recurrence following definitive resections of rectal cancer. Cancer. 1984;53:1354–62.

16. Wanebo HJ, Koness RJ, Vezeridis MP, Cohen SI, Wrobleski DE. Pelvic resection of recurrent rectal cancer. Ann Surg. 1994;220:586–97.

17. Suzuki K, Dozois RR, Devine RM, et al. Curative reoperations for locally recurrent rectal cancer. Dis Colon Rectum. 1996;39:730–6.

18. Maetani S, Onodera H, Nishikawa T, et al. Significance of local recurrence of rectal cancer as a local or disseminated disease. Br J Surg. 1998;85:521–5.

19. Magrini S, Nelson H, Gunderson LL, Sim FH. Sacropelvic resection and intraoperative electron irradiation in the management of recurrent anorectal cancer. Dis Colon Rectum. 1996;39:1–9.

20. Lowy AM, Rich TA, Skibber JM, Dubrow RA, Curley SA. Preoperative infusional chemoradiation, selective intraoperative radiation, and resection for locally advanced pelvic recurrence of colorectal adenocarcinoma. Ann Surg. 1996;223:1612–3.

21. Harrison LB, Minsky BD, Henker WE, et al. High dose rate intraoperative radiation therapy (HDR-IORT) as part of the management strategy for locally advanced primary and recurrent rectal cancer. Int J Radiat Oncol Biol Phys. 1998;42:325–30.

22. Hoffman JP, Riley L, Litwin S. Isolated locally recurrent rectal cancer: a review of incidence, presentation, and management. Semin Oncol. 1993;20:506–19.

23. Hayashi I, Shirai Y, Hatakeyama K. Complete remission after radiotherapy for recurrent rectal cancer. Hepatogastroenterology. 1997;44:1612–3.

24. Rominger CJ, Gelber R, Gunderson LL. Radiation therapy alone or in combination with chemotherapy in the treatment of residual or inoperable carcinoma of the rectum and rectosigmoid or pelvic recurrence following colorectal surgery. Am J Clin Oncol. 1985;8:118–27.

25. Wong CS, Cummings BJ, Keane TJ, O'Sullivan B, Catton CN. Results of external beam irradiation for rectal carcinoma locally recurrent after local excision or electrocoagulation. Radiother Oncol. 1991;22:145–8.

26. Minsky BD, Cohen AM, Enker WE, Sigurdson E, Harrison LB. Radiation therapy for unresectable rectal cancer. Int J Radiat Oncol Biol Phys. 1991;21:1283–9.

27. Dobrowsky W, Mitomycin C. 5-fluorouracil and radiation in advanced, locally recurrent rectal cancer. Br J Radiol. 1992;65:143–7.

28. Guiney MJ, Smith JG, Worotniuk V, Ngan S, Blakey D. Radiotherapy treatment for isolated loco-regional recurrents of rectosigmoid cancer following definitive surgery: Peter McCallum Cancer Institute experience, 1981–1990. Int J Radiat Oncol Biol Phys. 1997;38:1019–25.

29. Wong CS, Cummings BJ, Brierley JD, et al. Treatment of locally recurrent rectal carcinoma: results and prognostic factors. Int J Radiat Oncol Biol Phys. 1998;40:427–35.

30. Lingareddy V, Ahmad NR, Mohiuddin M. Palliative reirradiation for recurrent rectal cancer. Int J Radiat Oncol Biol Phys. 1997;38:785–90.

31. Bayer JR, von Heyden HW, Bartsch HH, et al. Intra-arterial perfusion therapy with 5-fluorouracil in patients with metastatic colorectal carcinoma and intractable pelvic pain. Recent Results Cancer Res. 1983;86:33–6.

32. Patt YZ, Peters RE, Chuang VP, Wallace S, Claghorn L, Mavligit G. Palliation of pelvic recurrence of colorectal cancer with intra-arterial 5-fluorouracil and mitomycin. Cancer. 1985;56:2175–80.

33. Estes NC, Morphis JG, Hornback NB, Jewell WR. Intraarterial chemotherapy and hyperthermia for pain control in patients with recurrent rectal cancer. Am J Surg. 1986;152:597–601.

34. Percivale P, Nobile MT, Vidili MG, et al. Treatment of colorectal cancer pelvic recurrences with hypogastric intraarterial 5-fluorouracil by means of totally implantable port systems. Reg Cancer Treat. 1990;3:143–6.

35. Muller H, Aigner KR. Palliation of recurrent rectal cancer with intraarterial mitomycin C/5-fluorouracil via Jet Port aortic bifurcation catheter. Reg Cancer Treat. 1990;3:147–51.

36. Tseng MH, Park HC. Pelvic intra-arterial mitomycin C infusion in previously treated patients with metastatic, unresectable pelvic colorectal cancer and angiographic determination of tumor vascularity. J Clin Oncol. 1985;3:1093–8.

37. Hafstorm L, Jonsson PE, Landberg T, Owman T, Sundkvist K. Intraarterial infusion chemotherapy (5-fluorouracil) in patients with inextirpable or locally recurrent rectal cancer. Am J Surg. 1979;137:757–62.

38. Carlsson C, Hafstrom L, Jonsson PE, Ask A, Kallum B, Lunderquist A. Unresectable and locally recurrent rectal cancer treated with radiotherapy or bilateral internal iliac artery infusion of 5-FU. Cancer. 1986;58:336–40.

39. Creech O, Krementz ET, Ryan RF, Winbald JN. Chemotherapy of cancer: regional perfusion utilizing an extracorporeal circuit. Ann Surg. 1958;148:616–32.

40. Wile AG, Stemmer EA, Andrews PA, Murphy MP, Abramson IS, Howell SB. Pharmacokinetics of 5-fluorouracil during hypothermic pelvic isolation-perfusion. J Clin Oncol. 1985;3:849–52.

41. Vaglini M, Cascinelli F, Chiti A, et al. Isolated pelvic perfusion for the treatment of unresectable primary or recurrent rectal cancer. Tumori. 1996;82:459–62.

42. Asten WA, Monaco AP, Richardson GS, Baker WH, Shaw RS, Raker JW. Treatment of malignant pelvic tumors by extracorporeal perfusion with chemotherapeutic agents. N Engl J Med. 1959;261:1037–45.

43. Ryan RF, Schramel RJ, Creech Jr O. Value of perfusion in pelvic surgery. Dis Colon Rectum. 1963;6:297–300.

44. Shingleton WW, Parker RT, Mahaley S. Abdominal perfusion for cancer chemotherapy with hypothermia and hyperthermia. Surgery. 1961;50:260–5.

45. Wile A, Smolin M. Hyperthermic pelvic isolation-perfusion in the treatment of refractory pelvic cancer. Arch Surg. 1987;122:1321–5.

46. Lawrence W, Kuehn P, Mori S, Poppel JW, Clarkson B. Regional perfusion of the pelvis: consideration of the "leakage" problem. Surgery. 1961;50:248–59.

47. Lathrop JC, Leone LA, Sodeberg CH, Colbert MP, Vargas LL. Perfusion chemotherapy for gynaecological malignancy. Trans N Engl Obstet Gynecol Soc. 1963;17:47–56.

48. Watkins E, Hering AC, Luna R, Adams HD. The use of intravascular balloon catheters for isolation of the pelvic vascular bed during pump-oxygenator perfusion of cancer chemotherapeutic agents. Surg Gynecol Obstet. 1960;111:464–8.

49. Lawrence W, Clarkson B, Kim M, Clapp P, Randall HT. Regional perfusion of pelvis and abdomen by an indirect technique. Cancer. 1963;16:567–82.

50. Turk PS, Belliveau JF, Darnowsky JW, Weinberg MC, Leenen L, Wanebo HJ. Isolated pelvic perfusion for unresectable cancer using a balloon occlusion technique. Arch Surg. 1993;128:533–9.
51. Wanebo HJ, Chung MA, Al L, Turk PS, Vezeridis MP, Belliveau JP. Preoperative therapy for advanced pelvic malignancy by isolated pelvic perfusion with the balloon-occlusion technique. Ann Surg Oncol. 1996;3:295–303.
52. Aigner KR, Kaevel K. Pelvic stopflow infusion (PSI) and hypoxic pelvic perfusion (HPP) with mitomycin and melphalan for recurrent rectal cancer. Reg Cancer Treat. 1994;7:6–11.
53. Thompson JF, Liu M, Waugh RC, et al. A percutaneous aortic "stop-flow" infusion technique for regional cytotoxic therapy of the abdomen and pelvis. Reg Cancer Treat. 1994;7:202–7.
54. Teicher BA, Lazo JS, Sartorelli AC. Classification of antineoplastic agents by their selective toxicities toward oxygenated and hypoxic tumor cells. Cancer Res. 1981;41:73–81.
55. Rockwell S. Effect of some proliferative and environmental factors on the toxicity of mitomycin to tumor cells in vitro. Int J Cancer. 1986;38:229–35.
56. Guadagni S, Aigner KR, Palumbo G, et al. Pharmacokinetics of mitomycin C in pelvic stop-flow infusion and hypoxic pelvic perfusion with and without hemofiltration: a pilot study of patients with recurrent unresectable rectal cancer. J Clin Pharmacol. 1998;38:936–44.
57. Suzuki K, Gunderson LL, Devine RM, et al. Intraoperative irradiation after palliative surgery for locally recurrent rectal cancer. Cancer. 1995;75:939–52.
58. Graham RA, Siddik ZH, Hohn DC. Extracorporeal hemofiltration: a model for degreasing systemic drug exposure with intraarterial chemotherapy. Cancer Chemother Pharmacol. 1990;26:210–4.
59. Door RT. New findings in the pharmacokinetic metabolic and drug resistance aspects of mitomycin C. Semin Oncol. 1998;15:32–41.
60. Guadagni S, Fiorentini G, Palumbo G, et al. Hypoxic pelvic perfusion with mitomycin C using a simplified balloon-occlusion technique in the treatment of patients with unresectable locally recurrent rectal cancer. Arch Surg. 2001;136:105–12.
61. Strocchi E, Iaffaioli RV, Facchini G, et al. Stop-flow technique for loco-regional delivery of high dose chemotherapy in the treatment of advanced pelvic cancers. EJSO. 2004;30:663–70.
62. Murata S, Onozawa S, Kim C, et al. Negative-balance isolated pelvic perfusion in patients with incurable symptomatic rectal cancer: results and drug dose correlation to adverse events. Acta Radiol. 2014;55:793–801.
63. Hengelberg H. Actions of heparin that may affect the malignant process. Cancer. 1999;85:257–72.
64. Fuchs CS, Moore MR, Harker G, Villa L, Rinaldi D, Hecht JR. Phase III comparison of two irinotecan dosing regimens in second-line therapy of metastatic colorectal cancer. J Clin Oncol. 2003;21:807–14.
65. Carrato A, Gallego J, Diaz-Rubio E. Oxaliplatin: results in colorectal carcinoma. Crit Rev Oncol Hematol. 2002;44:29–44.
66. Pilati P, Mocellin D, Miotto D, et al. Stop-flow technique for loco-regional delivery of antiblastic agents: literature review and personal experience. Eur J Surg Oncol. 2002;28:544–53.
67. Guadagni S, Fiorentini G, D'Alessandro V, et al. Intrahepatic artery high-dose chemotherapy with concomitant post-hepatic venous blood detoxification: comparison between drug removal systems. Reg Cancer Treat. 1995;8:140–50.
68. Aigner KR, Gailhofer S. High dose MMC: aortic stopflow infusion (ASI) with versus without chemofiltration: a comparison of toxic side effects (abstract). Reg Cancer Treat. 1993;6 Suppl 1:3.
69. Sauer R, Becker H, Hohemberger W, et al. Preoperative versus postoperative chemoradiotherapy for rectal cancer. N Engl J Med. 2004;351:1731–40.

70. Peeters KC, van de Velde CJ, Leer JW, et al. Late side effects of short-course preoperative radiotherapy combined with total mesorectal excision for rectal cancer: increased bowel dysfunction in irradiated patients – a Dutch colorectal cancer group study. J Clin Oncol. 2005;23:6199–206.
71. Marijnen CA, Kapiteijn E, van de Velde CJ, et al. Acute side effects and complications after short-term preoperative radiotherapy combined with total mesorectal excision in primary rectal cancer: report of a multicenter randomized trial. J Clin Oncol. 2002;20:817–25.
72. Fung-Kee-Fung S. Therapeutic approaches in the management of locally advanced rectal cancer. J Gastrointest Oncol. 2014;5:353–61.

Isolated Pelvic Perfusion with Chemofiltration for Pelvic Malignancies: Anal, Cervical, and Bladder Cancer

21

Karl Reinhard Aigner, Sabine Gailhofer, and Giuseppe Zavattieri

21.1 Introduction

Cancers in the pelvis are treated stage dependent according to guidelines. In early stages some cancers like cervical, bladder, or anal carcinoma may be cured; however, already after slight progression, local occult micro- or lymph node metastases may be present and be the source of later recurrence or even distant disseminated disease. In such cases radical resections are no longer radical because of microinvasion behind the resection margins, and the more local tumor progression becomes evident, the more therapies are intensified until a point is reached where therapy-related toxicity may outweigh clinical benefit and quality of life. Far advanced cervical, bladder, and anal cancers invading the pelvis may cause such problems.

21.2 Cervical Cancer

After breast cancer, cervical cancer is the second most common cause of cancer-related death, in women worldwide. In Western countries some 40,000 women die from advanced cervical cancer per year, in developing countries about six times as many. This dismal outcome in a highly preventable cancer can be improved by consistent early diagnosis in terms of Papanicolaou screening. Early-stage cervical cancer can be cured by surgery or radiotherapy alone. Advanced tumors, however, are at great risk of recurrence and account for the vast majority of deaths from cervical cancer. Therefore, the key to improve cure rates in cervical cancer consists of two components – first, enhancement of early diagnosis, which basically is manageable if resource settings are improved, and, second, improvement of treatments in

K.R. Aigner, MD (✉) • S. Gailhofer • G. Zavattieri
Department of Surgical Oncology, Medias Klinikum GmbH & Co KG, Krankenhausstrasse 3a, Burghausen 84489, Germany
e-mail: info@prof-aigner.de

© Springer-Verlag Berlin Heidelberg 2016
K.R. Aigner, F.O. Stephens (eds.), *Induction Chemotherapy*,
DOI 10.1007/978-3-319-28773-7_21

advanced cases with the goal to improve the therapeutic impact in terms of overall survival and quality of life. Another valuable endpoint might be therapy at reduced cost as compared to already existing treatments.

21.3   Therapy of Advanced Cervical Cancer

Therapy of advanced cervical cancer largely depends on the stage at the time of first diagnosis. Irradiation plays the major role in tumors restricted to the pelvic area. Concomitant chemotherapy with cisplatin reduces the relative risk of death by approximately 50 % by decreasing local pelvic failure and distant metastases [1–5]. Stage Ib2 lesions with tumors confined to the cervix can be treated with surgery alone, but the chances of adequate treatment are only 12 % [6]. As a consequence primary stage Ib2 tumors of more than 4 cm in diameter without invasion of the parametria are already considered advanced disease that requires postoperative adjuvant radiotherapy or radiochemotherapy. Thus there is an indication for radiochemotherapy in all stages from stage Ib2 with tumors of more than 4 cm in diameter to stage IVa with invasion of the bladder or/and rectum. Even if pelvic exenteration might be taken into account for stage IVa disease, not invading the pelvic side wall without evidence of spread beyond the pelvis, the standard of care for downsizing is induction chemotherapy combined with external beam irradiation and intracavitary brachytherapy, in order to minimize the risk of relapse [7].

21.4   Brachytherapy

Intracavitary brachytherapy is the unique tool that makes it possible to apply effective doses of radiotherapy to affect advanced cervical cancer, much more than with external beam irradiation. Depending on stage and pattern of metastatic dissemination in locally advanced disease, it is combined with external beam irradiation. Nevertheless, radiotherapy alone fails to control progression in 35–90 % [8].

In modern new dosimetric systems, the radioactive sources are distributed in an applicator in defined doses to a designated treatment volume. Since brachytherapy is the only means to induce substantial and long-lasting remission due to extremely high local exposure to radiotherapy, every attempt should be made to deliver tumoricidal doses, even if the vulnerable adjacent tissues receive a slightly higher dose [9, 10]. Risk-adapted dosimetry, however, is not safe or precise enough to exclude collateral damage to adjacent tissues, and after a tumoricidal local dose has been administered, the risk of collateral damage cannot be excluded. Irrespective of its firm position in treatment programs, until recently with no better alternative, brachytherapy, in terms of toxicity, should not be trivialized. As long as there is nothing less toxic, patients have to cope with the impact of radical radiation on bladder, rectal, psychosocial, and sexual function, with sometimes severe secondary effects like lymphedema of the legs; stenosis of the ureters, requiring stents or kidney fistulas; and, last but not least, rectovaginal or vesico-vaginal fistulas that reduce quality of life to a minimum [11, 12].

21.5 Intra-arterial Infusion Chemotherapy

The goal of regional chemotherapy is to improve the efficacy of cytostatic drugs without causing additional discomfort to the patient [13]. In chemosensitive tumors like cervical cancer, regional chemotherapy can generate much higher local drug exposure at low toxicity than systemic chemotherapy.

So far, there are only few studies addressing this concept. In a trial comprising 12 patients in clinical stages I–IIb with tumors beyond 4 cm in diameter, intra-arterial infusion via the uterine artery in 7 out of 12 cases induced a tumor mass reduction of more than 50 % of the initial volume after only two treatment cycles [14]. In another study, where intra-arterial infusion chemotherapy with cisplatin, adriamy-cin, and melphalan was administered via both internal iliac arteries, a remission induction of 65 % was achieved, 8.3 % (4/48 patients) of which were complete remissions and the remainder partial remissions. In two cases of complete remissions, this was also confirmed histologically [15].

A trial of intra-arterial infusion of cisplatin via hypogastric arteries was performed in 25 patients with advanced (14/25 patients) or recurrent (11/25 patients) cervical cancer. Forty milligrams of cisplatin was infused over 60 min on each side. Eleven of the 14 patients (78 %) showed a good response and had radical hysterectomy, lymph-adenectomy, and external beam radiation thereafter. In patients with recurrent disease, the overall response rate was 36 %. Pain relief was obtained in all patients. After a mean follow-up of 23 months, no pelvic recurrence had occurred [16].

Considering these data against the background of intensive radiotherapy, it seems obvious that achievement of optimal results without the threat of imminent toxicity is closely related to the optimal dosage and drug exposure in regional chemotherapy.

21.6 Isolated Pelvic Perfusion

Drug exposure can best be controlled with isolation perfusion techniques. Isolation of the pelvis is carried out via an arterial and venous femoral access. Both femoral vessels are cannulated with so-called stop-flow balloon catheters, which, after injec-tion of chemotherapeutics into the arterial catheter, are blocked above the bifurca-tion of the aorta and vena cava. Isolation of the pelvis is completed by means of upper thigh pneumatic cuffs (Fig. 21.1). After a 15 min isolation perfusion and deflation of the blocks, the drug levels in the systemic blood circulation are dimin-ished by means of chemofiltration. Consequently, by reducing systemic peak levels of drugs, systemic toxicity and side effects are alleviated. Local damage in pelvic organs does not occur and quality of life is usually undisturbed.

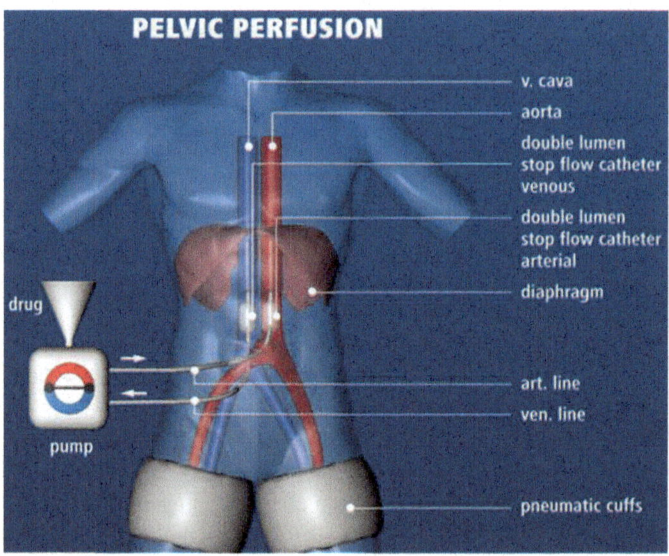

Fig. 21.1 Triple-channel balloon catheters are introduced via the femoral vessels, and the balloons blocked above the pelvic bifurcation of the aorta and vena cava. The upper thighs are blocked with pneumatic cuffs. After a 15 min drug exposure, chemofiltration is started via the deblocked arterial and venous catheters

In a patient with advanced stage IVa disease with tumor invasion of the bladder, lymph nodes, and both parametria, a histologically complete remission after hysterectomy was revealed after four courses of isolated pelvic perfusion with cisplatin, adriamycin, and mitomycin. There was no significant systemic or local toxicity, and the patient is in continuing complete remission after 10 years [17].

21.7 Bladder Cancer

Radical cystectomy is the recommended gold standard as primary treatment for patients with muscle-invasive bladder cancer. Alternative less invasive treatments are reserved only for patients with reduced performance status or extensive comorbid conditions. In patients with stage IV bladder cancers, the 5-year survival rate after radical cystectomy ranges from 0 % to 36 % [18]. In expert centers comparable outcomes are seen with bladder preservation using chemoradiotherapy protocols [21]. The rationale for giving induction chemotherapy before cystectomy or full-dose radiation therapy is to treat micrometastases present at diagnosis as 50 % of the patients in advanced stages develop metastatic disease within 2 years [19]. Thus induction chemotherapy provides a greater survival benefit than surgery or radiotherapy alone. Moreover, 50 % of patients who are considered to have undergone curative cystectomy develop local recurrence based on pathological examination [20, 22].

Regional chemotherapy with intra-arterial administration of drugs for advanced bladder cancer was reported already more than 30 years ago [23–25], but techniques and modes of application varied a lot, and new knowledge and experiences ever since have been continuously incorporated into the method [13, 17].

21.8   Hypoxic Pelvic Perfusion (HPP) with Chemofiltration (F) for Stage IIIb Bladder Cancer

In HPP-F chemotherapeutics are injected into the isolated circuit under hyperoxygenation and the isolated perfusion, as described herein, and then run under hypoxic condition. Advantage is taken from the increased cytotoxicity of adriamycin and mitomycin under hypoxic conditions. After 15 min of hypoxic perfusion, arterial and venous isolation blocks are released, and chemofiltration for systemic detoxification is started. Patients received four therapies in 4-week intervals each. The drug combination consisted of adriamycin, mitomycin, and cisplatin. Median survival in seven patients with stage IIIb cancers was 292 days (Fig. 21.2). One patient had two follow-up therapies for relapse after 1 year and has been disease-free ever since for 22 years.

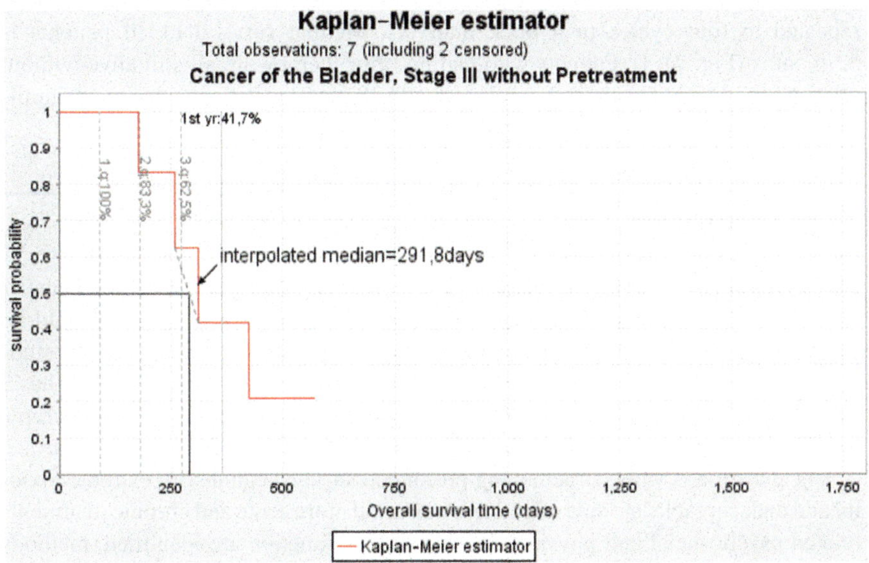

Fig. 21.2 Kaplan-Meier estimate. Total observations 7 (incl. two censored). Isolated hypoxic perfusion for bladder cancer stage IIIb

21.9 Muscle-Invasive Carcinoma of the Anal Canal

Concomitant chemoradiotherapy is the current standard of care [26]; however with regard to best clinical long-term results, several randomized clinical trials [28–31] define different primary and secondary endpoints such as disease-free survival (DFS), following surgery when there is no detectable tumor, progression-free survival with disease at baseline, or colostomy-free survival (CFS). Depending on clinical stage and tumor invasion, tumor-related colostomy rates amount to 26 % and treatment-related colostomy rates to 8 % [27]. Since CFS and DFS in the literature in times are mixed up and compared freely in the same way, along with variable endpoints, studies are not really comparable. One important parameter, quality of life (QoL), is not specifically reported in any trial. Especially, so far there is no pelvic radiotherapy-associated long-term QoL report from patient questionnaires. In a study by Petersen [32] on quality of life in palliative treatment, patients rated their quality of life worse than doctors did. As doctors may make a biased assessment, patients need to be interviewed too.

21.10 Isolated Hypoxic Pelvic Perfusion with Chemofiltration (HPP-F) for Advanced Carcinoma of the Anal Canal

Scheme of isolated perfusion is as described above. Seventeen patients (five were stage IV, four stage IIIb, one stage II, and two stage I and five had recurrent disease and 5/17 no prior therapy) underwent isolated perfusion with the three-drug combination CDDP, MMC, and ADM given as bolus into the isolated circuit. Therapy was repeated in four cycles in 4-week intervals. Median survival of all patients is 32 months (Fig. 21.3). Patients who had no prior therapy are all still alive without relapse for 271 (G3 tumor!), 197, 176, 42, and 28 months. Patients, due to chemofiltration, did not suffer side effects and no patient had a colostomy.

21.11 Discussion

The predominant role of radiotherapy in the treatment of advanced cervical cancer is derived from the unique tumoricidal effect of brachytherapy, which should be considered a "locoregional" therapy in terms of irradiation. So far, there are no studies of adequately effective treatment modalities, and therefore brachytherapy has a firm place in treatment protocols of cervical cancer. Locally enhanced radiotherapy, despite its effectiveness, bears a risk of severe local toxicity.

The question is whether achieving prolonged survival can justify extreme toxicity and unacceptable late side effects. As more and more acute and chronic treatment-related psychosocial and physical distress and dysfunction are identified, methods are desperately needed to reduce these adverse effects and toxicities [8]. If dose-intense radiotherapy could be completely or partially replaced by a less toxic but equally effective localized therapy, avoiding late irreversible side effects, patients would benefit greatly in terms of quality of life. This underscores the need for an equally potent but less toxic alternative.

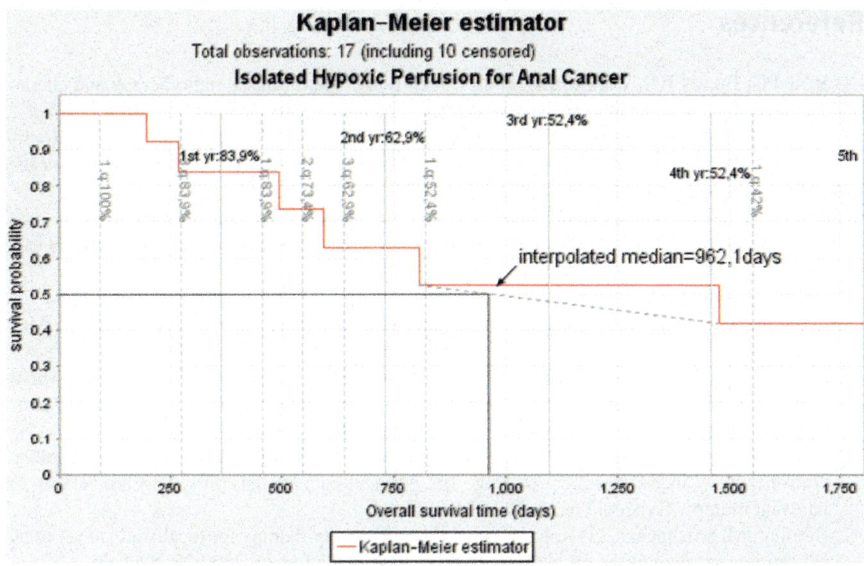

Fig. 21.3 Kaplan-Meier estimate. Total observations 17 (incl. ten censored). Isolated hypoxic perfusion for anal cancer

Regional chemotherapy might be an option, but so far there is little experience in small studies [14–16] that do report promising results in terms of response rates and survival. Until now, intra-arterial chemotherapy has not been performed with uniform evidence-based protocols; however, regardless of which mode of application is chosen, results have been remarkable. It is noteworthy that intra-arterial infusion of pelvic arteries, as reported in the de Dycker study, may induce a complete remission induction of 23 months and more without causing any major toxicity. Another most important aspect in regional induction chemotherapy for cervical cancer is immediate tumor shrinkage after one to two cycles [14, 15]. Downsizing of locally advanced cancers to operability is observed in most cases, which makes intra-arterial induction chemotherapy appear to be comparable to brachytherapy, however, without collateral damage to adjacent tissues.

It therefore remains a challenge to determine the optimal mode of administering regional induction chemotherapy as intra-arterial infusion or isolated perfusion. The latter certainly requires experience in vascular infusion and perfusion techniques, but can be extremely effective and induce total tumor necrosis.

Therefore, a controlled study, clarifying whether regional chemotherapy can induce the same long-term results as external beam radiation and brachytherapy without causing local damage and intolerable toxicity, is more than overdue.

There is a comparable situation with advanced bladder cancer and anal carcinoma. The latter tumor is treated according to firm evidence-based schedules, but this does not exclude innovative treatment modalities despite lack of large controlled studies. Especially in anal carcinoma which is highly responsive to high exposure of chemotherapy in an isolated circuit, there was no need for colostomy, and patients enjoy a long-lasting disease- and side-effect-free survival.

References

1. Rose PG, Bundy BN, Watkins EB, et al. Concurrent cisplatin-based radiotherapy and chemotherapy for locally advanced cervical cancer. N Engl J Med. 1999;340:1144–53.
2. Peters III WA, Liu PY, Barret Jr RJ, et al. Concurrent chemotherapy and pelvic radiation therapy compared with pelvic radiation therapy alone as adjuvant therapy after radical surgery in high-risk early-stage cancer of the cervix. J Clin Oncol. 2000;18:1606–13.
3. Keys HM, Bundy BN, Stehman FB, et al. Cisplatin, radiation and adjuvant hysterectomy compared with radiation and adjuvant hysterectomy for bulky stage IB cervical carcinoma. N Engl J Med. 1999;340:1154–61.
4. Morris M, Eifel PJ, Lu J, et al. Pelvic irradiation with concurrent chemotherapy compared with pelvic and para-aortic radiation for high-risk cervical cancer. N Engl J Med. 1999;340:1137–43.
5. Eifel PJ, Winter K, Morris M, et al. Pelvic irradiation with concurrent chemotherapy versus pelvic and para-aortic irradiation for high-risk cervical cancer: an update of Radiation Therapy Oncology Group trial (RTOG) 90–01. J Clin Oncol. 2004;22:872–80.
6. Yessaian A, Magistris A, Burger RA, et al. Radical hysterectomy followed by tailored postoperative therapy in the treatment of stage Ib2 cervical cancer: feasibility and indications for adjuvant therapy. Gynecol Oncol. 2004;94:61–6.
7. Bradley JM, Krishnansu ST, Koh W-J, et al. Multimodality therapy for locally advanced cervical carcinoma: state of the art and future directions. J Clin Oncol. 2007;25:2952–65.
8. Monk BJ, Tewari KS, Koh W-J. Multimodality therapy for locally advanced cervical carcinoma: state of the art and future directions. J Clin Oncol. 2007;25:2952–65.
9. Petereit DG, Pearcey R. Literature analysis of high dose rate brachytherapy fractionation schedules in the treatment of cervical cancer: is there an optimal fractionation schedule? Int J Radiat Oncol Biol Phys. 1999;43:359–66.
10. Mai J, Erickson B, Rownd J, et al. Comparison of four different dose specification methods for high-dose-rate intracavitary radiation for treatment of cervical cancer. Int J Radiat Oncol Biol Phys. 2001;51:1131–41.
11. Vistad I, Fossa SD, Dahl AA. A critical review of patient-rated quality of life studies of long-term survivors of cervical cancer. Gynecol Oncol. 2006;102:563–73.
12. Wenzel L, DeAlba I, Habal R, et al. Quality of life in long-term cervical cancer survivors. Gynecol Oncol. 2005;97:310–7.
13. Stephens FO. Why use regional chemotherapy? Principles and pharmacokinetics. Reg Cancer Treat. 1988;1:4–10.
14. Villena-Heinsen C, Mink D, Lung-Kurt S, et al. Preoperative intraarterial chemotherapy for bulky cervical carcinoma in stage Ib–IIb. Reg Cancer Treat. 1994;1:17–21.
15. Scarabelli C, Zarrelli A, Gallo A, et al. Pelvic recurrences in cervical cancer: multimodal treatment with sequential intra-arterial chemotherapy and surgery. Reg Cancer Treat. 1994;1:12–6.
16. de Dycker RP. Pelvic arterial chemotherapy in cervical cancer. Reg Cancer Treat. 1994;7:43–6.
17. Aigner KR, Gailhofer S. Six years disease free survival after isolated hypoxic pelvic perfusion with chemofiltration for advanced cervical carcinoma. J Nucl Med Radiat Ther. 2012. http://dx.doi.org/10.4172/2155-9619.S2-007.
18. Gore JL, Litwin MS, Lai J, et al. Use of radical cystectomy for patients with invasive bladder cancer. J Natl Cancer Inst. 2010;102(11):802–11.
19. Sternberg CN. Hospital San Camillo-Forlanini, Rome, Italy. Apolo AB. Centter for Cancer Research, National Cancer Institue, National Cancer Institues of Health, Bethesda, MD. Everythingt old is new again! Neoadjuvant chemotehrapy in the treatment of muscle-invasive bladder cancer. Clin Oncol. 2014;55:4055.
20. Mambrini A, Fiorentini G, Zamagni D et al. Intra-arterial chemiotherapy for invasive bladder Cancer J Exp Clin Cancer Res. 2003;22:4. Supplement.

21. Siegel R, Naishadham D, Jemal A. Cancer statistics, 2013. CA Cancer J Clin. 2013;63:11–30.
22. Ennis RD, Petrylak DP, Singh P, et al. The effect of cystectomy and perioperative methotrexate, vinblastine, doxorubicin and cisplatin chemotherapy on the risk and pattern of relapse in patients with muscle invasive bladder cancer. J Urol. 2000;163:1413–8.
23. Wallace S, Chuang VP, Samuels M, et al. Transcatheter intraarterial infusion of chemotherapy in advanced bladder cancer. Cancer. 1982;49:640–5.
24. Logothetis CJ, Samuels ML, Wallace S, et al. Management of pelvic complications of malignant urothelial tumors with combined intra-arterial and i.v. chemotherapy. Cancer Treat Rep. 1982;66:1501–7.
25. Nakazono M, Iwata S. Pre-operative intra-arterial chemotherapy for bladder cancer. Urol Exp. 1981;9:289–95.
26. Northover J, Glynne-Jones R, Sebag-Montefiore D, et al. Chemoradiation for the treatment of epidermoid anal cancer: 13-year follow-up of the first randomised UKCCCR Anal Cancer Trial (ACTI). Br J Cancer. 2010;102:1123–8.
27. Sunesen KG, Norgaard M, Lundby L, et al. Cause-specific colostomy rates after radiotherapy for anal cancer: a Danish multicentre cohort study. J Clin Oncol. 2011;29:3535–40.
28. UKCCCR. Anal cancer working party: epidermoid anal cancer: results from the UKCCCR randomised trial of radiotherapy alone versus radiotherapy, 5-fluorouracil and mitomycin. Lancet. 1996;348:1049–54.
29. Cartelink H, Roloefson F, Eschwege F, et al. Concomitant radiotherapy and chemotherapy is superior to radiotherapy alone in the treatment of locally advanced anal cancer: results of a phase III randomized trial of the European Organization for Research and Treatment of Cancer Radiotherapy and Gastrointestinal Cooperative Groups. J Clin Oncol. 1997;15:2040–9.
30. Flam M, John M, Pajak TF, et al. Role of mitomycin in combination with fluorouracil and radiotherapy, and of chemoradiation in the definitive nonsurgical treatment of epidermoid carcinoma of the anal canal: results of a phase III randomized intergroup study. J Clin Oncol. 1996;14:2527–39.
31. Ajani JA, Winter KA, Gunderson LL, et al. Fluorouracil, mitomycin and radiotherapy vs fluorouracil, cisplatin and radiotherapy for carcinoma of the anal canal: a randomised controlled trial. JAMA. 2008;199:1914–21.
32. Petersen MA, Larsen H, Pedersen L, et al. Assessing health-related quality of life in palliative care: comparing patient and physician assessments. Eur J Cancer. 2006;42:1159–66.

Penile Cancer Treated by Intra-arterial Infusion Chemotherapy

22

Maw-Chang Sheen

22.1 Introduction

Carcinoma of the penis is an uncommon malignancy in developed countries. However, it accounts for up to 20 % of all male cancers in some undeveloped countries [8, 19]. The penis is small in proportion to the rest of the body; however, it has very important functions and bears the symbol of manhood. For penile carcinoma the treatment most commonly employed is partial or total penectomy with or without inguinal lymphadenectomy. In most cases, the amputation of the penis is followed by difficult psychosexual problems and greatly affects the quality of life. Therefore, a lot of patients hesitated to seek treatment. As a result, the disease is advanced when the patient is first seen. Penile carcinoma spreads locally and disseminates mainly to lymph nodes in the groin and the pelvis. Distant metastases are rare and usually late. Lower abdominal aortic infusion chemotherapy has the main advantage of delivering a very high concentration of anticancer drug to the whole pelvic area to induce rapid shrinkage of the primary lesion and the metastatic lymph nodes. This is of major importance in the treatment of this localized lesion. In order to avoid anatomical and functional deficits, intra-arterial infusion chemotherapy was used in penile carcinoma.

22.2 Materials

From 1985 to 2009, 30 cases of previously untreated penile carcinoma were referred for intra-arterial infusion chemotherapy. They consisted of squamous cell carcinoma in 19 (63 %), verrucous carcinoma in 6 (20 %), carcinoma in situ in 3 (10 %),

M.-C. Sheen, MD
Division of Surgical Oncology, Department of Surgery, Faculty of Medicine, College of Medicine, Kaohsiung Medical University Hospital,
100 Tz You 1st Road, Kaohsiung 807, Taiwan
e-mail: sheenmc@kmu.edu.tw

© Springer-Verlag Berlin Heidelberg 2016
K.R. Aigner, F.O. Stephens (eds.), *Induction Chemotherapy*,
DOI 10.1007/978-3-319-28773-7_22

papillary adenocarcinoma in 1 (3 %), and Paget's disease in 1 (3 %). The median age was 56.5 years (range, 27–94 years; mean, 56.6 years). The anatomic site was distributed as follows: glans in 13 (43 %), glans and prepuce in 3 (10 %), coronal sulcus in 4 (13 %), shaft in 6 (20 %), and whole penis in 4 (13 %). The median duration of symptoms was 9 months, which varied from glans mass for 1 month to erythematous infiltrative plaque on the shaft for 30 years. All patients were classified according to the International Union Against Cancer (UICC) 2002 classification. Of the 18 evaluable cases of squamous cell carcinoma, 7 (39%) were T1 tumors, 6 (33%) T2, and 5 (28%) T4. Eight cases were grade 1 (44.5 %), eight (44.5 %) grade 2, and two grade 3 (11 %). The N-classification was distributed as follows: 7(37%) patients with N0, 1 (5 %) with N1, and 11 (58 %) with N2. The assessment of the extent of regional lymph node involvement was by physical examination and imaging procedures which were relatively inaccurate. Swelling of regional lymph nodes as a result of secondary infection is frequent, and lymphatic metastases are histologically detected in only about 45 % of such cases [8]. The distribution of patients by TNM stage was as follows: stage I, four patients (22 %); stage II, four patients (22 %); stage III, seven patients (39 %); and stage IV, three patients (17 %). Because penile verrucous carcinoma seldom metastasizes into regional nodes or distant areas, only the tumor character is shown in Table 22.3.

22.3 Methods

A 90-cm-long Jet Port Plus Allround catheter with an inner diameter of 0.60 mm and an outer diameter of 1.05 mm (PFM, Cologne, Germany) was used for catheterization. The catheter was inserted through the lateral circumflex branch of the profound femoral artery retrograde into the abdominal aorta with the tip of the catheter placed at the level of the third lumbar vertebra which was confirmed by X-ray. Patent blue V (Guebet, France) was injected through the catheter to further confirm the adequacy of tumor perfusion. After the catheter was properly placed and fixed, the distal end was connected to the port, which was implanted subcutaneously lateral and inferior to the umbilicus. Before 1990 when implantable arterial port-catheter was not available, Teflon catheters with an inner diameter of 0.5 mm and an outer diameter of 1 mm were used for catheterization.

Initially, the patients were infused continuously with 50 mg methotrexate every 24 h using a portable pump (CADD-1, Deltec, St. Paul, Minn, USA). Before 1990, Sharp MP 22 portable pumps made in Japan were used. Citrovorum factor (6 mg) was given intramuscularly every 6 h during the period of methotrexate infusion. Commencing in 2005, citrovorum factor (15 mg) was given intramuscularly every 12 h. The median continuous infusion period was 10 days (range 6–16 days). Then, all patients were followed closely at an outpatient clinic. After completion of continuous infusion, no further anticancer was given to complete responders. The partial responders subsequently received long-term, intermittent, intra-arterial infusion of 2 mg mitomycin C and 250 mg 5-fluorouracil or 50 mg methotrexate every 1–2 weeks until all tumors disappeared and all wounds had healed. Cisplatin, bleomycin, and Pharmorubicin which may cause more side effects were reserved for partial responders not responding to the above treatment. Only one case with carcinoma in situ received intermittent bleomycin infusion instead of continuous methotrexate infusion because of low WBC and PLT before treatment.

22.4 Results

The response was assessed by visual inspection and palpation during the treatment period. A complete response (CR) was defined as complete clinical disappearance of the tumor. A partial response (PR) was a greater than 50 % reduction in size of the tumor. Progressive disease (PD) was a greater than 25 % increase of the local tumor or appearance of new lesion. Local tumor responses that did not meet any of the preceding definitions were designated as stable disease (SD). After treatment, 29 cases were evaluable. In our early experience of treating penile carcinoma, one 42-year-old patient died suddenly and unexpectedly 3 days after discontinuing the 8-day continuous infusion. This case was excluded. The patient who received bleomycin infusion instead of methotrexate was evaluated separately. After methotrexate infusion, 14 (50 %) of 28 patients had complete response (CR), 11 (39 %) had partial response (PR), and three (11 %) had no response (NR) (Table 22.1). Of the 18 squamous cell carcinomas, eight (44 %) had complete response, eight (44 %) had partial response, and two (11 %) had no response (Table 22.2). Four (67 %) of the six verrucous carcinomas had complete response, and two had partial response (Table 22.3). For complete responders, the preservation of the organ and function was excellent. Needless amputations were avoided.

In this limited case study, verrucous carcinoma has a higher complete response rate than squamous cell carcinoma (67 % vs. 44 %). For squamous cell carcinoma, a lower grade and earlier stage tumor responded better to therapy. All complete responders except two were living recurrence-free between 1 year 7 months and 24 years 10 months after initial therapy at the time of follow-up (October 2010). One complete responder, a 36-year-old with squamous cell carcinoma (T1, G1),

Table 22.1 Results of intra-arterial infusion with methotrexate in penile carcinoma (1985–2010)

Tumor/response		CR	PR	NR
Squamous cell carcinoma	18[a]	8 (44 %)	8 (44 %)	2 (11 %)
Verrucous carcinoma	6	4 (67 %)	2 (33 %)	–
Carcinoma in situ	2[b]	2	–	–
Paget's disease	1	–	1	–
Papillary adenocarcinoma	1	–	–	1
Total	28	14 (50 %)	11 (39 %)	3 (11 %)

Follow-up October 2010
[a]One patient died suddenly 3 days after MTX infusion was excluded
[b]One case received bleomycin infusion was excluded

Table 22.2 Results of intra-arterial infusion with methotrexate in penile squamous cell carcinoma

Tumor/response	CR	PR	NR
Anatomic site			
Glans	3	6	1
Sulcus	2	1	
Shaft	1	1	
Whole penis	2		1
Histologic grade			
1	5	3	
2	3	3	2
3		2	
Tumor stage			
1	5	2	
2	1	4	1
3			
4	2	2	1
Stage I	3	1	
II	1	2	1
III	2	4	1
IV	2	1	
Total 18	8 (44 %)	8 (44 %)	2 (11 %)

Follow-up October 2010

One patient died suddenly 3 days after MTX infusion was excluded

Table 22.3 Results and side effects of intra-arterial infusion with methotrexate in penile verrucous carcinoma (1991–2010)

Case	Age year/old	Tumor location and size (cm)	Symptom duration	MTX (mg)	Results (survival)	Reasons to stop continuous infusion
1	27	Glans (5×5)	1 year	500	CR >19 years	Skin rash, itching
2	65	Glans (4×3)	3 months	600	CR >14 years 11 months	PLT 96×10³/UL (Nadir 62× 10³/ UL)
3	31	Shaft (5×5)	4 years	500	PR + penectomy >13 years 7 months	WBC 2.76×10³/ UL (Nadir)
4	75	Glans (2×2)	10 year	400	CR >9 years 10 months	Skin rash, itching,
5	47	Gland, prepuce (4×3)	3 months	550	PR + penectomy 3 years 1 month	Skin rash, itching,
6	28	Gland prepuce (5×4)	6 years	650	–	Skin rash, itching,
				450	–	GOT GPT increase
				800	CR >4 years 11 months	GOT GPT increase

Follow-up October 2010

developed recurrence 4 years and 5 months after complete response and showed partial response to further treatment. He died 2.5 years later. The other patient with carcinoma in situ died of a non-cancer-related disease 8 years and 2 months after treatment. Of eight squamous cell carcinomas, the survival time of complete responders was between 1 year 7 months and 24 years 10 months (three patients more than 20 years, two patients more than 10 years, two patients more than 5 years). Partial responses were not good enough; they were of short duration in spite of further continuous methotrexate infusions and intermittent infusion with various drugs including cisplatin (20–30 mg), epirubicin (20 mg), mitomycin C (4–8 mg), and bleomycin (15–30 mg) after initial therapy. Of the 14 penile carcinoma with partial or no response to methotrexate infusion, two were lost at follow-up, and seven patients died with a survival time ranging between 5 months and 2 and a half years (median 1 year). Four patients received penectomy subsequently. Two of them were still living: one verrucous carcinoma living 13 years 7 months and one squamous cell carcinoma 1 year 1 month after initial treatment. The other squamous cell carcinoma case died of a non-cancer-related disease 5 years after penectomy. One verrucous carcinoma transformed into invasive squamous cell carcinoma and died 3 years 1 month after treatment start. The 94-year-old patient with extramammary Paget's disease had partial response to methotrexate infusion (Fig. 22.7). Biopsy from the lesion still revealed residual cancer. He received intermittent infusion with mitomycin C (2 mg) plus 5 FU (250 mg) or methotrexate (25–50 mg) every 1–2 weeks at our outpatient clinic with stable disease until died of non-cancer-related disease at the age of 100 (2011). A 72-year-old man with carcinoma in situ that received bleomycin infusion rather than methotrexate had partial response to therapy. The tumor degenerated into squamous cell carcinoma (grade 2) 2 years after treatment. The tumor showed partial response to 5 FU infusions. The patient died of a non-cancer-related disease 1 year and 2 months later.

The observed drug side effects after continuous methotrexate infusion were skin rash (75 %), increase of GOT and GPT (36 %), leucopenia (36 %), thrombocytopenia (29 %), malaise (21 %), anorexia (18 %), nausea (14 %), fever (7 %), and diarrhea (7 %). The reasons to stop continuous methotrexate infusion were skin rash (21 %), thrombocytopenia (21 %), increase of GOT and GPT (21 %), leucopenia (18 %), wound infection (11 %), and malaise (7 %). Twenty-five cases (89 %) had grade 1–2 side effects according to WHO classification. Two cases (7 %) had grade 3 leucopenia and increase of GOT and GPT. One case (4 %) had grade 4 leucopenia. During the long-term intermittent infusions for partial responders, vomiting after cisplatin and palm erythema after bleomycin were noted. These side effects were mild and tolerable even to the old-aged patients. Nine (30 %) of our patients were over 70 years old (range, 70–94; median 75 years).

For patients with poor general condition or older age, methotrexate should be administered with caution. No major complications relating to port-catheter implantation during the treatment course were noted. However, inguinal wound infection and femoral arterial pseudoaneurysm were noted in a case of a 65-year-old verrucous carcinoma patient 4 months after treatment. The wound healed uneventfully after port-catheter removal, aneurysmectomy, and debridement.

22.5 Discussion

Surgery for penile carcinoma has ranged from partial (T1 >2 cm, T2, distal) to total (T2, proximal, T3, T4) penectomy which would be followed by anatomical, psychological, and functional disability [8, 19]. To avoid penile loss with extensive surgical resection, in the past a number of treatment modalities have been attempted including Mohs micrographic surgery, laser therapy (CO2 or neodymium:yttrium-aluminum-garnet (Nd-YAG) [7], cryosurgery [1], and interferon either systemically or intralesionally [5, 6]. However, the conservative organ-sparing treatments were recommended only for verrucous carcinoma and early-stage (T1) low- or intermediate-grade squamous cell carcinoma of the penis [8, 19]. Both external beam radiation therapy and brachytherapy have been used to preserve sexual function, but urethral stricture, skin change, and even penile atrophy or necrosis may ensue [2, 3]. Radiotherapy is controversial for verrucous carcinoma because of the potential malignant transformation and metastasis [4]. Systemic chemotherapy has had very limited application in advanced penile carcinoma due to its short duration of response and its occasional association with mobility and mortality [10]. Penile carcinoma spreads locally and disseminates mainly to lymph nodes in the groin and the pelvis. Distant metastases are rare and usually late.

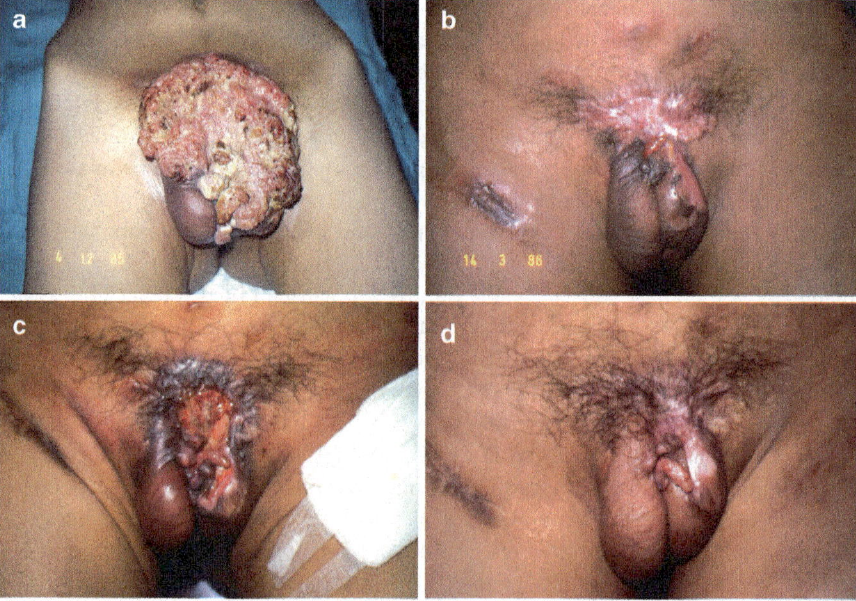

Fig. 22.1 Case 1: a 42-year-old patient with advanced penile squamous cell carcinoma (14×13 cm, T4N2M0, grade 2, stage IV). (**a**) Before treatment. (**b**) Three months after 450 mg methotrexate infusion. (**c**) Recurrent (8×4 cm) 9 months after complete response. (**d**) Three months after 700 mg methotrexate infusion. He is living recurrence-free 24 years and 10 months after treatment

Lower abdominal aortic infusion chemotherapy has the advantage of delivering a high concentration of anticancer drugs to the whole pelvic area to induce rapid shrinkage of the primary lesion and the metastatic lymph nodes. It was suitable even to T4 carcinoma [12, 15] (Figs. 22.1, 22.2 and 22.3). Our study of the serial light and electron microscopic changes of the primary tumor after initiation of intra-arterial infusion with methotrexate showed that the changes occurred early at the first day, both grossly and microscopically. The shrinkage of the mass is most obvious, on average, 1 week after initiation of the therapy. Under high local tissue methotrexate concentration by arterial infusion, a concurrent toxicity to the mitochondria may play an important role in the early stage of tumor necrosis [14, 15].

The well-defined hyperpigmentation of the infused region covering the external genitals and lower abdomen noted 17 days after the initiation of therapy showed the effect of a high methotrexate concentration to the skin (Fig. 22.4c). The skin over the port implantation area was less pigmented because of less vascularization after port insertion.

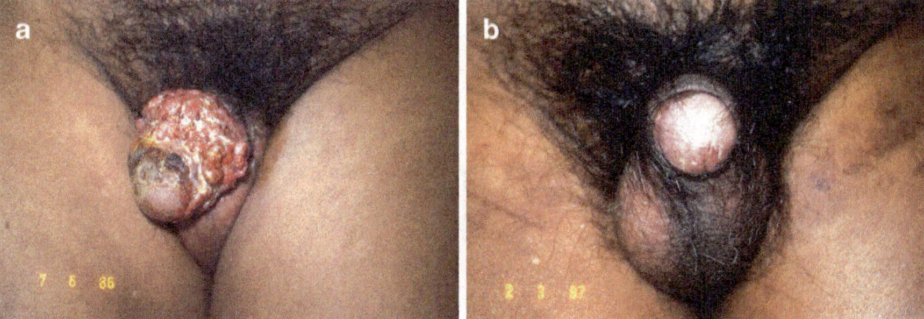

Fig 22.2 Case 2: a 52-year-old patient with penile squamous cell carcinoma (6×4 cm, T2N2M0, grade 2, stage III). (**a**) Before treatment. (**b**) Six months after treatment, the glans had healed with intact penis and intact sexual function. He is living recurrence-free 24 years and 2 months after treatment

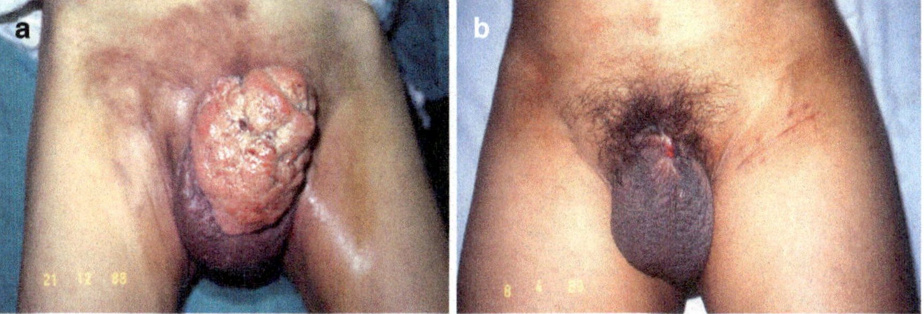

Fig. 22.3 Case 3: a 58-year-old patient with advanced penile squamous cell carcinoma (15×13 cm, T4N2M0, grade 1, stage IV). (**a**) Before treatment. (**b**) Three months after only 6 days of methotrexate (300 mg) infusion. No further anticancer drug was given. He is living recurrence-free 21 years and 10 months after treatment

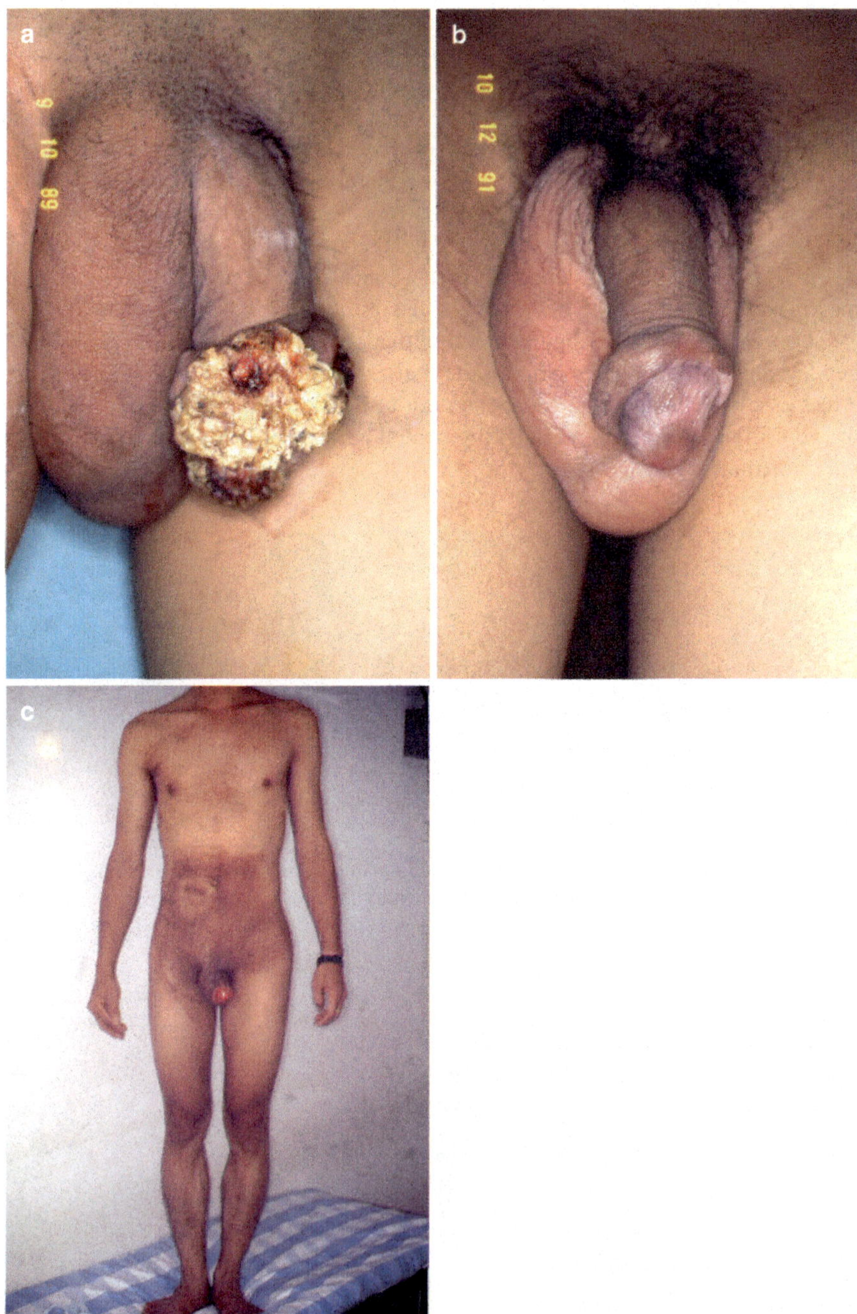

Fig. 22.4 Case 4: a 27-year-old single patient with penile glans verrucous carcinoma (5×5 cm). (**a**) Before treatment. (**b**) Two months after 10 days of methotrexate (500 mg) infusion. No further anticancer therapy was given. He got married 1 year and 10 months after treatment. He enjoyed a normal sexual life and has a child of 15 years. He is living recurrence-free 19 years after treatment. (**c**) Well-demarcated hyperpigmentation of the infusion region noted 17 days after therapy showed the effect of a high concentration to the skin

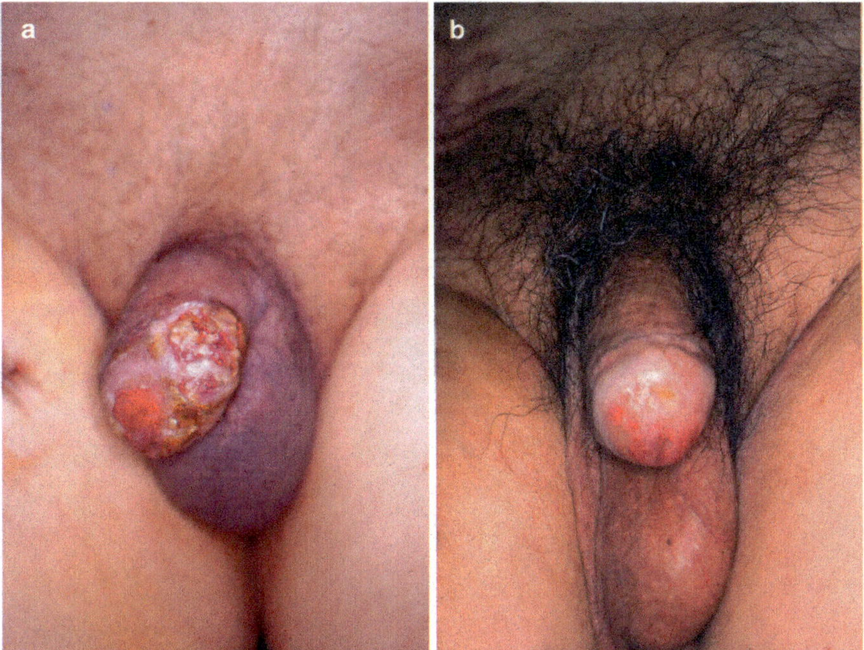

Fig. 22.5 Case 5: a 65-year-old patient with penile glans verrucous carcinoma (4×3 cm). (**a**) Before treatment. (**b**) 28 days after initiation of 10 days of methotrexate infusion. He is living recurrence-free 14 years and 11 month after treatment

Verrucous carcinoma is a distinctive variant of squamous cell carcinoma, characterized by slow growth and a locally aggressive nature, but it less commonly metastasizes into regional nodes or distant areas. From our previous studies, verrucous carcinoma of various sites including penis, oral cavity, and digit all showed excellent response to intra-arterial methotrexate infusion therapy [13, 16–18, 20]. After treatment, four of six patients with penile verrucous carcinoma had complete response. These four patients were living recurrence-free 19 years, 14 years 11 months, 9 years 10 months, and 4 years 11 months, respectively, after initial therapy (Table 22.3). Two patients aged 27 (case 4) and 28 (case 6) were both young and single. Case 4 was an only son and just engaged to be married. Their tumors were found accidentally following circumcision. These two patients refused penectomy and sought for penile-sparing therapy. Case 4 had complete response after only 10 days of methotrexate (500 mg) infusion. He got married 1 year and 10 months after treatment. He enjoyed a normal sexual life and has a child of 15 years [16]. The result of case 4 showed the uniqueness of not only the preservation of anatomic and sexual function integrity but also of fertility. In case 6 with prepuce verrucous carcinoma involving penile glans, the tumor regressed after 650 mg methotrexate continuous infusion and further 6 months weekly 50 mg methotrexate infusion so that circumcision became feasible ([17], Figs. 22.5 and 22.6a–e). Another course of 450 mg methotrexate infusion was given because there still an ulcerated mass on the glans. One year later a third course

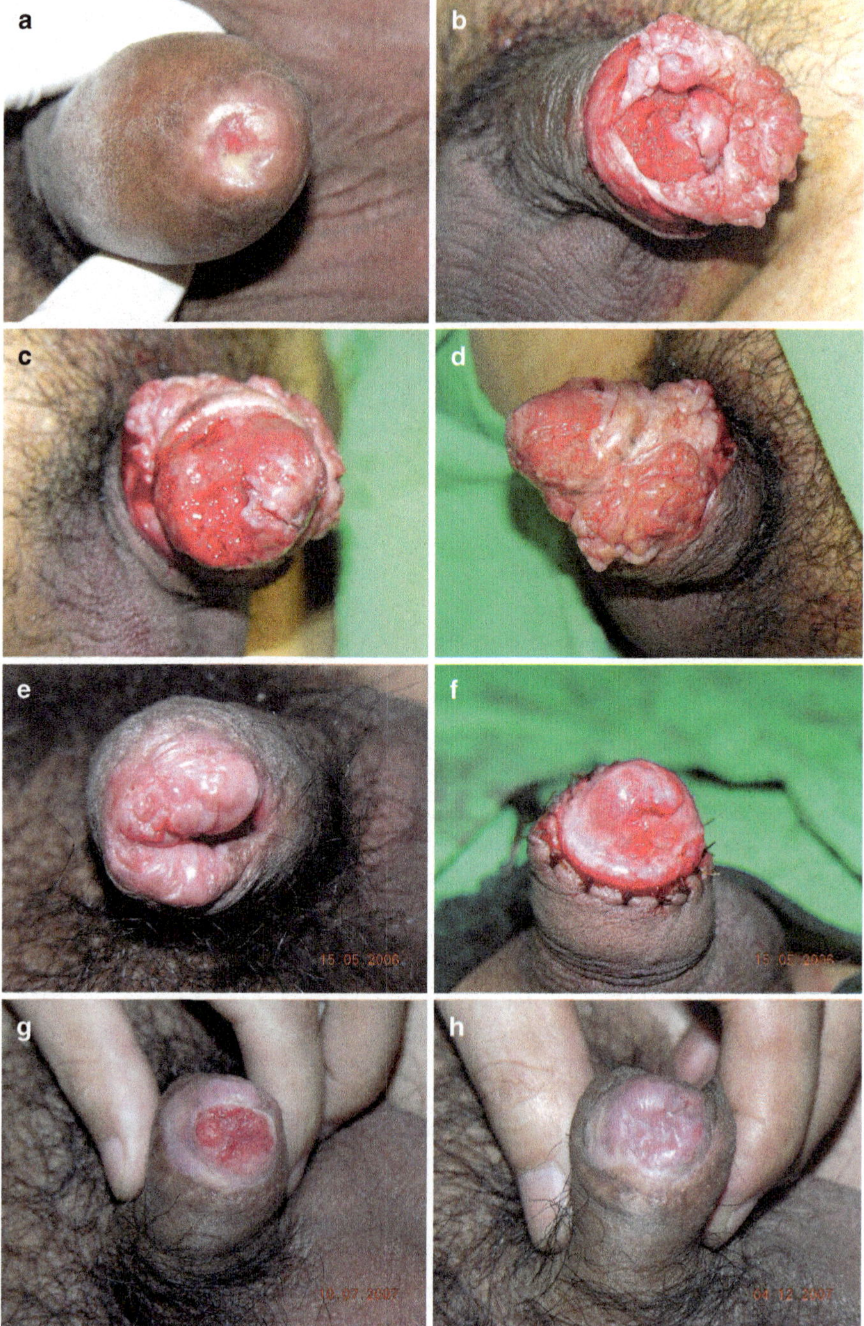

Fig. 22.6 Case 6: a 28-year-old single patient with prepuce verrucous carcinoma involving the whole glans (5×4 cm). (**a**) Penile tip on admission. (**b**) After dorsal slit. (**c, d**) After retraction of prepuce anterior and lateral view. (**e, f**) Before and after circumcision. (**g**) Well-circumscribed erosion on the penile glans. (**h**) Two years after treatment, follow-up evaluations including semen analysis and erectile function all proved to be normal. He is living recurrence-free 4 years and 11 month after treatment

of 800 mg methotrexate infusion was given because biopsy from the erosion on the glans revealed residual verrucous carcinoma (Fig. 22.6g). The entire wound healed 4 months later (Fig. 22.6h). The follow-up evaluations, including semen analysis and erectile function, all proved to be normal. The patient's sexual function was evaluated by international index of erectile function (IIEF-5), and the follow-up can keep within normal range (>21) [9, 11]. Now he is in sustained complete remission and has a functional penis 4 years 11 months after the start of treatment. Two partial responders showed no appreciable response in spite of various drugs given. Since a partial response is of no meaning to the patient, penectomy was performed subsequently. One of these two is still living 13 years 8 months after treatment. The other developed metastases of bilateral inguinal lymph nodes one and a half year after infusion chemotherapy. Penectomy was carried out. The histological examination of the mass on the glans of the penis revealed grade 2 squamous cell carcinoma. The patient's condition progressed rapidly and he died 11 months after penectomy. Whether that is a case of transformation following chemotherapy or just coincidence is unknown. So far no publications about malignant transformation of verrucous carcinoma following chemotherapy can be found.

Conclusion

Intra-arterial infusion chemotherapy is a simple and effective regional treatment for advanced penile carcinoma with the unique advantage of preservation of structure and function (Figs. 22.2, 22.4, 22.5, and 22.6). It is indicated for T1 to T4 tumors (Figs. 22.1 and 22.3). The drug side effects are mild and tolerable and even suitable to very old patients up to 98 years old. For young complete responders, this therapy showed the uniqueness of not only the preservation of anatomic and sexual function integrity but also fertility ([16], Figs. 22.4, 22.6 and 22.7). Because of a reasonable complete response rate of 50 % for penile carcinoma, 67 % for verrucous carcinoma ([16, 17], Figs. 22.4, 22.5, and 22.6), and 44 % for squamous cell carcinoma ([12, 14, 15], Figs. 22.1, 22.2, and 22.3), it may be considered as a penile-sparing therapy for penile carcinoma especially in the younger patients before amputation is considered. By using this simple method, many unnecessary penectomies could be avoided.

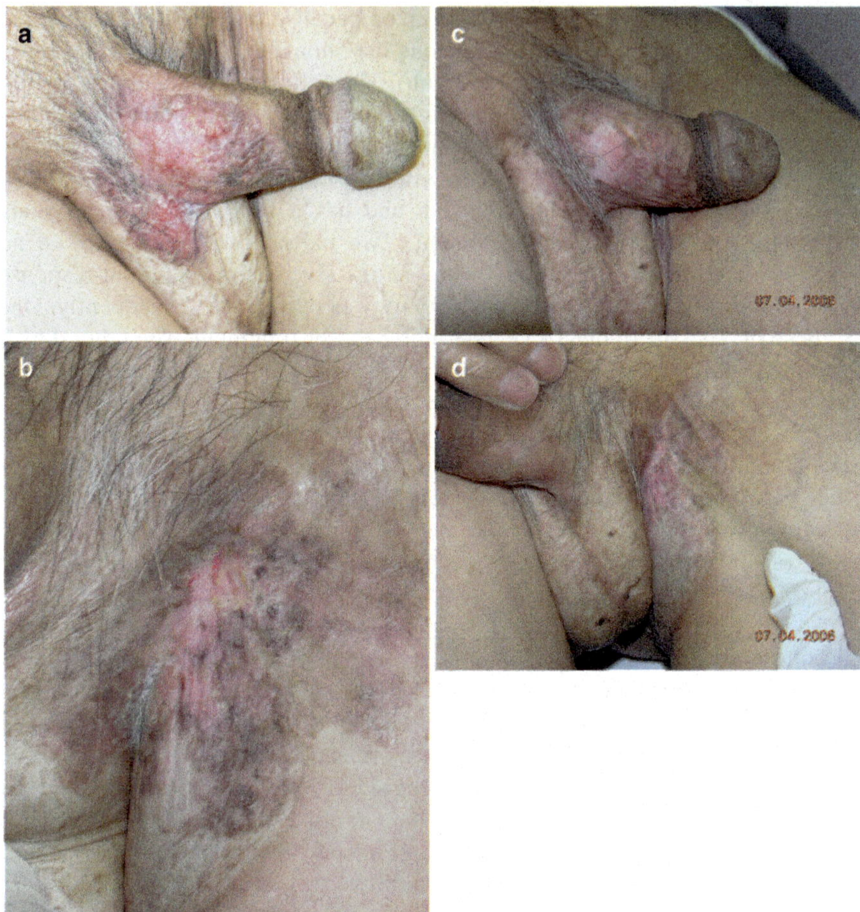

Fig. 22.7 Case 7: a 94-year-old patient with extramammary Paget's disease involving penile shaft, scrotum, and left inguinal area. (**a, b**) Before treatment. (**c, d**) After treatment. He received intermittent infusion regularly at our outpatient clinic with stable condition until he died of non-cancer-related disease at the age of 100 (2011)

References

1. Carson TE. Verrucous carcinoma of the penis: successful treatment with cryosurgery and topical fluorouracil therapy. Arch Dermatol. 1978;114:1546–7.
2. Culkin DJ, Beer TM. Advanced penile carcinoma. J Urol. 2003;170:359–65.
3. de Crevoisier R, Slimane K, Sanfilippo N, et al. Long-term results of brachytherapy for carcinoma of the penis confined to the glans (N-or NX). Int J Radiat Oncol Biol Phys. 2009;15:1150–6.
4. Fukunaga M, Yokoi K, Miyazawa Y, et al. Penile verrucous carcinoma anaplastic transformation following radiotherapy: a case report with human papillomavirus typing and flow cytometric DNA studies. Am J Surg Pathol. 1994;18:501–5.
5. Gomez De La Fuente E, Castuno Suarez E, Vanacolocha Sebastian F, et al. Verrucous carcinoma of the penis completely cured with shaving and intralesional interferon. Dermatology. 2000;200:152.
6. Maiche AG, Pyrhonen S. Verrucous carcinoma of the penis: three cases treated with interferon-alpha. Br J Urol. 1997;79:481–3.
7. Meijer RP, Boon TA, van Venrooij GE, et al. Long-term follow-up after laser therapy for penile carcinoma. Urology. 2007;69:759–62.
8. Micali G, Nasca MR, Innocenzi D. Penile cancer. J Am Acad. 2006;54:369–91.
9. Mulhall JP, King R, Kirby M, et al. Evaluating the sexual experience in men: validation of the sexual experience questionnaire. J Sex Med. 2008;5:365–76.
10. Protzel C, Hakenberg OW. Chemotherapy in patients with penile carcinoma. Urol Int. 2009;82:1–7.
11. Rosen RC, Riley A, Wagner G, et al. The international index of erectile function (IIEF): a multidimensional scale for assessment of erectile dysfunction. Urology. 1997;49:822–30.
12. Sheen MC. Intra-aortic infusion chemotherapy in previously untreated squamous cell carcinoma of the penis. Reg Cancer Treat. 1988;1:123–5.
13. Sheen MC, Sheen YS, Sheu HM, et al. Subungual verrucous carcinoma of the thumb treated by intra-arterial infusion with methotrexate. Dermatol Surg. 2005;31:787–9.
14. Sheen MC, Sheu HM, Chai CY, et al. Clinical and histological effects of aortic infusion of methotrexate for penile squamous cell carcinoma. Reg Cancer Treat. 1994;7:27–32.
15. Sheen MC, Sheu HM, Huang SL, et al. Serial clinical, light and electron-microscopic changes of penile squamous cell carcinoma after intra-aortic infusion chemotherapy. Reg Cancer Treat. 1990;3:185–91.
16. Sheen MC, Sheu HM, Huang CH, et al. Penile verrucous carcinoma successfully treated by intra-aortic infusion with methotrexate. Urology. 2003;61:1216–20.
17. Sheen MC, Sheu HM, Jang MY et al. Advanced penile verrucous carcinoma; treated with intra-aortic infusion chemotherapy. J Urol. 2010;183:1830–5.
18. Sheen MC, Sheu HM, Lai FJ, et al. A huge verrucous carcinoma of the lower lip treated with intra-arterial infusion of methotrexate. Br J Dermatol. 2004;51:727–9.
19. Solsona E, Algaba F, Horenblas S, et al. EAU guidelines on penile cancer. Eur Urol. 2004;46:1–8.
20. Wu CF, Chen CM, Shen YS, et al. Effective eradication of oral verrucous carcinoma with continuous infusion chemotherapy. Head Neck. 2008;30:611–7.

Systemic Induction Chemotherapy for Advanced-Stage Epithelial Ovarian Cancer

23

Maurie Markman

It is a well-established observation that epithelial ovarian cancer is the most sensitive solid tumor (excluding germ cell malignancies) to traditional cytotoxic chemotherapeutic agents. In fact, the inherent sensitivity of ovarian cancer has been known for more than 50 years since the publication of the initial results of human studies that examined anticancer drugs that were first developed as agents to be utilized in chemical warfare [1, 2].

In these studies it was identified that tumor regression was observed in as many as one-half of the treated population, and symptoms (particularly related to the presence of malignant ascites) were improved [3, 4]. However, compared to more recent efforts, it is difficult to accurately assess the overall impact of the therapy delivered in this era, and toxicity was inadequately quantified. This later point is emphasized by the subsequent reports that ovarian cancer patients treated with extended alkylating agent chemotherapy had a significant risk for the development of untreatable therapy-induced acute myelogenous leukemia [5–7].

Documentation of the benefits of cytotoxic chemotherapy in ovarian cancer was placed on a far more solid footing with the paradigm-changing establishment of randomized phase 3 trials as the definitive method to define the utility of such therapy [4, 8, 9]. In a series of phase 3 studies conducted over the past several decades by large cooperative groups throughout the world, the current standard of care has substantially changed from the era of single alkylating agents (Table 23.1).

In the early phase 3 studies, the combination of several (non-platinum) agents (e.g., 5-fluorouracil, doxorubicin, altretamine, methotrexate) was shown to improve the objective response rates and modestly impact measures of survival compared to single alkylating agents [9]. Impressive biological and clinical activity for the then "new" antineoplastic agent, cisplatin, in women who had progressed on their initial

M. Markman
Cancer Treatment Centers of America, Eastern Regional Medical Center,
1331 East Wyoming Avenue, Philadelphia, PA 19024, USA
e-mail: maurie.markman@ctca-hope.com

© Springer-Verlag Berlin Heidelberg 2016
K.R. Aigner, F.O. Stephens (eds.), *Induction Chemotherapy*,
DOI 10.1007/978-3-319-28773-7_23

Table 23.1 Historical development of primary (induction) ovarian cancer treatment paradigms

Single alkylating agents
Combination non-platinum containing chemotherapy
Combination platinum-based chemotherapy
Combination platinum/taxane-based chemotherapy
Combination platinum/taxane-based chemotherapy (IP cisplatin)
Combination platinum/taxane-based chemotherapy (weekly paclitaxel)
Combination platinum/taxane-based chemotherapy (plus bevacizumab)

Table 23.2 Defining the current standard of care in the induction chemotherapeutic management of ovarian cancer: superiority of cisplatin-paclitaxel compared to cisplatin-cyclophosphamide

	Progression-free survival (median)	Overall survival (median)
Study #1 [14]		
Cisplatin + paclitaxel	18 months	38 months
Cisplatin + cyclophosphamide	13 months	24 months
	$p<0.001$	$p<0.001$
Study #2 [15]		
Cisplatin + paclitaxel	15.5 months	35.6 months
Cisplatin + cyclophosphamide	11.5 months	25.8 months
	$p=0.0005$	$p=0.0016$

chemotherapy regimen led to the introduction of this agent into the frontline setting [10]. Subsequently conducted phase 3 studies revealed the survival advantage of treatment programs that included this agent, compared to non-platinum-based regimens [11–13].

The currently accepted standard of care in the management of ovarian cancer was established more than a decade ago based on the landmark study conducted by the Gynecologic Oncology Group (GOG) that compared the combination of cisplatin plus cyclophosphamide (one of the "gold standard" regimens employed at that time) to cisplatin plus paclitaxel (at that time an experimental agent) (Table 23.2) [14]. The cisplatin plus paclitaxel regimen was shown to result in an improved response rate, as well as superior progression-free and overall survivals. This study was subsequently confirmed in a second phase 3 randomized trial conducted in Canada and Europe [15].

Since that time a series of studies have modified treatment (e.g., substitution of carboplatin for cisplatin, based on toxicity considerations, acceptability of utilizing docetaxel instead of paclitaxel), but there is no evidence that any of these changes have further improved outcome, compared to the original cisplatin plus paclitaxel regimen (Table 23.3) [16–19]. In addition, a variety of options have been explored that have failed to demonstrate any benefit (improving efficacy or toxicity) compared to a standard platinum plus taxane approach (Table 23.4) [20–25].

A phase 3 trial conducted by the Japanese Gynecologic Oncology Group has challenged the traditional method of delivery of paclitaxel in epithelial ovarian

Table 23.3 Defining the current standard of care in the induction chemotherapeutic management of advanced ovarian cancer

	Progression-free survival (median)	Overall survival (median)
Study #1 [16]		
Cisplatin + paclitaxel	19.1 months	44.1 months
Carboplatin + paclitaxel	17.2 months	43.3 months
	NS	NS
Study #2 [17]		
Cisplatin + paclitaxel	19.4 months	48.7 months
Carboplatin + paclitaxel	20.7 months	57.4 months
	NS	NS
Study #3 [18]		
Carboplatin + paclitaxel	14.8 months	
Carboplatin + docetaxel	15.0 months	
	NS	

Table 23.4 Frontline (induction) chemotherapy strategies shown not to improve outcome in epithelial ovarian cancer

Doubling the dose intensity of platinum (cisplatin or carboplatin)
High-dose chemotherapy
Extending the duration of paclitaxel chemotherapy
Addition of a "third agent" to platinum/taxane chemotherapy

cancer. In this trial, patients with advanced-stage disease were randomized to either receive "standard" carboplatin plus paclitaxel, with the paclitaxel delivered on an every *3-week schedule*, versus the same dose/schedule of carboplatin but with the paclitaxel administered at a dose of 80 mg/m^2 on a *weekly schedule* [26]. The study revealed an improvement in objective response rate, time to disease progression, and 3-year survival in favor of the weekly regimen.

In general, more than one "positive trial" is suggested to be required in oncology to demonstrate a survival benefit before a new treatment is considered to become a new "standard of care." However, in this particular setting, it is reasonable to note that two phase 3 randomized trials in breast cancer, one each in the adjuvant and metastatic settings, have revealed a weekly schedule is superior to the traditional every 3-week treatment program [27, 28]. It is rational to consider these data as providing appropriate support for the conclusion that weekly delivery of paclitaxel is superior to more intermittent dosing.

One important follow-up issue relates to the question of the most likely biological explanation for this clinical outcome. Two hypotheses may reasonably be presented. First, it is possible that weekly delivery of this cycle-specific agent permits a higher percentage of relatively slowly dividing ovarian cancer cells to be susceptible to the cytotoxic effects of this important antineoplastic agent.

Alternatively, it may be proposed that weekly paclitaxel acts as a rather potent anti-angiogenic agent, consistent with data demonstrated in preclinical laboratory studies [29]. Understanding the relevance of angiogenesis in stimulating the growth of ovarian cancer and conversely the potential importance of inhibiting this process is one of the most exciting recent developments in the management of ovarian cancer.

It is uncertain if the results of the Japanese study will change the standard of care in the systemic administration of cytotoxic chemotherapy throughout the world. However, at a minimum, it is reasonable to state that weekly paclitaxel delivery along with every 3-week carboplatin represents an acceptable standard-of-care option in the management of this malignancy.

23.1 Maintenance Therapy

Despite the high objective response rate (70–80 %) of epithelial ovarian cancer to platinum-based induction (primary) chemotherapy, for the majority of patients, the disease will ultimately relapse. As a result, there has been a strong interest in determining if continuation of cytotoxic chemotherapy beyond the traditional five to six cycles would improve survival.

Prolongation of therapy raises concern for the potential risk of accentuating toxicities experienced during the initial treatment phase (e.g., emesis, neuropathy) or for the development of novel side effects (e.g., heart failure). The previously noted experience with the development of secondary acute leukemia in ovarian cancer patients treated during extended treatment regimens (e.g., 12–24 months) with alkylating agents emphasizes the potential serious implications of a "maintenance" chemotherapy strategy [5–7].

In fact, several phase 3 randomized trials have directly examined the utility of administering 5 or 6 cycles of cisplatin-based chemotherapy compared to 10 of 12 cycles, respectively [30–32]. Unfortunately, the studies failed to reveal evidence of an improvement in either the time to disease progression or overall survival associated with the longer treatment periods, but toxicity was increased.

However, reported non-randomized experience revealed surprising survival for a group of heavily pretreated ovarian cancer patients who were treated with single-agent paclitaxel [33]. In addition to the provocative survival of this population, there was no suggestion for the development of novel side effects associated with the extended use of the agent, compared to what has been observed with shorter treatment durations (e.g., alopecia until the completion of therapy, neutropenia with each cycle, peripheral neuropathy).

This non-randomized experience led to the initiation of a phase 3 trial conducted by the Southwest Oncology Group (SWOG) and the Gynecologic Oncology Group (GOG) that directly compared the monthly administration of 12 versus 3 cycles of single-agent paclitaxel in advanced ovarian cancer patients who had attained a clinically defined complete response to platinum/paclitaxel-based chemotherapy [34]. The study was stopped early by its Data Safety and Monitoring Committee at the time of a planned interim analysis based on a highly statistically significant improvement in progression-free survival in favor of the 12-cycle maintenance strategy. Follow-up of the study population confirmed the favorable impact on progression-free survival, but it was not possible to make a definitive statement regarding overall survival due to the ultimately limited total sample size [35].

It should be noted that a smaller phase 3 trial that employed quite a different study design failed to confirm the favorable impact of paclitaxel delivered in the maintenance setting [36]. An ongoing study conducted by the GOG reexamining the question of paclitaxel maintenance therapy will hopefully be able to provide a definitive answer to this highly clinically relevant question, particularly a beneficial effect on overall survival.

23.2 Re-induction Therapy of Ovarian Cancer

In the presence of recurrent ovarian cancer, multiple strategies have been employed, and a number of single agents are known to possess at least a modest level of biological and clinical activity in the malignancy [37]. Of particular interest to the topic of induction chemotherapy in ovarian cancer is the observation that patients who experience an initial response to the chemotherapy, and subsequently develop evidence of disease recurrence, may respond a second time to the identical (e.g., carboplatin plus paclitaxel) or a similar treatment regimen (e.g., carboplatin plus gemcitabine, carboplatin plus pegylated liposomal doxorubicin) [38–40].

The longer the duration of time from completion of primary treatment until the documentation of disease recurrence, the higher the statistical probability a patient will exhibit an objective response and/or clinically meaningful benefit. For example, with a treatment-free interval of 6–12 months, the anticipated objective response rate is 25–30 %, while with a treatment-free interval of >18–24 months, the response rate has been shown to be >50–60 % [41, 42].

This observation raises the question of whether any alteration in the induction chemotherapy strategy may be able to kill these potentially chemosensitive cells that remain quiescent but clearly viable. This is an important area for future research in ovarian cancer.

23.3 Induction (Neoadjuvant) Chemotherapy

Phase 2 trial and retrospective institutional experiences had suggested the potential utility of the delivery of cytotoxic chemotherapy prior to an attempt at maximal cytoreduction in women with very large volume intraperitoneal or stage IV ovarian cancer or where the presence of comorbid conditions (e.g., history of cardiac dysfunction) increased the risk of surgery [43–46]. Published data further highlighted the fact that a subsequently performed resection after several cycles of the initial induction ("neoadjuvant") chemotherapy was generally associated with reduced morbidity, compared to that anticipated with primary surgery in such patients, and a reasonable percentage of these individuals could be cytoreduced to no visible residual cancer [43–46].

The results of an international phase 3 randomized trial has confirmed the equivalent survival associated with an induction chemotherapy approach, followed by interval surgical cytoreduction, compared to primary surgery in women with large volume epithelial ovarian cancer [47]. While it remains unknown what impact these important study results will have on the routine management of ovarian cancer, it is reasonable to conclude primary chemotherapy followed by an attempt at maximal surgical cytoreduction should be considered an acceptable standard-of-care option in ovarian cancer patients considered to be unable to be optimally cytoreduced at initial presentation.

23.4 Future Directions in Induction Therapy of Epithelial Ovarian Cancer

Based on evidence of a somewhat surprising level of biological and clinical activity of single-agent bevacizumab in recurrent and platinum-resistant ovarian cancer (15–20 % objective response rate) [48, 49], several phase 3 trials were initiated to add this anti-angiogenic agent to carboplatin plus paclitaxel in the primary management of ovarian cancer. These trials have revealed that the addition of bevacizumab to chemotherapy improves progression-free survival in the frontline setting [50]. Of note, other studies have documented the utility of combining bevacizumab with chemotherapy in recurrent and resistant ovarian cancer [50].

It should be noted here that the cost of bevacizumab (and many novel agents recently introduced into clinical practice in oncology) may limit the widespread introduction of this, and other, drugs into the routine frontline management of ovarian cancer.

As is the case in oncology, in general, there has been significant interest in the introduction of a variety of "targeted agents" into the ovarian cancer treatment paradigm. Unfortunately, to date, a variety of such strategies have been unsuccessful, including targeting the epidermal growth factor receptor (EGFR) and HER-2 [51–53]. This outcome has become rather routine in small phase 2 studies exploring a variety of approaches despite the fact it is possible to demonstrate molecular abnormalities in ovarian cancer cells similar to that observed in tumor types (e.g., colon, lung, breast) where these strategies have been found to favorably impact survival. The most likely explanation for this rather disquieting and somewhat perplexing state of affairs is the increasingly understood fact that molecular pathways within the various tumor types, and individual cancer cells themselves, are remarkably complex and the expression (or lack of expression) of a particular marker on (or within) a cell provides a very limited view into the processes, which ultimately drive the malignant phenotype [54].

One important exception to this situation appears to be recent evidence for a potential role for poly (ADP-ribose) polymerase (PARP) inhibitors in the management of women with ovarian cancer who are known to have BRCA-1 and BRCA-2 abnormalities [55]. This class of drugs has been shown to inhibit the ability of cancer cells to repair DNA damage, and preclinical data demonstrate the impact of these agents is greatest against cancers which have intrinsic defects in their ability to repair such damage [56]. Importantly, this includes tumors with germ line or somatic mutations in BRCA 1 or 2.

Impressive single-agent biological and clinical activity, as well as striking improvement in progression-free survival in a phase 2 randomized trial, has been observed for this class of drugs in a population of previously treated patients with ovarian cancer [57, 58]. Phase 3 randomized trials examining several PARP inhibitors as single agents or in combination with platinum-based therapy are in progress. It is anticipated that induction chemotherapy studies employing these agents will be initiated in the near future likely targeting particularly relevant patient populations (e.g., documented presence of germ line or somatic mutations in BRCA-1 or BRCA-2).

References

1. Bateman JC. Chemotherapeutic management of advanced ovarian carcinoma. Med Ann Dist Columbia. 1959;28:537–44.
2. Kottmeier HL. Treatment of ovarian cancer with thiotepa. Clin Obstet Gynecol. 1968;11:428–38.
3. Thigpen T, Vance R, Lambuth B, et al. Chemotherapy for advanced or recurrent gynecologic cancer. Cancer. 1987;60:2104–16.
4. Omura GA, Morrow CP, Blessing JA, et al. A randomized comparison of melphalan versus melphalan plus hexamethylmelamine versus adriamycin plus cyclophosphamide in ovarian carcinoma. Cancer. 1983;51:783–9.
5. Greene MH, Boice Jr JD, Greer BE, Blessing JA, Dembo AJ. Acute nonlymphocytic leukemia after therapy with alkylating agents for ovarian cancer: a study of five randomized clinical trials: Gynecol Oncol. 1982;307:1416–21.
6. Travis LB, Curtis RE, Boice Jr JD, Platz CE, Hankey BF, Fraumeni Jr JF. Second malignant neoplasms among long-term survivors of ovarian cancer. Cancer Res. 1996;56:1564–70.
7. Travis LB, Holowaty EJ, Bergfeldt K, et al. Risk of leukemia after platinum-based chemotherapy for ovarian cancer. N Engl J Med. 1999;340:351–7.
8. Katz ME, Schwartz PE, Kapp DS, Luikart S. Epithelial carcinoma of the ovary: current strategies. Ann Intern Med. 1981;95:98–111.
9. Young RC, Chabner BA, Hubbard SP, et al. Advanced ovarian adenocarcinoma. A prospective clinical trial of melphalan (L-PAM) versus combination chemotherapy. N Engl J Med. 1978;299:1261–6.
10. Wiltshaw E, Subramarian S, Alexopoulos C, Barker GH. Cancer of the ovary: a summary of experience with cis-dichlorodiammineplatinum(II) at the Royal Marsden Hospital. Cancer Treat Rep. 1979;63:1545–8.
11. Advanced Ovarian Cancer Trialists Group. Chemotherapy in advanced ovarian cancer: four systematic meta-analyses of individual patient data from 37 randomized trials. Advanced Ovarian Cancer Trialists' Group. Br J Cancer. 1998;78:1479–87.
12. Advanced Ovarian Cancer Trialists Group. Chemotherapy in advanced ovarian cancer: an overview of randomised clinical trials. Br J Cancer. 1991;303:884–93.
13. Omura GA, Bundy BN, Berek JS, Curry S, Delgado G, Mortel R. Randomized trial of cyclophosphamide plus cisplatin with or without doxorubicin in ovarian carcinoma: a Gynecologic Oncology Group study. J Clin Oncol. 1989;7:457–65.
14. McGuire WP, Hoskins WJ, Brady MF, et al. Cyclophosphamide and cisplatin compared with paclitaxel and cisplatin in patients with stage III and stage IV ovarian cancer. N Engl J Med. 1996;334:1–6.

15. Piccart MJ, Bertelsen K, James K, et al. Randomized intergroup trial of cisplatin-paclitaxel versus cisplatin-cyclophosphamide in women with advanced epithelial ovarian cancer: three-year results. J Natl Cancer Inst. 2000;92:699–708.

16. du Bois A, Luck HJ, Meier W, et al. A randomized clinical trial of cisplatin/paclitaxel versus carboplatin/paclitaxel as first-line treatment of ovarian cancer. J Natl Cancer Inst. 2003;95:1320–9.

17. Ozols RF, Bundy BN, Greer BE, et al. Phase III trial of carboplatin and paclitaxel compared with cisplatin and paclitaxel in patients with optimally resected stage III ovarian cancer: a Gynecologic Oncology Group study. J Clin Oncol. 2003;21:3194–200.

18. Vasey PA, Jayson GC, Gordon A, et al. Phase III randomized trial of docetaxel-carboplatin versus paclitaxel-carboplatin as first-line chemotherapy for ovarian carcinoma. J Natl Cancer Inst. 2004;96:1682–91.

19. Covens A, Carey M, Bryson P, Verma S, Fung Kee FM, Johnston M. Systematic review of first-line chemotherapy for newly diagnosed postoperative patients with stage II, III, or IV epithelial ovarian cancer. Gynecol Oncol. 2002;85:71–80.

20. McGuire WP, Hoskins WJ, Brady MF, et al. Assessment of dose-intensive therapy in suboptimally debulked ovarian cancer: a Gynecologic Oncology Group study. J Clin Oncol. 1995;13:1589–99.

21. Gore M, Mainwaring P, A'Hern R, et al. Randomized trial of dose-intensity with single-agent carboplatin in patients with epithelial ovarian cancer. London Gynaecological Oncology Group. J Clin Oncol. 1998;16:2426–34.

22. Grenman S, Wiklund T, Jalkanen J, et al. A randomised phase III study comparing high-dose chemotherapy to conventionally dosed chemotherapy for stage III ovarian cancer: the Finnish Ovarian Cancer (FINOVA) study. Eur J Cancer. 2006;42:2196–9.

23. Schilder RJ, Brady MF, Spriggs D, Shea T. Pilot evaluation of high-dose carboplatin and paclitaxel followed by high-dose melphalan supported by peripheral blood stem cells in previously untreated advanced ovarian cancer: a Gynecologic Oncology Group study. Gynecol Oncol. 2003;88:3–8.

24. du Bois A, Weber B, Rochon J, et al. Addition of epirubicin as a third drug to carboplatin-paclitaxel in first-line treatment of advanced ovarian cancer: a prospectively randomized gynecologic cancer intergroup trial by the Arbeitsgemeinschaft Gynaekologische Onkologie Ovarian Cancer Study Group and the Groupe d'Investigateurs Nationaux pour l'Etude des Cancers Ovariens. J Clin Oncol. 2006;24:1127–35.

25. Bookman MA, Brady MF, McGuire WP, et al. Evaluation of new platinum-based treatment regimens in advanced-stage ovarian cancer: a Phase III Trial of the Gynecologic Cancer Intergroup. J Clin Oncol. 2009;27:1419–25.

26. Katsumata N, Yasuda M, Takahashi F, et al. Dose-dense paclitaxel once a week in combination with carboplatin every 3 weeks for advanced ovarian cancer: a phase 3, open-label, randomised controlled trial. Lancet. 2009;374:1331–8.

27. Seidman AD, Berry D, Cirrincione C, et al. Randomized phase III trial of weekly compared with every-3-weeks paclitaxel for metastatic breast cancer, with trastuzumab for all HER-2 overexpressors and random assignment to trastuzumab or not in HER-2 nonoverexpressors: final results of Cancer and Leukemia Group B protocol 9840. J Clin Oncol. 2008;26:1642–9.

28. Sparano JA, Wang M, Martino S, et al. Weekly paclitaxel in the adjuvant treatment of breast cancer. N Engl J Med. 2008;358:1663–71.

29. Miller KD, Sweeney CJ, Sledge Jr GW. Redefining the target: chemotherapeutics as antiangiogenics. J Clin Oncol. 2001;19:1195–206.

30. Lambert HE, Rustin GJ, Gregory WM, Nelstrop AE. A randomized trial of five versus eight courses of cisplatin or carboplatin in advanced epithelial ovarian carcinoma. A North Thames Ovary Group study. Ann Oncol. 1997;8:327–33.

31. Bertelsen K, Jakobsen A, Stroyer J, et al. A prospective randomized comparison of 6 and 12 cycles of cyclophosphamide, adriamycin, and cisplatin in advanced epithelial ovarian cancer: a Danish Ovarian Study Group trial (DACOVA). Gynecol Oncol. 1993;49:30–6.

32. Hakes TB, Chalas E, Hoskins WJ, et al. Randomized prospective trial of 5 versus 10 cycles of cyclophosphamide, doxorubicin, and cisplatin in advanced ovarian carcinoma. Gynecol Oncol. 1992;45:284–9.
33. Markman M, Hakes T, Barakat R, Curtin J, Almadrones L, Hoskins W. Follow-up of Memorial Sloan-Kettering Cancer Center patients treated on National Cancer Institute Treatment Referral Center protocol 9103: paclitaxel in refractory ovarian cancer. J Clin Oncol. 1996;14:796–9.
34. Markman M, Liu PY, Wilczynski S, et al. Phase III randomized trial of 12 versus 3 months of maintenance paclitaxel in patients with advanced ovarian cancer after complete response to platinum and paclitaxel-based chemotherapy: a Southwest Oncology Group and Gynecologic Oncology Group trial. J Clin Oncol. 2003;21:2460–5.
35. Markman M, Liu PY, Moon J, et al. Impact on survival of 12 versus 3 monthly cycles of paclitaxel (175 mg/m^2) administered to patients with advanced ovarian cancer who attained a complete response to primary platinum-paclitaxel: follow-up of a Southwest Oncology Group and Gynecologic Oncology Group phase 3 trial. Gynecol Oncol. 2009;114:195–8.
36. Pecorelli S, Favalli G, Gadducci A, et al. Phase III trial of observation versus six courses of paclitaxel in patients with advanced epithelial ovarian cancer in complete response after six courses of paclitaxel/platinum-based chemotherapy: final results of the after-6 protocol 1. J Clin Oncol. 2009;27:4642–8.
37. Markman M, Bookman MA. Second-line treatment of ovarian cancer. Oncologist. 2000;5:26–35.
38. Dizon DS, Hensley ML, Poynor EA, et al. Retrospective analysis of carboplatin and paclitaxel as initial second-line therapy for recurrent epithelial ovarian carcinoma: application toward a dynamic disease state model of ovarian cancer. J Clin Oncol. 2002;20:1238–47.
39. The ICON and AGO Collaborators. Paclitaxel plus platinum-based chemotherapy versus conventional platinum-based chemotherapy in women with relapsed ovarian cancer: the ICON4/AGO-OVAR-2.2 trial. Lancet. 2003;361:2099–106.
40. Pfisterer J, Plante M, Vergote I, et al. Gemcitabine plus carboplatin compared with carboplatin in patients with platinum-sensitive recurrent ovarian cancer: an intergroup trial of the AGO-OVAR, the NCIC CTG, and the EORTC GCG. J Clin Oncol. 2006;24:4699–707.
41. Gore ME, Fryatt I, Wiltshaw E, Dawson T. Treatment of relapsed carcinoma of the ovary with cisplatin or carboplatin following initial treatment with these compounds. Gynecol Oncol. 1990;36:207–11.
42. Markman M, Rothman R, Hakes T, et al. Second-line platinum therapy in patients with ovarian cancer previously treated with cisplatin. J Clin Oncol. 1991;9:389–93.
43. Vergote I, De Wever I, Tjalma W, Van GM, Decloedt J, van Dam P. Neoadjuvant chemotherapy or primary debulking surgery in advanced ovarian carcinoma: a retrospective analysis of 285 patients. Gynecol Oncol. 1998;71:431–6.
44. Kuhn W, Rutke S, Spathe K, et al. Neoadjuvant chemotherapy followed by tumor debulking prolongs survival for patients with poor prognosis in International Federation of Gynecology and Obstetrics Stage IIIC ovarian carcinoma. Cancer. 2001;92:2585–91.
45. Hou JY, Kelly MG, Yu H, et al. Neoadjuvant chemotherapy lessens surgical morbidity in advanced ovarian cancer and leads to improved survival in stage IV disease. Gynecol Oncol. 2007;105:211–7.
46. Markman M, Belinson J. A rationale for neoadjuvant systemic treatment followed by surgical assessment and intraperitoneal chemotherapy in patients presenting with non-surgically resectable ovarian or primary peritoneal cancers. J Cancer Res Clin Oncol. 2005;131:26–30.
47. Vergote I, Trope CG, Amant F, et al. Neoadjuvant chemotherapy or primary surgery in stage IIIC or IV ovarian cancer. N Engl J Med. 2010;363:943–53.
48. Burger RA, Sill M, Monk BJ, Greer BE, Sorosky JI. Phase II trial of bevacizumab in persistent or recurrent epithelial ovarian cancer or primary peritoneal cancer: a Gynecologic Oncology Group study. J Clin Oncol. 2007;25:5165–71.

49. Cannistra SA. Bevacizumab in patients with advanced platinum-resistant ovarian cancer. J Clin Oncol. 2006;34:5006.
50. Eskander RN, Tewari K. Incorporation of anti-angiogenesis therapy in the management of advanced ovarian carcinoma- mechanistics, review of phase III randomized clinical trials, and regulatory implications. Gynecol Oncol. 2014;132:496–505.
51. Bookman MA, Darcy KM, Clarke-Pearson D, Boothby RA, Horowitz IR. Evaluation of monoclonal humanized anti-HER2 antibody, trastuzumab, in patients with recurrent or refractory ovarian or primary peritoneal carcinoma with overexpression of HER2: a phase II trial of the Gynecologic Oncology Group. J Clin Oncol. 2003;21:283–90.
52. Schilder RJ, Sill MW, Chen X, et al. Phase II study of gefitinib in patients with relapsed or persistent ovarian or primary peritoneal carcinoma and evaluation of epidermal growth factor receptor mutations and immunohistochemical expression: a Gynecologic Oncology Group study. Clin Cancer Res. 2005;11:5539–48.
53. Coleman RL, Broaddus RR, Bodurka DC, et al. Phase II trial of imatinib mesylate in patients with recurrent platinum- and taxane-resistant epithelial ovarian and primary peritoneal cancers. Gynecol Oncol. 2006;101:126–31.
54. Lynch TJ, Bell DW, Sordella R, et al. Activating mutations in the epidermal growth factor receptor underlying responsiveness of non-small-cell lung cancer to gefitinib. N Engl J Med. 2004;350:2129–39.
55. Fong PC, Boss DS, Yap TA, et al. Inhibition of poly(ADP-Ribose) polymerase in tumors from BRCA mutation carriers. N Engl J Med. 2009;361:123–34 (published online June 24, 2009).
56. Farmer H, McCabe N, Lord CJ, et al. Targeting the DNA repair defect in BRCA mutant cells as a therapeutic strategy. Nature. 2005;434:917–21.
57. Lederman J, Harter P, Gourley C, et al. Olaparib maintenance therapy in platinum-sensitive relapsed ovarian cancer. N Engl J Med. 2012;366(15):1382–92.
58. Liu JF, Konstantinopoulso PA, Matulonis UA. PARP inhibitors in ovarian cancer: current status and future promise. 2014; 133:362–369.

Regional Chemotherapy in Recurrent Platinum-Refractory Ovarian Cancer

Karl Reinhard Aigner and Sabine Gailhofer

24.1 Introduction

The standard therapy with peritoneal metastatic ovarian cancer is extended cytoreduction, associated with combination chemotherapy based on platinum such as cisplatin or carboplatin and paclitaxel. Even though this tumor is very chemosensitive and the response rates range between 70 % and 80 %, recurrence appears within 2 years in almost half the patients who respond to the initial treatment well. The likelihood of a second response to chemotherapy after a recurrence is closely correlated with the recurrence-free interval. The shorter the time interval is to tumor progression, the less likely are the chances of a response to further chemotherapy [1, 2].

If a recurrence happens within 6 months, it is usually associated with a poor prognosis and the range of treatments available is very limited. A curative treatment is no longer possible [3]. Various attempts to overcome platinum resistance, such as increasing the dose [4–10], high-dose chemotherapy [11, 12] or various combination therapies [13, 14], were incapable of achieving any really relevant clinical survival advantage. Toxicity and side effects, however, are significantly worse under increased exposure to cytostatic agents and often intolerable.

Currently there is no cure for recurrent ovarian cancer, and objectively measurable response rates hardly exceed the 15 % limit. The treatment of platinum-resistant ovarian cancer continues to be a challenge. In relation to the studies, which could show an increase in response rate following dose-intensified therapies, an improvement in response and overall survival rates could be achieved in theory with an increase in exposure to cytostatic agents. However, this option is very limited due to its excessive toxicity. In a phase-III trial on maintenance therapy of 12 versus three

K.R. Aigner, MD (✉) • S. Gailhofer
Department of Surgical Oncology, Medias Klinikum GmbH & Co KG,
Krankenhausstrasse 3a, Burghausen 84489, Germany
e-mail: info@prof-aigner.de

© Springer-Verlag Berlin Heidelberg 2016
K.R. Aigner, F.O. Stephens (eds.), *Induction Chemotherapy*,
DOI 10.1007/978-3-319-28773-7_24

cycles of paclitaxel [15, 16], a clearly positive influence on progression-free survival among patients with 12 treatment cycles was observed. However, the study was canceled at this point so it was ultimately impossible to come to any conclusion about potentially prolonging overall survival. Due to the strong increase in toxicity in the form of neuropathies, the study was incapable of demonstrating any clinical benefit in terms of survival with quality of life.

Based on the observation that an increase in drug exposure is accompanied by an increased cytotoxic effect and consequently the clinical result could improve but is limited by the accompanying toxicity, there is an urgent need for a change or improvement in induction chemotherapy.

Based on this finding, it was an obvious step to investigate whether a further significant increase in the administered concentration of cytostatic agents could be achieved with an isolated perfusion procedure with extracorporeal circuit. Such a system is capable of generating a significantly higher cytostatic exposure, strong enough in some cases to break through chemoresistance and destroy all or at least a considerable amount of the residual tumor cell groups, possibly even tumor stem cells [17].

The hypothesis that chemoresistance could be breached with high drug exposure and that side effects could be minimized or prevented by extracorporeal chemofiltration at the same time has been investigated in a controlled study of patients with advanced and recurrent platinum-refractory FIGO IIIc and IV ovarian cancer [18].

## 24.2	Isolated Abdominal Perfusion

Isolated perfusion techniques are not new, but their clinical use has been limited so far.

There are two forms of isolated abdominal perfusion. In the perfusion system with a heart-lung machine and oxygenated extracorporeal circuit, the perfusion time may be extended to an hour and more, if cytostatic agents with increased cytotoxicity are used with hyperoxygenation [19, 20].

What is known as hypoxic abdominal perfusion (HAP) uses the increased cytotoxicity of several chemotherapeutic agents such as adriamycin and mitomycin under hypoxic conditions (Figs. 24.1 and 24.2). Cisplatin as the base substance in treating the ovarian cancer is equally effective under hypoxic as well as hyperoxic conditions [21].

## 24.3	Material and Methods

### 24.3.1	Technique of Hypoxic Abdominal Perfusion

The isolation of the abdominal segment in connection with an extracorporeal circuit is carried out under general anesthetic. A small longitudinal incision in the groin exposes the femoral or iliofemoral blood vessels below or above the inguinal

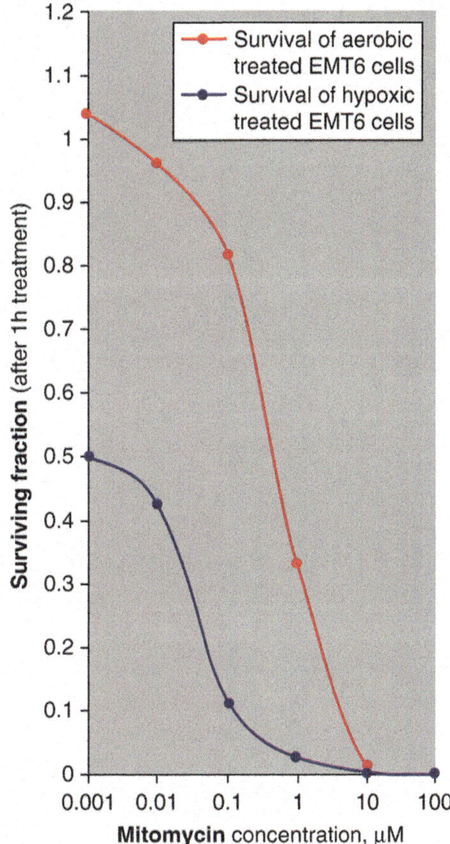

Fig. 24.1 Mitomycin toxicity to tumor cells in aerobic and hypoxic media [21]

ligament, and they are snared with tourniquets. A venous stop-flow catheter is inserted through a prolene purse-string suture and stab incision and fed forward. The femoral artery is cannulated through a transverse incision (Fig. 24.3). Both stop-flow catheters are placed with the balloon tips at diaphragm height, and the venous catheter is placed just above the confluence of the liver veins in the vena cava (Fig. 24.4). After being correctly positioned, both catheters are again unblocked to avoid immediate, prematurely occurring hypoxia in the abdominal segment. Both thighs are blocked with pneumatic cuffs. The chemotherapeutic agents are now administered with good oxygenation as a 1–2-min bolus through the arterial line. Immediately after this both stop-flow catheters are blocked, and the extracorporeal circuit maintained for 15 min (Fig. 24.5). As chemofiltration follows immediately, leakage control in the isolated circuit proves to be unnecessary. After both stop-flow balloon catheters have been unblocked, they start the chemofiltration (Fig. 24.6) and maintain it at a maximum capacity of 500 ml per minute until at least 4 l of filtrate is substituted. In a comparative study of intra-aortic chemotherapy with versus without chemofiltration, it was shown that post-therapeutic chemofiltration lowers

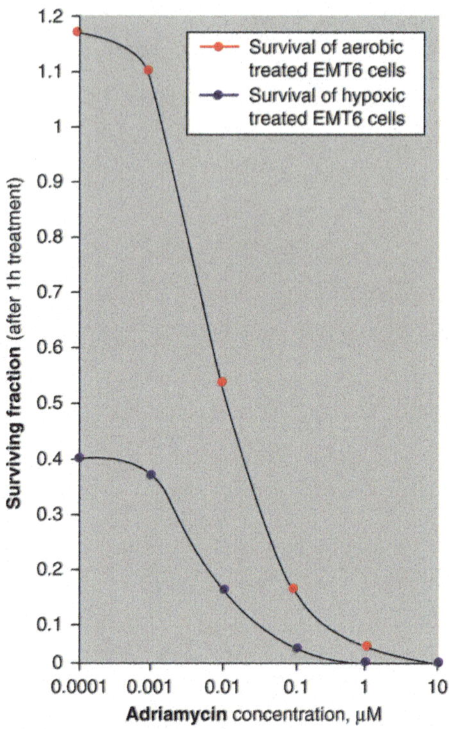

Fig. 24.2 Adriamycin toxicity to tumor cells in aerobic and hypoxic media [21]

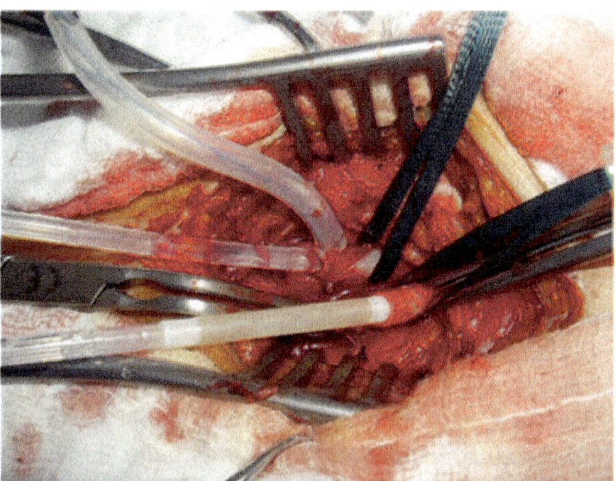

Fig. 24.3 Cannulation of the femoral vessels. The vein is cannulated by a purse-string suture, and the artery secured via a transverse incision and with a tourniquet. The arterial balloon is partially visible outside the artery in the photo. The perforations below the balloon drain the larger-diameter channel of the three lumens of the stop-flow catheter. A thinner channel is used to insufflate the balloon with a saline contrast medium mixture, and a second thin channel ends at the catheter tip and is used to feed in the guide wire to push up the catheter safely in the event of severely bent or twisted iliac arteries

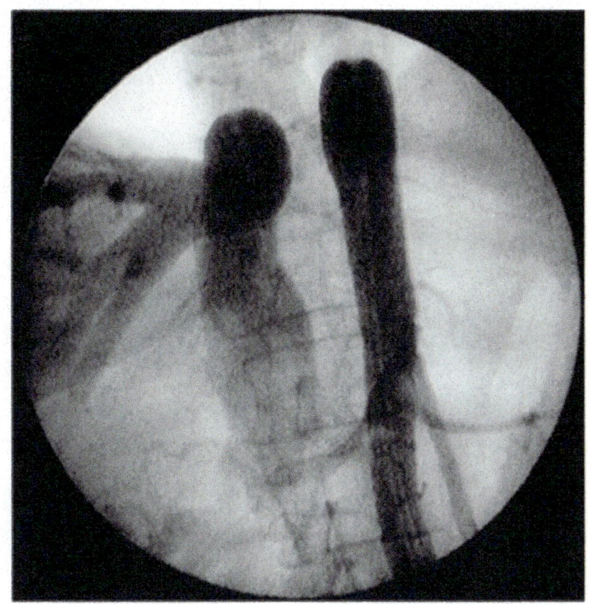

Fig. 24.4 Contrast imaging of the abdominal aorta and vena cava after contrast medium filling of both balloons with a saline contrast medium mixture and injection of contrast medium through the perforations of the stop-flow catheter's larger-diameter channel

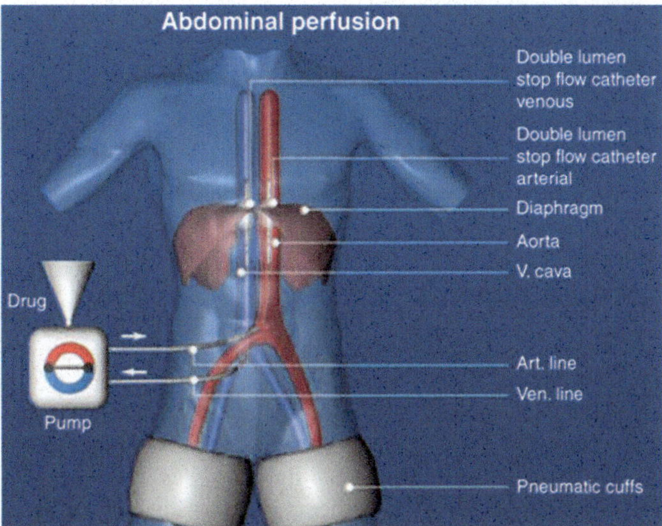

Fig. 24.5 Diagram of hypoxic abdominal perfusion. The larger-diameter channels of the aortic and venous stop-flow catheter are connected to an extracorporeal perfusion circuit. After 15 min of cytostatic exposure, the balloons are unblocked and chemofiltration begins through the same catheters

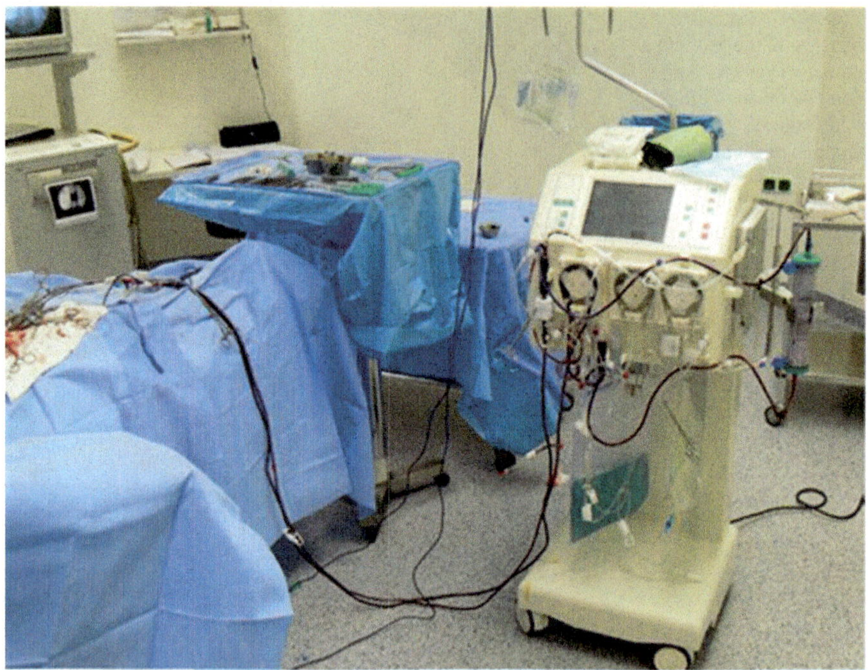

Fig. 24.6 Chemofiltration after local cytostatic exposure. The arterial and venous lines of the system are channeled out of the groin and connected to the chemoprocessor

cytostatic exposure by reducing the peak concentration so that both the immediate and subsequent cumulative toxicities are reduced, as in the case of mitomycin and adriamycin [22, 23]. After surgery and treatment, the catheters are removed and the vessels successively sutured.

24.4 Treatment Protocol

Four cycles of isolated hypoxic abdominal perfusion were conducted at 4-weekly intervals. Cisplatin, adriamycin, and mitomycin were prescribed, respectively [18]. After each treatment cycle, leukocytes and thrombocytes were monitored weekly, and monitoring occurred 2 weeks after therapy in the nadir range in 48-h intervals. The tumor marker CA 12-5 was determined immediately before each cycle and on the fifth day after, before the patient was discharged from inpatient treatment. After the second and fourth treatment session, imaging, computer tomographic monitoring was instigated.

Patients who had given their consent to it were subjected to laparotomy and explorative restaging and evaluation of their histological response rate after the final cycle. Particular importance was attached to the course of tumor marker CA 12-5 during the entire treatment, especially when a positive effect on the patient's general

Table 24.1 Patient characteristics

Stage	FIGO IIIb	4 % ($n=3$ patients)
	FIGO IIIc	71 % ($n=56$ patients)
	FIGO IV	25 % ($n=20$ patients)
Peritoneal carcinosis	4 quadrants	78 % ($n=62$ patients)
	2 quadrants	21.5 % ($n=17$ patients)
Grade of malignancy	G3	39 % ($n=31$ patients)

Table 24.2 Results

Response rates		
Clinical	CR 25 %/PR 39 %	Total 64 %
Histological	CR 13 %/PR 35 %	Total 48 %
Ascites		
Complete remission	43 %	Total 62 %
Reduction	19 %	
Survival rates	**PFS (months)**	**Overall survival (months)**
25 %	12	30
50 % (median)	8	14
75 %	4	8

condition was observed due to a reduction or complete disappearance of ascites and other symptoms.

Exclusion criteria were severe comorbidities such as cardiovascular insufficiency due to coronary heart disease or absolute arrhythmia, uncontrolled diabetes, or severe infections. The leukocyte figure should not be below 2,500/µl (not with a declining trend), and the thrombocyte figure should not fall below 150,000/µl. Cytostatic agents were chosen due to the hypoxic perfusion therapy in relation to their predominant toxicity under hypoxic conditions (Figs. 24.1 and 24.2), as described by B. Teicher [21]. The overall dose of cisplatin administered via the aorta in the abdominal segment did not exceed the 70 mg limit. For adriamycin the dose limit was 50 mg, and for mitomycin 20 mg.

The patients included in this study were mainly at FIGO stage IIIc (71 %) and FIGO IV (25 %). 87.5 % had a four-quadrant peritoneal carcinosis, and interestingly 39 % ($n=31$) showed a histologic grade of G3 malignancy (Table 24.1). 79 % of all patients were heavily pretreated; six of them had already undergone third-line and one patient fourth-line therapies [18].

24.5 Results

The study endpoints were quality of life, survival time, and response rate. The clinical response rate in terms of decline of the tumor marker CA 12-5, computer tomography, and quality of life, especially in the form of reduction or complete disappearance of ascites, pain, or general discomfort, was 64 %, in comparison to 48 % histological response after an explorative second-look surgery. A complete disappearance of ascites was observed in 43 % of patients after two treatments, and

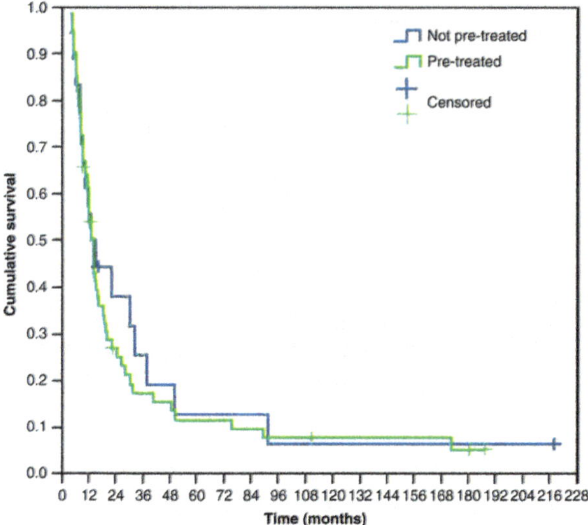

Fig. 24.7 Kaplan-Meier survival curve after hypoxic abdominal perfusion (HAP) with pretreated ($n = 63$) and non-pretreated ($n = 17$) FIGO III/IV ovarian cancer

a further 19 % of patients experienced a substantial decrease in abdominal fluid volume of an estimated more than 50 %. 74 % or three out of four patients reported a definite decrease in abdominal symptoms and a clear improvement in their pain situation (Table 24.2). Median progression-free survival was 8 months and median overall survival 14 months. Eight patients survived between 6 and 18 years. Of four patients who have currently survived between 11 and 19 years, three of them originally had G3 tumors. There was no statistical survival difference recorded between pretreated and non-pretreated patients (Fig. 24.7).

24.6 Toxicity

The bone marrow toxicity was not very pronounced and ranged between WHO grade 1 and 2. Only patients with previous severe third- or fourth-line chemotherapy had leukopenia and thrombocytopenia (WHO grade 3). Grade 4 toxicity or febrile neutropenia was never observed. Postoperative fatigue syndrome, whenever it occurred, was observed from the third day after surgery and was usually accompanied by post-therapeutic tumor necrosis and a temporary steep increase in LDH and CA 12-5. These syndromes are mainly observed during the first postoperative week with a focus on the second and third postoperative day, and this was the case with around 15–20 % of all patients. The predominant clinical symptom in these cases was fever and fatigue. A frequent accompanying symptom was postoperative lymphatic fistula in the groin in over 30 % of all cases. This ended without complications, however, if Redon drainage was concluded after only 14 days.

24.7   Discussion

The crucial point in treatment of ovarian cancer is that none of the cytostatic agent combinations – apart from the standard treatment with cisplatin and paclitaxel – have really produced a genuine improvement in progression-free survival (PFS), overall survival (OS), or quality of life (QoL). The limiting factor in all studies such as long-term chemotherapy, dose-intensive chemotherapy, or high-dose chemotherapy was toxicity as well as neuropathy (hand-foot syndrome), neutropenia, or fatigue and exhaustion. In addition, the lack of any formal assessment of quality of life in most studies did not allow for any conclusions about quality of life-related survival. In view of the fact that the mortality rate for ovarian cancer has hardly changed over the last 30 years, it seemed appropriate to investigate other treatment options. Based on the angiogenetic properties of ovarian cancer with extensive vascularization, the assumption was that targeted treatments that had the blood supply of neoplasia as their target would be capable of solving the problem by achieving a high tumor response rate while sparing healthy tissue at the same time. Apart from clinical effectiveness, usually in the form of prolonging progression-free survival (PFS), severe toxicity was also observed in the form of high blood pressure, bleeding, proteinuria, cardiotoxicity, and gastrointestinal toxicity with spontaneous perforations [32].

In a study of 32 patients, who had been pretreated with multiple chemotherapy regimens, positive results were observed with bevacizumab [24]. The median survival time was 6.9 months, with a median PFS of 5.5 months. These results are significantly lower compared to the isolated abdominal perfusion with a median survival time of 14 months and a PFS of 8 months. In a phase-II study to evaluate the efficacy and tolerability of bevacizumab, in patients with progressive ovarian cancer, a PFS of 4 months and an overall survival rate of 17 months were achieved. Toxicity and side effects were reported at grade 3 for hypertension and grade 4 for pulmonary embolism, vomiting, constipation, and proteinuria [25]. Even though these results appear promising, toxicity and side effects are definitely worse than after isolated perfusion and chemofiltration.

The first goal for any cancer drug or surgical treatment should be to increase the survival rate along with better quality of life. There should not actually be any other argument as the basis for recommended treatment [26]. However, thousands of patients in many studies [4–14] have been treated without any significant progress having been reported especially in relation to quality of life or survival with improved quality of life. Surgical tumor debulking and cytoreduction in advanced diseases prolong progression-free survival – but this is also limited to the early stages when what is seen as a curative operation is still possible [27].

Unfortunately, most therapeutic regimens aim for an improvement in progression-free survival (PFS) while accepting greater toxicity on the assumption that prolonged PFS will also involve prolonged overall survival. This is not always the case, however; instead prolonged overall survival is almost always associated with an extended PFS.

It is assumed that progress in the treatment of various types of cancer such as ovarian, colorectal, or testicular cancer correlates largely with the chemoresistance of tumor stem cells. During the last three decades, the cure rates for testicular cancer have risen dramatically (from 23 % to 81 %) and those of colorectal cancer at stage 3 likewise (from 29 % to 47 %) [17], while the cure rate for ovarian cancer has hardly changed during the same period (from 12 % to 14 %). The relatively very low cure rate for ovarian cancer patients may be associated with the low response rate of epithelial ovarian cancer stem cells, where the low increase in overall survival may be a result of the reduction in the non-stem cell proportion of the tumor. This could explain why further chemotherapy can bring about renewed remission after recurrences and under some circumstances even prolong life [26]. Such a strategy could even help in exposing patients to lower levels of toxicity. The problem with chemoresistant stem cells remains, however, and these patients have only limited therapeutic options.

A basic principle to avoid systemic "drug spill" and to increase the cytostatic effect in the target area is application via the arterial blood supply of tumors, where in particular the benefit of what is called first-pass extraction, cytostatic extraction, is used in the first pass through the tumor bed, which constitutes by far the most effective part of any cytostatic treatment [28–31]. The isolated perfusion technique may result in individually adapted drug exposure (area under the AUC curve) and may break through the chemoresistance of tumor stem cells in certain cases depending on the tumor and how pronounced the chemoresistance is. This is reflected in a few long-term surviving patients after regional therapy with initially very advanced G3 tumors. Despite highly concentrated regional therapy in the abdominal segment due to simultaneous chemofiltration, they had hardly any side effects and a very good quality of life even during therapy. Thoroughgoing relief from abdominal pain and discomfort for 74 % and the complete disappearance of ascites for 43 % of patients are essential components in relation to the value of isolated perfusion therapy. With the proposed treatment objective of prolonging life with good or improved quality of life, this may be a significant advance, considering that the patients who were usually suffering from the aftereffects of previous chemotherapy and the stress of pronounced ascites at the beginning of the treatment had a life expectancy of at best 6–12 weeks at that stage. Their survival benefits after isolated regional perfusion therapy are quite obvious with this tumor activity of the peritoneal metastatic and relapsed ovarian cancer mainly restricted to the abdominal segment, as their estimated life expectancy quadrupled and patients with recurrent G3 tumors in individual cases are still surviving free of recurrence after 11–19 years. In this constellation the systemically heavily pretreated or untreatable patient, who again experiences remission after regional chemotherapy often lasting for months and years, is her own monitor. It is impossible to conduct a prospective phase-III study on systemic versus regional chemotherapy with systemically untreatable patients, who still suffer from the aftereffects of toxicity, as their bone marrow reserves are often exhausted, the patients are considered untreatable, and they normally refuse further therapy.

The quality of life in cancer treatment is a parameter which should be focused on primarily, especially as newer treatment options only result in only minimal extensions of PFS or overall survival – 1, 2, or 3 months, if at all – and this at the expense of quite considerable toxicity and even a huge increase in the financial burden [33]. In this respect, a phase-III study, which investigates regional versus systemic chemotherapy among previously untreated patients, will be very important and could provide information about therapeutic options to be adopted in the future.

References

1. Gore ME, Fryatt I, Wiltshaw E, Dawson T. Treatment of relapsed carcinoma of the ovary with cisplatin or carboplatin following initial treatment with these compounds. Gynecol Oncol. 1990;36:207–11.
2. Markman M, Rothman R, Hakes T, et al. Second-line platinum therapy in patients with ovarian cancer previously treated with cisplatin. J Clin Oncol. 1991;9:389–93.
3. Ozols RF. Treatment of recurrent ovarian cancer: increasing options – "recurrent" results. J Clin Oncol. 1997;15:2177–80.
4. Dark GG, Calvert AH, Grimshaw R, Poole C, Swenerton K, Kaye S, et al. Randomized trial of two intravenous schedules of the topoisomerase I inhibitor liposomal lurtotecan in women with relapsed epithelial ovarian cancer: a trial of the National Cancer Institute of Canada Clinical Trials Group. J Clin Oncol. 2005;23:1859–66.
5. Gore M, Mainwaring P, A'Hern R, et al. Randomized trial of dose-intensity with single-agent carboplatin in patients with epithelial ovarian cancer. London Gynaecological Oncology Group. J Clin Oncol. 1998;16:2426–34.
6. Jodrell DI, Egorin MJ, Canetta RM, Langenberg P, Goldbloom EP, Burroughs JN, et al. Relationships between carboplatin exposure and tumor response and toxicity in patients with ovarian cancer. J Clin Oncol. 1992;10:520–8.
7. Levin L, Hryniuk WM. Dose intensity analysis of chemotherapy regimens in ovarian carcinoma. J Clin Oncol. 1987;5:756–67.
8. McGuire WP, Hoskins WJ, Brady MF, et al. Assessment of dose-intensive therapy in suboptimally ovarian cancer: a Gynecologic Oncology Group study. J Clin Oncol. 1995;13:1589–99.
9. Omura GA, Brady MF, Look KY, Averette HE, Delmore JE, Long HJ, et al. Phase III trial of paclitaxel at two dose levels, the higher dose accompanied by filgrastim at two dose levels in platinum-pretreated epithelial ovarian cancer: an intergroup study. J Clin Oncol. 2003;21:2843–8.
10. Thigpen JT. Dose-intensity in ovarian carcinoma: hold, enough? J Clin Oncol. 1997;15:1291–3.
11. Grenman S, Wiklund T, Jalkanen J, et al. A randomised phase III study comparing high-dose chemotherapy to conventionally dosed chemotherapy for stage III ovarian cancer: the Finnish Ovarian (FINOVA) study. Eur J Cancer. 2006;42:2196–9.
12. Möbus V, Wandt H, Frickhofen N, Bengala C, Champion K, Kimming R, et al. Phase III trial of high-dose sequential chemotherapy with peripheral blood stem cell support compared with standard dose chemotherapy for first-line treatment of advanced ovarian cancer: intergroup trial of the AGO-Ovar/AIO and EBMT. J Clin Oncol. 2007;25:4187–93.
13. du Bois A, Weber B, Rochon J, et al. Addition of epirubicin as a third drug to Carboplatin-paclitaxel in first-line treatment of advanced ovarian cancer: a prospectively randomized gynecologic cancer intergroup trial by the Arbeitsgemeinschaft Gynaekologische Onkologie Ovarian Cancer Study Group and the Groupe d'Investigateurs Nationaux pour l'Etude des Cancers Ovariens. J Clin Oncol. 2006;24:1127–35.
14. Fung MF, Johnston ME, Eisenhauer EA, Elit L, Hirte HW, Rosen B, et al. Chemotherapy for recurrent epithelial ovarian cancer previously treated with platinum – a systematic review of the evidence from randomized trials. Eur J Gynaecol Oncol. 2002;23:104–10.
15. Markman M, Liu PY, Moon J, et al. Impact on survival of 12 versus 3 monthly cycles of paclitaxel (175 mg/m^2) administered to patients with advanced ovarian cancer who attained a

complete response to primary platinum-paclitaxel: follow-up of a Southwest Oncology Group and Gynecologic Oncology Group phase 3 trial. Gynecol Oncol. 2009;114:195–8.

16. Markman M, Liu PY, Wilczynski S, et al. Phase III randomized trial of 12 versus 3 months of maintenance paclitaxel in patients with advanced ovarian cancer after complete response to platinum and paclitaxel-based chemotherapy: a Southwest Oncology Group and Gynecologic Oncology Group trial. J Clin Oncol. 2003;21:2460–5.

17. Huang L, Cronin Kathleen A, Johnson Karen A, Mariotto Angela B, Feuer Eric J. Improved survival time: what can survival cure models tell us about population-based survival improvements in late-stage colorectal, ovarian, and testicular cancer? Cancer. 2010;112:2289–300.

18. Aigner KR, Gailhofer S, et al. Hypoxic abdominal perfusion for recurrent platinum refractory ovarian cancer. Cancer Ther. 2008;6:213–20.

19. Creech O, Krementz ET, Ryan RF, Winbald JN. Chemotherapy of cancer: regional perfusion utilizing an extracorporeal circuit. Ann Surg. 1958;148:616–32.

20. Kroon BBR. Regional isolated perfusion in melanoma of the limbs; accomplishments, unsolved problems, future. Eur J Surg Oncol. 1988;14:101–10.

21. Teicher BA, Lazo JS, Sartorelli A. Classification of antineoplastic agents by their selective toxicities toward oxygenated and hypoxic tumor cells. Cancer Res. 1981;41:73–81.

22. Aigner KR, Gailhofer S. High dose MMC: aortic stopflow infusion (ASI) with versus without chemofiltration: a comparison of toxic side effects (abstract). Reg Cancer Treat. 1993;6 Suppl 1:3.

23. Muchmore JH, Aigner KR, Beg MH. Regional chemotherapy for advanced intraabdominal and pelvic cancer. In: Cohen AM, Winawer SJ, Friedman MA, Gunderson LL, editors. Cancer of the colon, rectum and anus. New York: McGraw Hill; 1995. p. 881–9. In Albert Cohn Colorectal Cancer.

24. Monk BJ, Han E, Joseph-Cowen CA, Pugmire G, Burger RA. Salvage bevacizumab (rhuMAB VEGF)-based therapy after multiple prior cytotoxic regimens in advanced refractory epithelial ovarian cancer. Gynecol Oncol. 2006;102:140–4.

25. Burger RA, Sill MW, Monk BJ, Greer BE, Sorosky JI. Phase II trial of Bevacizumab in persistent or recurrent epithelial ovarian cancer of primary peritoneal cancer: a Gynecologic Oncology Group Study. J Clin Oncol. 2007;25:5165–71.

26. Cannistra SA. The ethics of early stopping rules: who is protecting whom? J Clin Oncol. 2004;22:1542–5.

27. Crawford SC, Vasey PA, Paul J, Hay A, Davis JA, Kaye SB. Does aggressive surgery only benefit patients with less advanced ovarian cancer? Results from an international comparison within the SCOTROC-1 trial. J Clin Oncol. 2005;23:8802–11.

28. Stephens FO, Harker GJS, Crea P. The intra-arterial Infusion of chemotherapeutic agents as "basal" treatment of cancer: evidence of increased drug activity in regionally infused tissues. Aust N Z J Surg. 1980;50:597–602.

29. Stephens FO. Why use regional chemotherapy? Principles and pharmacokinetics. Reg Cancer Treat. 1988;1:4–10.

30. Stephens FO. Induction (neo-adjuvant) chemotherapy systemic and arterial delivery techniques and their clinical applications. Aust N Z J Surg. 1995;65:699–707.

31. Stephens FO. Induction (neo-adjuvant) chemotherapy: the place and techniques of using chemotherapy to downgrade aggressive or advanced localised cancers to make them potentially more curable by surgery and/or radiotherapy. Eur J Surg Oncol. 2001;27(7):627–88.

32. Stone Rebecca L, Sood Anil K, Coleman RL. Collateral damage: toxic effects of targeted antiangiogenic therapies in ovarian cancer. Lancet Oncol. 2010;11:465–75.

33. Aigner KR, Stephens FO. Guidelines and evidence-based medicine – evidence of what? EJCMO 2012. Published online. http://www.slm-oncology.com/Guidelines_and_Evidence_Based_Medicine_Evidence_of_What_,1,272.html.

Isolated Limb Perfusion for Melanoma

25

Bin B.R. Kroon, Hidde M. Kroon, Eva M. Noorda,
Bart C. Vrouenraets, Joost M. Klaase,
Gooike W. van Slooten, and Omgo E. Nieweg

25.1 Introduction

The technique of isolated limb perfusion, utilising an oxygenated extracorporeal circuit, was pioneered by Creech et al. at Tulane University, New Orleans, in 1957 [1]. A complete response was achieved in the 76-year-old male patient with extensive recurrent melanoma of his leg, and this lasted until he died at the age of 92. The advantage of this intriguing treatment modality is that a high dose of a cytostatic drug can be delivered to a tumour-bearing limb without the risk of systemic side effects. Isolated limb perfusion is a valuable therapeutic option in patients with an unresectable limb tumour and especially in lesions with a high tendency for locoregional recurrence, as is sometimes the case in melanoma [2].

B.B.R. Kroon, MD, PhD, FRCS (✉) • G.W. van Slooten, MSc
Department of Surgery, The Netherlands Cancer Institute – Antoni van Leeuwenhoek
Hospital, Plesmanlaan 121, Amsterdam 1066 CX, The Netherlands
e-mail: bbrkroon@gmail.com

H.M. Kroon, MD, PhD
Department of Surgery, Erasmus Medical Center,
s-Gravendijkwal 230, Rotterdam 3015 CE, The Netherlands

E.M. Noorda, MD, PhD
Department of Surgery, Isala Kliniek, Dr. Van Heesweg 2, Zwolle 8025 AB, The Netherlands

B.C. Vrouenraets, MD, PhD
Department of Surgery, Sint Lucas Andreas Hospital,
J. Tooropstraat 164, Amsterdam 1061 AE, The Netherlands

J.M. Klaase, MD, PhD
Department of Surgery, Medisch Spectrum Twente,
Haaksbergenstraat 55, Enschede 7500 KA, The Netherlands

O.E. Nieweg, MD, PhD
Melanoma Institute Australia, 40 Rocklands Road, North Sydney, NSW 2060, Australia

Sydney Medical School, The University of Sydney, North Sydney, NSW 2006, Australia

© Springer-Verlag Berlin Heidelberg 2016
K.R. Aigner, F.O. Stephens (eds.), *Induction Chemotherapy*,
DOI 10.1007/978-3-319-28773-7_25

25.2 Perfusion Methodology

25.2.1 Technique

Isolation of the blood circuit of a limb is achieved by open access to the major artery and vein supplying the limb and by ligating the collateral vessels. A tourniquet is applied around the limb proximal to the region to be perfused in order to compress the smaller vessels in the muscles and subcutaneous tissues. After insertion of a catheter in the major artery and vein, the isolated limb is perfused by an extracorporeal circulation, oxygenated and propelled by a heart-lung machine (Fig. 25.1). The cytostatic drug is administered into this circuit. The priming volume of the extracorporeal circuit is about 750 ml and is composed of 300 ml autologous whole blood diluted with physiological electrolyte solution to a haematocrit of about 30 %. The autologous blood is taken from the venous catheter, just before the start of the isolation. The flow-driven extracorporeal circulation aims for the highest flow rate possible without increasing the venous pressure more than 10 cm above the starting point. The venous pressure in the limb can be monitored in a subcutaneous vein at the distal end of the extremity. Physiological blood gas values can be obtained with flow rates of 30–40 ml/min/l tissue [3].

Perfusion may be conducted in the lower limb at the external iliac level, at the femoral or popliteal level and in the upper limb at the axillary or brachial level. For

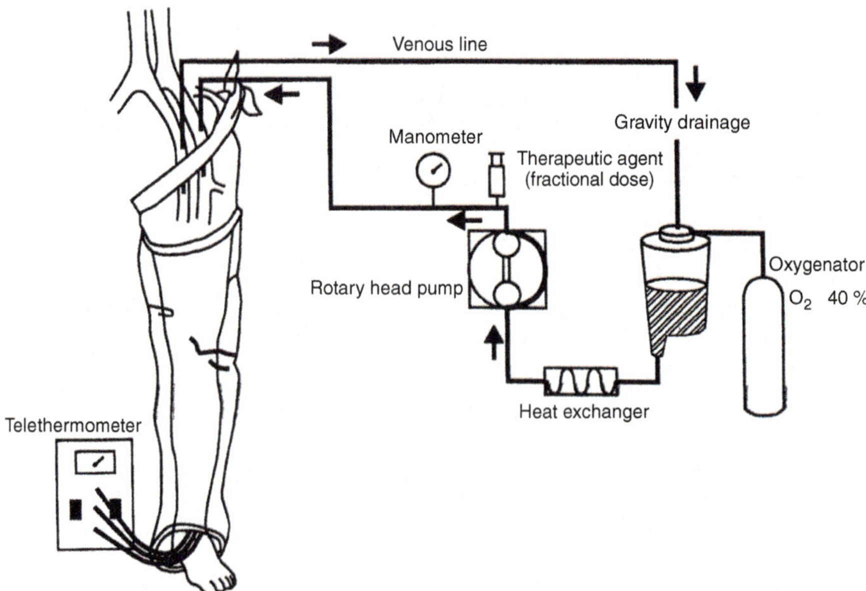

Fig. 25.1 Schematic drawing of the isolated perfusion circuit

iliac perfusion, the iliac and obturator lymph nodes are removed. Two recent descriptions of the surgical technique have been published [4, 5].

25.2.2 Drugs

Melphalan is the cytostatic drug of choice for melanoma. The dose of melphalan is guided by the limb volume to be perfused, and this volume can be determined by immersion of the limb in a cylinder filled with water [3]. The maximum dose associated with an acceptable risk of toxicity in the normal tissues is approximately 10 mg/l perfused tissue for the lower limb and 13 mg/l for the upper limb [6]. This difference in dosing is due to the change in drug concentration in the different circulating volumes that are used in upper and lower limb perfusions.

Recombinant tumour necrosis factor alpha (TNFα) is sometimes added to the melphalan in the circuit. The main indication for this biological response modifier is the presence of bulky, well-vascularised melanoma lesions, since TNFα has a selective destructive effect on newly formed vessels. This typically leads to thrombosis with acute necrosis of tumour tissue and to a selectively increased melphalan concentration in tumour tissue due to an enhanced permeability of the vessel walls [7–9]. Objective response data using other drugs like actinomycin D, cisplatin, vindesine, DTIC, fotemustine, interleukin-2 and lymphokine-activated killer cells are not encouraging [10–14]. It appears that none of these drugs is as effective as melphalan, neither as single agents nor in combination with other agents.

25.2.3 Monitoring Leakage

The extremely high cytostatic drug dosages in the limb could be fatal when they reach vital organs. The limbs, for example, can endure melphalan concentrations up to 20 times higher than would be tolerated in the rest of the body [6]. The potential leakage into the systemic circulation thus requires careful monitoring. To this end, a small dose of a radiopharmaceutical is administered into the extracorporeal circuit, and a detector placed over the heart registers radioactivity that reaches the main circulation. An experienced team can generally keep the leakage rate below 5 %. In 438 procedures, we measured a mean cumulative systemic leakage of 0.9 % (range 0.0–15.6 %) after 60 min of perfusion [15].

25.2.4 Tissue Temperatures

As we aim for physiological conditions, concentrating only on drug effectiveness, tissue temperatures of the limb are kept at normothermic levels between 37 and 38 °C during the whole drug circulation time. This is called "controlled" normothermia because special measures such as warming the perfusate and applying a warm water blanket around the limb must be taken to prevent the limb from cooling down during the preparative surgery [2]. The drug is added to the perfusate when a temperature of 37 °C is indicated by all four temperature probes inserted into proximal and distal subcutis and muscle. We question the benefit of the widely used so-called "mild" hyperthermia method (with tissue temperatures between 39 and 40 °C), since the specific cell-killing effect of heat is mainly obtained at temperatures exceeding 41.5 °C [16]. A retrospective analysis showed similar results for perfusions with normothermia and perfusions with mild hyperthermia [17]. "True" hyperthermia means heating the tissues to temperatures between 41.5 and 43 °C. Such high temperatures are no longer applied in perfusion because of unacceptable potentiation of melphalan toxicity by heat, although encouraging antitumour effects have been obtained [18]. The administration of true hyperthermia by a perfusion without cytostatics is, however, an option. Such a perfusion is based only on the cell-killing effect of high-dose hyperthermia [19]. To exploit this option, a double perfusion schedule was tested in our institute. A 2-h true hyperthermic (tissue temperatures between 42 and 43 °C) perfusion without melphalan was followed 1 week later by a 1-h normothermic perfusion with melphalan at a dose of 10 mg/l tissue [20]. The intention of the perfusion with high-dose hyperthermia was to kill cells in the hypoxic parts of the tumour, and the normothermic perfusion with high-dose melphalan was given to attack the residual well-perfused part of the tumour [21]. With this sequential schedule, both treatment modalities, high-dose hyperthermia and high-dose cytostatic, were given at their maximum dosage without an increase in toxicity, which the heat would have caused if used simultaneously with melphalan. Using this schedule, a high complete response rate (63 %) and a low limb recurrence rate (27 %) were seen in 17 patients with extensive, recurrent melanoma [22]. Toxicity was only mild. This regimen could be an alternative to perfusion with the combination of melphalan and TNFα in patients with extensive or bulky lesions.

25.3 Toxicity and Morbidity

25.3.1 Regional

Acute regional toxicity after isolated limb perfusion typically consists of slight oedema, erythema, and pain in a warm limb, commonly developing within 48 h after the procedure and resolving within 14 days (Fig. 25.2). The redness fades to a brown hue that gradually fades over a period of 3–6 months. Usually there is no visible evidence of any change after approximately 6 months. Other local manifestations are sometimes seen (e.g. temporary loss of nails (Fig. 25.3), drying or blistering of skin of the palm of the hand or sole of the foot, inhibition of hair growth on the extremity or transient neuralgia), but all subside over time. More severe toxicity may occur in the form of blistering and muscle damage. Damage to the deep tissues can cause permanent loss of function and may also result in a threatening or manifest compartment syndrome, which necessitates amputation on rare occasions. The grading system of these toxic reactions of the normal tissues after perfusion

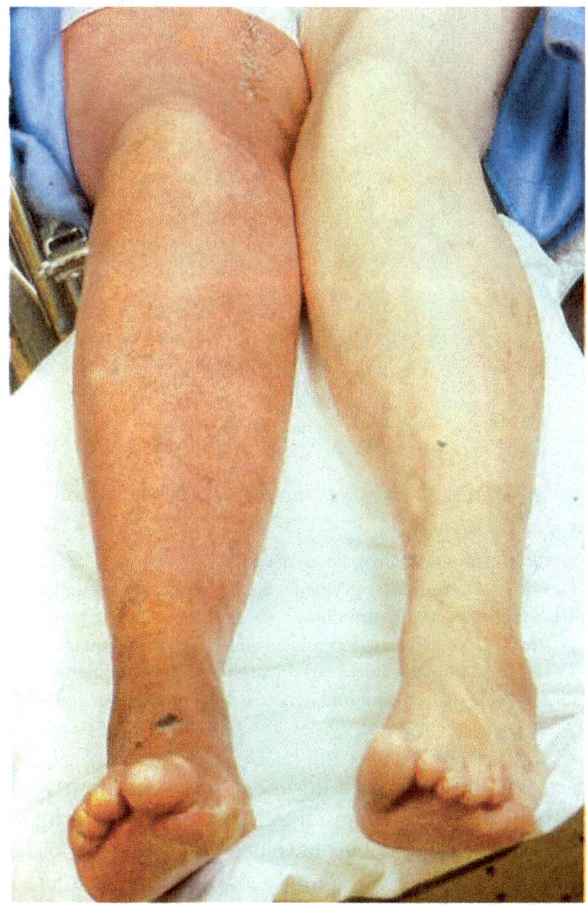

Fig. 25.2 Normal acute regional toxicity reaction after isolated limb perfusion (Grade II) (Reproduced from the Textbook of Melanoma, 2004, with permission of Taylor and Francis [86])

with melphalan was introduced by Wieberdink et al. in 1982 (Table 25.1) [3]. From published data of large series, one can conclude that moderate to severe acute skin or soft tissue reactions (grades III–V according to Wieberdink) occur in 7–37 % of patients. The degree of acute regional injury has a significant effect on the incidence of long-term morbidity [23]. This long-term morbidity mainly consists of stiffness, muscle atrophy and functional impairment. Restricted range of ankle motion is seen in 25 % of the patients [24–26]. Severe chronic pain as a result of the procedure is reported in 5–8 % of the patients [23, 26]. The occurrence of long-term neuropathy was studied at the authors' institute and was encountered in 20 % of the patients after perfusion at the axillary level and in 2 % after perfusion at the iliac level [27]. This morbidity is usually the result of the tourniquet being applied too tight during the procedure. The most important risk factors for severe acute regional toxicity are tissue temperatures over 40 °C, a high melphalan peak concentration in the perfusate, female gender and obesity [18, 28]. The reason why obese extremities are prone to develop toxicity is the higher melphalan uptake in muscle compared to fat.

Fig. 25.3 Normal acute regional toxicity reaction (Grade II) with loss of nails

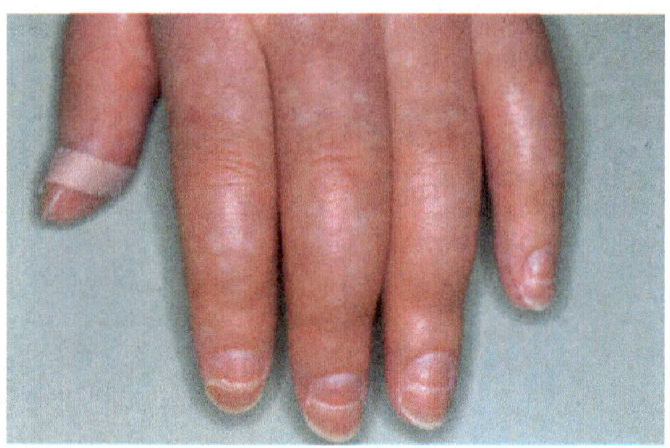

Table 25.1 Acute regional toxicity grading system according to Wieberdink et al. [3]

Grade I	No reaction
Grade II	Slight erythema and/or oedema
Grade III	Considerable erythema and/or oedema with some blistering; slightly disturbed motility permissible
Grade IV	Extensive epidermolysis and/or obvious damage to the deep tissues, causing definitive functional disturbances; threatening or manifest compartment syndrome
Grade V	Reaction which may necessitate amputation

Because the melphalan dosage is based on limb volume, muscle tissue in obese extremities is thus exposed to a relatively high drug dose [29]. Some strategies to lower the toxic reactions have been recommended. The melphalan peak concentration can be lowered without decreasing the absolute drug dose by using a larger priming volume and by prolonged or fractionated administration [30, 31]. Obese people often receive a 10 % reduction in melphalan dose [27].

25.3.2 Systemic

Systemic toxicity should be absent or mild, when leakage from the isolated limb is adequately controlled. Careful ligation of collateral vessels, the avoidance of high flow rates and high venous pressures and a thorough wash-out of the isolated circuit at the end of the procedure are particularly important in this respect. With these precautions, systemic toxicity was found to be absent or mild in patients perfused at the authors' institute, both after perfusions with melphalan alone and after perfusions in which the combination with TNFα was used [32, 33].

In the melphalan-alone group, nausea and vomiting were the most frequently encountered side effects. Fever immediately following the operation was common if TNFα was added. A systemic inflammatory response syndrome with hypotension and respiratory distress, as reported by others [34], was not observed in our TNFα-perfused patients.

25.4 Indications and Results

25.4.1 Locally Advanced Melanoma

Isolated perfusion with melphalan is the treatment of choice for patients with locally unresectable melanoma of a limb (Figs. 25.4, 25.5 and 25.6). In the past, these patients frequently had to undergo amputation, a mutilation that is now seldom necessary [35]. When the lesions are bulky and well vascularised, high response rates have been reported when melphalan is combined with TNFα [36, 37]. In a recent preclinical study in mice, selective targeting of VE-cadherin was found to be one of the mechanisms in which TNFα destroys the integrity of the tumour vasculature [38]. In our hands, a complete response rate of 59 % could be obtained with the combination of melphalan and TNFα in a group of 130 patients with truly unresectable lesions (i.e. more than ten nodules or nodules with a size larger than 3 cm) [39]. With melphalan alone, the complete response rate was 45 %. Approximately half of the patients with a complete response recurred in the perfused region after a median interval of 6 months after treatment. The recurrences could be managed by simple local treatment modalities, such as excision,

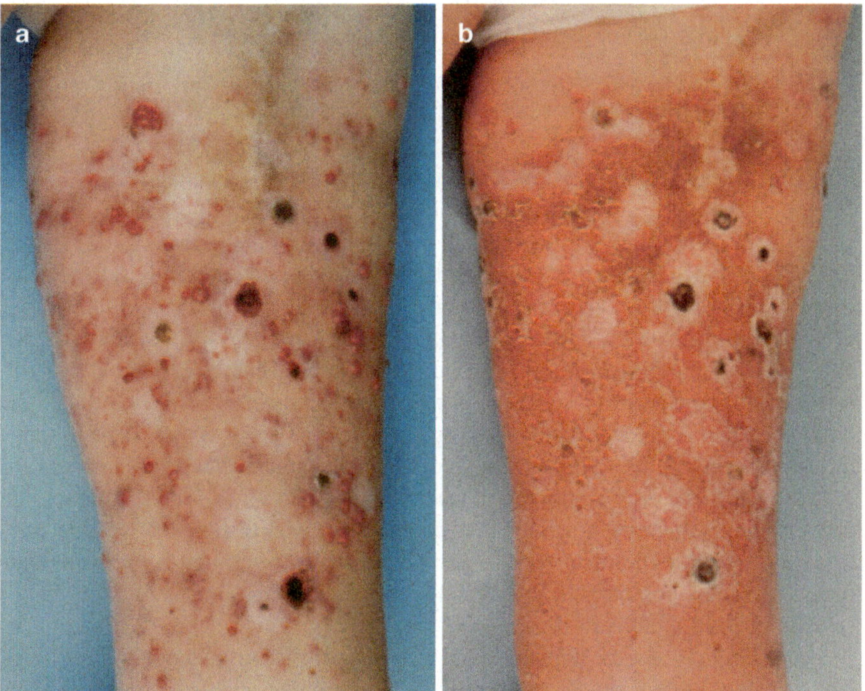

Fig. 25.4 (a) Multiple in-transit metastases of the left thigh. (b) Ongoing remission, 6 weeks after perfusion with melphalan. Complete remission was achieved some weeks later (Reproduced from the Textbook of Melanoma, 2004, with permission of Taylor and Francis [86])

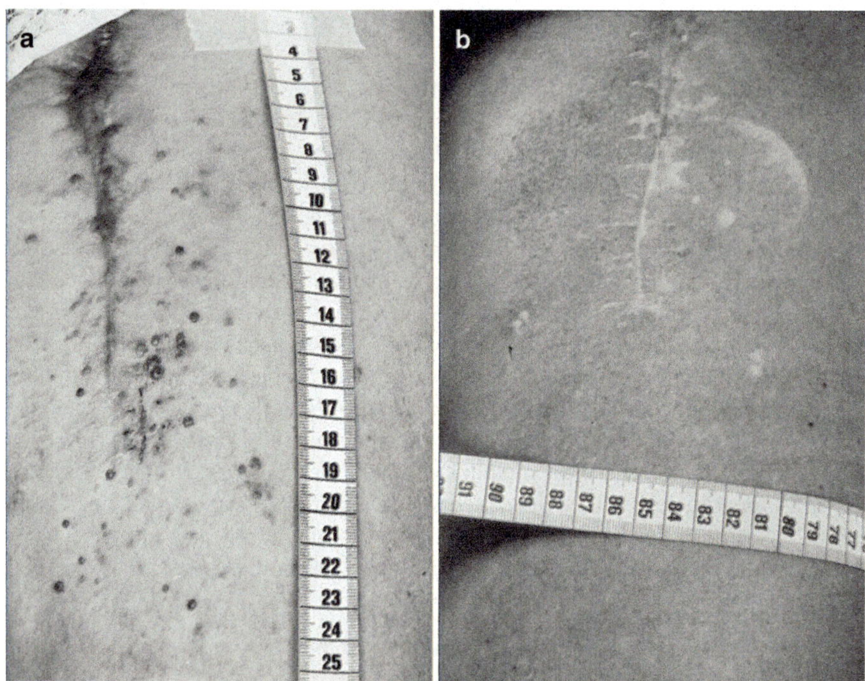

Fig. 25.5 (**a**) Multiple in-transit metastases around the scar of a left inguinal lymph node dissection. (**b**) Complete remission 3 months after perfusion

laser ablation or radiotherapy in 70 % of the patients. Approximately 50 % of the patients without a complete response could also be managed by simple local limb-sparing treatment. The limb-saving rate in the study population was 97 %, a satisfying percentage considering the fact that the disease had been truly unresectable in all cases. Literature shows the complete response rate after melphalan-alone perfusions for advanced limb melanoma to be on average 54 %, which is higher than the 45 % at our institution [40, 41]. This difference can be explained by a difference in tumour load. It has been shown that the number of lesions and the total tumour surface area are important prognostic factors for response after isolated limb perfusion [42, 43]. The published, complete response rates after isolated limb perfusion with the drug combination vary from 26 % to 90 %, with the higher percentages probably being attributable to a generally lower tumour load [37, 44–49]. In patients with a complete response, other investigators found subsequent limb recurrence rates comparable to ours: 44 % of the patients recur after a median interval of 5–10 months [40].

Perfusion may also be applied in the presence of distant melanoma metastases. Unresectable symptomatic locoregional limb melanoma is rare in these patients, but if present, perfusion can achieve satisfactory palliation [49]. The procedure has to be considered, especially in patients with distant skin metastases, distant subcutaneous metastases or distant nodal metastases, since these patients tend to survive longer than a year.

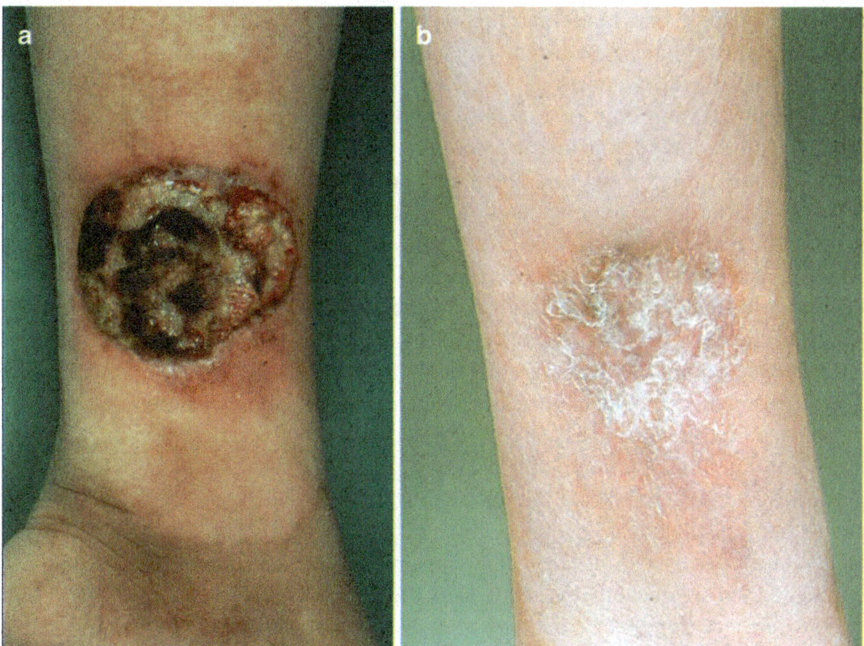

Fig. 25.6 (**a**) Neglected primary melanoma with bone involvement. (**b**) Complete remission 6 months after perfusion (Reproduced from the Textbook of Melanoma, 2004, with permission of Taylor and Francis [86])

A potential drawback of perfusion is the fact that it cannot be repeated frequently due to technical reasons. Still, a double perfusion schedule with intervals of 3–4 weeks between the treatments is feasible and has been investigated at the authors' institute [50]. Although 77 % of these patients obtained a complete response using such a schedule, half of them recurred in the perfused area after a median period of 5 months. It is noteworthy that in this study patients with a complete response had a significantly shorter time interval between their perfusions than patients without a complete response.

25.4.2 Isolated Limb Perfusion as an Adjunct in Primary and Recurrent Melanoma

Isolated limb perfusion as an adjunct after excision of high-risk primary melanoma (Breslow thickness ≥ 1.5 mm) was studied in a large multicentre randomised clinical trial, comprising 852 patients. The patients underwent either wide local excision or wide local excision and perfusion [51]. Locoregional recurrences occurred less frequently in the perfusion group (3.3 % versus 6.6 %, $P=0.05$). The disease-free survival was better in the perfusion group during the first 2–3 years after treatment ($P=0.02$), but no long-term effect was observed. There was no beneficial effect of perfusion on overall survival.

There is only one randomised prospective isolated limb perfusion study in patients with resectable recurrent melanoma [52]. In this rather small study, 69 patients with local recurrences, satellites and/or in-transit metastases were randomised to excision only or excision combined with perfusion. In the perfusion group, a lower locoregional recurrence rate of 45 % was seen versus 67 % in the excision-only group ($P=0.13$). The median disease-free interval was prolonged to 17 months after perfusion compared with 10 months after excision only ($P=0.04$). No significant difference in overall survival was observed, with 5-year survival rates of 44 % and 39 %, respectively ($P=0.28$).

The investigators of both studies concluded that isolated limb perfusion with all its costs and associated morbidity cannot be recommended as an adjunct treatment option, because no overall survival benefit was observed., However, it is interesting that perfusion reduced the number of recurrences and increased disease-free survival in both studies, suggesting a destructive effect on micrometastastic disease. Adjuvant perfusion may thus provide valuable locoregional disease control in patients with frequently recurring and multiple resectable lesions. This hypothesis was tested at the authors' institute in 43 patients, who had their first perfusion for a third or subsequent limb recurrence [53]. The median limb recurrence-free interval in these patients had decreased significantly over time from the primary excision to the third or fourth limb recurrence, for which perfusion was performed ($P<0.001$). After perfusion, the median limb recurrence-free interval was 4.7 times longer compared with the last interval before perfusion ($P<0.001$). The mean number of lesions was 2.6-fold lower compared with patients before perfusion ($P<0.001$). Perfusion in this study thus lengthened the limb recurrence-free interval and decreased the number of recurrences significantly. We concluded that perfusion is a valuable adjunct to excisional surgery of repeated locoregional melanoma recurrences in patients whose limb recurrence-free intervals tend to shorten over time [53].

25.5 Repeat Isolated Limb Perfusion

After successful treatment of locoregionally recurrent limb melanoma with isolated perfusion, further recurrences develop in 46–54 % of patients [54]. Treatment options in these situations vary depending on the extent of the disease and consist among others of further excision, CO_2 laser ablation, [55] intra-lesional chemo- or immunoablation, [56] and radiotherapy with or without local hyperthermia [57]. If lesions are too large or too numerous, repeat perfusion seems the only alternative to amputation. In 1996 the authors published their results of repeat isolated limb perfusion with melphalan, using various schedules, both single and multiple, normothermic and hyperthermic (tissue temperatures over 41.5 °C) [58]. A high complete response rate was obtained (74 %) with a limb recurrence-free interval of 9 months. The associated regional toxicity was substantial and was explained by the use of intensive schedules. Data on repeat perfusion using the combination of melphalan and TNFα were published in 2006 [59]. The complete response rate was 62 %, and the median limb recurrence-free survival was 13 months. Regional toxicity was mild and comparable with the first perfusion, a finding that was also reported by others [60]. Repeat isolated limb perfusion with melphalan and TNFα seems feasible with a relatively high complete response rate, a considerable limb recurrence-free survival and mild regional toxicity.

25.6 Isolated Limb Perfusion in Elderly Patients

The mean life expectancy at age 75 is 8.5 years for males and 11 years for females [61]. Maintaining and improving the quality of life in this age group is desirable. Therefore, effective perfusion with low morbidity is important also in this phase of life. A study of 202 patients was performed combining data from the authors' institute and from Erasmus Medical Center–Daniel den Hoed Cancer Center, Rotterdam, the Netherlands. Toxicity, complications and long-term morbidity were similar in patients younger than 75 years of age and patients over 75 years of age [62]. Responses were also similar with 56 % complete responses in the older patients and 58 % complete responses in the younger patients. Hospital stay was somewhat longer in the older patients. Approximately half of the patients with a complete response achieved long-term locoregional disease control in either age category. It was concluded that older patients can undergo perfusion safely and derive the same benefit as younger people. Age is not a contraindication for isolated limb perfusion.

25.7 Prognostic Factors for Poor Survival After Perfusion

Patients with recurrent melanoma have 5-year survival rates varying between 27 and 56 %. Some of these patients do not survive longer than 1 year after treatment. Considering the usual 3–6 months duration of locoregional toxicity after perfusion and the maximum response of the lesions at a median of 4 months after the procedure, identification of a tool to select patients who will live long enough to experience the benefits of perfusion would be desirable.

In an attempt to identify prognostic factors for short survival, a study was performed in 439 patients with recurrent melanoma at our institute [63]. Sixty-nine of them (16 %) died within 1 year, 64 of metastatic melanoma. Patients with regional lymph node metastases or with regional lymph node metastases combined with satellites and/or in-transit metastases had a relative risk of 4.6 (95 % CI 2.0–6.6) and 3.6 (95 % CI 2.1–10) of dying within 1 year from perfusion, respectively ($p < 0.001$). In patients with distant disease, the relative risk was 22 (95 % CI 3.8–127, $p = 0.001$). Therefore, patients with limb melanoma have an increased risk of dying within 1 year after perfusion when regional lymph node or distant metastases are present. In these patients, the indication for perfusion should be carefully considered.

25.8   Quality of Life in Long-Term Survivors After Perfusion

Isolated limb perfusion can result in long-term morbidity in up to 40 % of the patients. We examined the impact of long-term morbidity on the quality of life. Fifty-one long-term disease-free survivors, perfused for recurrent melanoma (mean age 71 (38–90), median time after perfusion 14 (3–25) years), were selected from our database [64]. Quality of life assessment in this group was compared with an age- and gender-matched group of the Dutch population. It was demonstrated that the study group scored better on all domains of quality of life. The difference was statistically significant regarding bodily pain, general health perception, and overall mental and physical health scores. Nevertheless, the perfused patients reported considerable disease- and treatment-related morbidity, fear of recurrent disease and cosmetic problems. This counterintuitive outcome can be due to the composition of the study group, a favourable selection of long-term survivors, and "response shift", meaning that patients have changed their perspectives over time and accommodated these to their complaints.

25.9   Isolated Limb Infusion as an Alternative to Isolated Limb Perfusion

Isolated limb *infusion* was designed as a simplified and minimally invasive alternative to isolated limb perfusion [65]. Similar to isolated limb perfusion, it involves a method of vascular isolation to be able to distribute high concentrations of cytotoxic drugs to the extremity (Fig. 25.7).

During isolated limb infusion, arterial and venous access are obtained percutaneously using a standard Seldinger technique, obviating the need for an open surgical procedure [66]. Via the contralateral femoral artery and vein, the tips of the catheters are placed in the disease-bearing limb. In the operating room, the catheters are connected to an extracorporeal circuit primed with saline solution, incorporating a heat exchanger but no mechanical pump or oxygenator. In order to achieve reliable isolation, a pneumatic tourniquet is inflated proximally around the affected limb. A low blood flow can be achieved in this isolated circuit by repeated aspiration from the venous catheter and reinjection into the arterial catheter, using a syringe. This results in a lower blood flow compared to isolated limb perfusion (150–1,000 ml/min for isolated limb perfusion vs. 50–100 ml/min for isolated limb infusion). The lack of oxygenation during isolated limb infusion results in a hypoxic and acidotic environment, rendering the melphalan more potent [67]. Great care is given to heating the limb with the goal to raise the temperature to mild hyperthermia, which is achieved by a heat exchanger in the external circuit, a warm air blanket placed around the limb and a radiant heater placed above it. The cytotoxic drug combination of choice for isolated limb infusion is melphalan and actinomycin D [68]. A relatively short circulation time of 30 min is sufficient given the 15–20 min half-life of melphalan and the quick tissue absorption of both melphalan and actinomycin D [68–70]. Real-time leakage control of the cytotoxic drugs to the systemic

ISOLATED LIMB INFUSION
CIRCUIT

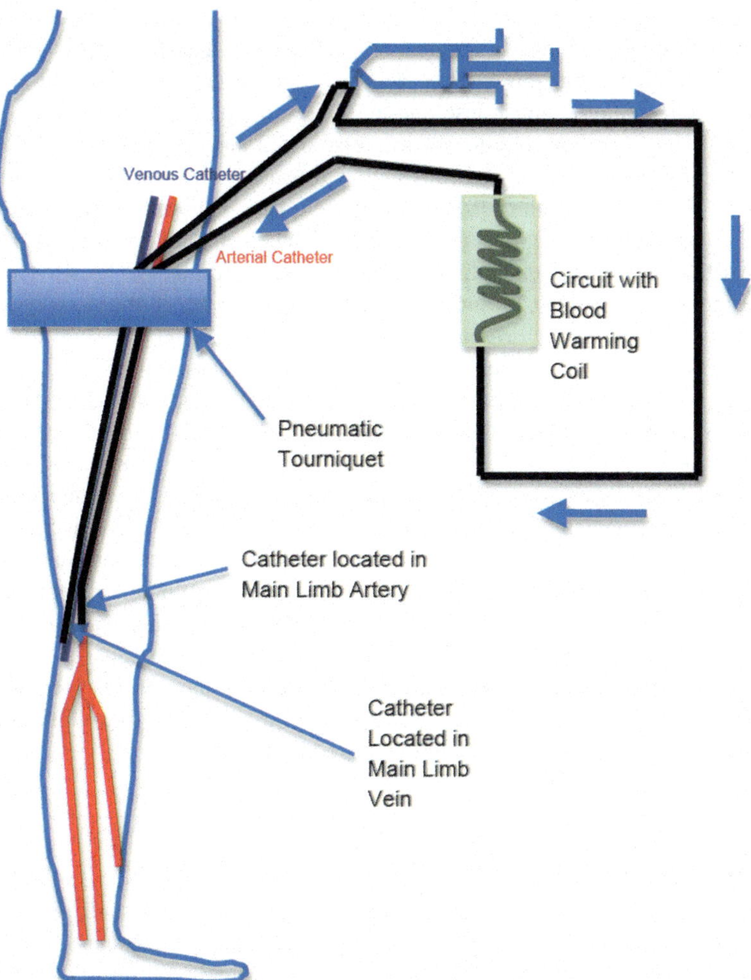

Fig. 25.7 Schematic drawing of the isolated infusion circuit (Reproduced from Cancer Management and Research, 2013, with permission of Dove Press [87])

circulation is not required because the flow and the pressure in the isolated limb circuit are low and the pneumatic tourniquet secures effective isolation. After 30 min, the limb vasculature is flushed, and the normal circulation to the limb is restored by removing the tourniquet and the catheters.

Local toxicity following isolated limb infusion is also scored according to the Wieberdink classification [3]. On average, toxicity following infusion is limited and manageable [71]. A systematic review revealed that 2 % of the patients suffered from a threatening or manifest compartment syndrome after infusion [72]. Isolated limb infusion can also safely be performed in elderly patients, and repeat procedures are possible without increased toxicity [73, 74].

Isolated infusion limb was pioneered at the Melanoma Institute Australia, and their response percentages appear somewhat less than those achieved by isolated limb perfusion, but this may be due to patient selection. Following isolated limb infusion, a complete response rate of 38 % and a partial response rate of 46 % are seen with a median duration of response of 22 and 13 months, respectively [75]. Recent reports from other centres show a somewhat lower fraction of responders [76, 77]. A multicenter US study achieved a 31 % complete response rate and a 33 % partial response rate [78]. Another multicenter study reported the responses in Australian centres, excluding the Melanoma Institute Australia. The complete response rate was 27 % and the partial response 36 % [79]. A recent systematic review including all original isolated limb infusion papers showed a complete response in 33 % of the patients and a partial response in 40 % [72]. Patient selection, slight technical differences and difficulties of standardising a response reporting system for in-transit metastases may play a role in the differences between the various reports [72, 80, 81]. Isolated limb infusion, for instance, is frequently performed in older and medically more compromised patients, both of which are statistically independent prognostic factors for an inferior response [75]. Similarly to isolated limb perfusion, isolated limb infusion does not alter survival as this is mostly dictated by tumour biology. Patients with a complete response to isolated limb infusion have a median survival of 53 months. Median survival times are significantly shorter in those with a partial response or stable disease [75]. More additional mature data from centres other than the Melanoma Institute Australia are needed to define the exact place of isolated limb infusion as a minimally invasive alternative procedure compared to isolated limb perfusion.

25.10 Future

Isolated limb perfusion has a significant effect on micrometastatic disease. Its application in resectable primary and recurrent melanoma lesions may therefore be useful. Tools to identify patients with a high risk of limb recurrence and a limited risk of distant metastases whose disease is susceptible to perfusion are desirable. Perhaps, genetic testing can select such patients. To lengthen the limb recurrence-free interval after perfusion, promising preliminary results of consolidation systemic biotherapy have been published. This combined regional and systemic approach deserves further study [82, 83].

Since 2010, a number of targeted systemic therapies and immunotherapies, such as B-Raf, MEK and KIT inhibitors, anti-CTLA4 antibodies and PD-1 pathway inhibitors, have become available and result in considerable response rates and improved survival in patients with inoperable stage III and IV melanoma [84]. Currently, however, the high 54 % complete response rate of perfusion and its modest morbidity compare favourably to the limited complete response rates and the substantial morbidity of these new drugs. We feel that perfusion (and infusion) is still the first choice of treatment for patients with extensive disease confined to a limb [85]. For patients who also have distant metastases, systemic therapy with the new drugs may be a more attractive option. Combining systemic targeted therapy with high drug concentrations administered by isolated limb perfusion in these patients is another interesting option to be explored.

References

1. Creech OJ, Krementz ET, Ryan RF, Winbald JN. Chemotherapy of cancer: regional perfusion utilizing an extracorporeal circuit. Ann Surg. 1958;148:616–32.
2. Kroon BBR. Regional isolation perfusion in melanoma of the limbs; accomplishments, unsolved problems, future. Eur J Surg Oncol. 1988;14:101–10.
3. Wieberdink J, Benckhuijsen C, Braat RP, van Slooten EA, Olthuis GAA. Dosimetry in isolation perfusion of the limbs by assessment of perfused tissue volume and grading of toxic tissue reactions. Eur J Cancer Clin Oncol. 1982;18:905–10.
4. Nieweg OE, Imhof O, Kroon BBR. Isolated limb perfusion. In: Mulholland MW, Hawn MT, Hughes SJ, Albo D, Sabel MS, Dalman RL, editors. Operative techniques in surgery. Riverwoods: Wolters Kluwer; 2014. p. 1647–55.
5. Boesch CE, Meyer T, Waschke L, et al. Long-term outcome of hyperthermic isolated limb perfusion (HILP) in the treatment of locoregionally metastasized malignant melanoma of the extremities. Int J Hyperthermia. 2010;26:16–20.
6. Benckhuijsen C, Kroon BBR, van Geel AN, Wieberdink J. Regional perfusion treatment with melphalan for melanoma in a limb: an evaluation of drug kinetics. Eur J Surg Oncol. 1988;14:157–63.
7. Lejeune FJ. High dose recombinant tumour necrosis factor (rTNF alpha) administered by isolation perfusion for advanced tumours of the limbs: a model for biochemotherapy of cancer. Eur J Cancer. 1995;31A:1009–16.
8. De Wilt JH, ten Hagen TL, de Boeck G, et al. Tumour necrosis factor alpha increases melphalan concentration in tumour tissue after isolated limb perfusion. Br J Cancer. 2000;82:1000–3.
9. Van Etten B, de Vries MR, van IJken MG, et al. Degree of tumour vascularity correlates with drug accumulation and tumour response upon TNF-alpha-based isolated hepatic perfusion. Br J Cancer. 2003;88:314–9.
10. Aigner K, Hild P, Henneking K, Paul E, Hundeiker M. Regional perfusion with cis-platinum and dacarbazine. Recent Results Cancer Res. 1983;86:239–45.
11. Vaglini M, Belli F, Marolda R, Prada A, Santinami M, Cascinelli N. Hyperthermic antiblastic perfusion with DTIC in stage IIIA–IIIAB melanoma of the extremities. Eur J Surg Oncol. 1987;13:127–9.
12. Vaglini M, Belli F, Santinami M, et al. Isolation perfusion in extracorporeal circulation with interleukin-2 and lymphokine-activated killer cells in the treatment of in-transit metastases from limb cutaneous melanoma. Ann Surg Oncol. 1995;2:61–70.
13. Hoekstra HJ, Schraffordt Koops H, de Vries LG, van Weerden TW, Oldhoff J. Toxicity of hyperthermic isolated limb perfusion with cisplatin for recurrent melanoma of the lower extremity after previous perfusion treatment. Cancer. 1993;72:1224–9.
14. Bonenkamp JJ, Thompson JF, de Wilt JH, Doubrovsky A, de Faria Lima R, Kam PC. Isolated limb infusion with fotemustine after dacarbazine chemosensitisation for inoperable locoregional melanoma recurrence. Eur J Surg Oncol. 2004;30:1107–12.
15. Klaase JM, Kroon BBR, van Geel AN, Eggermont AMM, Franklin HR. Low frequency of isotopically measured systemic leakage in a flow and venous pressure controlled isolated perfusion methodology of the limbs. Br J Surg. 1993;80:1124–6.
16. Hahn GM, editor. Hyperthermia and cancer. New York: Plenum Press; 1982.

17. Klaase JM, Kroon BBR, Eggermont AMM, et al. A retrospective comparative study evaluating the results of mild hyperthermic versus controlled normothermic perfusion for recurrent melanoma of the extremities. Eur J Cancer. 1995;31A:58–63.
18. Vrouenraets BC, Klaase JM, Nieweg OE, et al. Toxicity and morbidity of isolated limb perfusion: a review. Semin Surg Oncol. 1998;14:224–31.
19. Van der Zee J, Kroon BBR, Nieweg OE, van de Merwe SA, Kampinga HH. Rationale for different approaches to combined melphalan and hyperthermia in regional isolated perfusion. Eur J Cancer. 1997;33:1546–50.
20. Kroon BBR, Klaase JM, van Geel AN, Eggermont AMM. Application of hyperthermia in regional isolated perfusion for melanoma of the limbs. Reg Cancer Treat. 1992;4:223–6.
21. der Zee V, Kroon BBR. Isolated limb perfusion for malignant melanoma; possibly better results with high dose hyperthermia. Int J Hyperthermia. 2008;24:602–3.
22. Noorda EM, Vrouenraets BC, Nieweg OE, Klaase JM, van der Zee J, Kroon BBR. Long-term results of a double perfusion schedule using high-dose hyperthermia and melphalan sequentially in extensive melanoma of the lower limb. Melanoma Res. 2003;13:395–9.
23. Vrouenraets BC, Klaase JM, Kroon BBR, van Geel AN, Eggermont AMM, Franklin HR. Long-term morbidity after regional isolated perfusion with melphalan for melanoma of the limbs. The influence of acute regional toxic reactions. Arch Surg. 1995;130:43–7.
24. Van Geel AN, van Wijk J, Wieberdink J. Functional morbidity after regional isolated perfusion of the limb for melanoma. Cancer. 1989;63:1092–6.
25. Olieman AF, Schraffordt Koops H, Geertzen JH, Kingma H, Hoekstra JH, Oldhoff J. Functional morbidity of hyperthermic isolated regional perfusion of the extremities. Ann Surg Oncol. 1994;15:382–8.
26. Knorr C, Melling N, Goehl J, Drachsler T, Hohenberger W, Meyer T. Long-term functional outcome after hyperthermic isolated limb perfusion (HILP). Int J Hyperthermia. 2008;24:409–14.
27. Vrouenraets BC, Eggermont AMM, Klaase JM, van Geel AN, van Dongen JA, Kroon BBR. Long-term neuropathy after regional isolated perfusion with melphalan for melanoma of the limbs. Eur J Surg Oncol. 1994;20:681–5.
28. Vrouenraets BC, Kroon BBR, Klaase JM, et al. Severe acute regional toxicity after normothermic or 'mild' hyperthermic isolated limb perfusion with melphalan for melanoma. Melanoma Res. 1995;5:425–31.
29. Klaase JM, Kroon BBR, Beijnen JH, et al. Melphalan tissue concentrations in patients treated with regional isolated perfusion for melanoma of the lower limb. Br J Cancer. 1994;70:151–3.
30. Klaase JM, Kroon BBR, van Slooten GW, et al. Relation between calculated melphalan peak concentrations and toxicity in regional isolated perfusion for melanoma. Reg Cancer Treat. 1992;4:309–12.
31. Scott RN, Blackie R, Kerr DJ, et al. Melphalan in isolated limb perfusion for malignant melanoma, bolus or divided dose, tissue levels, the pH effect. In: Jakesz R, Rainer H, editors. Progress in regional cancer therapy. Berlin: Springer; 1990. p. 195–20017.
32. Sonneveld EJA, Vrouenraets BC, van Geel BN, et al. Systemic toxicity after isolated limb perfusion with melphalan for melanoma. Eur J Surg Oncol. 1996;22:521–7.
33. Vrouenraets BC, Kroon BBR, Ogilvie AC, et al. Absence of severe systemic toxicity after leakage-controlled isolated limb perfusion with high-dose TNFα + melphalan. Ann Surg Oncol. 1999;6:405–12.
34. Liénard D, Lejeune F, Ewalenko P. In transit metastases of malignant melanoma treated by high dose rTNF in combination with interferon-γ and melphalan in isolation perfusion. World J Surg. 1992;16:234–40.
35. Kapma MR, Vrouenraets BC, Nieweg OE, et al. Major amputation for intractable extremity melanoma after failure of isolated limb perfusion. Eur J Surg Oncol. 2005;31:95–9.

36. Fraker DL, Alexander HR, Andrich M, Rosenberg SA. Palliation of regional symptoms of advanced extremity melanoma by isolated limb perfusion with melphalan and high-dose tumour necrosis factor. Cancer J Sci Am. 1995;1:122–30.
37. Rossi CR, Foletto M, Mocelli S, Pilati P, Lise M. Hyperthermic isolated limb perfusion with low-dose tumor necrosis factor-α and melphalan for bulky in-transit melanoma metastases. Ann Surg Oncol. 2004;11:173–7.
38. Menon C, Ghartey A, Canter R, Feldman M, Fraker DL. Tumor necrosis factor-alpha damages tumor blood vessel integrity by targeting VE-cadherin. Ann Surg. 2006;244:781–91.
39. Noorda EM, Vrouenraets BC, Nieuweg OE, et al. Isolated limb perfusion for unresectable melanoma of the extremities. Arch Surg. 2004;139:1237–42.
40. Vrouenraets BC, Nieweg OE, Kroon BBR. 35 years of isolated limb perfusion for melanoma: indications and results. Br J Surg. 1996;83:1319–28.
41. Sanki A, Kam CA, Thompson JF. Long-term results of hyperthermic isolated perfusion for melanoma. A reflection of tumor biology. Ann Surg. 2007;245:591–6.
42. Di Filippo F, Calabro, Giannarelli D, et al. Prognostic variables in recurrent limb melanoma treated with hyperthermic antiblastic perfusion. Cancer. 1989;63:2551–61.
43. Klaase JM, Kroon BBR, van Geel AN, et al. Prognostic factors for tumor response and limb recurrence-free interval in patients with advanced melanoma of the limbs treated with regional isolated perfusion with melphalan. Surgery. 1994;115:39–45.
44. Cornett WR, McCall LM, Petersen RP, et al. Randomized multicenter trial of hyperthermic isolated limb perfusion with melphalan alone compared with melphalan plus tumor necrosis factor: American College of Surgeons Oncology Group Trial Z0020. J Clin Oncol. 2006;25:4196–201.
45. Grünhagen DJ, Brunstein F, Graveland WJ, van Geel AN, de Wilt JH, Eggermont AM. One hundred consecutive isolated limb perfusions with TNF-alpha and melphalan in melanoma patients with multiple in-transit metastases. Ann Surg. 2004;240:939–47.
46. Fraker D, Alexander H, Ross M, et al. A phase III trial of isolated limb perfusion for extremity melanoma comparing melphalan alone versus melphalan plus tumor necrosis factor (TNF) plus interferon gamma. Ann Surg Oncol. 2002;9:S8.
47. Alexander HR, Fraker DL, Bartlett DL, et al. Analysis of factors influencing outcome in patients with in-transit malignant melanoma undergoing isolated limb perfusion using modern treatment parameters. J Clin Oncol. 2010;28:114–8.
48. Deroose JP, Grünhagen DJ, van Geel AN, de Wilt JH, Eggermont AM, Verhoef C. Long-term outcome of isolated limb perfusion with tumour necrosis factor-α for patients with melanoma in-transit metastases. Br J Surg. 2011;98:1573–80.
49. Takkenberg RB, Vrouenraets BC, van Geel AN, et al. Palliative isolated limb perfusion for advanced limb disease in stage IV melanoma patients. J Surg Oncol. 2005;91:107–11.
50. Kroon BBR, Klaase JM, van Geel AN, Eggermont AMM, Franklin HR, van Dongen JA. Results of a double perfusion schedule with melphalan in patients with melanoma of the lower limb. Eur J Cancer. 1993;29A:325–8.
51. Schraffordt Koops H, Vaglini M, Suciu S, et al. Prophylactic isolated limb perfusion for localized, high-risk limb melanoma: results of a multicenter randomized phase III trial. J Clin Oncol. 1998;16:2906–12.
52. Hafström L, Rudenstam CM, Blomquist E, et al. Regional hyperthermic perfusion with melphalan after surgery for recurrent malignant melanoma of the extremities. J Clin Oncol. 1991;9:2091–4.
53. Noorda EM, Takkenberg B, Vrouenraets BC, et al. Isolated limb perfusion prolongs the limb recurrence-free interval after several episodes of excisional surgery for locoregional recurrent melanoma. Ann Surg Oncol. 2004;11:491–9.
54. Thompson JF, Hunt JA, Shannon KF, Kam PC. Frequency and duration of remission after isolated limb perfusion for melanoma. Arch Surg. 1997;132:903–7.

55. Strobbe LJA, Nieweg OE, Kroon BBR. Carbon dioxide laser for cutaneous melanoma metastases: indications and limitations. Eur J Surg Oncol. 1997;23:2435–8.

56. Thompson JF, Hersey P, Wachter E. Chemoablation of metastatic melanoma using intralesional Rose Bengal. Melanoma Res. 2007;18:405–11.

57. Overgaard J, Gonzalez Gonzalez D, Hulshoff MC, et al. Randomised trial of hyperthermia as adjuvant to radiotherapy for recurrent or metastastic malignant melanoma. Society for Hyperthermic Oncology. Lancet. 1995;345:540–3.

58. Klop WM, Vrouenraets BC, van Geel AN, et al. Repeat isolated limb perfusion with melphalan for recurrent melanoma of the limbs. J Am Coll Surg. 1996;182:467–72.

59. Noorda EM, Vrouenraets BC, Nieweg OE, et al. Repeat isolated limb perfusion with TNF-alpha and melphalan for recurrent limb melanoma after failure of previous perfusion. Eur J Surg Oncol. 2006;32:318–24.

60. Grünhagen DJ, van Etten B, Brunstein F, et al. Efficacy of repeat isolated limb perfusions with tumor necrosis factor alpha and melphalan for multiple in-transit metastases in patients with prior isolated limb perfusion failure. Ann Surg Oncol. 2005;12:609–15.

61. Zenilman ME. Surgery in the elderly. Curr Probl Surg. 1998;35:99–179.

62. Noorda EM, Vrouenraets BC, Nieweg OE, van Geel AN, Eggermont AMM, Kroon BBR. Safety and efficacy of isolated limb perfusion in elderly melanoma patients. Ann Surg Oncol. 2002;9:968–74.

63. Noorda EM, Vrouenraets BC, Nieweg OE, Van Geel AN, Eggermont AMM, Kroon BBR. Prognostic factors for poor survival after isolated limb perfusion for malignant melanoma. Eur J Surg Oncol. 2003;29:916–21.

64. Noorda EM, van Kreij RH, Vrouenraets BC, et al. The health-related quality of life of long-term survivors of melanoma treated with isolated limb perfusion. Eur J Surg Oncol. 2007;33:776–8.

65. Thompson JF, Kam PC, Waugh RC, et al. Isolated limb infusion with cytotoxic agents: a simple alternative to isolated limb perfusion. Semin Surg Oncol. 1998;14:238–47.

66. Kroon HM, Huismans A, Waugh RC, et al. Isolated limb infusion: technical aspects. J Surg Oncol. 2014;109:352–6.

67. Siemann DW, Chapman M, Beikirch A. Effects of oxygenation and pH on tumor cell response to alkylating chemotherapy. Int J Radiat Oncol Biol Phys. 1991;20:287–9.

68. Kroon HM, Thompson JF. Isolated limb infusion: a review. J Surg Oncol. 2009;100:169–77.

69. Wu ZY, Smithers BM, Parsons PG, et al. The effects of perfusion conditions on melphalan distribution in the isolated perfused rat hindlimb bearing a human melanoma xenograft. Br J Cancer. 1997;75:1160–6.

70. Wu ZY, Smithers BM, Roberts MS. Tissue and perfusate pharmacokinetics of melphalan in isolated perfused rat hindlimb. J Pharmacol Exp Ther. 1997;282:1131–8.

71. Kroon HM, Moncrieff M, Kam PCA, Thompson JF. Factors predictive of acute regional toxicity after isolated limb infusion with melphalan and actinomycin D in melanoma patients. Ann Surg Oncol. 2009;16:1184–92.

72. Kroon HM, Huismans AM, Kam PC, et al. Isolated limb infusion with melphalan and actinomycin D for melanoma: a systematic review. J Surg Oncol. 2014;109:348–51.

73. Kroon HM, Lin DY, Kam PC, Thompson JF. Efficacy of repeat isolated limb infusion with melphalan and actinomycin D for recurrent melanoma. Cancer. 2009;115:1932–40.

74. Kroon HM, Lin DY, Kam PC, Thompson JF. Safety and efficacy of isolated limb infusion with cytotoxic drugs in elderly patients with advanced locoregional melanoma. Ann Surg. 2009;246:1008–13.

75. Kroon HM, Moncrieff M, Kam PCA, Thompson JF. Outcomes following isolated limb infusion for melanoma. A 14-year experience. Ann Surg Oncol. 2008;15:3003–13.

76. Barbour AP, Thomas J, Suffolk J, et al. Isolated limb infusion for malignant melanoma. Predictors of response and outcome. Ann Surg Oncol. 2009;16:3463–72.

77. Beasley GM, Petersen RP, Yoo J, et al. Isolated limb infusion for in-transit malignant melanoma of the extremity: a well tolerated but less effective alternative to hyperthermic isolated limb perfusion. Ann Surg Oncol. 2008;15:2195–205.
78. Beasley GM, Caudle A, Petersen RP, et al. A multi-institutional experience of isolated limb infusion: defining response and toxicity in the United States. J Am Coll Surg. 2009;208:706–15.
79. Coventry BJ, Kroon HM, Giles MH, et al. Australian multi-center experience outside of the Sydney Melanoma Unit of isolated limb infusion chemotherapy for melanoma. J Surg Oncol. 2014;109:780–5.
80. Tyler D. Regional therapeutic strategies in melanoma: not just local disease control, but an opportunity to develop novel therapeutic strategies with potential implications for systemic therapy. Ann Surg Oncol. 2008;15:2987–90.
81. Huismans AM, Kroon HM, Kam PC, Thompson JF. Does increased experience with isolated limb infusion for advanced limb melanoma influence outcome? A comparison of two treatment periods at a single institution. Ann Surg Oncol. 2011;18:1877–83.
82. Rossi CR, Russano F, Mocellin S, et al. TNF-based isolated limb perfusion followed by consolidation biotherapy with systemic low-dose interferon alpha 2b in patients with in-transit melanoma metastases: a pilot trial. Ann Surg Oncol. 2008;15:1218–23.
83. Beasley GM, Riboh JC, Augustine CK, et al. Prospective multicenter phase II trial of systemic ADH-1 in combination with melphalan via isolated limb infusion in patients with advanced extremity melanoma. J Clin Oncol. 2011;29:1210–5.
84. Menzies AM, Long GV. Systemic treatment for BRAF-mutant melanoma: where do we go next? Lancet Oncol. 2014;15:e371–81.
85. Nieweg OE, Kroon BBR. Isolated limb perfusion with melphalan for melanoma. J Surg Oncol. 2014;109:132–7.
86. Kroon BBR, Fraker DL, Vrouenraets BC, Thompson JF. Isolated limb perfusion: results and complications. In: Thompson JF, Morton DL, Kroon BBR, editors. Textbook of melanoma. London: Taylor & Francis; 2004. p. 410–28.
87. Giles MH, Coventry BJ. Isolated limb infusion chemotherapy for melanoma: an overview of early experience at the Adelaide Melanoma Unit. Cancer Manag Res. 2013;5:243–9.

Anna M. Huismans, Hidde M. Kroon, Peter C.A. Kam, and John F. Thompson

26.1 Introduction

The treatment of patients with locally advanced or recurrent malignancies in a limb is often challenging due to the size and number of the satellite and/or in-transit metastases in those who have melanomas, or the invasion of tumour into adjacent structures in those with sarcomas. Before the mid-1950s, amputation of the affected limb was usually recommended, but following the introduction of the isolated limb perfusion (ILP) technique, this mutilating procedure was avoided in the majority of melanoma patients and many with limb sarcomas [1]. Using this technique, high-dose cytotoxic drugs are administered into the affected limb after it has been isolated from the systemic circulation, resulting in complete response (CR) rates of 46 % (7–90 %) in melanoma and 29 % (8–40 %) in sarcoma [2, 3]. Leakage of cytotoxic drugs from the isolated circuit, which can cause systemic toxicity, is low because effective vascular isolation of the affected limb is achieved with a tourniquet [3, 4].

The ILP technique, however, is a technically complex procedure and involves an invasive surgical approach. In the past, various attempts were made to design a simplified and less invasive alternative to ILP. Procedures such as intra-arterial infusion [5]

A.M. Huismans, MD, PhD • H.M. Kroon, MD, PhD
Melanoma Institute Australia, 40 Rocklands Road, North Sydney, NSW 2060, Australia

P.C.A. Kam, MD
Sydney Medical School, The University of Sydney, Sydney, NSW, Australia

Department of Anaesthetics, Royal Prince Alfred Hospital, Camperdown, NSW, Australia

J.F. Thompson, MD (✉)
Melanoma Institute Australia, 40 Rocklands Road, North Sydney, NSW 2060, Australia

Sydney Medical School, The University of Sydney, Sydney, NSW, Australia

Department of Melanoma and Surgical Oncology, Royal Prince Alfred Hospital, Camperdown, NSW, Australia
e-mail: John.Thompson@melanoma.org.au

© Springer-Verlag Berlin Heidelberg 2016
K.R. Aigner, F.O. Stephens (eds.), *Induction Chemotherapy*,
DOI 10.1007/978-3-319-28773-7_26

and 'tourniquet infusion' with partial venous outflow occlusion [6, 7] were used for this purpose, but these techniques failed to achieve response rates comparable to those obtained by ILP. In the early 1990s, Thompson and colleagues at Melanoma Institute Australia (MIA; formerly the Sydney Melanoma Unit) developed a simplified, minimally invasive procedure that they called isolated limb infusion (ILI). Using the ILI technique, they were able to obtain the benefits of ILP without incurring its major disadvantages [8, 9]. ILI is essentially a low-flow ILP, performed via percutaneously placed catheters under hypoxic conditions (i.e. without oxygenation of the perfusate). This simplified technique, now in use at many centres around the world, produces response rates similar to those achieved by ILP for both melanoma and sarcoma [10–13].

Until now, ILI with cytotoxic drugs has been used predominantly as a therapeutic procedure, but its simplicity and low morbidity suggest that it has great potential as induction therapy for advanced limb tumours. Limited clinical experience with ILI as induction therapy (described later in this chapter) indicates that it is indeed useful in reducing the size of large limb tumours and rendering operable many that were previously considered inoperable.

26.2 Isolated Limb Infusion

26.2.1 ILI Technique

A schematic overview of the procedure is shown in Fig. 26.1 [14]. In the radiology department, standard radiological catheters with additional side holes near their tips

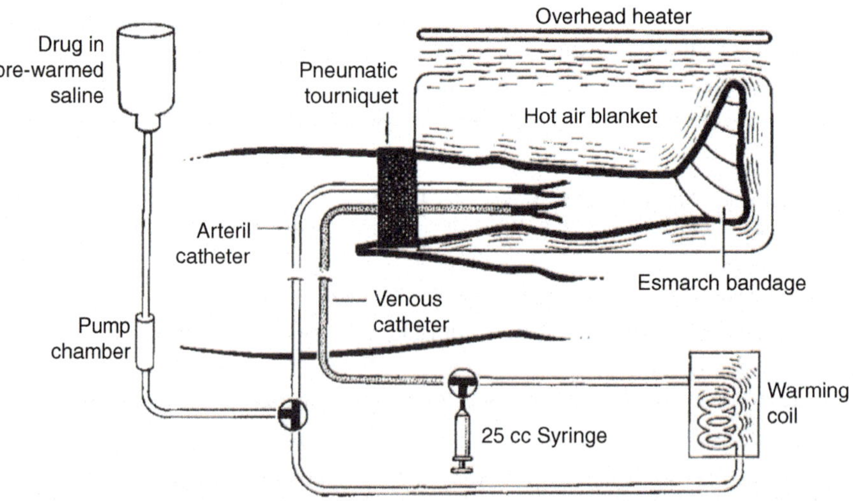

Fig. 26.1 Schematic illustration of the circuit used for isolated infusion of a lower limb (Adapted from Thompson et al.) [14]

are inserted percutaneously into the axial artery and vein of the disease-bearing limb via the contralateral groin using the Seldinger technique. For lower limb ILIs, the catheter tips are positioned in the popliteal artery and vein just above the knee; for upper limb ILIs, the catheter tips are positioned in the brachial artery and basilic vein, just above the elbow. Tissues located more proximally in the limb but distal to the level of the tourniquet are perfused in a retrograde fashion via collateral vascular channels.

Because of the synergistic antitumour effects of hyperthermia and melphalan, and the fact that melphalan is ineffective when administered to a hypothermic limb, strenuous efforts are made to maintain limb temperatures preoperatively and increase limb temperatures intraoperatively [15]. To achieve mild limb hyperthermia (ideally 38–39 °C), special precautions are necessary to avoid body and limb cooling in the immediate preoperative period. These include the placement of a hot-air blanket over the patient as soon as the vascular catheters have been inserted. This measure is very effective because the patient's body temperature decreases rapidly after the insertion of the catheters in the radiology department, during the transportation to the operating suite and while awaiting the ILI procedure in the anaesthetic room. Intraoperatively, special precautions to maintain limb temperature are used, including use of an overhead radiant heater, placement of a hot-air blanket around the disease-bearing limb to form a cocoon around it [8, 11] and placement of a blood-warming device in the extracorporeal vascular circuit (Fig. 26.1).

The patient is given a general anaesthetic, and heparin (3 mg/kg) is administered to achieve full systemic heparinization. Then intra-arterial papaverine (30–60 mg) is injected directly into the popliteal or brachial artery via the arterial catheter after a pneumatic tourniquet has been inflated around the root of the disease-bearing limb. If the foot or hand is not involved in the tumour process, it is excluded by applying an Esmarch rubber bandage tightly around it to prevent local toxicity [13, 16]. When there is no tumour in the distal leg or forearm either, a second pneumatic tourniquet can be applied around the distal limb tissue to exclude a larger volume of tissue that does not require drug exposure. To determine an appropriate drug dosage, the volume of limb tissue distal to the thigh or arm tourniquet and proximal to the distal tourniquet or Esmarch bandage (if either is used) is then estimated, based on volume measurements made preoperatively and marked on the limb. Limb volume can be determined using several techniques; the simplest is the water-displacement method, first described by Wieberdink et al. [17]. Another method involves performing calculations based on measurements of the patient's leg or arm circumference at 1.5-cm intervals up to the level of the tourniquet, encompassing the entire area to be infused [10]. Both methods are subject to a certain margin of error, however, and a simple but more precise method suitable for everyday clinical use has not yet been reported.

When all is in readiness, the cytotoxic drug solution is infused into the isolated limb via the arterial catheter. For the duration of the ILI procedure (usually 30 min), the cytotoxic infusate is continually circulated by repeated aspiration from the venous catheter and reinjection into the arterial catheter using a syringe attached to

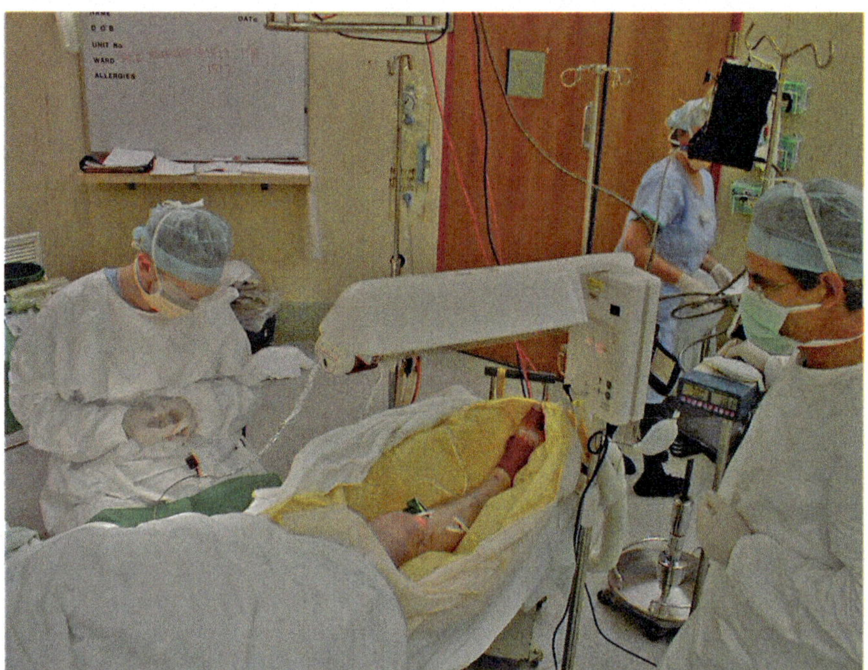

Fig. 26.2 Photograph of an isolated limb infusion procedure in progress in the operating suite. Note the Esmarch bandage around the foot to protect the acral region from developing postoperative toxicity

a three-way tap in the external circuit. Figure 26.2 shows an overview photograph of the operating room during an ILI. Subcutaneous and intramuscular limb temperatures are monitored continuously during the ILI procedure, and blood samples are taken at regular intervals to measure the cytotoxic drug concentrations and blood gases in the limb. The drug leakage rate from the isolated limb into the systemic circulation is evaluated after the procedure. Intraoperative systemic leakage monitoring, as performed routinely during ILP, is not performed during ILI since early studies demonstrated that systemic leakage is invariably minimal [11, 16]. As previously mentioned, mild hyperthermia of the limb (38–39 °C) is achieved by incorporating a blood-warming coil in the extracorporeal circuit and by encasing the limb in a hot-air blanket, with a radiant heater placed over it.

After 30 min, the limb is flushed with 1 l of Hartmann's solution via the arterial catheter, and the venous effluent is discarded. The limb tourniquet is then deflated to restore the normal limb circulation, the effect of heparin is reversed with intravenous (IV) protamine, and the venous and arterial catheters are removed. For patients with metastatic disease in the groin or axilla requiring a regional lymph node dissection as well as an ILI, this is undertaken directly after completion of the ILI procedure (and after reversal of the heparin), while the patient is still under general anaesthesia.

Postoperatively, the serum creatine phosphokinase (CK) level is measured daily as an indicator of muscle and tissue damage. CK levels exceeding 1000 IU/l after ILI correlate with increased and potentially serious limb toxicity [18, 19]. Therefore, all patients whose CK levels exceed 1000 IU/l and those who develop clinically severe limb toxicity are treated promptly with systemic corticosteroids (initially dexamethasone 4 mg IVq6h) until CK levels have fallen below 1000 IU/l and clinical evidence of toxicity has subsided. Postoperative limb toxicity and systemic toxicity are assessed daily, and tumour response is assessed at regular intervals. The peak reaction in the infused limb normally occurs 3–5 days after the ILI procedure, and patients are routinely observed in hospital until this peak has passed.

The ILI technique as described above is the result of progressive modifications based on accumulated experience over time [20]. Initially, a dose of 5–7 mg/l melphalan, with a circulation time of 15–20 min, was used. Subsequently, the melphalan dosage was gradually increased to the current 7.5 mg/l. In 1998, when it became apparent that drug uptake was not complete after 20 min and satisfactory limb temperatures had often not yet been reached, the drug circulation time was prolonged to 30 min [11]. This prolonged drug circulation increased the total tourniquet time to over 60 min, resulting in an increase of limb ischaemia [20]. This, however, has not been a problem, bearing in mind that in orthopaedic surgery even longer tourniquet times are used routinely without adverse effects. Indeed, the greater hypoxia and acidosis resulting from prolonged tourniquet times are likely to be beneficial, since in vitro studies have shown that increased hypoxia and acidosis produce up to a threefold increase in the cytotoxic effects of melphalan on tumour deposits [21–24].

Intra-arterial administration of papaverine prior to drug infusion is an important part of the protocol, to enhance early blood flow through the capillary vessels into cutaneous and subcutaneous tumour deposits when the cytotoxic drugs are infused, the 'first-pass' effect. This results in higher concentrations of melphalan to the tumour deposits early in the drug exposure period, which is important since there is a rapid decline in melphalan concentration thereafter because of the short half-life of the drug melphalan [25, 26].

Increased stage of disease is a predictive factor for a less favourable response [11, 27]. However, following the above-mentioned modifications and increased experience with the procedure, the response rates remain similar to those following conventional ILP, despite the greater tumour load in many patients treated with ILI, and the fact that many more of them also have systemic disease [20].

26.2.2 Similarities and Differences Between ILI and ILP

Both ILP and ILI involve vascular isolation and perfusion of an extremity with high doses of cytotoxic agents. The major differences between the procedures are the lower flow rate and shorter circulation time in the isolated extremity during ILI (150–1000 ml/min for 60 min during ILP versus 50–100 ml/min for 30 min during ILI) [11, 28]. As mentioned above, ILI is a hypoxic procedure, which leads to marked

Table 26.1 Differences between isolated limb perfusion and isolated limb infusion

Isolated limb perfusion	Isolated limb infusion
Technically complex	Technically simple
Open surgical exposure of vessels for catheter insertion	Percutaneous vascular catheter insertion in radiology department
4–6-h duration	Approximately 1 h
Perfusionist and ancillary staff required	No perfusionist required and fewer total staff
Complex and expensive equipment needed	Equipment requirements modest
Magnitude of procedure excludes patients	Well tolerated by medically compromised, frail and elderly patients
Not possible in occlusive vascular disease	Can be performed in occlusive vascular disease
Technically challenging to perform a repeat procedure	Not difficult to perform a repeat procedure
Systemic metastases normally a contraindication	Systemic metastases not a contraindication
Higher perfusion pressures predispose to systemic leakage	Low pressure system, effective vascular isolation with tourniquet
Limb tissues oxygenated, with normal blood gases maintained	Progressive hypoxia and acidosis
Hyperthermia (>41 °C can be achieved)	Usually not possible to raise limb temperature above 40 °C
General anaesthesia required	Possible with regional anaesthesia

acidosis in the isolated circuit, in contrast to ILP where full oxygenation in the limb is maintained by including a membrane oxygenator in the external circuit. Obtaining vascular access with an open surgical procedure to perform a repeat ILP procedure, or after groin or axillary lymph node dissection, can be technically difficult due to the presence of scar tissue, resulting in a considerably increased risk of morbidity. A repeat ILI, on the other hand, is normally straightforward because the catheters are placed percutaneously, are smaller in diameter and are inserted via the contralateral groin [29, 30]. Also, blood transfusion, or more recently the use of autologous blood, is required for ILP to prime the perfusion circuit, but is unnecessary during ILI. A 400-ml infusion of normal saline into the limb is sufficient for ILI, due to the small volume of the circuit. Finally, ILP is a technically demanding procedure that requires complex and expensive equipment, occupies many hours of operating room time and involves numerous surgical, anaesthetic and nursing personnel plus ancillary technical staff. Compared to this ILI is a much simpler procedure which requires more modest equipment, much less time in the operating room and fewer personnel. The main differences between ILI and conventional ILP are listed in Table 26.1.

26.2.3 Drugs Used in Isolated Limb Infusion

Melphalan remains the cytotoxic agent of choice to treat patients by either ILP or ILI [11, 31]. In our centre and most other centres, actinomycin-D is used in addition to melphalan in ILI procedures because of the good response rates without any apparent increase in toxicity when it is administered with melphalan during ILP or ILI [4, 8, 19]. As mentioned above, the melphalan dose that is normally administered for an ILI procedure is 7.5 mg/l of infused tissue, with a maximum dose of 100 mg for large tissue volumes and a minimum dose of 15–20 mg for very small tissue volumes. The melphalan is infused in a warmed, heparinized normal saline solution. Infusion fluids containing albumin should be avoided because albumin binds melphalan and reduces melphalan uptake into the tissues by a factor of three [32]. The dose of actinomycin-D is usually 75 μg/l of infused tissue, with a minimum of 200 μg for smaller limb volumes and a maximum of 500 μg for larger limb volumes.

The relationship between infused melphalan dose in mg/L and outcome remains unclear [10, 17, 19]. Using a rat model, Roberts et al. demonstrated in a dose-response study that increasing the melphalan tissue concentration above a threshold of 25 μg/ml did not further improve the response rate, whereas higher melphalan concentrations caused more severe toxicity [33]. In other words, increasing melphalan dose above a certain threshold only increased toxicity without improving outcome. However, melphalan concentrations are quite variable in individual patients, and the factors that determine them are not yet fully understood [34, 35].

In an attempt to decrease toxicity without compromising outcome, clinicians at Duke University Medical Center adjusted the melphalan dose according to ideal body weight (IBW) [36]. This adjustment was based primarily on the observation that the strongest predictor of toxicity in patients undergoing conventional ILP is the ratio of estimated limb volume (Vesti) to steady-state limb drug volume of distribution (Vss) [34, 35]. Hypothetically, patients with a weight greater than their IBW are likely to have a high Vesti/Vss since melphalan uptake is lower in fat compared to muscle [37]. The Duke University group reported that dose adjustment according to IBW did decrease the number of patients with grade III toxicity, but at the expense of a lower partial response (PR) rate, while the CR rate remained unchanged [10, 35]. Grade IV toxicity was already rare without dose adjustment. Although it might be argued that the achievement of a CR is clinically most important, any reduction in the PR rate due to the administration of a lower melphalan dose is clinically relevant since a PR following an ILI greatly improves the quality of life in most patients [38]. Moreover, in many cases a PR can be followed by resection of the remaining lesions, thus using ILI as an induction therapy, often resulting in a disease-free limb after this palliative surgery [39]. A retrospective study at Melanoma Institute Australia showed a correlation between larger limb volume (and therefore higher total melphalan dose) and toxicity; BMI was not correlated with toxicity [40]. Therefore, dose adjustment to IBW is not expected to lower toxicity at least in patients with larger limbs. This seeming contradiction was described 30 years ago by Wieberdink et al. who pointed out that regional volumes as a percentage of body weight showed a ±30 % variability from the mean [17]. It is clear that to further lower toxicity following ILI without compromising outcome, more research is required, focusing on optimizing melphalan concentrations in the individual patient.

The simplicity of ILI makes it an ideal model in which to test other drugs. For example, the alkylating agent fotemustine was tested in a pilot study in patients with advanced melanoma confined to a limb. In this study, a high response rate was achieved after ILI, with a CR rate of 31 % and a PR rate of 61 %. However, the pilot was discontinued because of unexpectedly severe local toxicity, with 4 of 13 patients (31 %) developing Wieberdink grade V toxicity requiring amputation of the infused limb [17, 41].

More recently, the alkylating agent temozolomide (TMZ) was studied as a regional cytotoxic agent to treat melanoma. The effect of this agent is thought to be dependent on the activity of the DNA repair enzyme O6-methylguanine-DNA methyltransferase (MGMT) in tumour cells. In an animal model, regional therapy with TMZ was more effective than melphalan for a xenograft tumour with low MGMT activity, whereas melphalan was more effective than temozolomide in another xenograft tumour with high MGMT activity [42]. Unfortunately, a multicentre phase I trial could not confirm this association between the level of MGMT activity and tumour response. The response rates after ILI with TMZ were modest (CR 10.5 %) in patients who had already experienced treatment failure or disease recurrence after previous melphalan-based regional chemotherapy. However, the low toxicity of TMZ administered by ILI may allow for repeated treatments to increase the response rate [43].

Another approach to increasing tumour response is by using systemic modulators of drug-resistance proteins to overcome regional chemotherapy resistance. TMZ chemomodulation with O6-benzylguanine (O6BG), an inhibitor of the DNA repair enzyme AGT, significantly improved the tumour response in a melanoma xenograft model using TMZ in ILI [44]. Tumour resistance to melphalan was associated with elevated intracellular GSH levels. In an animal model, short-term systemic therapy with butathione sulfoximine (BSO), an inhibitor of the rate-limiting enzyme in GSH synthesis, enhanced the effects of regional melphalan without increasing toxicity [45]. Phase I clinical trials of these agents have not yet been performed. More drug modulators are currently under development [46, 47].

26.3 Toxicity and Side Effects Following ILI

Following ILI with melphalan and actomyocin-D, regional toxicity is normally mild [9, 10, 19, 36, 48, 49]. Toxicity is mostly reported using the Wieberdink toxicity scale (Table 26.2) [17]. Alternatively, some study groups use the 'common terminology criteria for adverse events' version 3.0 (CTCAE v. 3.0) to report toxicity following ILI. Slight erythema and oedema is seen in approximately 46 % of patients following an ILI, and in about 19 %, this is accompanied by the formation of blisters, corresponding to Wieberdink toxicity grades II and III, respectively. The toxic reaction normally reaches its peak after 3–5 days and then begins to subside. In most cases, conservative treatment involving bed rest, limb elevation and sometimes the administration of systemic corticosteroids is sufficient. In 2 % of patients, the muscle and other deeper tissues are involved, and in order to prevent a compartment syndrome from occurring, a prophylactic fasciotomy is performed in these cases. To date, except for the toxicity after fotemustine in an experimental setting, as described previously, it has not been necessary in our centre to amputate a limb due to severe regional toxicity following ILI [50].

Table 26.2 Wieberdink toxicity grading [17]

Grade I	No visible effect
Grade II	Slight erythema and/or oedema
Grade III	Considerable erythema and/or oedema with blistering
Grade IV	Extensive epidermolysis and/or obvious damage to deep tissues with a threatened or actual compartment syndrome
Grade V	Severe tissue damage necessitating amputation

Minor side effects of ILI include superficial desquamation of the skin, which if it occurs does so after 2–3 weeks. Hair growth in drug-exposed sites of the treated limb normally ceases for up to 3 months after ILI, and some residual pigmentation of the limb is common. If the foot or hand is not excluded by an Esmarch bandage or pneumatic tourniquet, loss of the superficial layers of the epidermis of the sole or palm may occur, leaving a delicate and sensitive new skin surface exposed. If this occurs, it can take many weeks until the area is again covered by normal, heavily keratinized plantar or palmar skin. Additionally, loss of toenails or fingernails can occur 3–4 months after the treatment [19]. These side effects are identical to those observed after conventional ILP [29].

26.4 Indications and Results

As for ILP, the primary indications for therapeutic ILI are the presence of inoperable in-transit melanoma confined to an extremity, and advanced, inoperable extremity sarcoma [11, 13, 51]. ILI has also been used successfully in patients with refractory warts of the hands [52], refractory chromomycosis [53], localized cutaneous T-cell lymphoma [54], squamous cell carcinoma and Merkel cell carcinoma [55].

26.4.1 Melanoma

Since the introduction of ILI in the early 1990s, a multitude of studies reporting results following this procedure have been published. The range of response rates reported is wide, probably due to the small numbers of patients in some studies and the inclusion of results from the physicians' 'learning curves' before they had fully mastered the technique. Furthermore, different institutions have used protocols that vary in small but potentially important ways. A study performed at MIA showed that increased experience and small modifications that were made to the ILI protocol over a 14-year period resulted in a positive effect on outcome [20]. Another possible explanation for the wide range in results is that the response to the procedure has been assessed at different time points; some studies have used the best response exactly 3 months following the treatment, while others have reported the outcome according to the WHO system for reporting responses to treatment, allowing a larger time window to detect the best response [56–58].

In 2014, a systematic review was published, combining the published results of ILI for melanoma using melphalan and actinomycin-D [49]. In this study including 576 patients, 33 % experienced a complete response (CR) and 40 % a partial response (PR). In total 27 % of the patients had a less favourable response to ILI, with stable disease (SD) seen in 14 % and progressive disease (PD) in 13 % (Table 26.3). Figure 26.3 shows a bulky melanoma metastasis in the calf of a leg before and after ILI.

Table 26.3 Meta-analysis of response rates following isolated limb infusion for melanoma with melphalan and actinomycin-D [49]

Author, year	No. of patients	Response criteria	CR (%)	PR (%)	SD (%)	PD (%)
Mian, 2001	9	Best response	44	56	0	0
Kroon, 2008	185	Best response	38	46	10	6
Marsden, 2008	13	Unknown	31	53	0	16
Beasley, 2009	128	3 months	31	33	7	29
Duprat Neto, 2012	31	Best response	26	53	21	0
Wong, 2013	79	3 months	37	37	8	18
Coventry, 2014	131	Best response	27	36	29	8
Total	**576**		**33**	**40**	**14**	**13**

CR complete response, *PR* partial response, *SD* stable disease, *PD* progressive disease

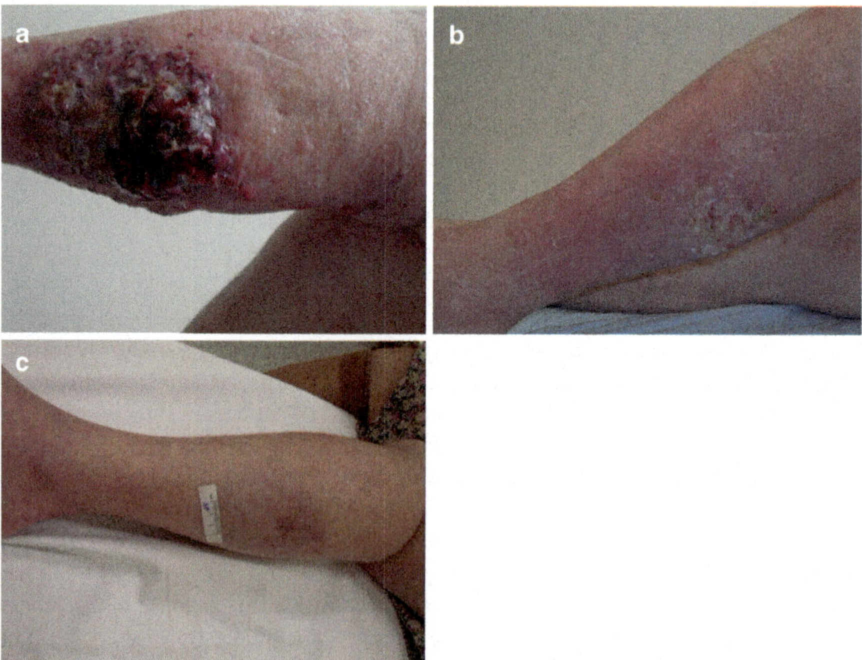

Fig. 26.3 (**a**) Extensive in-transit melanoma metastases of the left lower leg before ILI. (**b**) Remission 4 weeks post-ILI. (**c**) Complete response 4 months post-ILI

As the reported response rates have varied quite widely, so too have the published survival rates. In 2008, Kroon et al. reported a median survival after a CR of 53 months (IQR 28–120) for patients treated at MIA [11]. Coventry et al. more recently published results from a multicentre study and reported that patients had a median survival following CR of 101 months (range 5 to >120) [59]. In 2011, Raymond et al. reported that patients treated in the period 1995–2010 at Duke Medical Center had a median survival of 31 months after a CR [50]. All these studies report less favourable survival rates for those patients with a PR (27–41 months) or stable or progressive disease (13–33 months).

26.4.2 Sarcoma and Other Non-melanoma Skin Malignancies

Experience using ILI for inoperable sarcoma is limited. A study conducted at MIA involved the use of ILI in a cohort of 21 patients with soft tissue sarcomas. In 14 of these patients, ILI was performed as induction therapy, and in the other 7 patients, ILI was used as a palliative measure [13]. The OR was 90 % (CR 57 %, PR 33 %). The response rate in the induction therapy group was 100 %, with a histologically confirmed CR rate of 65 % (i.e. in 65 % of the surgical resection specimens, no tumour cells were found). After a median follow-up of 28 months, the limb salvage rate was 76 %. Turaga et al. described a cohort of 22 patients: 14 with sarcoma, 7 with Merkel cell carcinoma and 1 with squamous cell carcinoma, all treated with ILI [55]. The overall response rate in this report was 79 % (CR 21 %, PR 58 %). In 86 % of the patients, limb preservation was achieved. Interestingly, four of the five patients who underwent resection of residual disease after their ILI remained disease free after a median follow-up of 8.6 months.

26.5   Isolated Limb Infusion as Induction Therapy

As well as using ILI to test new drugs and to find systemic modulators to overcome resistance to known cytotoxic agents, the technique can also be used as an induction therapy [46].

The goals of 'therapeutic' ILI are to achieve satisfactory palliation and limb salvage. Achieving a CR improves the quality of life markedly, but achieving a PR or even SD can substantially improve the patient's quality of life also [38, 60]. After a PR or when recurrent lesions appear following ILI, simple local treatments of the remaining or recurrent lesions by excision, laser ablation, electrodessication, injection with rose bengal or radiotherapy can be effective in controlling the disease [61]. Resection of residual disease after ILI leads to similar DFS and OS as a complete response after ILI alone [39]. If recurrent disease is too extensive to be treated with simple local measures, a repeat ILI can be considered and can usually be performed without difficulty due to the minimally invasive character of the initial procedure [62]. Over a 15-year period, only 14 of 235 patients treated with an ILI at MIA eventually needed an amputation to control persistent or recurrent limb disease [63].

In patients with inoperable sarcoma, ILI can be used as a neoadjuvant therapy, prior to surgical excision or radiotherapy, similarly to ILP. Using this approach, limb salvage rates of 76–86 % have been reported [13, 51, 55]. Another approach has been to combine preoperative ILI with doxorubicin and external beam radiotherapy to obtain local control and make limb-sparing surgery feasible. This approach led to a limb salvage rate of 82.5 % [51].

An interesting induction strategy is the use of systemic modulators to augment the cytotoxic effects of regional chemotherapy administered by ILI. In a phase II study designed to test whether systemic ADH1 enhanced the response of metastatic melanoma to ILI with melphalan, an overall response rate of 60 % was achieved without increasing toxicity, compared with an overall response rate of 40 % achieved with melphalan alone at the same institution previously [64, 65]. Along similar lines, following the promising results of systemic therapy with sorafenib (a non-specific BRAF inhibitor) combined with systemic dacarbazine (DTIC) [66, 67], the effect on melanoma of systemic sorafenib in combination with regional melphalan or TMZ was studied. Unfortunately, despite the encouraging results in preclinical studies [68], a phase I clinical trial showed that this combination only increased toxicity without increasing response rates [69]. Because a phase III trial with systemic sorafenib also turned out to be disappointing, this drug has not been registered for the treatment of advanced melanoma [70]. However, more specific second-generation BRAF inhibitors such as vemurafenib and dabrafenib have lived up to expectations [71–73]. Possibly, these new targeted drugs, administered systemically by themselves or as combination therapy with melphalan or TMZ, may further improve responses following ILI. Finally, immunotherapy may also be a potential systemic modulator of regional chemotherapy administered by ILI [74]. Both the use of adjuvant ipilimumab following melphalan ILI (as induction therapy) and neoadjuvant ipilimumab before ILI with melphalan is currently being investigated in phase I/II trials (NCT01323517, NCT02115243).

26.6 Conclusions

By using ILI with therapeutic intent or as induction therapy, amputation of an affected limb with inoperable melanoma or sarcoma can be avoided in almost all patients. When used for palliation of extensive or recurrent limb disease, satisfactory control can be achieved in the majority of them. ILI is an excellent model to test new drugs or new treatment regimens. A number of studies are currently investigating new strategies for treating melanoma and sarcoma using the ILI technique, and innovative methods of using ILI as induction therapy, not yet fully exploited, are being developed.

References

1. Creech Jr O, Krementz ET, Ryan RF, Winblad JN. Chemotherapy of cancer: regional perfusion utilizing an extracorporeal circuit. Ann Surg. 1958;148(4):616–32.
2. Noorda EM, Vrouenraets BC, Nieweg OE, Van Coevorden F, Kroon BB. Isolated limb perfusion: what is the evidence for its use? Ann Surg Oncol. 2004;11(9):837–45.
3. Thompson JF, Hunt JA, Shannon KF, Kam PC. Frequency and duration of remission after isolated limb perfusion for melanoma. Arch Surg. 1997;132(8):903–7.
4. Vrouenraets BC, Nieweg OE, Kroon BB. Thirty-five years of isolated limb perfusion for melanoma: indications and results. Br J Surg. 1996;83(10):1319–28.
5. Karakousis CP, Kanter PM, Lopez R, Moore R, Holyoke ED. Modes of regional chemotherapy. J Surg Res. 1979;26(2):134–41.
6. Bland KI, Kimura AK, Brenner DE, et al. A phase II study of the efficacy of diamminedichloroplatinum (cisplatin) for the control of locally recurrent and intransit malignant melanoma of the extremities using tourniquet outflow-occlusion techniques. Ann Surg. 1989;209(1):73–80.
7. Karakousis CP, Kanter PM, Park HC, Sharma SD, Moore R, Ewing JH. Tourniquet infusion versus hyperthermic perfusion. Cancer. 1982;49(5):850–8.
8. Thompson JF, Kam PC, Waugh RC, Harman CR. Isolated limb infusion with cytotoxic agents: a simple alternative to isolated limb perfusion. Semin Surg Oncol. 1998;14(3):238–47.
9. Thompson JF, Waugh RC, Saw RP, Kam PC. Isolated limb infusion with melphalan for recurrent limb melanoma: a simple alternative to isolated limb perfusion. Reg Cancer Treat. 1994;7:188–92.
10. Santillan AA, Delman KA, Beasley GM, et al. Predictive factors of regional toxicity and serum creatine phosphokinase levels after isolated limb infusion for melanoma: a multi-institutional analysis. Ann Surg Oncol. 2009;16(9):2570–8.
11. Kroon HM, Moncrieff M, Kam PC, Thompson JF. Outcomes following isolated limb infusion for melanoma. A 14-year experience. Ann Surg Oncol. 2008;15(11):3003–13.
12. Lindner P, Doubrovsky A, Kam PC, Thompson JF. Prognostic factors after isolated limb infusion with cytotoxic agents for melanoma. Ann Surg Oncol. 2002;9(2):127–36.
13. Moncrieff MD, Kroon HM, Kam PC, Stalley PD, Scolyer RA, Thompson JF. Isolated limb infusion for advanced soft tissue sarcoma of the extremity. Ann Surg Oncol. 2008;15(10):2749–56.
14. Thompson JF, Kam PC. Isolated limb infusion for melanoma: a simple but effective alternative to isolated limb perfusion. J Surg Oncol. 2004;88(1):1–3.
15. Kroon BB. Regional isolation perfusion in melanoma of the limbs; accomplishments, unsolved problems, future. Eur J Surg Oncol. 1988;14(2):101–10.
16. Thompson JF, Lai DT, Ingvar C, Kam PC. Maximizing efficacy and minimizing toxicity in isolated limb perfusion for melanoma. Melanoma Res. 1994;4 Suppl 1:45–50.
17. Wieberdink J, Benckhuysen C, Braat RP, van Slooten EA, Olthuis GA. Dosimetry in isolation perfusion of the limbs by assessment of perfused tissue volume and grading of toxic tissue reactions. Eur J Cancer Clin Oncol. 1982;18(10):905–10.
18. Lai DT, Ingvar C, Thompson JF. The value of monitoring serum creatine phosphokinase values following hyperthermic isolated limb perfusion for melanoma. Reg Cancer Treat. 1993;6:36–9.
19. Kroon HM, Moncrieff M, Kam PC, Thompson JF. Factors predictive of acute regional toxicity after isolated limb infusion with melphalan and actinomycin D in melanoma patients. Ann Surg Oncol. 2009;16(5):1184–92.

20. Huismans AM, Kroon HM, Kam PC, Thompson JF. Does increased experience with isolated limb infusion for advanced limb melanoma influence outcome? A comparison of two treatment periods at a single institution. Ann Surg Oncol. 2011;18(7):1877–83.
21. Skarsgard LD, Skwarchuk MW, Vinczan A, Kristl J, Chaplin DJ. The cytotoxicity of melphalan and its relationship to pH, hypoxia and drug uptake. Anticancer Res. 1995;15(1):219–23.
22. de Wilt JH, Manusama ER, van Tiel ST, van Ijken MG, ten Hagen TL, Eggermont AM. Prerequisites for effective isolated limb perfusion using tumour necrosis factor alpha and melphalan in rats. Br J Cancer. 1999;80(1–2):161–6.
23. Siemann DW, Chapman M, Beikirch A. Effects of oxygenation and pH on tumor cell response to alkylating chemotherapy. Int J Radiat Oncol Biol Phys. 1991;20(2):287–9.
24. Chaplin DJ, Acker B, Olive PL. Potentiation of the tumor cytotoxicity of melphalan by vasodilating drugs. Int J Radiat Oncol Biol Phys. 1989;16(5):1131–5.
25. Thompson JF, Ramzan I, Kam PCA, Yau DF. Pharmacokinetics of melphalan during isolated limb infusion for melanoma. Reg Cancer Treat. 1996;9:13–6.
26. Roberts MS, Wu ZY, Siebert GA, Anissimov YG, Thompson JF, Smithers BM. Pharmacokinetics and pharmacodynamics of melphalan in isolated limb infusion for recurrent localized limb malignancy. Melanoma Res. 2001;11(4):423–31.
27. Muilenburg DJ, Beasley GM, Thompson ZJ, Lee JH, Tyler DS, Zager JS. Burden of disease predicts response to isolated limb infusion with melphalan and actinomycin D in melanoma. Ann Surg Oncol. 2015;22(2):482–8.
28. Schraffordt Koops H, Lejeune FJ, Kroon BBR, Klaase JM, Hoekstra HJ. Isolated limb perfusion for melanoma: technical aspects. In: Thompson JF, Morton DL, Kroon BBR, editors. Textbook of melanoma. London: Martin Dunitz; 2004. p. 404–9.
29. Vrouenraets BC, Klaase JM, Nieweg OE, Kroon BB. Toxicity and morbidity of isolated limb perfusion. Semin Surg Oncol. 1998;14(3):224–31.
30. Thompson JF, Kam PC, De Wilt JH, Lindner P. Isolated limb infusion for melanoma. In: Thompson JF, Morton DL, Kroon BBR, editors. Textbook of melanoma. London: Martin Dunitz; 2004. p. 429–37.
31. Kroon BB, Noorda EM, Vrouenraets BC, Nieweg OE. Isolated limb perfusion for melanoma. J Surg Oncol. 2002;79(4):252–5.
32. Wu ZY, Smithers BM, Parsons PG, Roberts MS. The effects of perfusion conditions on melphalan distribution in the isolated perfused rat hindlimb bearing a human melanoma xenograft. Br J Cancer. 1997;75(8):1160–6.
33. Roberts MS, Wu ZY, Siebert GA, Thompson JF, Smithers BM. Saturable dose-response relationships for melphalan in melanoma treatment by isolated limb infusion in the nude rat. Melanoma Res. 2001;11(6):611–8.
34. Cheng TY, Grubbs E, Abdul-Wahab O, et al. Marked variability of melphalan plasma drug levels during regional hyperthermic isolated limb perfusion. Am J Surg. 2003;186(5):460–7.
35. McMahon N, Cheng TY, Beasley GM, et al. Optimizing melphalan pharmacokinetics in regional melanoma therapy: does correcting for ideal body weight alter regional response or toxicity? Ann Surg Oncol. 2009;16(4):953–61.
36. Beasley GM, Petersen RP, Yoo J, et al. Isolated limb infusion for in-transit malignant melanoma of the extremity: a well-tolerated but less effective alternative to hyperthermic isolated limb perfusion. Ann Surg Oncol. 2008;15(8):2195–205.
37. Klaase JM, Kroon BB, Beijnen JH, van Slooten GW, van Dongen JA. Melphalan tissue concentrations in patients treated with regional isolated perfusion for melanoma of the lower limb. Br J Cancer. 1994;70(1):151–3.
38. Jiang BS, Speicher PJ, Thomas S, Mosca PJ, Abernethy AP, Tyler DS. Quality of life after isolated limb infusion for in-transit melanoma of the extremity. Ann Surg Oncol. 2015;22(5):1694–700.
39. Wong J, Chen YA, Fisher KJ, Beasley GM, Tyler DS, Zager JS. Resection of residual disease after isolated limb infusion (ILI) is equivalent to a complete response after ILI-alone in advanced extremity melanoma. Ann Surg Oncol. 2014;21(2):650–5.

40. Huismans AM, Kroon HM, Haydu LE, Kam PCA, Thompson JF. Is melphalan dose adjustment according to ideal body weight useful in isolated limb infusion for melanoma? Ann Surg Oncol 2012;19(9):3050–6.
41. Bonenkamp JJ, Thompson JF, de Wilt JH, Doubrovsky A, de Faria Lima R, Kam PC. Isolated limb infusion with fotemustine after dacarbazine chemosensitisation for inoperable locoregional melanoma recurrence. Eur J Surg Oncol. 2004;30(10):1107–12.
42. Yoshimoto Y, Augustine CK, Yoo JS, et al. Defining regional infusion treatment strategies for extremity melanoma: comparative analysis of melphalan and temozolomide as regional chemotherapeutic agents. Mol Cancer Ther. 2007;6(5):1492–500.
43. Beasley GM, Speicher P, Augustine CK, et al. A multicenter phase I dose escalation trial to evaluate safety and tolerability of intra-arterial temozolomide for patients with advanced extremity melanoma using normothermic isolated limb infusion. Ann Surg Oncol. 2015;22(1):287–94.
44. Ueno T, Ko SH, Grubbs E, et al. Modulation of chemotherapy resistance in regional therapy: a novel therapeutic approach to advanced extremity melanoma using intra-arterial temozolomide in combination with systemic O6-benzylguanine. Mol Cancer Ther. 2006;5(3):732–8.
45. Grubbs EG, Ueno T, Abdel-Wahab O, et al. Modulation of resistance to regional chemotherapy in the extremity melanoma model. Surgery. 2004;136(2):210–8.
46. Lidsky ME, Speicher PJ, Jiang B, Tsutsui M, Tyler DS. Isolated limb infusion as a model to test new agents to treat metastatic melanoma. J Surg Oncol. 2014;109(4):357–65.
47. Beasley GM, Tyler DS. Standardizing regional therapy: developing a consensus on optimal utilization of regional chemotherapy treatments in melanoma. Ann Surg Oncol. 2011;18(7):1814–8.
48. Brady MS, Brown K, Patel A, Fisher C, Marx W. Isolated limb infusion with melphalan and dactinomycin for regional melanoma and soft-tissue sarcoma of the extremity: final report of a phase II clinical trial. Melanoma Res. 2009;19(2):106–11.
49. Kroon HM, Huismans AM, Kam PC, Thompson JF. Isolated limb infusion with melphalan and actinomycin D for melanoma: a systematic review. J Surg Oncol. 2014;109(4):348–51.
50. Raymond AK, Beasley GM, Broadwater G, et al. Current trends in regional therapy for melanoma: lessons learned from 225 regional chemotherapy treatments between 1995 and 2010 at a single institution. J Am Coll Surg. 2011;213(2):306–16.
51. Hegazy MA, Kotb SZ, Sakr H, et al. Preoperative isolated limb infusion of Doxorubicin and external irradiation for limb-threatening soft tissue sarcomas. Ann Surg Oncol. 2007;14(2):568–76.
52. Damian DL, Barnetson RS, Rose BR, Bonenkamp JJ, Thompson JF. Treatment of refractory hand warts by isolated limb infusion with melphalan and actinomycin D. Australas J Dermatol. 2001;42(2):106–9.
53. Damian DL, Barnetson RS, Thompson JF. Treatment of refractory chromomycosis by isolated limb infusion with melphalan and actinomycin D. J Cutan Med Surg. 2006;10(1):48–51.
54. Elhassadi E, Egan E, O'Sullivan G, Mohamed R. Isolated limb infusion with cytotoxic agent for treatment of localized refractory cutaneous T-cell lymphoma. Clin Lab Haematol. 2006;28(4):279–81.
55. Turaga KK, Beasley GM, Kane 3rd JM, et al. Limb preservation with isolated limb infusion for locally advanced nonmelanoma cutaneous and soft-tissue malignant neoplasms. Arch Surg. 2011;146(7):870–5.
56. World Health Organization: WHO handbook for reporting results of cancer treatments (WHO offset publication no. 48). Geneva; 1979.
57. Wong J, Chen YA, Fisher KJ, Zager JS. Isolated limb infusion in a series of over 100 infusions: a single-center experience. Ann Surg Oncol. 2013;20(4):1121–7.
58. Beasley GM, Caudle A, Petersen RP, et al. A multi-institutional experience of isolated limb infusion: defining response and toxicity in the US. J Am Coll Surg. 2009;208(5):706–15.
59. Coventry BJ, Kroon HM, Giles MH, et al. Australian multi-center experience outside of the Sydney Melanoma Unit of isolated limb infusion chemotherapy for melanoma. J Surg Oncol. 2014;109(8):780–5.

60. Giles MH, Coventry BJ. Isolated limb infusion chemotherapy for melanoma: an overview of early experience at the Adelaide Melanoma Unit. Cancer Manag Res. 2013;5:243–9.
61. Feldman AL, Alexander Jr HR, Bartlett DL, Fraker DL, Libutti SK. Management of extremity recurrences after complete responses to isolated limb perfusion in patients with melanoma. Ann Surg Oncol. 1999;6(6):562–7.
62. Kroon HM, Lin DY, Kam PC, Thompson JF. Efficacy of repeat isolated limb infusion with melphalan and actinomycin D for recurrent melanoma. Cancer. 2009;115(9):1932–40.
63. Kroon HM, Lin DY, Kam PC, Thompson JF. Major amputation for irresectable extremity melanoma after failure of isolated limb infusion. Ann Surg Oncol. 2009;16(6):1543–7.
64. Beasley GM, McMahon N, Sanders G, et al. A phase 1 study of systemic ADH-1 in combination with melphalan via isolated limb infusion in patients with locally advanced in-transit malignant melanoma. Cancer. 2009;115(20):4766–74.
65. Beasley GM, Riboh JC, Augustine CK, et al. Prospective multicenter phase II trial of systemic ADH-1 in combination with melphalan via isolated limb infusion in patients with advanced extremity melanoma. J Clin Oncol. 2011;29(9):1210–5.
66. Eisen T, Marais R, Affolter A, et al. Sorafenib and dacarbazine as first-line therapy for advanced melanoma: phase I and open-label phase II studies. Br J Cancer. 2011;105(3):353–9.
67. McDermott DF, Sosman JA, Gonzalez R, et al. Double-blind randomized phase II study of the combination of sorafenib and dacarbazine in patients with advanced melanoma: a report from the 11715 Study Group. J Clin Oncol. 2008;26(13):2178–85.
68. Augustine CK, Toshimitsu H, Jung SH, et al. Sorafenib, a multikinase inhibitor, enhances the response of melanoma to regional chemotherapy. Mol Cancer Ther. 2010;9(7):2090–101.
69. Beasley GM, Coleman AP, Raymond A, et al. A phase I multi-institutional study of systemic sorafenib in conjunction with regional melphalan for in-transit melanoma of the extremity. Ann Surg Oncol. 2012;19(12):3896–905.
70. Hauschild A, Agarwala SS, Trefzer U, et al. Results of a phase III, randomized, placebo-controlled study of sorafenib in combination with carboplatin and paclitaxel as second-line treatment in patients with unresectable stage III or stage IV melanoma. J Clin Oncol. 2009;27(17):2823–30.
71. McArthur GA, Chapman PB, Robert C, et al. Safety and efficacy of vemurafenib in BRAF(V600E) and BRAF(V600K) mutation-positive melanoma (BRIM-3): extended follow-up of a phase 3, randomised, open-label study. Lancet Oncol. 2014;15(3):323–32.
72. Chapman PB, Hauschild A, Robert C, et al. Improved survival with vemurafenib in melanoma with BRAF V600E mutation. N Engl J Med. 2011;364(26):2507–16.
73. Hauschild A, Grob JJ, Demidov LV, et al. Dabrafenib in BRAF-mutated metastatic melanoma: a multicentre, open-label, phase 3 randomised controlled trial. Lancet. 2012;380(9839):358–65.
74. Turley RS, Fontanella AN, Padussis JC, et al. Bevacizumab-induced alterations in vascular permeability and drug delivery: a novel approach to augment regional chemotherapy for in-transit melanoma. Clin Cancer Res. 2012;18(12):3328–39.

Maurice Matter, Antonia Digklia, Béatrice Gay,
Berardino De Bari, Manuel Diezi, and Eric Raymond

27.1 Introduction

Soft tissue sarcomas (STSs) account for 1 % of all human cancers and consist of at least 50 different histological subtypes. STSs are known as rare tumours that can primarily localise in many organs with various presentations. Although their rarity more than 200,000 people annually are diagnosed worldwide. Expected new cases and death-related estimates from the American Cancer Society in 2015 represent 11,930 and 4870 patients, respectively [218]. There is a clinical common behaviour of STSs with a symptomatic growing mass, however in some cases such as the retroperitoneal localization, they typically produce only few symptoms until they become large and compress surrounding structures. Currently, the origin of the sarcoma tumourigenesis is largely unknown although STSs are thought to arise de

All the authors are members of the multidisciplinary sarcoma board.

M. Matter, (✉)
Department of Visceral Surgery, Centre Hospitalier Universitaire Vaudois, CHUV,
Rue du Bugnon 46, Lausanne 1011, Switzerland
e-mail: Maurice.Matter@chuv.ch; http://www.chirurgieviscerale.ch

A. Digklia • B. Gay • E. Raymond
Department of Oncology, Centre Hospitalier Universitaire Vaudois, CHUV,
Rue du Bugnon 46, Lausanne 1011, Switzerland
e-mail: Antonia.Digklia@chuv.ch; Eric.Raymond@chuv.ch

B. De Bari
Department of Radio-Oncology, Centre Hospitalier Universitaire Vaudois, CHUV,
Rue du Bugnon 46, Lausanne 1011, Switzerland
e-mail: Berardino.De-Bari@chuv.ch

M. Diezi
Department of Paediatrics, Centre Hospitalier Universitaire Vaudois, CHUV,
Rue du Bugnon 46, Lausanne 1011, Switzerland
e-mail: Manuel.Diezi@chuv.ch

© Springer-Verlag Berlin Heidelberg 2016
K.R. Aigner, F.O. Stephens (eds.), *Induction Chemotherapy*,
DOI 10.1007/978-3-319-28773-7_27

novo. Nevertheless, several predisposing factors have been identified including genetic predisposition (neurofibromatosis type 1, Li Fraumeni), previous exposure to radiotherapy or chemotherapy as well as virus infection (e.g. HHV8 for Kaposi sarcoma). Interestingly, some STSs are associated with specific chromosomal translocations (alveolar, synovial, myxoid chondrosarcoma) leading to protein expression of the fusion gene but for the moment without any therapeutic implication. Recently, using the TCGA (The Cancer Genome Atlas), a possible role of deregulation Hippo pathway leading to tumourigenesis of fibrosarcoma and pleomorphic sarcoma had been shown in a murine model, suggesting a new attractive therapeutic target [64]. Tumour size, histologic grade and tumour stage are the most important prognostic factors at the time of diagnosis, with the risk of developing distant metastasis that increases substantially as tumour size and grade increases. So-called pleomorphic sarcomas accounting for about 40 % of STSs have been reclassified in various subtypes of undifferentiated pleomorphic sarcomas according to new WHO classification [49, 72]. The relationship between histologic subtype and prognosis was also well illustrated with synovial sarcoma and MPNST (malignant peripheral nerve sheath tumours) to have been proven to be among the more aggressive. Another difficulty for STS treatment is illustrated by hemangiopericytoma/solitary fibrous tumour, which may disclose malignancy according to histopathology characteristics (size, number of mitotic figures, cellular atypia, necrosis/haemorrhage), or according to retroperitoneal and pelvic location, where induction radiotherapy may be recommended [184].

Following new immunohistochemical, cytogenetic and molecular developments, the 2013 WHO classification of STS has included several changes (several new entities and reclassification of others) that were reviewed by Jo and Fletcher [118].

Diagnosis, staging and grading are essential for pretreatment assessment. Investigations include imaging (contrast-enhanced CT scan, MRI) and Tru-Cut biopsy, which may be guided by ultrasound or CT scan. Core needle biopsy has a high accuracy of 68–100 %. The tumour grade can be determined in 76–87 % and histologic subtypes in 68–78 % [247].

Positron emission tomography has been evaluated in diagnosis and treatment response. A review of early studies concluded that ^{18}F-FDG-PET use could not be recommended [17, 18]. A recent review however showed a promising future to PET (combined with CT), which may correlate with tumour grade (and orientate biopsy), help in staging, in assessing tumour response to induction therapy and act as a prognostic factor [20].

According to the 7th 2010 edition of the AJCC staging manual, a three-grade system is now combined with T stage ($\leq$5 or >5 cm) used to differentiate stage IA/B-IIA/B. Stage III includes G3 or N1 (previously stage IV disease) and M1 only now defines stage IV [2]. FNCLCC grading with the best reproducibility and prognostic predictive value for metastatic disease [36] has now replaced AJCC and NIH grading systems. Despite different histologic subtypes, tumour size and grade (according to the FNCLCC scoring system) are the best two prognostic factors [94].

27.2 Induction Therapy in Sarcomas: Rationale and General Principles

Due to rarity and the complexity of treatment, the best therapeutic approach has to be individualised for each patient after a multidisciplinary team discussion [96]. A multimodal treatment concept, including surgery, radiotherapy and chemotherapy, aims at increasing overall survival, local control and functional outcome with minimal morbidity. The rationale for administering induction chemotherapy is based on lessons learned from the treatment of osteosarcoma in association with some efficacy mentioned by the Italian Sarcoma Group in a meta-analysis and a randomised trial [196]. The use of induction therapy in STS is still controversial and is a matter of debate. Theoretical advantages of preoperative chemotherapy include cytoreduction (reduction in tumour volume and cellular viability in order, e.g. to facilitate limb-salvage surgery), treatment of micrometastatic disease [208] and assessment of treatment efficacy and responsiveness in vivo (drug sensitivity). A low tumour proliferative activity (identified by mitotic count, proliferative index and apoptosis) after isolated limb perfusion (ILP) is correlated with a significantly better OS [199]. As microscopically positive surgical margins are an increased risk for subsequent local recurrence and tumour-specific mortality [76, 89, 194, 211, 228], induction therapy aims ideally at decreasing risk and extent of positive margins. It has also been postulated that response to chemotherapy provides prognostic information [48, 191]. Treatment-induced pathologic necrosis is considered as an independent prognostic variable in bone sarcomas. Eilber et al. have observed that pathologic response to induction radiochemotherapy was also highly prognostic for intermediate-to-high-grade extremity STS patients [61]. Patients responding with ≥95 % pathologic necrosis had a lower recurrence rate. Five- and 10-year overall survival rates were 80 % and 71 %, respectively, and 62 % and 55 %, respectively, for patients with less than 95 % necrosis [61]. MacDermed observed that response to induction chemoradiotherapy had a prognostic predictive value and could guide postoperative systemic therapy [150]. But in another retrospective study focusing only on systemic neoadjuvant doxorubicin and ifosfamide without radiotherapy post-treatment tumour necrosis, fibrosis/hyalinisation and cellular degeneration did not correlate with the outcome [149].

Response to chemotherapy is, however, not predicted by the same factors as is overall survival [250]. Several prognostic factors have been identified in STS and include primary site of tumour, histologic type, grade, stage of disease, patient's age and some molecular factors. Definition and selection of the so-called "high-risk" STS is difficult. Poor prognosis factors identified by Pisters included age >60 years, tumours >5 cm and high-grade histology, whereas recurrence was associated with positive margins, age >50 years and some histologic subtypes (fibrosarcomas and malignant peripheral nerve sheath tumours). Significant factors for distant metastases were high grade, deep localisation, intermediate tumour size and leiomyosarcoma and nonliposarcoma histology [194]. But in a randomised study of Gortzak et al., while selecting high-risk STSs (tumours ≥8 cm of any grade or grade II/III tumours <8 cm or grade II/III locally recurrent tumours or grade II/III tumours with inadequate surgery performed in the previous 6 weeks and therefore requiring further surgery), failed to significantly improve time to relapse or overall survival [81]. Badellino and Toma suggested guidelines according to tumour stage [10] adapted to STS patients, which is precisely the task of multidisciplinary sarcoma boards.

Three possible indications for induction chemotherapy are recognised [22]:

1. Tumours that could not be resected R0 or R1 (microscopically positive margins)
2. Tumours which would be treated by a mutilating surgery

    It is sometimes possible to perform conservative surgery after induction chemotherapy in patients initially considered for non-conservative surgery (amputation). There is no superiority of one treatment over the other (radiation, chemotherapy and combined chemoradiation), because there is no prospective randomised trial that has investigated this model.
3. Tumours which could be resected by a conservative surgery

    The EORTC trial comparing induction treatment followed by locoregional treatment, versus locoregional treatment only, found no differences between the two arms regarding amputation, recurrence-free survival and overall survival [196].

Disadvantages of induction chemotherapy are perioperative complications with wound complications, myelosuppression, immunosuppression [237] and delayed definitive surgery. One retrospective study evaluated this morbidity by including 309 patients: 105 patients received induction chemotherapy versus 204 who had surgery first. The incidence of surgical complications was not different for patients with induction chemotherapy compared with patients having surgery first: both in those with extremity sarcomas (34 % vs. 41 %) and in those with retroperitoneal/visceral sarcomas (29 % vs. 34 %). Nevertheless, preoperative radiation, autologous flap coverage and extremity tumours were associated with increased wound complications [159].

Outcomes observed in non-randomised phase II studies seem to suggest that induction chemotherapy delivered in not-metastatic patients allows higher response rates than chemotherapy delivered in metastatic settings [153, 208]. Similar data are available from treatment in the head and neck, osteosarcoma and breast cancers [219]. Overall, patients with induction therapy are fitter and thus tolerate such treatment better than those with metastatic disease. Moreover, it could not be excluded that metastatic cancers present a more aggressive intrinsic behaviour. This potential bias should be taken into account when the results of available studies are analysed.

Chapter 27 will review the different opportunities of neoadjuvant treatment in sarcomas. We will focus on some type of sarcomas, including sarcomas in limbs, osteosarcomas, soft tissue sarcomas (mainly body wall and retroperitoneal) and primary metastatic sarcoma. We will not review the treatment of Ewing's sarcoma, GIST (gastrointestinal stromal tumours) and some kind of paediatric sarcomas, like alveolar or embryonal rhabdomyosarcomas, unless they are located in the retroperitoneum or intra-abdominal.

Overall treatment may differ according to location. AJCC classification sites for STS include head and neck, extremities (limbs), superficial trunk (abdominal and chest) wall, gastrointestinal, genitourinary, visceral retroperitoneal, gynaecologic, breast, lung pleura and mediastinum and others [2].

27.3 STS in Limbs and Isolated Limb Perfusion (ILP)

27.3.1 Chemotherapy

The use of induction chemotherapy treatment was studies in several clinical trials since the mid-1990s.

The therapeutic objective in STS of the extremities is to improve local control with adequate surgical margins with a good functional outcome and to reduce the risk of distant metastases for better survival. Risk of distant metastases increases with tumour grade and size [63]. For some patients with intermediate- or high-grade, large tumours, induction therapy may allow achieving this goal with possibly adequate resection margins.

Eilber reported in 1984 the results of a multimodality treatment for high-grade STS with intra-arterial doxorubicin (30 mg total dose over 24 h for each of three consecutive days) followed by radiotherapy (3500 rad in ten fractions) and 7–14 days later en bloc resection [59]. Local recurrence was observed in only 3/100 patients with a high rate of primary limb salvage. Similar results were published with the same regimen by other authors [146, 222, 256]. Most frequently reported complication was wound healing requiring subsequent amputation in some cases. Fractures and lymphoedema were less frequent. So far, no significant differences in local control, limb salvage and complications have been demonstrated between intra-arterial and intravenous route [60]. Induction therapy associating multiple chemotherapy agents and radiotherapy showed a higher response rate. In large (≥ 8 cm) high-grade tumours, a preoperative MAID regimen (mesna, adriamycin, ifosfamide and dacarbazine) interdigitated with 44 Gy of radiotherapy followed by resection, and postoperative chemotherapy (16 Gy only for patients with positive margins) was reported in 48 patients [45]. The outcome was superior when compared with a control group from the investigator database. The median necrosis rate of resected tumours was 95 % with only a 10 % partial response using RECIST criteria. The treated group showed a significant reduction in 5-year distant metastasis freedom (75 % versus 44 %, $P=0.0016$), disease-free survival (70 % versus 42 %, $P=0.0002$) and overall survival (87 % versus 58 %, $P=0.0003$). No significant relationship was noted between tumour necrosis and distant metastases and disease-free or overall survival in univariate analysis. Toxicity was not negligible with febrile neutropenia in 25 % and wound complications in 29 % of patients. One patient developed a fatal myelodysplasia. Higher toxicities and worse outcomes were reported lately with the same regimen [131]. Role of induction systemic chemotherapy was retrospectively examined in extremity sarcoma larger than 5 cm by Pezzi et al. [191]. Preoperative chemotherapy of CYADIC (cyclophosphamide, adriamycin, dacarbazine, ± vincristine) was administered from 1 to 16 cycles (mean = 4.4 cycles).

Radiotherapy was delivered in the preoperative (16 patients) or in the postoperative setting (seven patients). Limb-preserving resections were performed in 31 of the 45 patients (67 %). Sixty per cent of patients did not respond, 11 % had a complete response, 13 % a partial response and 15 % a minor response. Distant metastatic disease-free survival ($p=0.006$) and median overall survival (>60 months versus 32.7 months, $p=0.002$) were significantly higher in responder patients. A retrospective analysis of induction chemotherapy for tumours larger than 10 cm was reported by the MSKCC and Dana Farber Cancer Institute. Three-year disease-free survival was significantly improved from 62 % with surgery alone, to 83 % for doxorubicin- and ifosfamide-containing chemotherapy [87]. In 2001, a randomised phase II study published after 7 years of follow-up failed to show OS benefit for the induction chemotherapy group (3 cycles of adriamycin/ifosfamide) versus surgery alone although was not powered for this endpoint. The authors concluded that preoperative chemotherapy did not seem to add major survival benefits [81]. In 2004, a cohort analysis of 674 patients with stage III of extremity treated at the Memorial Sloan-Kettering Cancer Center (MSKCC) and the University of Texas M.D. Anderson Cancer Center (MDACC) from 1984 to 1999 showed that combining perioperative chemotherapy and surgery did not give a sustained benefit beyond 1 year [37].

At the moment, the use of induction chemotherapy is still controversial although the preoperative chemotherapy offers several theoretical advantages including cytoreduction, elimination of micrometastatic disease and assessment of treatment efficacy.

27.3.1.1 Isolated Limb Perfusion (ILP)

Thirty to forty per cent of all STS are located in limbs [28, 155]. Treatment modalities include chemotherapy, radiation therapy (including brachytherapy and intraoperative radiotherapy), ILP and amputation, depending on the size, location and tumour grade. Surgery remains the mainstay of treatment, combined or not with adjuvant or neoadjuvant approaches. The ultimate goal is limb preservation. Limb STS may present either as a directly resectable disease according to compartment surgery, disease where margins are deemed to be increased by induction therapy, unresectable disease where multimodality treatment may help limb salvage and finally disease threatening life (necrosis, infection) or quality of life (pain, impotence) leading directly to amputation [34]. Definition of limb non-resectable STS is subjective, which enhances the importance of multidisciplinary sarcoma board. Some non-resectability criteria for primary or recurrent STS are tumour burden (size and number of lesions) and proximity of vital structures like motor nerves, main blood vessels and bone. This is mainly related to the possibility of getting or not getting an ideal safe margin of 1–3 cm.

Isolated limb perfusion (ILP) was initiated by Creech, Ryan and Krementz in 1957 [38]. Potential neoadjuvant use of this therapy was soon recognised [133], while observing some kind of response rate in 83 % of patients after melphalan alone. The concept was to allow chemotherapy in a limb only, controlled by a tourniquet. Many experiments and reviews have assessed the indications for melanoma and STS [141]. Main advantages are high-dose chemotherapy in the limb only (up to ten times the maximal systemic tolerated dose), sparing systemic toxicity, provided a secure isolation and a systemic control during the procedure [128]. This latter condition, among others, explains why ILP is limited to only about 50 certified centres in Europe. ILP for melanoma and STS patients with carboplatin [40], doxorubicin [127, 178], cisplatin [99] or other agents had comparable efficacy but higher local or general toxicity compared with melphalan, an alkylating agent, that remains the drug of choice [216], and is the chemotherapy more commonly perfused.

Combination of interferon gamma and TNF alpha dramatically increased melphalan efficacy [148]. Recombinant tumour necrosis factor (TNFα-1a, Tasonermin, Beromun®, Boehringer Ingelheim GmbH, Germany) is a proapoptotic molecule for angiogenic endothelial tumour cells [142]. TNF induces vasoplegia, increasing drug uptake and destruction of tumour vasculature [107], and has synergy with interferon gamma (*IFNχ*). In combination, up to 80–90 % CR can thus be achieved in melanoma patients and 20–40 % in limb STS [100, 141]. The effect of melphalan is potentiated by mild hyperthermia (38–41.5 °C) [163]. Due to its higher toxicity without significantly adding to the efficacy of combination of TNF with melphalan, INF use has been cancelled in many STS protocols.

As limb-sparing surgery is the main goal, even if resection does not take place (ILP as exclusive therapy [140]), quality of life may be better compared with amputation [71]. It is well recognised that amputation may achieve local control but does not improve survival, neither in primary treatment [3, 204, 264], nor in recurrent STS [227]. Survival is conditioned by tumour size, grade and distant metastasis. Limited distant metastatic disease does not represent an absolute contraindication to ILP, and an 84 % response rate with a 97 % limb salvage have been reported by Grünhagen et al. in 37 stage IV patients (18 primary and 19 recurrent STS) [92]. At this point, therefore, a randomised study comparing ILP and amputation with survival as the end point would be ethically difficult and not acceptable to patients.

27.3.1.2 Indication for ILP

Indication for isolated limb perfusion can be summarised in four groups of patients:

(A) Group 1: limb salvage for primary sarcoma, anticipated narrow margins (case report in Fig. 17.1) or local recurrence in order to spare functionally mutilating surgical resection
(B) Group 2: local recurrence in a previously irradiated limb. ILP is still feasible for recurrent STS in previously irradiated limbs: Lans et al. reviewed 26 patients (30 ILPs) with an overall response rate of 70 % (20 % complete and 50 % partial) and limb salvage of 65 % [136].
(C) Group 3: multicentric sarcoma of the limb [135]. Sixty-four ILPs in 53 patients with multifocal primary sarcomas (28 patients) or multiple sarcoma recurrences (36 patients) have been reviewed by Grünhagen, who demonstrated an overall response of 88 % (42 % complete and 45 % partial response) with a 39 % 5-year survival rate [91].
(D) Group 4: patient with distant metastatic disease and local limb-threatening disease [92]. As amputation will not prolong survival, ILP acts as a limb salvage procedure for quality of life.

The last three indications represent clear palliative options directed to limb salvage, whereas the first group of patients represents the main indication for induction therapy. Even if ILP may help to get free margins in further resection, clinical and radiological response after ILP must be evaluated in the multidisciplinary STS board: ILP may become exclusive because of progression, unresectability anyway, or because of worsening of patient's condition (case report in Fig. 17.2). In this setting, efficacy of induction ILP is difficult to evaluate, and limb salvage rate [57] is often a better surrogate marker. Moreover, no randomised trial has compared to date induction chemotherapy, radiation therapy and induction ILP.

27.3.1.3 Surgical Technique for ILP

Patients are selected in multidisciplinary sarcoma tumour boards. Complete surgical technique has been described elsewhere in the most recent comprehensive review to date by Seinen of all published ILP for STS [216]. Basically, a vascular access for introducing venous and arterial cannulas is performed through subclavian, axillary or brachial dissection for the upper limb and through iliac, femoral or popliteal dissection for lower limb. A simultaneous radical lymph node dissection is performed or not, according to the vascular access and centres.

This point has never been evaluated when dealing with induction ILP efficacy. When nodes are evaluated in STS patients, lymph node metastasis can be observed in up to 15 % overall. This incidence varies according to histology: 0.6 % in undifferentiated sarcoma and 10–32 % in epithelioid sarcoma, rhabdomyosarcoma, angiosarcoma and clear cell sarcoma [39, 74, 203, 217]. Synchronous metastatic lymph nodes have a bad prognosis when associated with distant metastatic disease [19]. When considering other procedures than ILP, radical lymph node dissection may improve survival and must be discussed in patients with rhabdomyosarcoma, epithelioid sarcoma, clear cell sarcoma and grade III angiosarcoma and synovial sarcomas [39, 70, 157]. It must be underlined that in the new 2010 AJCC TNM classification, N1 disease has been reclassified as stage III rather than stage IV [2].

Following secured cannulation, a tourniquet is applied at the root of the limb and secured by a Steinman pin inserted in the iliac crest. A heart-lung machine provides vascularisation, oxygenation and treatment delivery. Systemic leakage is checked by injection of technetium 99 m-labelled albumin in the extra-corporeal circulation (ECC) with systemic monitoring by a precordial gamma probe. Uninvolved hands or feet are wrapped in order to decrease toxicity. When steady-state hyperthermia >38.0 °C is reached, sequential therapy is injected. TNF (dosage is discussed below) and INF (depending on centres) are injected for 30 min. Melphalan is injected (according to the limb volume: 10 mg/l for leg or 13 mg/l arm) for 60 min. These original timings have been reduced in many centres (simultaneous injection and 60 min duration). The limb is then rinsed with physiologic solutions, the vessels closed and circulation re-established. Regional monitoring during ILP includes tissue temperature (needle probes) and in some centre compartmental tissue pressure [101], in order to detect compartmental syndrome. Usually, recovery in the intensive care unit is preferred for 24-h surveillance but is not mandatory in all teams. Post-operative limb survey is essential in order to diagnose compartment syndromes or vascular problems. The patient starts rehabilitation after a mean hospital stay of 7–10 days: full recovery may necessitate assistance and physiotherapy up to 3 months. Re-evaluations of tumour status by local examination, MRI or PET-CT decide if limb salvage surgery can be performed or if STS is still unresectable.

27.3.1.4 Toxicity

Severe systemic toxicity depends mainly on the dose of TNF and the efficacy of the leakage control [23]. Historically, it included vasoplegia and shock (3 % grade III–IV [57]), myelotoxicity, heart, liver, kidney and lung failures. These were due to leakage of tourniquet during ILP [216] and are nowadays rarely encountered. Limb toxicity includes skin burns, rhabdomyolisis, neurotoxicity and rare septic necrosis leading to amputation (less than 3 % after ILP). Locoregional toxicity is usually reported according to Wiberdink grading [262], but "severe" toxicity, for example, does not correspond to the same gradings among studies. Severe local and systemic morbidity induced by ILP can be lowered by the following adjuncts to original procedure:

1. Avoiding hyperthermia above 39–40 °C.
2. Decreasing TNF dosage (1–2 mg for upper/lower limb instead of 3–4 mg) which should not change tumour response or overall survival [52, 106, 207]. This was demonstrated in a multi-institutional randomised trial with 100 patients [23] and later confirmed in a cohort study of 100 patients with 1 mg TNF [24], but challenged in another retrospective study with 41 patients [165]. This study showed that the overall response rate was 65.2 % in the high-dose group (3–4 mg TNF) versus 30.7 % in the low-dose group (1 mg).
3. Prophylactic fasciotomy as advocated by Hoven-Gondrie et al. [105], creatinine kinase value surveillance [255] or at least intra- and post-operative compartment pressure monitoring as proposed by Hohenberger, who avoided fasciotomy [101].
4. A specific rehabilitation programme.
5. We advocate preoperative ultrasonographic identification of femoral bifurcation (variable anatomy) in order to avoid straight placement of the tip of cannula in deep femoral artery. We currently use early fluorescein injection in the ECC and Wood lamp for showing and confirming the skin territory and corresponding muscle group really perfused.

27.3.1.5 Results

Noorda et al. reviewed evidence-based facts supporting the use of isolated limb perfusion in STS (and in melanoma) [174]. Due to different regimens of combined treatments (TNFα dosage, ± interferon, melphalan or other chemotherapy), different assessment of response (clinical/radiological/pathology) and type of patients' study (retrospective cohort, prospective observational, rarely randomised studies), direct comparison between all trials is difficult [23, 33, 50, 58, 93, 95, 97, 140, 145, 173, 178, 190, 206, 207, 212, 249], but was attempted in Table 27.1. Globally, combination of melphalan and TNF resulted in an 8–80 % partial and 8–56 % complete

Table 27.1 ILP as induction therapy

Author	Year/reference	N patients	Drugs[a]	Overall CR	N (%) patients with resection	Delay ILP-resection (weeks) (mean/ median)	Tumour involved margins	Limb salvage %[g]
Eggermont	1996 [57]	187	TM±I	29 %	126/186 (68 %)	4–24 (mean 10)	NA	152/186 (82 %)
Gutman	1997 [95]	35	TIM	37 %	9/35 (26 %)[e]	6–8	NA	29/34 (85 %)
Olieman	1998 [179]	9	TM	44.4 %	6/9 (67 %)	NA	58 %	8/9 (89 %)
Rossi	1999 [206]	67	TD	27.7 %	65/67 (97 %)	4–6	NA	60/67 (92.3)
Lejeune	2000 [140]	22	TIM	18 %	17/22 (77 %)	6–31 (mean 17)	NA	19/22 (86 %)
Noorda	2003 [173]	49	TM±I	8 %	31/49 (63 %)	1.5–35 (median 17)	48 %	36/49 (73 %)
Bonvalot	2005 [23]	100	TM	36 %	71/100 (71 %)	NA	51 % R0: 35, R1: 32, R2: 4	87/100 (87 %)
Rossi	2005 [207]	21	TD	55 %	17/20 (85 %)	6–8	NA	15/21 (71 %)
Grünhagen	2006 [93]	197	TM±I	26 %	130/197 (66 %)	NA	NA	171/197 (87 %)
Pennacchioli	2007 [191]	51	TD/M	41 %	NA[f]	NA	NA	42/51 (82 %)
Van Ginkel	2007 [206]	73	TM±I	26 %	68/73 (93 %)	2–15 (mean 8)	NA (CR: 17/68)	59/73 (81 %)
Hayes	2007 [97]	16	TM	20 %	NA	NA	NA	15/16 (94 %)
Cherix	2008 [33]	51	TM±I	25 %	33/51 (65 %)	NA	70 % R0: 10, R1: 20, R2: 3	44/51 (86 %)
Grabellus	2009 [82]	65	TM	54 %[b]	47/65 (72 %)	6	30 %[b] R0: 33, R1: 10, R2: 4	40/47 (85 %)
Nachmany	2009 [165]	43	TM	15 %	37/43 (86 %)	8–12	NA	28/43 (65 %)
Bonvalot	2009 [24]	100	TM	30 %/19 %[c]	83/100 (83 %)	mean 8	R0: 47, R1: 23, R2: 1	87/100 (87 %)
Di Filippo	2009 [55]	75	TD	34 %	64/75 (85 %)	4–6	NA	64/75 (85 %)

Author	Year/reference	N patients	Drugs[a]	Overall CR	N (%) patients with resection	Delay ILP-resection (weeks) (mean/median)	Tumour involved margins	Limb salvage %[g]
Deroose	2011 [50]	208	TM±I	18 %	109/208 (52 %)	12	R0: 63, R1: 43	167/208 (80 %)
Olofsson	2012 [179]	54	TM	21 %	30/54 (56 %)	0–14 (median 8)	R0: 4, R1: 24, R2: 1	40/54 (74 %)
Jakob	2014 [116]	90	TM	37 %[d]	86/90 (96 %)	6–10	R0: 70, R1: 16	8/90 (89 %)
Andreou	2014 [8]	35	TM	NA	35/35 (100 %)	5–10 (median 7)	R0: 27, R1: 6, R2: 2	3/35 (86 %)

T TNF, *I* interferon, *M* melphalan, *D* doxorubicin, *NA* not assessed, *CR* complete response: clinical/radiological, biopsy proven or resection

[a]Variable dosages of TNF: 0.5–4 mg according to limb, team or study

[b]25 patients were considered with <10 % viable cells as CR

[c]CR assessed by MRI (30/100) and by histopathology after surgery (16/83)

[d]33/86 had ≥90 % necrosis

[e]Resection only in 9/13 patients with CR

[f]Study included non TNF ILP, with overall 61/88 (69 %) limb-sparing resections

[g]Primary amputation rate

pathology response rates. Limb salvage was observed in 57–100 % of patients [100, 103, 141]. This is remarkable, knowing that previous experience before TNF era showed only 0–7 % complete response [100]. Because ILP is a regional therapy, overall survival will not be prolonged [141]. The review of ILP performed in Lausanne for STS patients showed 25 % CR [33]. Resection of tumour remnants was performed in 65 % and final amputation rate was 24 % with a mean follow-up of 38.9 months (4–159). Regular reviews of ILP in STS have confirmed efficacy and safety over the years [216], despite no randomised study comparing or associating ILP with or without combined radiotherapy or chemotherapy (induction or adjuvant). Relation between tumour grade and treatment response has been observed: high-grade STS showed a better response to ILP [57, 199]. Prognostic factors for local recurrence after ILP are grade and R1-positive margins [24, 205], and possibly STS histology [83]. Most STSs are hypervascularised tumours (Fig. 27.1a) (ii);. TNF selectively destroys tumour microvasculature, while sparing normal tissues and acts in synergy with chemotherapy [142]. Olieman et al. compared in 25 patients angiographies before and after ILP: return to a normal angiography in 18 patients was associated with complete anatomopathological response [177] (which was not the case in patient in Fig. 27.1b despite complete pathology response). Treatment response is hard to assess on imaging: Grabellus et al. showed that size changes based on MRI and RECIST criteria did not correspond to pathology and clinical response [84]. In another study, the histopathology tumour regression correlated with the kind of tumour vascularisation (reflected by microvessel density) and was associated with a better prognosis [83]. Treatment response was investigated with FDG PET-CT by comparing SUV before and after ILP by Andreou et al. They observed that high/low SUV_{max} after ILP and high/low ΔSUV_{max} (before – after ILP) significantly correlated with 2-year metastatic-free survival (80 % / 31 % $p < 0.01$ and 76 %/42 % $p < 0.05$, respectively) [8] (Fig. 27.2).

27.3.1.6 ILP as Induction Therapy

In STS patients, limb-sparing surgery combined or not combined with external beam radiotherapy is feasible in up to 90 % of patients [35]. With the advent of TNF-melphalan ILP, complete regression is more often observed with an overall response rate of 63–100 % [100] so that unresectable STS may be more prone to resection. Low-grade small well-defined compartmental STS may be directly resected without induction therapy. According to Enneking's recognition of the importance of compartments in limbs [66], resectability can be expected when STS respects fascia, for example. Extracompartmental STS may arise where boundaries are less well defined, in the axilla, subcutaneously in the limb or popliteal fossa, for example. Turcotte et al. reported 18 patients with popliteal STS (2–21 cm). Induction chemotherapy was administered in two unresectable tumours (one with postoperative chemotherapy), induction radiotherapy in eight patients with high-grade STS (50 Gy, six with postoperative boost of 13 Gy) and six patients with postoperative radiotherapy (63 Gy). This resulted in limb salvage for 15 patients with no secondary amputation in this group [246].

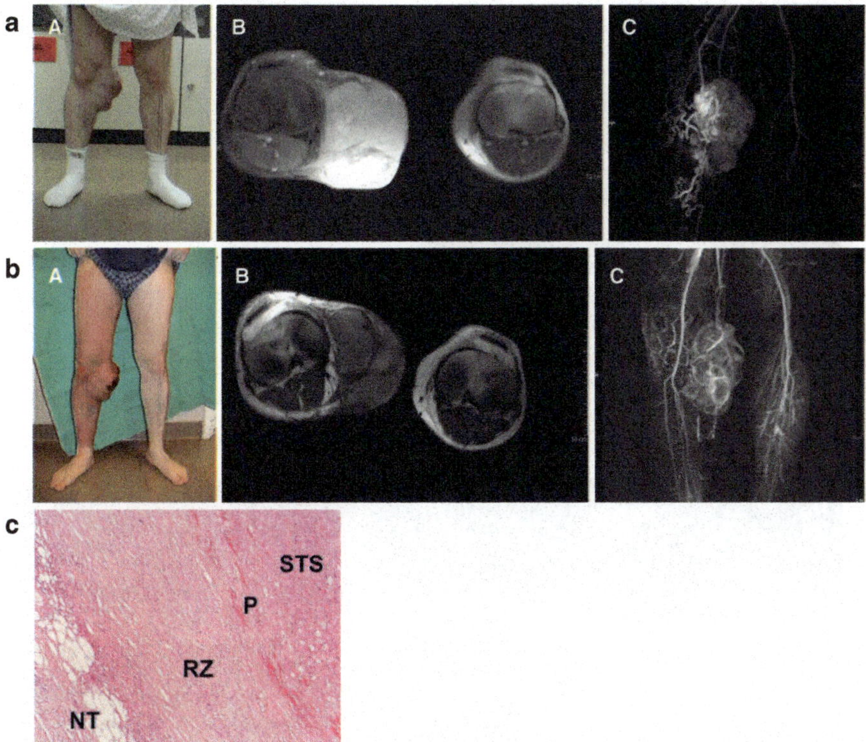

Fig. 27.1 (**a**) A 25-year-old man with no specific past medical history presented with a painless 17×10×10 cm right knee tumour (**aA**). Core biopsy diagnosed an unclassified fusiform and pleiomorphic FNCLCC grade II sarcoma, without distant metastatic disease on thoraco-abdominal CT scan. Preoperative MRI (**bA**) before ILP demonstrated a heterogeneous STS with necrotic and hypervascularised regions (**cA**). A primary resection would be at risk for narrow margins regarding knee joint and neighbouring muscular fascia. ILP was planned as induction therapy. (**b**) Thirteen days after ILP: the thin skin overlying the tip of the tumour started to necrotise (**aB**). MRI 1 month after ILP estimated 85 % necrosis (**bB**, **cB**). Radical resection surgery was realised 6 weeks following ILP. Anatomopathology showed a complete necrosis. Nine days later the 12×12 cm defect was reconstructed by mobilising an intern gastrocnemius muscle flap with proximal vascular pedicle covered with a skin meshed graft. Four cycles of adjuvant chemotherapy were planned (IFOS-adriamycin). MRI at 4 years showed no evidence of local or distant disease. (**c**) Histopathology of wide surgical margins. *STS* tumour, *P* pseudocapsule (fibrous tissue), *RZ* reactive zone (haemorrhage, inflammation, necrosis, regression), *NT* normal tissues

Histologically, STS are surrounded by a pseudocapsule and a so-called reactive zone. These may contain isolated or clusters of cells that may even skip to neighbouring normal tissues in high-grade STS. Based on his anatomopathological observations, Enneking defined four types of surgical margins: intralesional, marginal, wide and radical [65, 66]. ILP as induction therapy may be considered as a means to destroy this marginal zone between tumour and normal tissues. Grabellus

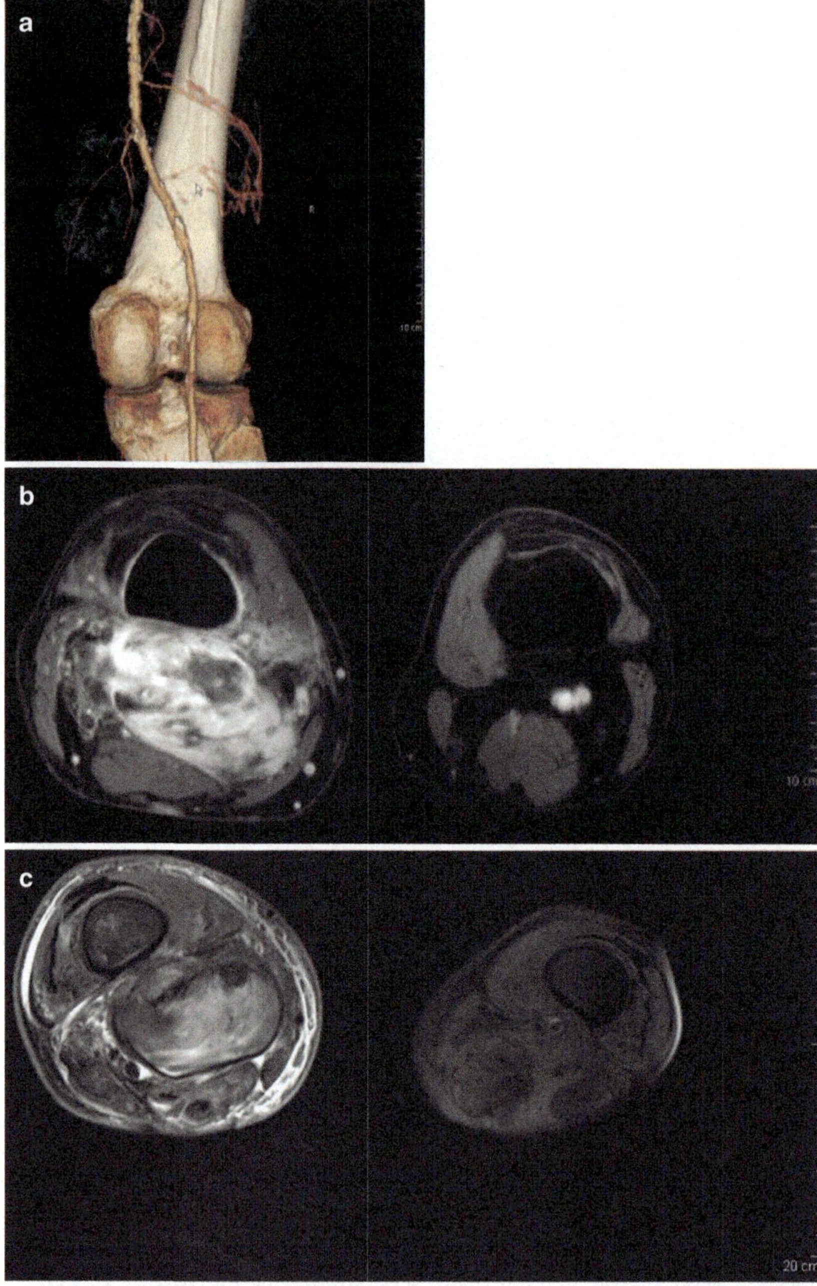

Fig. 27.2 A 74-year-old man was referred for a grade II liposarcoma of the right thigh deeply located against the neurovascular femoral bundle (**a, b**). He was a heavy smoker with symptomatic arteriopathy (claudication but no critical ischemia) on the contralateral limb and respiratory insufficiency. Sarcoma board decided for induction ILP that was performed with no specific morbidity. MRI (**c**) 3 months later demonstrated more than 80 % radiological response. Because the patient's general condition was deteriorating, the multidisciplinary team reconsidered the patient's treatment and final decision was to accept ILP as an exclusive limb salvage therapy

et al. have systematically analysed histopathologically surgical margins in 47 STS (44 grade II or III) patients after TNF-melphalan ILP [82]. A complete resection (wide or radical) according to Enneking's classification was achieved in only 23.4 % of tumours. Marginal margins were observed in 42.6 %, intralesional margins in 27.7 % and not classifiable due to extensive fibrosis in 6.4 % of patients. Tumour regression throughout margins was graded as % viable cells: 7 patients had complete regression and 18 had less than 10 % viable cells. Histological necrotic or regressive nonviable tumour cells at the margins improved their clearance for an average of 0.57 mm in three patients (otherwise with intralesional margin). Poor margins (including patients with viable tumour cells only at resection margins) were associated with local and distant recurrences and limited disease-specific survival. As none of 12 patients with "improved margins" subsequently recurred locally, the authors concluded that ILP may improve margins, corresponding to a better outcome [82]. This confirms previous publications on quality of margins [89, 228]. Interestingly, following ILP, no major definitive histological changes are seen in the surrounding normal tissues [110]. In another study, Grabellus analysed the effectiveness of induction therapy in a group of 39 patients compared with 37 patients with direct surgery. Histopathology response (assessed by increased pseudo-capsule and reactive zone) was in ascending order: radiotherapy alone, chemotherapy alone, combination of chemotherapy and ILP, chemoradiotherapy and ILP alone [85]. Effectiveness of combining modalities has prompted the University Medical Centre in Groningen (The Netherlands) to start a prospective trial investigating induction with ILP plus radiotherapy and delayed surgery [216].

Limb sparing is the major surrogate marker in ILP and Table 27.1 underlines results of induction effect of ILP. With 8–55 % CR, surgery was performed in 26–100 % of previously unresectable limb STS within a mean delay of 6 weeks. Involved margins were encountered in 30–70 % of patients. This is higher than what is generally seen after primary resection for extremity STS with up to 26 % positive margins [76, 89, 194, 228]. A majority of centres will suggest adjuvant radiotherapy in this setting [76, 89, 211, 216] as well as adjuvant chemotherapy. This may translate in a decreasing local recurrence rate. No definitive conclusion can be drawn in patients with free margins after ILP and may also because of conflicting results: Thijssens et al. observed the same benefit in R0 patients [236] but Deroose did not [51].

27.3.1.7 Amputation

As multiple phase of treatment and multiple modalities are available, amputation is still a choice or a mandatory option [3, 71, 249, 252]. It is estimated that nowadays 70 % of patients with osteosarcoma or STS can be treated by limb-saving surgery with adequate oncological result. Amputation may be due to ILP severe toxicity (around 3 % of patients) [161], following relapse or other treatments' toxicity. Kapma et al. reviewed 451 patients who underwent 505 ILP from two centres for melanoma patients and reported 11 amputations due to disease progression, loss of function, infection or intractable pain [122] and a number may be similar for STS. Post-therapy and long-term vascular limb morbidity after ILP and adjuvant radiotherapy were reviewed by Hoven-Gondrie and van Ginkel from the same team. Amputation risk was observed in three time periods in a group of 73 patients after

ILP: post-operative risk (toxicity) with a 1-year limb salvage rate of 80.1 %, a second-time period with late local recurrence (5-year limb salvage rate of 68.2 %) and a third for critical ischemia [249]. No patient was known with vascular disease before ILP and radiotherapy. Clinicians and patients should be informed of this increased late peripheral vascular risk (arterial and venous) and be convinced to avoid known vascular risk factors [104].

27.3.1.8 ILP and Age: Children and Elderly

Patients 12–18 years old have been included but not always detailed in ILP publication for STS [24, 50, 95, 102, 173, 179]. Hohenberger detailed two synovial sarcoma patients. First, an 8-year-old boy with a complete clinical response (MRI) and a partial response after resection at pathology (>90 %), who had a 6 years survival (lung metastasis) without local recurrence. Second is a 14-year-old girl with recurrent synovial sarcoma with a past adjuvant chemoradiation. She had no recurrence after 1-year follow-up. Both children received 2 mg TNF-α [102]. A 10 year-old-girl was included in a specific analysis of 14 patients with ILP for synovial sarcoma, showing a 100 % regression but R1 status following surgery [215]. There is only one article dedicated to ILP in six children and eight adolescent with melanoma, showing 5-year and 10-year survivals of 93 % and 81 %, respectively. Prophylactic fasciotomy was the rule; no local or general morbidity and no growth disturbance were observed [9]. Clearly ILP, like in adults, belongs to the armamentarium of therapy aiming limb salvage, with less morbidity than radiotherapy (wound problems, fracture, joint disturbance and risk for secondary induced cancer).

Old age (>75) is not a contraindication: results are similar when compared with younger patients [172].

27.3.1.9 Isolated Limb Infusion (ILI)

Another technique promoted by Thompson is isolated limb infusion (ILI) where cannulation is performed through a direct or a contralateral intravascular route in the radiology department: small catheters are inserted percutaneously [134, 239]. ILI can be performed for upper and lower limbs. At least in melanoma patients, similar (but overall slightly lower) results are obtained compared with ILP [119]. However, an ILP placement of an Esmarch wrap tourniquet at the root of the limb instead of a pneumatic tourniquet around the thigh allows treatment of more proximally located STS than with ILI. As ILP is an open surgical procedure, collateral vessels are ligated, which may assure a better leakage control, and a regional lymphadenectomy is added [182].

Hegazy et al. combined ILI which followed 3–7 days after by radiotherapy (35 Gy) as induction treatment within 40 patients. Response assessed by MRI was partial (>50 % volume reduction) in 12, minimal (<50 %) in 22 and stable in 6. Response based on histopathology necrosis was regarded as good (>90 %) in 15 patients, fair (60–90 %) in 17 and poor (<60 %) in 8. No severe toxicity was observed [98]. Moncrieff et al. performed 21 ILI, of which 14 as induction therapy: 9 of these had a complete response. Severe toxicity observed in three patients was attributed to the addition of mitomycin C to the protocol. Additional radiotherapy in ten patients

Table 27.2 ILI as induction therapy

Author	Year/ reference	N patients	Drugs[a]	Overall CR (%)	N (%) patients with resection	Delay ILI-resection (weeks) (mean/median)	Tumour involved margins	Limb salvage %[g]
Hegazy	2007 [98]	40	D	38[c]	40/40 (100 %)	3–7[f]	NA	33/40 (84 %)
Moncrieff	2008 [162]	21	MA[b]	57	14/21 (67 %)	NA	NA	16/21 (76 %)
Turaga	2011 [245]	12	MA	17[d]	3/12 (25 %)	NA	NA	11/14 (78 %)
Vohra	2013 [253]	22	MA	24[e]	2/22 (9 %)	NA	NA	16/22 (73 %)

T TNF, *I* interferon, *M* melphalan, *D* doxorubicin, *A* actinomycin D, *NA* not assessed, *CR* complete response: clinical/radiological, biopsy proven or resection
[a]Variable dosages of TNF: 0.5–4 mg according to limb, team or study
[b]Three patients had mitomycin C in addition to melphalan
[c]Response with >90 % necrosis
[d]Clinically and with imaging
[e]RECIST criteria
[f]Delay after completion of radiotherapy
[g]Primary amputation rate

did not significantly improve the outcome [162]. Two other papers showed limited experience with ILI as induction therapy [245, 253] (Table 27.2). No child was included in these studies.

A pharmacokinetic and drug resistance evaluation comparing ILP and ILI showed that to date there is no clear indication that one procedure is superior to the other, but ILI is definitively a less invasive technique. ILP may be somewhat more effective than ILI, but it has a higher toxicity [182]. ILI like ILP can be repeated.

27.3.1.10 Induction Thermochemotherapy

A phase II trial investigated the efficacy of combining regional hyperthermia (electromagnetic regional heating device, temperature $\geq$42 °C) with chemotherapy EIA (etoposide, ifosfamide and doxorubicin) in 47 patients with high-risk (deeply situated, $\geq$5 cm and grade II–III) STS. According to response, surgery was performed and followed by EIA ± radiotherapy. Response rate (21 %) was complete in only one patient. In the 35 patients (74 %) who had surgery, 12 showed any response. The 5-year relapse-free survival was 48 % [214].

In conclusion, ILP is a challenging therapy for specialised centres and multidisciplinary teams. As a regional therapy, ILP has found its place as a limb-sparing surgery for STS patients. TNFα dose reduction has decreased postoperative toxicity and morbidity, but questions regarding best (STS orientated) chemotherapy agents and ideal combinations with systemic induction chemotherapy or radiotherapy are still under investigation.

27.4 Osteosarcomas

Osteosarcoma is the most common primary bone sarcoma. There are several histological subtypes including conventional with its classic form or less often fibroblastic or chondroblastic form. Conventional OS (often referred to simply as osteosarcoma) is a high-grade tumour by definition and most of the times is accompanied by a soft tissue extension. The OS is staging using the Enneking staging system which is appropriate for skeletal tumours taking into account histologic grade, anatomic location and the presence or without metastases. The lungs are the main organ of metastasisation and elevated LDH has been shown to have prognostic value. Patients with an elevated ALP at diagnosis are more likely to have pulmonary metastases [12, 13].

Induction chemotherapy is a standard of care since it has been found not only to eradicate micrometastasis leading to better prognosis but also to facilitate subsequent surgical removal. It is well established that a good histopathologic response to induction chemotherapy (>95 %) is a major prognostic factor leading to better prognosis (5-year OS rates 71–80 % vs. 45–60 %, respectively) [12, 13]. Postoperative chemotherapy has demonstrated OS benefit, but the optimal drug regimen remains unclear. In the recent EURAMOS randomised trial modification of adjuvant chemotherapy based on the pathological response, (good or bad responders) did not lead to any OS benefit in paediatric-young adult patients [261]. On the other hand, data from Bacci et al. are suggesting the opposite [11].

In case of patients with synchronous metastatic lung, nodules cured can be achieved by complete surgical resection (most often wedge resection) which should be performed at the time of the primary tumour resection. In case of metachronous lung metastases, PFS is important. Based on retrospective data, for an osteosarcoma that recurs as one or more lung lesions only more than 1 year after the initial therapy, surgical resection alone can be curative [54]. However, chemotherapy is warranted if recurrence occurs earlier since the risk of other micrometastatic disease is high.

Chemotherapy is the main treatment in case of metastatic disease although recent data are showing that the bone-seeking radioisotope samarium (153-samarium ethylene diamine tetramethylene phosphonate) has an interesting activity since selectively delivers high doses of radiation to the osteosarcoma cells [7].

Lifelong follow-up of patients with OS including not only radiological assessment but monitoring also of complete blood count (CBC), as well as cardiologic evaluation since these patients are treated with high-dose alkylating agents leading to higher risk for myelodysplasia and leukaemia as well as heart dysfunction.

27.5 Induction Therapy in STS

27.5.1 Induction Chemotherapy in STS (Other Than Limbs)

The role of induction chemotherapy has been actively studied in clinical investigations. For several malignancies, like bladder cancer, osteosarcoma, head and neck cancer and inflammatory breast cancer, induction therapy is the standard of care. There are several kinds of administrations, including intra-arterial, isolated limb perfusion and systemic chemotherapy, with or without concomitant radiation, or combined with locoregional hyperthermia. Despite the evidence that induction chemotherapy may not have a negative impact on the perioperative management and may not negatively affect patients, there has been little evidence to support the use of induction chemotherapy in STS [81, 237]. The most popular chemotherapy protocols contain doxorubicin (Adriamycin) + ifosfamide or doxorubicin + ifosfamide + dacarbazine (DTIC), doxorubicin alone and doxorubicin + cisplatin + ifosfamide or doxorubicin + cisplatin. Whether combinations of polychemotherapy provide a better antitumoral activity than doxorubicin alone remains unclear. Nowadays, there is no prospective randomised trial comparing two different chemotherapy regimens in an induction setting.

27.5.2 Systemic Chemotherapy

With the aim of downstaging unresectable STS, Rouesse et al. and Maree et al. observed objective response rates of 25–40 % and 2-year OS of 65 %. All patients who could not achieve a complete response died of the sarcoma [153, 208]. Other non-randomised phase II studies used more toxic regimens [185, 224]. Like two other studies with metastatic patients [138, 171], results showed that an increasing dose (and subsequent toxicity) did not improve outcome.

An EORTC randomised controlled trial comparing surgery alone versus three cycles of induction chemotherapy with doxorubicin/ifosfamide in high-risk adult STS, histiocytoma, synovial sarcoma, liposarcoma and leiomyosarcoma, located in the limbs, head and neck, trunk or pelvis, failed to show an improvement in DFS (56 % vs. 52 %) and OS (65 % vs. 64 %). The study closed early after completion of phase II, because of poor accrual [81].

From that time, various therapeutic designs have been investigated in the search for the best treatment sequence without any success. The last decades, several attempts have been made in order to progress in the cure rate of STS when they present without clinically detectable metastatic disease by adding adjuvant chemotherapy. However, although several controlled trials and a recent pooled meta-analysis suggest an improvement of relapse-free survival, data did not show any clearly statistical OS benefit, and in this context adjuvant chemo stays experimental [213].

In 2010, a large cohort-based analysis with a median of 9-year follow-up indicates that patients with FNCLCC grade 3 sarcoma may benefit from adjuvant chemo. This analysis including 1513 patients showed a statistically significant improvement for the postoperative chemotherapy, with a difference of a median 5-year survival of 58 % vs. 45 % ($P=0.0002$), respectively, in FNCLCC grade 3 sarcoma. On the other hand, in patients with grade 2 was not significantly better (75 vs. 65 %, $P=0.15$) [114].

A recent pooled individual patient data from two consecutive EORTC trials comparing adjuvant chemotherapy to simply follow up was published in completed resected STS. In this analysis, CYVADIC and doxorubicin/ifosfamide failed to show any OS benefit [139].

Despite an extensive scientific literature on sarcoma, high-level evidences for the benefit of adjuvant chemo are spare and the decision should be tailored according to tumour characteristics especially pathological subtype, grade, site and age of the patients.

For example, in high-grade uterus LMS, a very aggressive subtype with poor prognosis, a recent phase II showed that adjuvant gemcitabine plus docetaxel followed by doxorubicin leads to an impressive 78 % and 58 % progression-free survival at 2 and 3 years, respectively. Currently, a phase III comparing this regimen versus surgery alone is ongoing.

To date, regarding the regimen choice is an open question. Anthracycline plus ifosfamide should be regarded as standard mostly due to the superiority in terms of RR and PFS in the metastatic setting comparing to monotherapy and in the absence of data for histology-driven regimen such as trabectedin in myxoid liposarcoma.

27.5.3 Combined Chemotherapy and Radiotherapy

There is a growing interest in combining induction chemotherapy with concomitant radiotherapy as a possible treatment modality, especially in limbs and retroperitoneal STS. Trials investigated the optimal way of chemotherapy administration: intravenous (iv) versus intra-arterial (ia), advantage of continuous infusion versus brief administration, efficacy, feasibility and toxicity of concomitant treatment or sequential treatments. Limb and retroperitoneal STS were studied separately because toxicity and treatment are substantially different. Retroperitoneal sarcomas have a worse outcome because of their larger volume at presentation. Even with complete resection, they do worse, independently of size, grade or surgical margins. Moreover, surrounding tissues (i.e. bowel, kidney) have a lower radiation tolerance. Eilbers' results already presented in Chap. 27.3.1. confirmed Goodnight et al. results [78], who used i.a. doxorubicin and 30 Gy in limb sarcomas. Based on Eilber's protocol, most groups switched to i.v. administration of chemotherapy during concurrent chemoradiation. Published studies most commonly used short duration of administration (3 days) combined with hyperfractionation of radiation. Continuous infusion over 5 days repeated every 2–3 weeks, to maximise radiosensitisation, was used by Toma et al. in a phase II study. Toxicity was acceptable and overall response rate was 67 % [241].

An RTOG study [131] initiated a phase II study to evaluate the efficacy and toxicity of a modified MAID combination (mesna, doxorubicin, ifosfamide and dacarbazine) in large (>8 cm) limbs and trunk STS patients. Three chemotherapy cycles were administrated with interdigitated radiotherapy with split courses of 44 Gy in 11 daily fractions of 2 Gy between the first and second, and the second and third cycles followed by surgery. Significant toxicity was observed. Long-term follow-up from this study confirmed the activity regarding local control and overall survival with 5-year disease-free survival and overall survival of 56.1 % and 71.2 %, respectively. However, this regimen was associated with short-term grade 3 or higher toxicities in all patients [132].

27.5.4 Combined Chemotherapy with Regional Hyperthermia

A complete review of the role of regional hyperthermia is beyond the scope of this paragraph and another chapter of the textbook is dedicated to this treatment modality (Chap. 5. Local and regional hyperthermia) and we will focus on specific STS indications.

Heat exposure increases tumour cell death and sensitisation of tumour to chemotherapy [53]. However, hyperthermia does not translate into distant control or survival benefit. Issels et al. carried out a first phase I/II study combining second-line chemotherapy with ifosfamide and etoposide with hyperthermia on day 1 and 5 of each cycle, every 4 weeks, in patients with locally advanced chemoresistant sarcomas. Radiologic and/or pathologic response was in the range of 30–35 %. Temperature mapping identified high intratumoral temperature. Toxicity remained modest [111]. In a second phase II study, Issels et al. investigated in 59 patients with primary advanced or recurrent high-risk STS, the efficacy and safety of combined regional hyperthermia and chemotherapy with ifosfamide, etoposide and doxorubicin, followed by surgery for resectable tumours. Patients with signs of response completed the treatment with four cycles of ifosfamide + etoposide with hyperthermia and patients with positive margins received external beam radiation. Sixty-one per cent of patients were rendered disease-free (radiologic and/or pathological tumour response). Toxicity was acceptable. OS did not differ in limb sarcoma versus non-limb sarcoma patients, but was better for those responding to induction treatment [112]. In another study, Wendtner et al. investigated response to induction chemotherapy, using the same regimen as Issels [112], with regional hyperthermia followed by surgery, adjuvant chemotherapy and irradiation. Objective response rate was 13 %, and radiographic response and histological response were, respectively, 33 % and 42.5 %. Patients responding to induction thermochemotherapy had a better 5-year probability of local failure-free survival (LFFS) than patients not responding (LFFS 59 % versus 0 %, $p < 0.001$), same for OS (60 % versus 10 %; $p < 0.001$). Heating quality was associated to chemotherapy response. As the study did not include a control arm, it was impossible to demonstrate what hyperthermia was adding to induction chemotherapy alone [259].

A multicentric randomised trial included 341 M0 patients with grade 2 or 3 STSs ≥ 5 cm. It compared 172 patients with induction chemotherapy alone (EIA-etoposide, ifosfamide, doxorubicin) with 169 patients with combination of induction EIA and regional hyperthermia (RHT - radiofrequency energy up to 42 °C). Surgery performed in 91 % of patients was R0 in 42 % and 51 %, respectively. According to response and/or surgery, radiotherapy was added (50–60 Gy) and then the same groups had adjuvant EIA or EIA + RHT. Two-year progression-free survival was 61 % in the EIA-alone group versus 76 % for the EIA+RHT group. Overall survival was not different, but when only patients who completed treatments were compared, those in the EIA+RHT had better overall survival compared with those in the EIA alone group ($p = 0.038$). Toxicity was higher for the former regarding thrombocytopenia and leucopoenia [113].

In conclusion, all these approaches emphasise the need for further randomised phase III trials. The significant efficacy of combined induction chemoradiation for *resectable* STS has not been proven to date in any randomised trial and for *unresectable* tumours; there is no randomised trial evaluating preoperative chemoradiation and induction chemotherapy alone. This clearly underlines that for a rare disease STS management must be performed in large reference centres with expertise in these fields and emphasises the need for further studies [22]. Jansen-Landheer et al. have shown that national guidelines and centralisation of treatments in expertise teams in the Netherlands have improved diagnosis and treatment of sarcoma patients over time [117].

27.5.5 Induction Radiotherapy (RT) in STS: Radiotherapy (Treatment Options)

Given STS rarity, treatments have evolved over the years. Up to now, few prospective trials have been published. Available data are reported by some institutions and/or by international collaborative groups active in rare diseases [75, 194]. Surgery in combination with radiotherapy has been used for nearly half a decade to achieve the goal of limb preservation in extremity soft tissue sarcoma, with success rates in excess of 80–90 % [160, 198]. In most modern series, radiotherapy (delivered in the preoperative and/or in the adjuvant setting), with or without intraoperative techniques (IORT, brachytherapy), local control rates in excess of 80 % are reported [160], depending on a number of factors such as tumour location, size, grade and resection margins [200]. Practical and theoretical advantages support both the preoperative and the postoperative approaches. Preoperative RT allows direct tumour visualisation and then a more precise target delineation. Moreover, preoperative RT includes smaller treatment volumes, lower doses, immediate RT after biopsy, no seeding from surgery and more oxygenated tissue. One may expect less fibrosis and tissue damage [42]. Moreover, some studies showed that treatment fields in the preoperative setting could be smaller than in the postoperative one, with a reduction of the normal tissues exposed to radiation. Disadvantages of this approach mainly consist of a potential risk of delayed wound healing and smaller biopsy samples for diagnosis, thus limiting the knowledge of the disease [180]. Advantages of postoperative RT are the availability of full pathologic review and then more precise information to take a decision about the indication of adjuvant therapy. The postoperative approach seems to be also associated with fewer acute wound complications, especially for thigh sarcomas [181]. On the other hand, for patients who develop acute wound complications following surgical resection, there can be a delay in the initiation of RT [31]. The issue of the correct timing of radiotherapy has been addressed in only one trial. The primary end point was rate of wound complications within 4 months of surgery. Wound complications were recorded in 35 % of patients in preoperative arm and 17 % in postoperative arm ($p = 0.01$). There was no difference in local recurrence rate ($p = 0.7119$). Overall survival was slightly better in preoperative arm

($p=0.0481$) [180, 181]. Late radiation morbidity (at 2 years) of this trial was reported by Davis et al. Rate of fibrosis (grade 2 or greater) was slightly higher in the postoperative arm (48.2 % vs. 31.5 %, $p=0.07$). Oedema and joint stiffness were more frequent in postoperative arm, but not significantly: 23.2 % versus 15.5 % and 23.2 % versus 17.8 %, respectively (p=NS) [43]. Patients treated with postoperative RT had a not-significant tendency to greater fibrosis due to larger field size.

Currently, conservative surgery (wide excision) and adjuvant RT enable achieving good local cure (80–90 %) with moderate risk of impaired function (5–15 %) in patients with STS. High conformal techniques (as intensity modulated radiation therapy (IMRT), helical tomotherapy, volumetric arc radiotherapy, proton therapy) allow to safely deliver larger RT doses while sparing normal tissue as far as possible [73, 121, 124]. Preoperative RT may be a good approach to reduce long-term morbidity if new technologies are also integrated, such as conformal RT and/or IMRT.

Looking at the clinical results of postoperative radiotherapy, Rosenberg et al. published a randomised study (43 patients) of amputation versus wide local excision followed by radiotherapy (60–70 Gy) [204]. This approach of limb preservation resulted in good rates of local control (four local recurrences occurred in limb-sparing surgery and none in the amputation arm), without any statistically significant change in overall or disease-free survival. Patients with positive resection margins presented a higher risk of local recurrence compared with those with negative margins ($p<0.0001$), even after postoperative radiotherapy. The same group lately showed, in another randomised study, that the addition of adjuvant irradiation to limb-sparing surgery was significantly associated with improved local control but not overall survival [266]. Pisters et al. from MSKKC compared in a series of 164 patients wide excision with or without adjuvant brachytherapy [195]. High differences regarding local control in high-grade tumours were observed (89 % vs. 66 %, $p=0.0025$), but no difference in low-grade STS ($p=0.49$). Yang et al. evaluated prospectively in a series including 91 patients with high-grade STS and 50 patients with low-grade STS if RT could be omitted after wide excision [266]. Local recurrence-free survival was significantly higher in the RT group, both for high-grade ($p=0.0028$) and low-grade STS ($p=0.016$), but without any impact on overall survival. Many retrospective studies have been published reporting prognostic factors for local recurrence (margin status, grade, direct extension, age at diagnosis, central location, delayed RT and the lack of dedicated sarcoma unit [62, 77, 200]). Delaney et al. evaluated the efficacy of adjuvant RT after wide excision in a series of 154 patients. The 5-year actuarial local control was at 76 %. Higher local control was observed in extremity tumours, radiation dose more than 64 Gy, positive margin R1 and superficial lesions [46]. Alektiar et al. have shown that upper extremity STSs were associated with a greater rate of local failure compared with lower extremity STS [5]. This can be explained by more limited surgery and difficulty of administering full total radiation doses in upper extremity.

The morbidity of adjuvant RT after surgery is well recognised in the literature and may result in functional disability and reduced quality of life for patients [41, 42].

27.6 Sarcomas in Other Situations

27.6.1 Thoracic, Trunk and Breast STS

27.6.1.1 Truncal STS: Abdominal (AWSTS) and Chest Wall (CWSTS) STS

Truncal sarcomas represent about 10 % of all STS [28] and their work-up includes treatment modalities according to histology and problems of complex reconstructions. Salas analysed 343 trunk wall STSs and found that 5- and 10-year disease-free survival (local and distant) were 58.4 % and 55.5 %, respectively, much lower than extremity STS, despite induction radiotherapy, suggesting difficulties in R0 completion [209]. Moreover, a past medical history of radiotherapy (PHR) (not only radiation induced STS) complicated treatment planning and was an adverse prognostic factor for local and distant recurrence (hazard ratio RR 4.2 and 2.2, respectively), followed by tumour size (>10 cm) and FNCLCC high grade [209]. A possible induction therapy in case of PHR and large size was only suggested by the authors. CWSTSs are often analysed with RPSTS, but as CWSTSs are more superficial than the latter, the diagnosis is easier, allowing a better local control and more favourable prognosis with nearly 90 % 5-year survival [244]. By analogy with other STS localisations, Wilder et al. recommend induction chemotherapy in specific groups of CWSTS patients: Ewing's sarcoma and rhabdomyosarcoma, ≥5 cm liposarcoma, synovial sarcoma, round cell liposarcoma and ≥10 cm myxofibrosarcoma, undifferentiated pleomorphic sarcoma and leiomyosarcoma. Overall, they observed in their heterogeneous cohort of 543 patients with truncal STS a 5-year and 10-year disease-specific survival of 83 % and 74 %, respectively. Chest and breast had a worse prognosis compared with their abdominal wall corresponding histology subtypes, including desmoids [263]. Managements of spine STS are similar; induction therapy is proposed according to histology and aggressive patterns [156].

Reconstruction of the abdominal wall [123] and the thoracic wall [14, 151] can use autologous (non-irradiated) flaps, meshes or combination. Induction radiotherapy can impair healing and bioprosthetic materials or autologous reconstruction should be preferred.

Breast STSs include a large variety of rare aggressive sarcoma [229], and definitive conclusions regarding induction and adjuvant therapies are hampered by the variety and rarity of them [254]. Pencavel et al. reviewed the 10 years' experience of The Royal Marsden Hospital with 57 patients. *Primary breast STSs* are best treated in tertiary centres with better margins control translating in improved 5-year disease-free survival when compared with non-specialised centres (58 % versus 37 %) [187].

In the absence of specific data on breast sarcoma, indications for adjuvant chemotherapy and/or radiotherapy should follow those for soft tissue sarcomas in general (higher grade – II or III, size >5 cm and resection with positive margins that cannot be re-excised) [16]. Adjuvant radiotherapy decreased local failure from 34 to 13 % in a series of 59 patients, although this did not reach statistical significance probably due to the small number of patients [16].

Radical surgery can be challenged by more breast conservative surgery including tumourectomy according to the series of 77 patients reviewed by Toesca et al., who observed similar oncologic results when compared with radical mastectomies [240].

These two authors agree that *secondary (radio-induced) breast STS* showed a worse prognosis compared with primary breast STS with 5-year disease-free survival of 14 % versus 50 % [240] and 26 % versus 55 % [187].

Induction chemotherapy or radiotherapy is empirically proposed in high-grade STS or when a primary resection seems not feasible [254]. Neuhaus et al. reviewed 67 patients with radio-induced STS of which 34, following breast cancer. Overall, seven patients received chemotherapy either as induction or adjuvant setting [170]. Aggressive behaviour translated in 65 % local recurrence and 45 % 5-year overall survival. Like primary breast sarcoma, radical surgery (R0) is the main significant survival factor. De Jong et al. presented a promising technique of combined hyperthermy (electromagnetically) and reirradiation (32–36 Gy) in 16 patients (13 unresectable and 3 in adjuvant setting). Response evaluated in 12 patients was complete in 7 and partial in 2. Median survival was 9.5 months (0–68) [44].

27.6.2 Retroperitoneal Sarcomas (RPSTSs) and Abdominal STS

RPSTSs account for 10–15 % of STSs [232]. Radical surgery remains the cornerstone of therapy: complete R0 resection is feasible in 28–64 % of patients, with a 5-year disease free survival of about 44 % (according to histology and grade) and a 5-year disease-specific survival of 35–63 % [226, 232]. An increasing rate up to 80 % R0 surgery observed in the USA could be explained by referring more patients in expert centres. This translated in a 5-year disease-free survival of 50–70 % and a 5-year disease-specific survival of 40–50 % [232]. Bonvalot et al. reported in a retrospective study of 382 RPSTS the advantage of "compartmental resection" (wide margins en bloc with surrounding organs) that resulted in 10 % 3-year recurrence rate against 47 % for simple complete resection [25]. Gronchi et al. reported the same concept with same conclusion in 288 RPSTS [88]. Due to their location, they are usually misdiagnosed and inappropriately treated: preoperative STS diagnosis offered a better radical resection rate compared with the group of patients with undiagnosed tumour having smaller size in the retrospective study of van Dalen [248]. Multifocal RPSTSs behave significantly worse, mainly those with >7 tumours: the 5-year overall survival rate was 7 % versus 37 % for those patients with less tumours. The authors proposed to consider these sarcomatosis criteria in classifications and studies and to discuss systemic chemotherapy in these patients [6]. Inadequate surgery and frequently encountered positive margins are of utmost importance: recurrence expose to the risk of dedifferentiation [69] in the recurrent tumour burden with consecutive risk for distant metastatic disease [226, 230] and also sarcomatosis [242].

As local recurrence is the main form of relapse related to tumour grade, induction therapy may be introduced in selective STS patients. Induction radiotherapy in a phase I trial [186] improved R0/R1 resection rate of intermediate- or high-grade retroperitoneal STS (95 % versus 65–95 % in other studies), 5-year relapse-free survival (60 % versus 53–58 %) and 5-year overall survival rate (61 % versus 24–48 %). Planned 50.4 Gy was achieved in 89 % of patients (in 11 % lower dose due to rapid disease progression, proximity with the liver, grade 3 anorexia or patient refusal), following which a phase III trial (ACOSOG Z9031) was activated aiming inclusion of 370 patients randomised either on surgery alone or preoperative radiation plus resection [186]. It had to be closed early due to lack of accrual [109]. The results of the pooled data of two prospective data showed 5-year local recurrence-free, disease-free and overall survival rates of 60 %, 46 % and 61 %, respectively, for patients undergoing R0 or R1 resection after preoperative radiotherapy [186].

The MD Anderson Cancer Center investigated preoperative chemoradiation in localised retroperitoneal sarcomas with continuous doxorubicin infusion (Bolus 4 mg/m^2 followed by 4 mg/m^2 in a continuous infusion over 4 days), and escalating radiation therapy of 18, 30.6, 36, 41.4, 46.8 or 50.4 Gy (in 1.8 Gy/fraction), as well as intraoperative electron-beam therapy, to the bed of the resected tumour. This treatment seemed to be feasible with acceptable toxicity, and the planned treatment could be completed in 80 % of patients [197]. An RTOG phase II trial by Pisters et al. followed investigating preoperative combined modality treatment with preoperative doxorubicin and ifosfamide followed by preoperative radiotherapy and surgery, as well as intraoperative radiotherapy for patient with high- or intermediate-grade retroperitoneal sarcomas. The trial, unfortunately, had to close in 2003 because of poor accrual, reflecting again difficulties in including patients in such trials.

The Italian Sarcoma Group enrolled 83 patients in a phase I–II study (ITASARC_*II_2004_003) and confirmed the feasibility of combining high-dose long-infusion ifosfamide (HLI) and radiotherapy (50.4 Gy) as induction treatment for resectable RPSTS. Sixty patients had a complete treatment and 79 had surgery after 4–6 weeks. Response based on RECIST showed partial response in seven patients, stable disease in 66 and progression in 10. Five-year disease-free and overall survival was 44 % and 59 %, respectively [90].

The introduction of intra-operative electron beam radiation (IOERT) or brachytherapy (BRT) provided encouraging results in patients with RPSTS [4, 221]). A prospective observational study of Pierie et al. showed that the delivery of IOERT in high-risk RPSTS patients receiving also pre- or post-operative radiotherapy improved the recurrence-free and overall survival, compared to patients receiving only one of these treatment modalities [193]. These data has been lately confirmed in a study by Stucky et al.: these authors reported data results of surgical resection combined with preoperative external beam radiation therapy with or without IOERT. IOERT was the only variable associated with a lower risk of LR (HR 0.19; CI 0.05–0.69, $P = 0.003$) [231].

Postoperative radiotherapy is valuable treatment option in high-risk RPSTS patients. A comparative non-randomised study evaluated 110 patients operated for RPSTS: 62 had surgery only and 42 patients had adjuvant conformal postoperative radiotherapy. The relapse-free survival was 47 % and 60 % ($P = 0.02$), respectively, without overall survival benefit [144].

In the 2015 consensus guidelines from a panel of international radiation oncologists, the definitive role of induction radiotherapy in retroperitoneal sarcoma patients is still pending [15]. Answers should come from a phase III randomised study of preoperative radiotherapy plus surgery versus surgery alone for patients with retroperitoneal sarcoma (EORTC 69092-22092). The study started in 2012 and will include 256 patients (https://clinicaltrials.gov/ct/show/NCT01344018).

In conclusion, RPSTSs are a heterogeneous group of tumours. Although surgery is the mainstay of treatment and it is well demonstrated its quality is critical for the outcome of the patients, their prognosis depends mostly on the histologic subtype, the stage and on the grade leading to a more personalising approach. In this context, all this patients should be addressed on centres of expertise [26].

27.6.2.1 Pelvic Sarcoma

Pelvic STSs are rare and bear a poor prognosis with a median survival of few months. Lewis reported 18 consecutive patients over 8 years, 15 out of which received induction radio- and/or chemotherapy. Eleven had surgery: complication rate was high, and treatment was hampered by pelvic anatomy with radiation-sensitive organs. Eleven patients died with a mean survival of 15 months (2–58). Large tumours, and high grade, are commonly encountered, and despite induction therapy and mutilating surgery, margins are frequently positive with an overall bad survival [147]. In an interesting phase II study based on the concept of ILP (TNF 300 µg and melpahalan), Bonvalot et al. performed an isolated hyperthermic pelvic perfusion in 28 patients with unresectable pelvic and inguinal carcinomas including three STSs [27]. Response according to RECIST criteria was complete in eight patients, eight partial, five stable and four had progressive disease. Median overall survival was 17 months in this difficult-to-treat population. The challenge of pelvic STS was reviewed in 90 patients with surgery: 84 had excision and 6 hindquarter amputation. Resection was radical in 21, marginal in 33 and intralesional in 3. Adjuvant radiotherapy was used for all high-grade tumours. Local recurrence was 23 % and 5-year disease-specific survival was 53 % [166].

Primary liver sarcomas are rare representing less than 1 % of all liver malignancies and present a first challenge regarding diagnosis [267]. Their management is also problematic as shown by Weitz' review of 30 patients with liver STS: 16 had a laparotomy, with 5 R1/R2 resections and 11 with R0 resection. No induction chemotherapy has been discussed to date [260].

Uterine STSs include a large variety of histology subtypes. Adjuvant chemotherapy and radiotherapy are performed accordingly and no induction treatment is generally advocated [143, 175]. A recent phase II in high-grade uterus LMS showed that adjuvant gemcitabine plus docetaxel followed by doxorubicin leads to an impressive 78 % and 58 % progression-free survival at 2 and 3 years, respectively. Currently, a phase III comparing this regimen versus surgery alone is ongoing. Surgery includes total abdominal hysterectomy and bilateral salpingo-oophorectomy. According to Tsikouras et al., a radical lymphadenectomy is an important prognostic factor for a not so rare lymph node metastatic risk (15/35 patients with pelvic or para-aortic metastatic lymph nodes). Recurrence was observed in 14/25 patients (56 %) who did not receive lymphadenectomy, but in only 10/35 35 patients (29 %) who did [243].

The role of adjuvant radiotherapy is controversial, as retrospective series showed a potential improvement in local control, without any impact on overall survival [210, 258]. In the largest retrospective analysis of uterine sarcoma, adjuvant radiotherapy conferred a 53 % reduction in the risk of LRF at 5 years [210].

Prostate and bladder STSs encompass rare aggressive histology subtypes: mainly leiomyosarcoma and rhabdomyosarcoma [164, 233]. The review of the Memorial Sloan Kettering Experience with 38 patients showed an overall median cancer-specific survival of 2.9 years (but 7.7 years for localised disease). In the 27 seven patients who had surgery, 7 received induction systemic combined chemotherapy and radiation [164].

27.6.3 ENT Sarcomas

Between 4 and 10 % of adult STSs occur in the head and neck region [188, 189], with about half of patients surviving at 5 years. Two main overall survival prognostic factors are tumour grade and surgery (number of procedure for cure and clear margins). Neoadjuvant therapy could be considered in the context of multidisciplinary tumour board, but neither specific recommendations nor randomised studies exist regarding induction versus adjuvant therapy.

There is an increasing interest in combined modality for cutaneous angiosarcoma of the face. Demartelare et al. reported a cohort of 21 patients, where 6 patients were treated by surgery followed by radiotherapy and/or chemotherapy, 15 underwent initial chemotherapy with different regimens followed by radiotherapy in 9 and with delayed resection with postoperative radiotherapy in 6 patients. The 5-year rates of disease-specific survival and recurrence-free survival in the entire cohort were, respectively, 60 % and 32 % [47]. Paclitaxel seemed to be associated with better disease-specific survival. Koontz et al. reported two head and neck angiosarcoma patients with combined induction radiotherapy of 50 Gy with three doses of bevacizumab (every other week during radiotherapy). Following surgery, complete pathology response was observed [130]. These excellent results could be explained by the vascular origin of angiosarcoma. In a large SEER database, Peng observed that disease-specific survival was not significantly modified by radiotherapy in a multivariate analysis. ENT STS differed between adults and children with histologic subtype distribution and with 10-year cancer-specific survival of 61 % and 71 %, respectively [189]. Radical surgery with clear margins is the only chance for prolonged survival and induction or adjuvant chemo-/radiotherapy is proposed according to histology, in the absence of any randomised clinical trial due to rarity of ENT STS [68, 158]. In a retrospective study of 111 patients with osteosarcomas of the mandible, induction chemotherapy (cisplatin, anthracycline, methotrexate, ifosfamide, etoposide and other combined drugs) improved disease-free and metastatic-free survival and increased cleared margins rates from 50 to 68 % [234].

Radiation-induced ENT STSs have a worse prognosis compared with primary STS (5-year disease-free survival rates: 10–30 % versus 54 %). Induction or adjuvant therapy can play a role in selected cases [235].

27.7 Multidisciplinary Management of Metastatic STS Patient

27.7.1 Lung Metastases

Most sarcomas of the extremity, chest wall, and head and neck, metastasise first to the lung (invaded in 20–38 % of STS patients) with pulmonary surgery offering 21–51 % 5-year survival [201]. Indeed sarcoma is the second most frequent primary following colorectal cancer to produce lung metastases [67].

Some exceptions are seen in myxoid/round cell liposarcoma which have metastases in spine, retroperitoneum or soft tissue. Abdominal and pelvic STSs predominantly metastasise to the liver. As previously discussed in Chap. 27.3.1.1. lymph node metastases are seen in angiosarcomas, rhabdomyosarcomas and epithelioid sarcomas.

Metastatic propensity depends on STS grade (low: 10 %, intermediate: 30 % and high grade: >50 %). Medium overall survival of lung STS metastatic patients is 12–14 months [220].

The place of perioperative chemotherapy in synchronous or metachronous metastases in sarcomas is not well defined. There are limited data on how to integrate metastasectomy and chemotherapy [192]. Before the era of ifosfamide, Lanza et al. found no survival benefit in 26 metastatic STS patients treated with doxorubicin as induction therapy [137].

There is a lack of prospective randomised trials studying the perioperative chemotherapy in metastatic STS. EORTC recently tried to conduct a randomised phase III trial (EORTC 62933) in patients with lung metastasis comparing metastasectomy alone versus induction chemotherapy followed by metastasectomy. The trial was conducted from 1996 to 2000 and had unfortunately to be closed due to poor accrual (unpublished data). Reported outcomes of patients with synchronous metastatic disease cannot be analysed separately from those who develop metachronous metastases [126]. Median survival for metastatic STS patients ranges from 8 to 15 months. Several factors have been associated with the survival of these patients: age, surgery for metastases, local recurrence and primary tumour size. After having analysed multiple prognostic factors, Kane et al. showed that survival of patients with STS and synchronous metastases was comparable to those with metachronous metastases [120]. Billingsey et al. found an improved survival for patients with surgically resected metachronous pulmonary metastases [21]. Therefore, the management of patients with pulmonary metastases (metachronous or synchronous) remains a challenge. Canter et al. analysed in a retrospective study the impact of perioperative chemotherapy in metastatic STS patients. Median post-metastasectomy disease-specific survival was not statistically significantly different: 24 months in patients treated with chemotherapy and surgery, versus 33 months in patients treated with surgery alone ($p=0.19$). In 38 patients treated with induction chemotherapy, there was no association between radiological response and post-metastasectomy survival. But the study sample was too small to detect a possible difference [32]. Despite evidence of some benefit of perioperative chemotherapy in retrospectives studies, no randomised trial is available yet [220].

When metastatic disease has occurred, surgery can be applied with curative intent in selected patients combined or not with chemotherapy and radiation therapy [21, 67, 129, 238]. A review of published series showed that radical surgery showed a 5-year overall survival of 23–43 % [220]. Burt et al. proposed in a phase I study an isolated lung perfusion (ILuP) for patients with unresectable metastases from sarcoma, which was well tolerated by patients, and effectively delivers high doses of doxorubicin to the lung and tumour tissues while minimising systemic toxicities. The median follow-up was 11 months and the longest, 31 months. There were no partial or complete responses in patients perfused with doxorubicin at the maximum tolerated dose of 40 mg/m². One patient had stabilisation of disease in the perfused lung [30]. Recently, Van Schil et al. published a review about many phase I trials with isolated lung perfusion (ILuP) in patients with carcinomas and sarcomas with lung metastases. This seems to be feasible, but further studies are necessary to determine the effect on local recurrence, survival and pulmonary function as well as its place in induction or adjuvant therapy [251].

Due to the lack of definitive trials helping to guide the treatment of metastatic soft tissue sarcomas, Porter et al. analysed the cost-effectiveness of resection and systemic chemotherapy. They found that systemic chemotherapy alone compared with no treatment was not cost-effective. Pulmonary resection alone was the most cost-effectiveness treatment [201].

Stereotactic body radiation therapy (SBRT) has been recently evaluated in the treatment of lung metastases from soft tissue sarcoma [168, 223] in these series. After a median follow-up of 51–95 months, 5-year local control and overall survival ranged between 96 % and 100 % and between 50 % and 60 %, respectively (from start of SBRT). The treatment was well tolerated with minimal, mainly skin toxicity.

Lung radiofrequency ablation in pulmonary metastases from sarcomas may be also a safe and useful therapeutic option [56]. Three-year survival rate was 59.2 % (95 % CI; 10.2–100 % [167].

To date, current uncontrolled data show that there are some long-term survivors among those who have local ablation therapy. Furthermore, retrospective data showed that multiple operations in select patients with recurrent disease may improve survival [125]. Some authors conclude that the decision whether to proceed at local ablation therapy with or without perioperative chemotherapy depends on the disease-free survival (more or less than 2 years) and on the number of metastasis.

27.7.2 Other Metastases

Optimal management of patients with metastatic osteosarcomas has not been defined in randomised trials either. Long-term survival is possible in about 30 % of patients with isolated pulmonary metastases treated with chemotherapy and local treatments; those with *bone* metastases seem to have a worse prognosis. The POG (paediatric oncology group) proposed the combination of ifosfamide + etoposide as induction chemotherapy followed by postoperative therapy of a combination of high-dose methotrexate alternating with doxorubicin + cisplatin and ifosfamide + etoposide. The 2-year PFS were, respectively, 39 % and 58 % for patients with lung-only and bone metastases [79].

Systemic chemotherapy in patients with *liver* metastases is not effective, except for GIST (gastrointestinal stromal tumour). Therefore, whenever possible, an attempt to resect liver metastases should be tried because it may offer the possibility of long-term survival [202]. The review of Adam et al. showed that surgery could achieve a 5-year survival of 31 % with a median survival of 32 months in a group of 125 metastatic sarcoma patients [1]. In the retrospective study of Marudanayagam, the 5-year overall survival (from the time of metastasectomy) was 48.0 % and the median survival 24 months [154]. Adjuvant (but not induction) chemotherapy has been proposed in selected patients.

All these approaches emphasise again the need for further randomised studies. Therefore, due to complexity of treatments in metastatic STS patients, management should be performed in large centres with expertise in the field.

27.8 Paediatric Sarcomas

Paediatric sarcomas account for around 20 % of all paediatric solid malignant cancers (i.e. excluding leukaemia and lymphomas) and represent less than 1 % of all adult solid malignant cancers. Around 7 % of diagnosed sarcomas in children will be soft tissue sarcomas, while malignant bone tumours make up just over 10 % of them [29, 108, 176, 183, 257].

The incidence of the different forms of sarcoma in childhood is variable according to age. In children younger than 5 years, the most common histological subtypes are, in decreasing order of incidence: (1) rhabdomyosarcoma (RMS), (2) other non-rhabdo soft tissue sarcomas (NRSTSs) such as synovial sarcoma, malignant peripheral nerve sheet tumours or fibrosarcoma, (3) osteosarcomas (OS) and (4) Ewing's tumours (ES). In older children and adolescents, NRSTSs tend to be more frequent than RMS.

Although the prognosis has dramatically improved over the last decades for children and adolescents with localised tumours, it remains poor for the 15–25 % of patients presenting with a metastatic or recurrent disease.

Although the separation between induction and adjuvant chemotherapy is not as clear cut as it might be in the adult patients, the ultimate goals remain the same, namely obtaining an optimal local control and preventing distant recurrence. This is accomplished using a multimodality approach including surgery, chemotherapy and radiotherapy. The optimal timing and intensity of these modalities is usually planned according to different prognostic factors and possible late effects of treatment. Several strategies of these multimodality approaches including various chemotherapy regimens have been tested in multiple clinical trials run by cooperative groups in Europe or the USA.

27.8.1 Rhabdomyosarcomas (RMSs)

Local control is necessary to cure children with RMS and this may be achieved with surgery and/or radiotherapy. A conservative approach is usually used, avoiding as much as possible debulking, R2, initial resection. Tumour resection or irradiation is planned in consideration of tumour response to chemotherapy.

Different drug combinations have been used and proved to be effective in RMS. The most widely used regimens are VAC (vincristine, actinomycin-D, cyclophosphamide), VACA (vincristine and cyclophosphamide plus adriamycin alternating with actinomycin-D), IVA (ifosfamide, vincristine, actinomycin-D), VAIA (ifosfamide and vincristine with adriamycin alternating with actinomycin-D) and CEVAIE (carboplatin, epirubicin, vincristine, actinomycin-D, ifosfamide, etoposide).

Prognostic factors in paediatric RMS include (1) pathological subtype (embryonal, spindle cells and botryoid versus alveolar), (2) post-surgical stage (IRS I (R0, pT1), II (R1, N1), III (R2), (3) site (extremities, parameningeal and bladder/prostate localisation having a poorer prognosis), (4) Lymphatic node invasion (N1), (5) tumour size (<5 cm having a better prognosis) and (6) patient age (patients younger than 10 years doing better than older ones).

Based on these risk factors, patients are categorised in risk groups, whose definition is slightly different in the USA or Europe. In the system used in the USA by the Children's Oncology Group (COG), stage (defined by site and size of the tumour), clinical group (post-surgical status) and histology are combined to obtain three risk groups (low-, standard- and high-), whereas the system used in European cooperative groups such as the Cooperative Weichteilsarkom Study Group (CWS) or the European Paediatric Soft Tissue Sarcoma Study Group (EpSSG) assigns patients to four risk groups, adding a very-high-risk group to the system used by COG [152].

Comparing outcomes of therapies based on these different risk-group classifications is beyond the scope of this chapter, and for the sake of simplicity, only the treatments according to the European Collaborative Groups (CWS/EpSSG) are mentioned here.

Patients with low-risk RMS usually have an upfront resection followed by chemotherapy including vincristine and actinomycin-D, without radiotherapy.

Standard-risk group comprises favourable histology and localised disease patients. In these cases, surgical re-excision is considered in R1 or R2 patients after induction chemotherapy of IVA and a response evaluation done after 9 weeks of treatment. Secondary local therapy, surgery or radiotherapy, is done between week 9 and 13, before adjuvant chemotherapy. Radiotherapy is omitted in patients with upfront or delayed R0 resection, but administered at doses between 36 and 50.4 Gy, depending on resection margins, in others.

High-risk patients, mainly R1 or R2 patients with unfavourable histology, tumour size greater than 5 cm, unfavourable localisation or N1 status, are treated with similar chemotherapy regimens (IVA) and considered for re-resection after 25 weeks (i.e. the end of chemotherapy) to achieve R0 if it was not possible after the initial 4 cycles (11 weeks). These patients are all irradiated with doses between 36 and 50.4 Gy, depending on resection margins.

The very high-risk group of patients includes those with unfavourable histology, i.e. alveolar subtype, and N1 status. These patients receive a VAIA type of chemotherapy, followed by radiotherapy at doses between 41.4 and 50.4 Gy, depending on resection margins.

27.8.1.1 Metastatic Patients

Metastatic patients receive a CEVAIE chemotherapy regimen, with response assessment at the end of induction chemotherapy (week 9) to rate for the possibility of local control. After an intensive phase of chemotherapy administered over 25 weeks, a maintenance phase consisting of oral administration of trofosfamide, idarubicin and etoposide is proposed. Metastatic patients with other unfavourable risk factors (i.e. age, tumour size or localisation) are included in early phase trials if available.

27.8.1.2 Non-rhabdomyosarcoma STS (NRSTS)

NRSTSs are a heterogeneous group of biologically distinct tumours, with variable response to chemotherapy [225]. Because of the rarity of each individual tumour type, studies evaluating systematically the efficacy of chemotherapy regimen are scarce. In general, induction chemotherapy is recommended for patients not amenable to upfront complete resection, for those with high grade tumours greater than 5 cm and for those with metastatic disease at diagnosis. Drugs include ifosfamide and doxorubicin (such as in the recently closed COG study ARST0332), while some add vincristine and actinomycin D to that regimen (such as in the CWS current recommendations). In all cases, as in other types of STS, the goal of chemotherapy is to increase the possibility of an optimal local control, with surgery, radiotherapy or both.

27.8.1.3 Osteosarcoma (OS)

Before the chemotherapy era, 5-years survival rates rarely exceeded 20 % [115]. The introduction of drug combinations, primarily the association of methotrexate, doxorubicin and cisplatin (MAP regimen), in an induction setting offered several advantages beside taking care of clinically and radiologically undetectable micro-metastatic disease present at diagnosis. These advantages included improved surgical planning and customisation of the endoprosthesis, better resectability and, importantly, histological evaluation of the tumour response to chemotherapy, an important prognostic factor [80]. Unfortunately, since then, no real, clinically significant, progress has been made, the results of the EURAMOS/AOST0331 studies showing no statistically significant effect of the post surgery addition of ifosfamide and etoposide in the poor responder group to the induction chemotherapy.

27.8.1.4 Ewing Sarcoma (ES)

As with other types of childhood sarcomas, induction chemotherapy plays an important role in the management of ES, with regimen including vincristine (V), oxazaphosphorines such as ifosfamide (I) or cyclophosphamide (C), doxorubicin (D) and etoposide (E) administered in several different ways (VIDE or VDC alternating with IE) and usually administered in a neoadjuvant fashion before local control is performed with surgery and/or radiotherapy [86, 169]. Interval compression of chemotherapy administered every 2 weeks instead of 3 weeks has been showed to improve survival in patients with localised disease as reported in a recent COG study [265]. As in OS, histological response to induction chemotherapy and taking into account the metastatic status at diagnosis allows the stratification in several subgroups and customisation of adjuvant chemotherapy.

Acknowledgements We thank Dr Essia Saiji for the anatomopathology imaging.

References

1. Adam R, Chiche L, Aloia T, et al. Hepatic resection for noncolorectal nonendocrine liver metastases. Analysis of 1452 patients and development of a prognostic model. Ann Surg. 2006;244:524–35.
2. AJCC. Soft tissue sarcoma. In: Edge SB, Byrd DR, Compton C, Fritz AG, Greene FL, Trotti 3rd A, editors. Cancer staging Manuel. 7th ed. New York: Springer; 2010.
3. Alamanda VK, Crosby SN, Archer KR, et al. Amputation for extremity soft tissue sarcoma does not increase overall survival: a retrospective study. Eur J Surg Oncol. 2012; 38:1178–83.
4. Alektiar KM, Hu K, Anderson L, Brennan MF, Harrison LB. High-dose-rate intraopertaive radiation therapy (HDR-IORT) for retroperitoneal sarcomas. Int J Radiat Oncol Biol Phys. 2000;47:157–63.
5. Alektiar KM, Brennan MF, Singer S. Influence of site on the therapeutic ratio of adjuvant radiotherapy in soft tissue sarcoma of the extremity. Int J Radiat Oncol Biol Phys. 2005;63:202–8.
6. Anaya DA, Lahat G, Liu J, et al. Multifocality in retroperitoneal sarcoma. A prognostic factor critical to surgical decision-making. Ann Surg. 2009;249:137–42.
7. Anderson PM, Subbiah V, Rohren E, et al. Bone-seeking radiopharmaceuticals as targeted agents of osteosarcoma: samarium-153-EDTMP and radium-223. Adv Exp Med Biol. 2014;804:291–304.
8. Andreou D, Boldt H, Pink D, et al. Prognostic relevance of 18F-FDG PET uptake in patients with locally advanced, extremity soft tissue sarcomas undergoing neoadjuvant isolated limb perfusion with TNF-α and melphalan. Eur J Nucl Med Mol Imaging. 2014;41:1076–83.
9. Baas PC, Hoekstra HJ, Schraffordt H, et al. Hyperthermic isolated regional perfusion in the treatment of extremity melanoma in children and adolescents. Cancer. 1989;63:199–203.
10. Badellino F, Toma S. Treatment of soft tissue sarcoma: a European approach. Surg Oncol Clin N Am. 2008;17:649–72.
11. Bacci G, Picci P, Ferrari S, et al. Primary chemotherapy and delayed surgery for nonmetastatic osteosarcoma of the extremities. Results in 164 patients preoperatively treated with high doses of methotrexate followed by cisplatin and doxorubicin. Cancer. 1993;72:3227–38.

12. Bacci G, Longhi A, Ferrari S, et al. Prognostic significance of serum alkaline phosphatase in osteosarcoma of the extremity treated with neoadjuvant chemotherapy: recent experience at Rizzoli Institute. Oncol Rep. 2002;9:171–5.

13. Bacci G, Longhi A, Versari M, et al. Prognostic factors for osteosarcoma of the extremity treated with neoadjuvant chemotherapy: 15-year experience in 789 patients treated at a single institution. Cancer. 2006;106:1154–61.

14. Bakri K, Mardini S, Evans KK, Carlsen BT, Arnold PG. Workhorse flaps in chest wall reconstruction: the pectoralis major, latissimus dorsi, and rectus abdominis flaps. Semin Plast Surg. 2011;25:43–54.

15. Baldini EH, Wang D, Haas RLM, et al. Treatment guidelines for preoperative radiation therapy for retroperitoneal sarcoma: preliminary consensus of an international expert panel. Int J Radiat Oncol Biol Phys. 2015;92:602–12.

16. Barrow BJ, Janjan NA, Gutman H, et al. Role of radiotherapy in sarcoma of the breast – a retrospective review of the M.D. Anderson experience. Radiother Oncol. 1999;52:173–8.

17. Bastiaannet E, Groen H, Jager PL, et al. The value of FDG-PET in the detection, grading and response to therapy of soft tissue and bone sarcomas; a systematic review and meta-analysis. Cancer Treat Rev. 2004;30:83–101.

18. Becher S, Oskouei S. PET imaging in sarcoma. Orthop Clin N Am. 2015;46:409–15.

19. Behranwala KA, A'Hern R, Omar AM, Thomas JM. Prognosis of lymph node metastasis in soft tissue sarcoma. Ann Surg Oncol. 2003;11:714–9.

20. Benz MR, Tchekmedyian N, Eilber FC, et al. Utilization of positron emission tomography in the management of patients with sarcoma. Curr Opin Oncol. 2009;21:345–51.

21. Billingsley KG, Burt ME, Jara E, et al. Pulmonary metastases from soft tissue sarcoma: analysis of patterns of diseases and postmetastasis survival. Ann Surg. 1999;229:602–10.

22. Blay JY, Bonvalot S, Fayette J, et al. Neoadjuvant chemotherapy in sarcoma. Bull Cancer. 2006;93:1093–8.

23. Bonvalot S, Laplanche A, Lejeune F, et al. Limb salvage with isolated perfusion for soft tissue sarcoma: could less TNF-α be better? Ann Oncol. 2005;16:1061–8.

24. Bonvalot S, Rimareix F, Causeret S, et al. Hyperthermic isolated limb perfusion in locally advanced soft tissue sarcoma and progressive desmoid-type fibromatosis with TNF 1 mg and Melphalan (T1-M HILP) is safe and efficient. Ann Surg Oncol. 2009;16:3350–7.

25. Bonvalot S, Rivoire M, Castaing M, et al. Primary retroperitoneal sarcomas: a multivariate analysis of surgical factors associated with local control. J Clin Oncol. 2009;27:31–8.

26. Bonvalot S, Raut CP, Pollock RE, et al. Technical considerations in surgery for retroperitoneal sarcomas: position paper from E-Surge, a master class in sarcoma surgery, and EORTC–STBSG. Ann Surg Oncol. 2012;19:2981–91.

27. Bonvalot S, de Baere T, Mendiboure J, et al. Hyperthermic pelvic perfusion with tumor necrosis factor-α for locally advanced cancers. Encouraging results of a phase II study. Ann Surg. 2012;255:281–6.

28. Brennan MF, Antonescu CR, Moraco N, Singer S. Lessons learned from the study of 10,000 patients with soft tissue sarcoma. Ann Surg. 2014;260:416–22.

29. Burningham Z, Hashibe M, Spector L, Schiffman JD. The epidemiology of sarcoma. Clin Sarcoma Res. 2012;2:14.

30. Burt ME, Liu D, Abolhoda A, et al. Isolated lung perfusion for patients with unresectable metastases from sarcoma: a phase I trial. Ann Thorac Surg. 2000;69:1542–9.

31. Cannon CP, Ballo MT, Zagars GK, et al. Complications of combined modality treatment of primary lower extremity soft-tissue sarcomas. Cancer. 2006;2006(107):2455–61.

32. Canter RJ, Qin LX, Downey RJ, et al. Perioperative chemotherapy in patients undergoing pulmonary resection for metastatic soft-tissue sarcoma of the extremity. A retrospective analysis. Cancer. 2007;110:2050–60.

33. Cherix S, Speiser M, Matter M, et al. Isolated limb perfusion with tumor necrosis factor and melphalan for non-resectable soft tissue sarcomas: long-term results on efficacy and limb salvage in a selected group of patients. J Surg Oncol. 2008;98:148–55.

34. Clark MA, Thomas JM. Amputation for soft-tissue sarcoma. Lancet Oncol. 2003;4:335–42.

35. Clark MA, Fisher C, Judson I, Thomas JM. Soft tissue sarcomas in adults. N Engl J Med. 2005;353:701–11.
36. Coindre JM, Terrier P, Guillou L, et al. Predictive value of grade for metastasis development in the main histologic types of adult soft tissue sarcomas. A study of 1240 patients from the French Federation of Cancer Centers Sarcoma Group. Cancer. 2001;91:1914–26.
37. Cormier JN, Huang X, Xing Y, et al. Cohort analysis of patients with localized, high-risk, extremity soft tissue sarcoma treated at two cancer centers: chemotherapy-associated outcomes. J Clin Oncol. 2004;22:4567–74.
38. Creech Jr O, Krementz ET, Ryan RF, Winblad JN. Chemotherapy of cancer: regional perfusion utilizing an extracorporeal circuit. Ann Surg. 1958;148:616–32.
39. Daigeler A, Kuhnen C, Moritz R, et al. Lymph node metastases in soft tissue sarcomas- a single center analysis of 1597 patients. Langenbecks Arch Surg. 2009;394:321–9.
40. Daryanani D, de Vries EGE, Guchelaar HJ, et al. Hyperthermic isolated regional of the limb with carboplatin. Eur J Surg Oncol. 2000;26:792–7.
41. Davis AM, Sennik S, Griffin AM, et al. Predictors of functional outcomes following limb salvage surgery for lower-extremity soft tissue sarcoma. J Surg Oncol. 2000;73:206–11.
42. Davis AM, O'Sullivan B, Bell RS, et al. Function and health status outcomes in a randomized trial comparing preoperative and postoperative radiotherapy in extremity soft tissue sarcoma. J Clin Oncol. 2002;20:4472–7.
43. Davis AM, O'Sullivan B, Turcotte R, et al. Late radiation morbidity following randomization to preoperative versus postoperative radiotherapy in extremity soft tissue sarcoma. Radiother Oncol. 2005;75:48–53.
44. De Jong MAA, Oldenborg S, Oei SB, et al. Reirradiation and hyperthermia for radiation-associated sarcoma. Cancer. 2012;118:180–7.
45. DeLaney TF, Spiro IJ, Suit HD, et al. Neoadjuvant chemotherapy and radiotherapy for large extremity soft-tissue sarcomas. Int J Radiat Oncol Biol Phys. 2003;56:1117–27.
46. Delaney TF, Kepka L, Goldberg SI, et al. Radiation therapy for control of soft-tissue sarcoma resected with positive margins. Int J Radiat Oncol Biol Phys. 2007;67:1460–9.
47. DeMartelaere SL, Roberts D, Burgess MA, et al. Neoadjuvant chemotherapy-specific and overall treatment outcomes in patients with cutaneous angiosarcomas of the face with periorbital involvement. Head Neck. 2008;30:639–46.
48. Demetri GD, Pollock R, Baker L, et al. NCCN sarcoma practice guidelines. National Comprehensive Cancer Network. Oncology (Williston Park). 1998;12:183–218.
49. Dei Tos AP. Classification of pleomorphic sarcomas: where are we now? Histopathology. 2006;48:51–62.
50. Deroose JP, Eggermont AMM, van Geel AN, et al. Long-term results of tumor necrosis factor α- and melphalan-based isolated limb perfusion in locally advanced extremity soft tissue sarcomas. J Clin Oncol. 2011;29:4036–44.
51. Deroose JP, Burger JWA, van Geel AN, et al. Radiotherapy for soft tissue sarcomas after isolated limb perfusion and surgical resection: essential for local control in all patients? Ann Surg Oncol. 2011;18:321–7.
52. Deroose JP, Grünhagen DJ, de Wilt JHW, et al. Treatment modifications in tumour necrosis factor-α (TNF)-based isolated limb perfusion in patients with advanced extremity soft tissue sarcomas. Eur J Cancer. 2015;51:367–73.
53. Dewey WC. Interaction of heat with radiation and chemotherapy. Cancer Res. 1984;44:4714–20.
54. Diemel KD, Klippe HJ, Branseheid D, et al. Pulmonary metastasetomy for osteosarcoma: is it justified? Recent Results Cancer Res. 2009;179:183–208.
55. Di Filippo F, Giacomini P, Rossi CR, et al. Hyperthermic isolated perfusion with tumor necrosis factoralpha and doxorubicin for the treatment of limb-threatening soft tissue sarcoma: the experience of the Italian Society of Integrated Locoregional Treatment in Oncology (SITILO). In Vivo. 2009;23:363–8.
56. Ding JH, Chua TC, Glenn D, Morris DL. Feasibility of ablation as an alternative to surgical metastasectomy in patients with unresectable sarcoma pulmonary metastases. Interact Cardiovasc Thorac Surg. 2009;9:1051–3.

57. Eggermont AM, Shraffordt Koops H, Klausner JM, et al. Isolated limb perfusion with tumor necrosis factor and melphalan for limb salvage in 186 patients with locally advanced soft tissue extremity sarcomas. The cumulative multicenter European experience. Ann Surg. 1996;224:756–65.

58. Eggermont AMM, Schraffordt Koops H, Liénard D, et al. Isolated limb perfusion with high-dose tumor necrosis factor-α in combination with Interferon-χ and melphalan for nonresectable extremity soft tissue sarcomas: a multicenter trial. J Clin Oncol. 1996;14:2653–65.

59. Eilber FR, Morton DL, Eckardt J, et al. Limb salvage for skeletal and soft tissue sarcomas. Multidisciplinary preoperative therapy. Cancer. 1984;53:2579–84.

60. Eilber FR, Giulano AE, Huth JF, et al. Intravenous (IV) vs. intraarterial (IA) adriamycin, 2800r radiation and surgical resection for extremity soft-tissue sarcomas: a randomized prospective trial. Proc Am Soc Clin Oncol. 1990;9:309 (abstr 1194).

61. Eilber FC, Rosen G, Eckardt J, et al. Treatment-induced pathologic necrosis: a predictor of local recurrence and survival in patients receiving neoadjuvant therapy for high-grade extremity soft tissue sarcomas. J Clin Oncol. 2001;19:3203–9.

62. Eilber FC, Brennan MF, Riedel E, et al. Prognostic factors for survival in patients with locally recurrent extremity soft tissue sarcomas. Ann Surg Oncol. 2005;12:228–36.

63. Eilber FC, Tap WD, Nelson SD, et al. Advances in chemotherapy for patients with extremity soft tissue sarcoma. Orthop Clin N Am. 2006;37:15–22.

64. Eisinger-Mathasona TSK, Mucaja V, Kevin M, Bijua KM, et al. Deregulation of the Hippo pathway in soft-tissue sarcoma promotes FOXM1 expression and tumorigenesis. PNAS. 2015;112(26):E3402–11.

65. Enneking WF, Spanier SS, Goodman MA. A system for the surgical staging of musculoskeletal sarcoma. Clin Orthop Relat Res. 1980;153:106–20.

66. Enneking WF, Spanier SS, Malawer MM. The effect of the anatomic setting on the results of surgical procedures for soft parts sarcoma of the thigh. Cancer. 1981;47:1005–22.

67. Ehrhunmwunsee L, D'Amico TA. Surgical management of pulmonary metastases. Ann Thorac Surg. 2009;88:2052–60.

68. Fayda M, Aksu G, Yaman Agaoglu F, et al. The role of surgery and radiotherapy in treatment of soft tissue sarcomas of the head and neck region: review of 30 cases. J Cranio-Maxillofac Surg. 2009;37:42–8.

69. Ferguson PC, Deshmukh N, Abudu A, et al. Change in histological grade in locally recurrent soft tissue sarcomas. Eur J Surg Oncol. 2004;40:2237–42.

70. Ferguson PC, Deheshi BM, Chung P, et al. Soft tissue sarcoma presenting with metastatic disease. Outcome with primary surgical resection. Cancer. 2011;117:372–9.

71. Ferrone ML, Raut CP. Modern surgical therapy: limb salvage and the role of amputation for extremity soft-tissue sarcomas. Surg Oncol Clin N Am. 2012;21:201–13.

72. Fletcher CDM. The evolving classification of soft tissue tumours: an update based on the new WHO classification. Histopathology. 2006;48:3–12.

73. Folkert MR, Singer S, Brennan MF, et al. Comparison of local recurrence with conventional and intensity-modulated radiation therapy for primary soft-tissue sarcomas of the extremity. J Clin Oncol. 2014;32:3236–41.

74. Fong Y, Coit DG, Woodruff JM, Brennan MF. Lymph node metastasis from soft tissue sarcoma in adults. Analysis of data from a prospective database of 1772 sarcoma patients. Ann Surg. 1993;217:72–7.

75. Frustaci S, Gherlinzoni F, De Paoli A, et al. Adjuvant chemotherapy for adult soft tissue sarcomas of the extremities and girdles: results of the Italian randomized cooperative trial. J Clin Oncol. 2001;19:1238–47.

76. Gerrand CH, Wunder JS, Kandel RA, et al. Classification of positive margins after resection of soft-tissue sarcoma of the limb predicts the risk of local recurrence. J Bone Joint Surg (Br). 2001;83-B:1149–55.

77. Gerrand CH, Bell RS, Wunder JS, et al. The influence of anatomic location on outcome in patients with soft tissue sarcoma of the extremity. Cancer. 2003;97:485–92.

78. Goodnight JE, Bargar W, Voegeli T, Blaisdell FW. Limb-sparing surgery for extremity sarcomas after preoperative intraarterial doxorubicin and radiation therapy. Am J Surg. 1985;150:109–13.

79. Goorin AM, Harris MB, Bernstein M, et al. Phase II/III trial of etoposide and high-dose ifosfamide in newly diagnosed metastatic osteosarcoma: a pediatric oncology group trial. J Clin Oncol. 2002;20:426–33.

80. Goorin AM, Schwartzentruber DJ, Devidas M, et al. Presurgical chemotherapy compared with immediate surgery and ajudvant chemotherapy for nonmetastatic osteosarcoma: Pediatric Oncology Group Study POG-8651. J Clin Oncol. 2003;21:1574–80.

81. Gortzak E, Azzarelli A, Buesa J, et al. A randomised phase II study on neo-adjuvant chemotherapy for "high-risk" adult soft-tissue sarcoma. Eur J Cancer. 2001;37:1096–103.

82. Grabellus F, Kraft C, Sheu SY, et al. Evaluation of 47 soft tissue sarcoma resection specimens after isolated limb perfusion with TNF-α and melphalan: histologically characterized improved margins correlate with absence of recurrences. Ann Surg Oncol. 2009;16:676–86.

83. Grabellus F, Kraft C, Sheu-Grabellus SYS, et al. Tumor vascularization and histopathologic regression of soft tissue sarcomas treated with isolated limb perfusion with TNF-α and melphalan. J Surg Oncol. 2011;103:371–9.

84. Grabellus F, Stylianou E, Umutlu L, et al. Size-based clinical response evaluation is insufficient to assess clinical response of sarcomas treated with isolated limb perfusion with TNF-a and melphalan. Ann Surg Oncol. 2012;19:3375–85.

85. Grabellus F, Podleska LE, Sheu SY, et al. Neoadjuvant treatment improves capsular integrity and the width of the fibrous capsule of high grade soft-tissue sarcomas. Eur J Surg Oncol. 2013;39:61–7.

86. Grier HE, Krailo MD, Tarbell NJ, et al. Addition of ifosfamide and etoposide to standard chemotherapy for Ewing's sarcoma and primitive neuroectodermal tumor of bone. N Engl J Med. 2003;348:694–701.

87. Grobmyer SR, Maki RG, Demetri GD, et al. Neo-adjuvant chemotherapy for primary high-grade extremity soft tissue sarcoma. Ann Oncol. 2004;15:1667–72.

88. Gronchi A, La Vulla S, Fiore M, et al. Aggressive surgical policies in a retrospectively reviewed single-institution case series of retroperitoneal soft tissue sarcoma patients. J Clin Oncol. 2009;27:24–40.

89. Gronchi A, Casali PG, Mariani L, et al. Status of surgical margins and prognosis in adult soft tissue sarcomas of the extremities: a series of patients treated at a single institution. J Clin Oncol. 2005;23:96–104.

90. Gronchi A, De Paoli A, Dani C, et al. Preoperative chemo-radiation therapy for localised retroperitoneal sarcoma: a phase I–II study from the Italian Sarcoma Group. Eur J Cancer. 2014;50:784–92.

91. Grünhagen DJ, Brunstein F, Graveland WJ, et al. Isolated limb perfusion with tumor necrosis factor and melphalan prevents amputation in patients with multiple sarcomas in arm or leg. Ann Surg Oncol. 2005;12:1–7.

92. Grünhagen DJ, de Wilt JHW, Graveland WJ, et al. The palliative value of tumor necrosis factor α-based isolated limb perfusion in patients with metastatic sarcoma and melanoma. Cancer. 2006;106:156–62.

93. Grünhagen DJ, de Wilt JH, Graveland WJ, et al. Outcome and prognostic factor analysis of 217 consecutive isolated limb perfusion with tumor necrosis factor-alpha and melphalan for limb-threatening soft tissue sarcoma. Cancer. 2006;106:1776–84.

94. Guillou L, Coindre JM, Bonichon F, et al. Comparative study of the National Cancer Institute and French federation of Cancer Centers Sarcoma Group Grading systems in a population of 410 adult patients with soft tissue sarcoma. J Clin Oncol. 1997;15:350–62.

95. Gutman M, Inbar M, Lev-Shlush D, et al. High dose tumor necrosis factor-α and melphalan administered via isolated limb perfusion for advanced limb soft tissue sarcoma results in a >90% response rate and limb preservation. Cancer. 1997;79:1129–37.

96. Ham SJ, van der Graaf WTA, Pras E, et al. Soft tissue sarcoma of the extremities. A multimodality diagnostic and therapeutic approach. Cancer Treat Rev. 1998;24:373–91.

97. Hayes AJ, Neuhaus SJ, Clark MA, Thomas JM. Isolated limb perfusion with melphalan and tumor necrosis factor α for advanced melanoma and soft-tissue sarcoma. Ann Surg Oncol. 2007;14:230–8.

98. Hegazy MAF, Kotb SZ, Sakr H, et al. Preoperative isolated limb infusion of doxorubicin and external irradiation for limb-threatening soft tissue sarcomas. Ann Surg Oncol. 2007;14: 568–76.

99. Hoekstra HJ, Schraffordt Koops H, de Vries LGE, et al. Toxicity of hyperthermic isolated limb perfusion with cisplatin for recurrent melanoma of the lower extremity after previous perfusion treatment. Cancer. 1993;72:1224–9.

100. Hoekstra HJ. Extremity perfusion for sarcoma. Surg Oncol Clin N Am. 2008;17:805–24.

101. Hohenberger P, Finke LH, Schlag PM. Intracompartmental pressure during hyperthermic isolated limb perfusion for melanoma and sarcoma. Eur J Surg Oncol. 1996;22:147–51.

102. Hohenberger P, Tunn PU. Isolated limb perfusion with rhTNF-α and melphalan for locally recurrent childhood synovial sarcoma of the limb. J Pediatr Hematol Oncol. 2003;25:905–9.

103. Hohenberger P, Wysocki WM. Neoadjuvant treatment of locally advanced soft tissue sarcoma of the limbs: which treatment to choose? Oncologist. 2008;13:175–86.

104. Hoven-Gondrie ML, Thijssens KM, Van den Dungen JJAM. Long-term locoregional vascular morbidity after isolated limb perfusion and external-beam radiotherapy for soft tissue sarcoma of the extremity. Ann Surg Oncol. 2007;14:2105–12.

105. Hoven-Gondrie ML, Thijssens KMJ, Geertzen JHB, et al. Isolated limb perfusion and external beam radiotherapy for soft tissue sarcomas of the extremity: long-term effects on normal tissue according to the LENT-SOMA scoring system. Ann Surg Oncol. 2008;15:1502–10.

106. Hoven-Gondrie ML, Bastiaannet E, Van Ginkel RJ, et al. TNF dose reduction and shortening of duration of isolated limb perfusion for locally advanced soft tissue sarcoma of the extremities is safe and effective in terms of long-term patient outcome. J Surg Oncol. 2011;103:648–55.

107. Hoving S, Seynhaeve ALB, van Tiel ST, et al. Early destruction of tumor vasculature in tumor necrosis factor-α-based isolated limb perfusion is responsible for tumor response. Anticancer Drugs. 2006;17:949–59.

108. Howlader N, Noone AM, Krapcho M, et al., editors. SEER cancer statistics review, 1975–2012. Bethesda: National Cancer Institute; 2015. http://seer.cancer.gov/csr/1975_2012/.

109. Hueman MT, Herman JM, Ahuja N. Management of retroperitoneal sarcomas. Surg Clin N Am. 2008;88:583–97.

110. Issakov J, Merimsky O, Gutman M, et al. Hyperthermic isolated limb perfusion with tumor necrosis factor-α and melphalan in advanced soft-tissue sarcomas: histopathological considerations. Ann Surg Oncol. 2000;7:155–9.

111. Issels RD, Prenninger SW, Nagele A, et al. Ifosfamide plus etoposide combined with regional hyperthermia in patients with locally advanced sarcomas: a phase II study. J Clin Oncol. 1990;8:1818–29.

112. Issels RD, Abdel-Rahman S, Wendtner C. Neoadjuvant chemotherapy combined with regional hyperthermia (RHT) for locally advanced primary or recurrent high-risk adult soft-tissue sarcomas (STS) of adults: long-term results of a phase II study. Eur J Cancer. 2001;37:1599–608.

113. Issels RD, Lindner LH, Verweij J, et al. Neo-adjuvant chemotherapy alone or with regional hyperthermia for localised high-risk soft-tissue sarcoma: a randomised phase 3 multicentre study. Lancet Oncol. 2010;11:561–70.

114. Italiano A, Delva F, Mathoulin-Pelissier S, et al. Effect of adjuvant chemotherapy on survival in FNCLCC grade 3 soft tissue sarcomas: a multivariate analysis of the French Sarcoma Group Database. Ann Oncol. 2010;21:2436–41.

115. Jaffe N. Historical perspective on the introduction and use of chemotherapy for the treatment of osteosarcoma. Adv Exp Med Biol. 2014;804:1–30.

116. Jakob J, Tunn PU, Hayes AJ, et al. Oncological outcome of primary non-metastatic soft tissue sarcoma treated by neoadjuvant isolated limb perfusion and tumor resection. J Surg Oncol. 2014;109:786–90.

117. Jansen-Landheer MLEA, Krijnen P, Oostindiër MJ, et al. Improved diagnosis and treatment of soft tissue sarcoma patients after implementation of national guidelines: a population-based study. Eur J Surg Oncol. 2009;35:1326–32.

118. Jo VY, Fletcher CD. WHO classification of soft tissue tumours: an update based on the 2013 (4th) edition. Pathology. 2014;46:95–104.
119. Kam PCA, Thompson JF. Pharmacokinetics of regional therapy: isolated limb infusion and other low flow techniques for extremity melanoma. Surg Oncol Clin N Am. 2008;17:795–804.
120. Kane 3rd JM, Finley JW, Driscoll D, et al. The treatment and outcome of patients with soft tissue sarcomas and synchronous metastases. Sarcoma. 2002. doi:10.1080/13577140210000 22168.
121. Kantor G, Mahé MA, Giraud P, et al. French national evaluation of helicoidal tomotherapy: description of indications, dose constraints and set-up margins. Cancer Radiother. 2007;11:331–7.
122. Kapma MR, Vrouenraets BC, Nieweg OE, et al. Major amputation for intractable extremity melanoma after failure of isolated limb perfusion. Eur J Surg Oncol. 2005;31:95–9.
123. Khansa I, Janis JE. Modern reconstructive techniques for abdominal wall defects after oncologic resection. J Surg Oncol. 2015;111:587–98.
124. Kim BK, Chen YLE, Kirsch DG, et al. An effective preoperative three-dimensional radiotherapy target volume for extremity soft tissue sarcoma and the effect of margin width on local control. Int J Radiat Oncol Biol Phys. 2010;77:843–50.
125. Kim S, Ott HC, Wright CD, et al. Pulmonary resection of metastatic sarcoma: prognostic factors associated with improved outcomes. Ann Thorac Surg. 2011;92:1780–6.
126. King JJ, Fayssoux RS, Lackman RD, Ogilvie CM. Early outcomes of soft tissue sarcomas presenting with metastases and treated with chemotherapy. Am J Clin Oncol. 2009;32:308–13.
127. Klaase JM, Kroon BBR, Benckhuijsen C, et al. Results of regional isolation perfusion with cytostatics in patients with soft tissue tumors of the extremities. Cancer. 1989;64:616–21.
128. Klaase JM, Kroon BBR, van Geel AN, et al. Systemic leakage during isolated limb perfusion for melanoma. Br J Surg. 1993;80:1124–6.
129. Komdeur R, Hoekstra HJ, van den Berg E, et al. Metastasis in soft tissue sarcomas: prognostic criteria and treatment perspectives. Cancer Metastasis Rev. 2002;21:167–83.
130. Koontz BF, Miles EF, Rubio MA, et al. Preoperative radiotherapy and bevacizumab for angiosarcoma of the head and neck: two case studies. Head Neck. 2008;30:262–6.
131. Kraybill WG, Harris J, Spiro IJ, et al. Phase II study of neoadjuvant chemotherapy and radiation therapy in the management of high-risk, high-grade, soft tissue sarcomas of the extremities and body wall: Radiation Therapy Oncology Group Trial 9514. J Clin Oncol. 2006;24:619–25.
132. Kraybill WG, Harris J, Spiro IJ, et al. Long-term results of a phase 2 study of neoadjuvant chemotherapy and radiotherapy in the management of high-risk, high-grade, soft tissue sarcomas of the extremities and body wall: Radiation Therapy Oncology Group Trial 9514. Cancer. 2010;116:4613–21.
133. Krementz ET, Carter RD, Sutherland CM, Hutton I. Chemotherapy of sarcomas of the limbs by regional perfusion. Ann Surg. 1977;185:556–63.
134. Kroon HM, Huismans A, Waugh RC, et al. Isolated limb infusion: technical aspects. J Surg Oncol. 2014;109:352–6.
135. Lans TE, de Wilt JHW, van Geel AN, Eggermont AMM. Isolated limb perfusion with tumor necrosis factor and melphalan for nonresectable Stewart-Treves lymphangiosarcoma. Ann Surg Oncol. 2002;9:1004–9.
136. Lans TE, Grünhagen DJ, de Wilt JHW, et al. Isolated limb perfusion with tumor necrosis factor and melphalan for locally recurrent soft tissue sarcoma in previously irradiated limbs. Ann Surg Oncol. 2005;12:1–6.
137. Lanza LA, Putnam JB, Benjamin RS, Roth JA. Response to chemotherapy does not predict survival after resection of sarcomatous pulmonary metastases. Ann Thorac Surg. 1991;51:219–24.
138. Le Cesne A, Judson I, Crowther D, et al. Randomized phase III study comparing conventional dose doxorubicin plus ifosfamide versus high dose doxorubicin plus ifosfamide plus rhGMCSF in advanced soft tissue sarcomas: an EORTC Soft Tissue and Bone Sarcoma Group trial. J Clin Oncol. 2001;18:2676–84.

139. Le Cesne A, Ouali M, Leahy MG, et al. Doxorubicin-based adjuvant chemotherapy in soft tissue sarcoma: pooled analysis of two STBSG-EORTC phase III clinical trials. Ann Oncol. 2014;25:2425–32.
140. Lejeune FJ, Pujol N, Liénard D, et al. Limb salvage by neoadjuvant isolated perfusion with TNFα and melphalan for non-resectable soft tissue sarcoma of the extremities. Eur J Surg Oncol. 2000;26:669–78.
141. Lejeune FJ, Kroon BBR, Di Filippo F, et al. Isolated limb perfusion. The European experience. Surg Oncol Clin N Am. 2001;10:821–32.
142. Lejeune FJ, Lienard D, Matter M, Rüegg C. Efficiency of recombinant human TNF in human cancer therapy. Cancer Immun. 2006;6:1–17.
143. Le Péchoux C, Pautier P, Delannes M, et al. Clinical practice guideline: 2006 update of recommendations for the radiotherapeutic management of patients with soft tissue sarcoma (sarcoma of the extremity, uterin sarcoma and retroperitoneal sarcoma). Cancer Radiothér. 2006;10:185–207.
144. Le Péchoux C, Musat E, Baey C, et al. Should adjuvant radiotherapy be administered in addition to front-line aggressive surgery (FAS) in patients with primary retroperitoneal sarcoma? Ann Oncol. 2013;24:832–7.
145. Lev-Chelouche D, Abu-Abeid S, Kollander Y, et al. Multifocal soft tissue sarcoma: limb salvage following hyperthermic isolated limb perfusion with high-dose tumor necrosis factor and melphalan. J Surg Oncol. 1999;70:185–9.
146. Levine EA, Trippon M, Das Gupta TK. Preoperative multimodality treatment for soft tissue sarcomas. Cancer. 1993;71:3685–9.
147. Lewis SJ, Wunder JS, Couture J, et al. Soft tissue sarcomas involving the pelvis. J Surg Oncol. 2001;77:8–14.
148. Lienard D, Ewalenko P, Delmotte JJ, et al. High-dose recombinant tumor necrosis factor alpha in combination with interferon gamma and melphalan in isolation perfusion of the limbs for melanoma and sarcoma. J Clin Oncol. 1992;10:52–60.
149. Lucas DR, Kshirsagar MP, Biermann JS, et al. Histologic alterations from neoadjuvant chemotherapy in high-grade extremity soft tissue sarcoma: clinicopathological correlation. Oncologist. 2008;13:451–8.
150. MacDermed DM, Miller LL, Peabody TD et al. Primary tumor necrosis predicts distant control in locally advanced soft-tissue sarcomas after preoperative concurrent chemoradiotherapy. Int J Radiat Oncol Biol Phys, 1–7. 2009. doi:10.1016/j.ijrobp.2009.03.015.
151. Mahabir RC, Butler CE. Stabilization of the chest wall: autologous and alloplastic reconstructions. Semin Plast Surg. 2011;25:34–42.
152. Malempati S, Hawkins DS. Rhabdomyosarcoma: review of the Children's Oncology Group (COG) soft-tissue sarcoma committee experience and rationale for current COG studies. Pediatr Blood Cancer. 2012;59:5–10.
153. Maree D, Hocke C, Bui NB, et al. Conservative loco-regional treatment of soft tissue sarcoma in adults after induction chemotherapy. Presse Med. 1985;14:1069–72.
154. Marudanayagam R, Sandhu B, Perera MTPR, et al. Liver resection for metastatic soft tissue sarcoma: an analysis of prognostic factors. Eur J Surg Oncol. 2011;37:87–92.
155. Mastrangelo G, Coindre JM, Ducimetiere F, et al. Incidence of soft tissue sarcoma and beyond. A population-based prospective study in 3 European regions. Cancer. 2012;118:5339–48.
156. Mattei TA, Teles AR, Mendel AE. Modern surgical techniques for management of soft tissue sarcomas involving the spine: outcomes and complications. J Surg Oncol. 2015;111:580–6.
157. Mazeron JJ, Suit HD. Lymph nodes as sites of metastases from sarcomas of soft tissue. Cancer. 1987;60:1800–8.
158. Mendenhall WM, Mendenhall CM, Werning JW, et al. Adult head and neck soft tissue sarcomas. Head Neck. 2005;27:916–22.
159. Meric F, Milas M, Hunt KK, et al. Impact of neoadjuvant chemotherapy on postoperative morbidity in soft tissue sarcomas. J Clin Oncol. 2000;18:3378–83.
160. Miller ED, Xu-Welliver M, Haglund KE. The role of modern radiation therapy in the management of extremity sarcomas. J Surg Oncol. 2015;111:599–603.

161. Möller MG, Lewis JM, Dessureault S, Zager JS. Toxicities associated with hyperthermic isolated limb perfusion and isolated limb infusion in the treatment of melanoma and sarcoma. Int J Hyperth. 2008;24:275–89.

162. Moncrieff MD, Kroon HM, Kam PC, et al. Isolated limb infusion for advanced soft tissue sarcoma of the extremity. Ann Surg Oncol. 2008;15:2749–56.

163. Moyer HR, Delman KA. The role of hyperthermia in optimizing tumor response to regional therapy. Int J Hyperth. 2008;24:251–61.

164. Musser JE, Assel M, Mashni JW, Sjoberg DD, Russo P. Adult prostate sarcoma: the memorial sloan kettering experience. Urology. 2014;84:624–8.

165. Nachmany I, Subhi A, Meller I, et al. Efficacy of high vs low dose TNF-isolated limb perfusion for locally advanced soft tissue sarcoma. Eur J Surg Oncol. 2009;35:209–14.

166. Nakamura T, Abudu A, Murata H, et al. Oncological outcome of patients with deeply located soft tissue sarcoma of the pelvis: a follow up study at minimum 5 years after diagnosis. Eur J Surg Oncol. 2013;39:1030–5.

167. Nakamura T, Matsumine A, Yamakado K, et al. Lung radiofrequency ablation in patients with pulmonary metastases from musculoskeletal sarcomas. Cancer. 2009;115:3774–81.

168. Navaria P, Ascolese AM, Cozzi L, et al. Stereotaxic body radiation therapy for lung metastases from soft tissue sarcoma. Eur J Cancer. 2015;51:668–74.

169. Nesbit ME, Gehan EA, Burgert EO, et al. Multimodal therapy for the management of primary, nonmetastatic Ewing's sarcoma of bone: a long-term follow-up of the First Intergroup study. J Clin Oncol. 1990;8:1664–74.

170. Neuhaus SJ, Pinnock N, Giblin V, et al. Treatment and outcome of radiation-induced soft-tissue sarcomas at a specialist institution. Eur J Surg Oncol. 2009;35:654–9.

171. Nielsen OS, Judson I, van Hoesel Q, et al. Effect of high-dose ifosfamide in advanced soft tissue sarcomas. A multicentre phase II study of the EORTC Soft Tissue and Bone Sarcoma Group. Eur J Cancer. 2000;36:61–7.

172. Noorda EM, Vrouenraets BC, Nieweg OE, et al. Safety and efficacy of isolated limb perfusion in elderly melanoma patients. Ann Surg Oncol. 2002;9:968–74.

173. Noorda EM, Vrouenraets BC, Nieweg OE, et al. Isolated limb perfusion with tumor necrosis factor-α and melphalan for patients with unresectable soft tissue sarcoma of the extremities. Cancer. 2003;98:1483–90.

174. Noorda EM, Vrouenraets BC, Nieweg O, et al. Isolated limb perfusion: what is the evidence for its use? Ann Surg Oncol. 2004;12:837–45.

175. Novetsky AP, Powell MA. Management of sarcomas of the uterus. Curr Opin Oncol. 2013;25:546–52.

176. Ognjanovic S, Linabery AM, Charbonneau B, Ross JA. Trends in childhood rhabdomyosarcoma incidence and survival in the United States, 1975–2005. Cancer. 2009;115:4218–26.

177. Olieman AFT, van Ginkel RJ, Hoekstra HJ, et al. Angiographic response of locally advanced soft-tissue sarcoma following hyperthermic isolated limb perfusion with tumor necrosis factor. Ann Surg Oncol. 1997;4:64–9.

178. Olieman AFT, van Ginkel RJ, Molenaar WM, et al. Hyperthermic isolated limb perfusion with tumour necrosis factor α and melphalan as palliative limb-saving treatment in patients with locally advanced soft-tissue sarcomas of the extremities with regional or distant metastases. Is it worthwhile? Arch Orthop Trauma Surg. 1998;118:70–4.

179. Olofsson R, Bergh P, Berlin Ö, et al. Long-term outcome of isolated limb perfusion in advanced soft tissue sarcoma of the extremity. Ann Surg Oncol. 2012;19:1800–7.

180. O'Sullivan B, Wylie J, Catton C, et al. The local management of soft tissue sarcoma. Semin Radiat Oncol. 1999;9:328–48.

181. O'Sullivan B, Davis AM, Turcotte R, et al. Preoperative versus postoperative radiotherapy in soft tissue sarcoma of the limbs: a randomized trial. Lancet. 2002;359:2235–41.

182. Padussis JC, Steerman SN, Tyler DS, Mosca PJ. Pharmakokinetics & drug resistance of melphalan in regional chemotherapy: ILP versus ILI. Int J Hyperth. 2008;24:239–49.

183. Pappo AS, Pratt CB. Soft tissue sarcomas in children. Cancer Treat Res. 1997;9:205–22.
184. Park MS, Araujo DM. New insights into the hemangiopericytoma/solitary fibrous tumor spectrum of tumors. Curr Opin Oncol. 2009;21:327–31.
185. Patel SR, Vadhan-Raj S, Burgess MA, et al. Preoperative chemotherapy with dose-intensive adriamycin and ifosfamide for high risk primary soft-tissue sarcomas of extremity origin. Proc Conn Tissue Oncol Soc. 1995;5:16.
186. Pawlik TM, Pisters PWT, Mikula L, et al. Long-term results of two prospective trials of preoperative external beam radiotherapy for localized intermediate- or high-grade retroperitoneal soft tissue sarcoma. Ann Surg Oncol. 2006;13:508–17.
187. Pencavel T, Allan CP, Thomas JM, Hayes AJ. Treatment for breast sarcoma: a large, single-centre series. Eur J Surg Oncol. 2011;37:703–8.
188. Penel N, Mallet Y, Robin YM, et al. Prognostic factors for adult sarcomas of head and neck. Int J Oral Maxillofac Surg. 2008;37:428–32.
189. Peng KA, Grogan T, Wang MB. Head and neck sarcomas: analysis of the SEER database. Otolaryngol Head Neck Surg. 2014;151:627–33.
190. Pennacchioli E, Deraco M, Mariani L, et al. Advanced extremity soft tissue sarcoma: prognostic effect of isolated limb perfusion in a series of 88 patients treated at a single institution. Ann Surg Oncol. 2007;14:553–9.
191. Pezzi CM, Pollock RE, Evans HL, et al. Preoperative chemotherapy for soft-tissue sarcomas of the extremities. Ann Surg. 1990;211:476–81.
192. Pfannschmidt J, Hoffmann H, Schneider T, et al. Pulmonary metastasectomy for soft tissue sarcomas: is it justified? Recent Results Cancer Res. 2009;179:321–36.
193. Pierie JPEN, Betensky RA, Choudry U, et al. Outcomes in a series of 103 retroperitoneal sarcomas. Eur J Surg Oncol. 2006;32:1235–41.
194. Pisters PW, Leung DH, Woodruff J, et al. Analysis of prognostic factors in 1,041 patients with localized soft tissue sarcomas of the extremities. J Clin Oncol. 1996;14:1679–89.
195. Pisters PW, Harrison LB, Leung DH, et al. Long-term results of a prospective randomized trial of adjuvant brachytherapy in soft-tissue sarcoma. J Clin Oncol. 1996;14:859–68.
196. Pisters PW, Ballo MT, Patel SR. Preoperative chemoradiation treatment strategies for localized sarcoma. Ann Surg Oncol. 2002;9:535–42.
197. Pisters PW, Ballo MT, Fenstermacher MJ, et al. Phase I trial of preoperative concurrent doxorubicin and radiation therapy, surgical resection, and intraoperative electron-beam radiation therapy for patients with localized retroperitoneal sarcoma. J Clin Oncol. 2003;21:3092–7.
198. Pisters PWT, O'Sullivan B, Maki RG. Evidence-based recommendations for local therapy for soft tissue sarcomas. J Clin Oncol. 2007;25:1003–8.
199. Plaat BEC, Molenaar WM, Mastik MF, et al. Hyperthermic isolated limb perfusion with Tumor Necrosis Factor-α and melphalan in patients with locally advanced soft tissue sarcomas: treatment response and clinical outcome related to changes in proliferation and apoptosis. Clin Cancer Res. 1999;5:1650–7.
200. Pollack A, Zagars GK, Goswitz MS, et al. Preoperative vs. Postoperative radiotherapy in the treatment of soft tissue sarcomas: a matter of presentation. Int J Radiat Oncol Biol Phys. 1998;42:563–72.
201. Porter GA, Cantor SB, Walsh GL, et al. Cost-effectiveness of pulmonary resection and systemic chemotherapy in the management of metastatic soft tissue sarcoma: a combined analysis from the University of Texas M.D. Anderson and Memorial Sloan-Kettering Cancer Centers. J Thorac Cardiovasc Surg. 2004;127:1366–72.
202. Rehders A, Peiper M, Stoecklein NH, et al. Hepatic metastasectomy for soft-tissue sarcomas: is it justified? World J Surg. 2009;33:111–7.
203. Riad S, Griffin AM, Libermann B, et al. Lymph node metastasis in soft tissue sarcoma in an extremity. Clin Orthop. 2004;426:129–34.
204. Rosenberg SA, Tepper J, Glatstein E, et al. The treatment of soft-tissue sarcomas of the extremities. Prospective randomized evaluations of (1) limb-sparing surgery plus radiation

therapy compared with amputation and (2) the role of adjuvant chemotherapy. Ann Surg. 1982;196:305–14.

205. Rossi CR, Foletto M, Alessio S, et al. Limb-sparing treatment for soft tissue sarcomas: influence of prognostic factors. J Surg Oncol. 1996;63:3–8.

206. Rossi CR, Foletto M, Di Filippo F, et al. Soft tissue limb sarcomas. Italian clinical trials with hyperthermic antiblastic perfusion. Cancer. 1999;86:1742–9.

207. Rossi CR, Mocellin S, Pilati P, et al. Hyperthermic isolated perfusion with low-dose tumor necrosis factor α and doxorubicin for the treatment of limb-threatening soft tissue sarcomas. Ann Surg Oncol. 2005;12:398–405.

208. Rouesse JG, Friedman S, Sevin DM, et al. Preoperative induction chemotherapy in the treatment of locally advanced soft tissue sarcomas. Cancer. 1987;60:296–300.

209. Salas S, Bui B, Stoeckle E, et al. Soft tissue sarcomas of the trunk wall (STS-TW): a study of 343 patients from the French Sarcoma Group (FSG) database. Ann Oncol. 2009;20:1127–35.

210. Sampath S, Schultheiss TE, Ryu JK, Wong JYC. The role of adjuvant radiation in uterine sarcomas. Int J Radiat Oncol Biol Phys. 2010;76:728–34.

211. Sampo M, Tarkkanen M, Huuhtanen R, et al. Impact of the smallest surgical margin on local control in soft tissue sarcoma. Br J Surg. 2008;95:237–43.

212. Santinami M, Deraco M, Azzarelli A, et al. Treatment of recurrent sarcoma of the extremities by isolated limb perfusion using tumor necrosis factor alpha and melphalan. Tumori. 1996;82:579–84.

213. Sarcoma Meta-analysis Collaboration. Adjuvant chemotherapy for localised resectable soft-tissue sarcoma of adults: meta-analysis of individual data. Lancet. 1997;350:1647–54.

214. Schlemmer M, Wendtner CM, Lindner L, et al. Thermochemotherapy in patients with extremity high-risk soft tissue sarcomas (HR-STS). Int J Hyperth. 2010;26:127–35.

215. Schwindenhammer B, Podleska LE, Kutritz A, et al. The pathologic response of resected synovial sarcomas to hyperthermic isolated limb perfusion with melphalan and TNF-α: a comparison with the whole group of resected soft tissue sarcomas. World J Surg Oncol. 2013;11:185–91.

216. Seinen JM, Hoekstra HJ. Isolated limb perfusion of soft tissue sarcomas: a comprehensive review of literature. Cancer Treat Rev. 2013;39:569–77.

217. Sherman KL, Kinnier CV, Farina DA, et al. Examination of national lymph node evaluation practices for adult extremity soft tissue sarcoma. J Surg Oncol. 2014;110:682–8.

218. Siegel R, Miller KD, Jemal A. Cancer statistics, 2015. CA Cancer J Clin. 2015;65:5–29.

219. Simon MA, Nachman J. The clinical utility of preoperative therapy for sarcomas. J Bone Joint Surg Am. 1986;68:1458–63.

220. Smith R, Demmy TL. Pulmonary metastasectomy for soft tissue sarcoma. Surg Oncol Clin N Am. 2012;21:269–86.

221. Sindelar WF, Kinsella TJ, Chen PW. Intraoperative radiotherapy in retroperitoneal sarcomes. Arch Surg. 1993;128:402–10.

222. Soulen MC, Weissmann JR, Sullivan KL, et al. Intraarterial chemotherapy with limb-sparing resection of large soft-tissue sarcomas of the extremities. J Vasc Interv Radiol. 1992;3:659–63.

223. Soyfer V, Corn BW, Shtraus N, et al. Single-institution experience of SBRT for lung metastases in sarcoma patients. Am J Clin Oncol. 2014. http://dx.doi.org/10.1097/COC.0000000000000103

224. Spiro IJ, Suit H, Gebhardt M, et al. Neoadjuvant chemotherapy and radiotherapy for large soft tissue sarcomas. Proc Am Soc Clin Oncol. 1996;15:5243.

225. Spunt SL, Skapek SX, Coffin CM. Pediatric nonrhabdomyosarcoma soft tissue sarcomas. Oncologist. 2008;13:668–78.

226. Stoeckle E, Coindre JM, Bonvalot S, et al. Prognostic factors in retroperitoneal sarcoma. A multivariate analysis of a series of 165 patients of the French Cancer Center Federation Sarcoma Group. Cancer. 2001;92:359–68.

227. Stojadinovic A, Jaques DP, Leung DHY, et al. Amputation for recurrent soft tissue sarcoma of the extremity: indications and outcome. Ann Surg Oncol. 2001;8:509–18.
228. Stojadinovic A, Leung DHY, Hoos A, et al. Analysis of the prognostic significance of microscopic margins in 2,084 localized primary adult soft tissue sarcomas. Ann Surg. 2002;235:424–34.
229. Stolnicu S, Moldovan C, Podoleanu C, Georgescu R. Mesenchymal tumors and tumor-like lesions of the breast: a contemporary approach review. Ann Pathol. 2015;35:15–31.
230. Strauss DC, Hayes AJ, Thway K, et al. Surgical management of primary retroperitoneal sarcoma. Br J Surg. 2010;97:698–706.
231. Stucky CCH, Wasif N, Ashman JB, et al. Excellent local control with preoperative radiation therapy, surgical resection, and intra-operative electron radiation therapy for retroperitoneal sarcoma. J Surg Oncol. 2014;109:798–803.
232. Swallow CJ, Catton CN. Improving outcomes for retroperitoneal sarcomas: a work in progress. Surg Oncol Clin N Am. 2012;21:317–31.
233. Tavora F, Kryvenko ON, Epstein JI. Mesenchymal tumours of the bladder and prostate: an update. Pathology. 2013;45:104–15.
234. Thariat J, Schouman T, Brouchet A, et al. Osteosarcomas of the mandible: multidisciplinary management of a rare tumor of the young adult a cooperative study of the GSF-GETO, Rare Cancer Network, GETTEC/REFCOR and SFCE. Ann Oncol. 2013;24:824–31.
235. Thiagarajan A, Iyer NG. Radiation-induced sarcomas of the head and neck. World J Clin Oncol. 2014;5:973–81.
236. Thijssens KMJ, van Ginkel RJ, Pras E, et al. Isolated limb perfusion with tumor necrosis factor α and melphalan for locally advanced soft tissue sarcoma: the value of adjuvant radiotherapy. Ann Surg Oncol. 2006;13:518–24.
237. Thornton K. Chemotherapeutic management of soft tissue sarcoma. Surg Clin N Am. 2008;88:647–60.
238. Thornton K, Pesce CE, Choti MA. Multidisciplinary management of metastatic sarcoma. Surg Clin N Am. 2008;88:661–72.
239. Thompson JF, Kam PCA, Waugh RC, Harman CR. Isolated limb infusion with cytotoxic agents: a simple alternative to isolated limb perfusion. Semin Surg Oncol. 1998;14:238–47.
240. Toesca A, Spitaleri G, De Pas T, et al. Sarcoma of the breast: outcome and reconstructive options. Clin Breast Cancer. 2012;12:438–44.
241. Toma S, Canavese G, Grimaldi A, et al. Concomitant chemo-radiotherapy in the treatment of locally advanced and/or metastatic soft tissue sarcomas: experience of the national cancer Institute of Genoa. Oncol Rep. 2003;10:641–7.
242. Toulmonde MP, et al. Retroperitoneal sarcomas: patterns of care at diagnosis, prognostic factors and focus on main histological subtypes: a multicenter analysis of the French Sarcoma Group. Ann Oncol. 2014;25:735–42.
243. Tsikouras P, Dafopoulos A, Ammari A, et al. Should lymphadenectomy be performed in early stage I and II sarcomas of the corpus uteri. J Obstet Gynaecol Res. 2011;37:1588–95.
244. Tsukushi S, Nishida Y, Sugiura H, et al. Soft tissue sarcomas of the chest wall. J Thorac Oncol. 2009;4:834–7.
245. Turaga KK, Beasley GM, Kane III JM, et al. Limb preservation with isolated limb infusion for locally advanced nonmelanoma cutaneous and soft-tissue malignant neoplasms. Arch Surg. 2011;146:870–5.
246. Turcotte RE, Ferrone M, Isler MH, Wong C. Outcomes in patients with popliteal sarcomas. Can J Surg. 2009;52:51–5.
247. Tuttle R, Kane III JM. Biopsy techniques for soft tissue and bowel sarcomas. J Surg Oncol. 2015;111:504–12.
248. Van Dalen T, Van Geel AN, Van Coevorden F, et al. Soft tissue sarcoma in the retroperitoneum: an often neglected diagnosis. Eur J Surg Oncol. 2001;27:74–9.
249. Van Ginkel RJ, Thijssens KMJ, Pras E, et al. Isolated limb perfusion with tumor necrosis factor alpha and melphalan for locally advanced soft tissue sarcoma: three time periods at risk for amputation. Ann Surg Oncol. 2007;14:1499–506.

250. Van Glabbeke M, van Oosterom AT, Oosterhuis JW, et al. Prognostic factors for the outcome of chemotherapy in advanced soft tissue sarcoma: an analysis of 2,185 patients treated with anthracycline-containing first-line regimens- a European Organization for Research and Treatment of Cancer Soft Tissue and Bone Sarcoma Group Study. J Clin Oncol. 1999;17:150–7.
251. Van Schil PE, Hendriks JM, van Putte BP, et al. Isolated lung perfusion and related techniques for the treatment of pulmonary metastases. Eur J Cardiothorac Surg. 2008;33:486–95.
252. Veth R, van Hoesel R, Pruszczynski M, et al. Limb salvage in musculoskeletal oncology. Lancet Oncol. 2003;4:343–50.
253. Vohra NA, Turaga KK, Gonzalez RJ, et al. The use of isolated limb infusion in limb threatening extremity sarcomas. Int J Hyperth. 2013;29:1–7.
254. Voutsadakis IA, Zaman K, Leyvraz S. Breast sarcomas: current and future perspectives. Breast. 2011;20:199–204.
255. Vrouenraets BC, Kroon BBR, Klaase JM, et al. Value of laboratory tests in monitoring acute regional toxicity after isolated limb perfusion. Ann Surg Oncol. 1997;4:88–94.
256. Wanebo HJ, Temple WJ, Popp MB, et al. Preoperative regional therapy for extremity sarcoma. A tricenter update. Cancer. 1995;75:2299–306.
257. Weihkopf T, Blettner M, Dantonello T, et al. Incidence and time trends of soft tissue sarcomas in German children 1985–2004 – a report from the population-based German Childhood Cancer Registry. Eur J Cancer. 2008;44:432–40.
258. Weitmann HD, Knocke TH, Kucera H, Pötter R. Radiation therapy in the treatment of endometrial stromal sarcoma. Int J Radiat Oncol Biol Phys. 2001;49:739–48.
259. Wendtner CM, Abdel-Rahman S, Krych M, et al. Response to neoadjuvant chemotherapy combined with regional hyperthermia predicts long-term survival for adult patients with retroperitoneal and visceral high-risk soft tissue sarcomas. J Clin Oncol. 2002;20:3156–64.
260. Weitz J, Klimstra DS, Cymes K, et al. Management of primary liver sarcomas. Cancer. 2007;109:1391–6.
261. Whelan JS, Bielack S, Marina N, et al. EURAMOS-1, an international randomised study for osteosarcoma: results from pre-randomisation treatment. Ann Oncol. 2015;26:407–14.
262. Wieberdink J, Benckhuysen C, Braat RP, et al. Dosimetry in isolation perfusion of the limbs by assessment of perfused tissue volume and grading of toxic tissue reactions. Eur J Cancer Clin Oncol. 1982;18:905–10.
263. Wilder F, D'Angelo S, Crago AM. Soft tissue tumors of the trunk: management of local disease in the breast and chest and abdominal walls. J Surg Oncol. 2015;111:546–52.
264. Williard WC, Hajdu SI, Casper ES, Brennan MF. Comparison of amputation with limb-sparing operations for adult soft tissue sarcoma of the extremity. Ann Surg. 1992;215:269–75.
265. Womer RB, West DC, Krailo MD, et al. Randomized controlled trial of interval-compressed chemotherapy for the treatment of localized Ewing sarcoma: a report from the Children's Oncology Group. J Clin Oncol. 2012;30:4148–54.
266. Yang JC, Chang AE, Baker AR, et al. A randomized prospective study of the benefit of adjuvant radiation therapy in the treatment of soft tissue sarcomas of the extremity. J Clin Oncol. 1998;16:197–203.
267. Yu RS, Chen Y, Jiang B, et al. Primary hepatic sarcomas: CT findings. Eur J Radiol. 2008;18:2196–205.

Isolated Limb Perfusion for Locally Advanced Soft Tissue Sarcoma

28

Harald J. Hoekstra and Jojanneke M. Seinen

28.1 Introduction

Soft tissue sarcoma (STS) represents a heterogeneous group of mesenchymal tumors accounting for about 1 % of all cancers. Approximately 40 % of these patients will ultimately die of their disease [1, 2]. Half of the patients are at the time of diagnosis over the age of 65 years; however, the median age varies significantly by histologic type and subtype [3]. STS are classified according to the WHO classification in 9 types, and even over 50 subtypes might be distinguished [4]. The soft tissue tumors are graded according to the FNCLCC (French Fédération Natiionale des Centres de Lutte Contre le Cancer) system. This so-called French grading system is based on tumor differentiation, mitotic rate, and necrosis [5]. Half of the STS are located at the limbs, and roughly 10 % of the grade III STS are already metastasized at the time of initial diagnosis [3].

The overall aggressive oncological behavior of STS, the low incidence, the heterogeneity among the (sub)types, and the changes in the classification, grading, and staging systems in combination with the lack of large randomized clinical trials made it difficult to get a real insight in the progress achieved in the treatment of these tumors during the last two decades.

Multislice computer tomography (CT) can rule out metastatic disease, while magnetic resonance (MR) imaging provides excellent insight in the local growth pattern of these tumors [6]. There is no role for FDG-PET in the standard diagnostic and/or treatment of STS [7]. So, today the majority of STS can adequately be preoperatively staged: locally, regionally, and distantly.

The most effective STS treatment is planned in a multidisciplinary manner, including the individual patient's clinical and pathologic characteristics. Surgery

H.J. Hoekstra (✉) • J.M. Seinen
Division of Surgical Oncology, University Medical Center Groningen,
University of Groningen, PO Box 30.001, Groningen 9700 RB, The Netherlands
e-mail: h.j.hoekstra@umcg.nl

© Springer-Verlag Berlin Heidelberg 2016
K.R. Aigner, F.O. Stephens (eds.), *Induction Chemotherapy,*
DOI 10.1007/978-3-319-28773-7_28

remains the principal therapeutic modality in STS. MR might have contributed to define the extent of required surgery, particularly the pattern of spread expected for the patient's histologic subtype and therefore increase in the percentage of R0 resections.

The indication for adjuvant radiation is based on the tumor grade, the resection margins, and the possibility for a second surgical procedure in case of local recurrence. Overall, the local tumor control improved through increased use of combined treatment of surgery and radiation treatment, especially after R1 resections with the aim of minimizing local recurrence, maximizing function, and improving overall survival [8]. Since adjuvant radiotherapy has become the golden standard of care of STS in case of marginal resection margins, local control rates have improved up to 80–95 %, with a 5-year survival rate up to 60–70 % [9, 10]. Although brachytherapy (BRT) was advocated in the late 1980s and early 1990s, today it is hardly used in the treatment of STS, since local control with intensity-modulated radiation therapy (IMRT) was significantly better than BRT. Despite the higher rates of adverse features for IMRT, IMRT should be further examined as the treatment of choice for primary high-grade extremity sarcoma [11]. In the radiation treatment, there is a trend toward preoperative radiation treatment, although no randomized trial showed a real benefit in local tumor control or survival, but an increased treatment-related morbidity [12]. The idea behind preoperative radiation treatment with IMRT is a smaller radiation volume and a more precise radiation field, lower total radiation dose, and no tumor boost, which should result in a more effective radiation treatment with a decrease in treatment-related morbidity and improved functional outcome [13].

There is no role for adjuvant systemic chemotherapy in the treatment of STS. Adjuvant systemic treatment had only a small benefit on decreasing the risk of local failure without improving overall survival with an exception for the rhabdomyosarcomas and Ewing sarcomas of the soft tissues [14]. Gastrointestinal stromal tumor (GIST) is the most common sarcoma of the intestinal tract. Imatinib is an effective first-line drug targeting treatment of metastatic gastrointestinal stromal tumor. Adjuvant imatinib therapy is safe and improved recurrence-free survival after the resection of primary gastrointestinal stromal tumor [15]. Since targeted therapies can eventually develop resistance, adjuvant surgery is performed if possible in responders to improve overall survival. During the last few years, numerous innovative agents have been discovered as a result of the understanding of the molecular basis of cancer. Targeted cancer therapies are more selective for cancer cells than normal cells and therefore reduce side effects and improve quality of life. Today, already of over 35 drug targeting therapies for various other malignancies are approved and over 39 drugs are investigated [16]. There is still no breakthrough in the systemic or drug targeting treatment of STS, although currently new promising drugs are explored [17].

Overall STS survival might be improved through the improved local control rate, surgery performed for recurrent disease (local, regional, and/or distal), and possibly, in case of metastatic disease, the improved palliative care. Research is now focused on the identification of new pathways and their correspondent inhibitors to improve the outcome of STS patients.

One of the major challenging treatments for the surgical oncologist is still the primary, irresectable locally advanced STS of the limb, e.g., the limb salvage opportunity with the use of regional chemotherapy.

28.2 Development of Regional Chemotherapy for Limb Sarcomas

Klop described in 1950 the effectiveness of the intra-arterial administration of nitrogen mustard for the treatment of various malignancies [18]. Attempts to reduce the systemic toxicity associated with intra-arterial chemotherapy led Creech, Ryan, and Krementz to develop the technique of isolated limb perfusion (ILP) utilizing an oxygenated extracorporeal circuit for the treatment of melanoma and sarcoma confined to the limbs [19]. ILP with melphalan ± actinomycin-D was successfully applied in the therapeutic or adjuvant treatment of melanoma of the limbs [20]. Lebrun performed after these reports, in 1960, in Belgium the first perfusion in Europe [21]. Oldhoff initiated together with Schraffordt Koops in 1964 an ILP program at the University Medical Center Groningen in the Netherlands. Shortly afterward, ILP treatment was introduced with various success in other cancer centers, mainly in Europe.

Initially, perfusions were performed under normothermia (37–38 °C). Cavaliere showed that mild hyperthermic ILP (39–40 °C) could enhance tumor kill with less serious local toxicity [22]. The pressure-regulated perfusion technique was introduced, leakage monitoring was improved, and dose calculation of the cytostatic agent was no longer based on the bodyweight (BW) but on the perfused limb volume to reduce regional toxicity [23–26].

ILP with melphalan was effective in the therapeutic setting of locally advanced melanomas of the limbs, but ineffective in the adjuvant setting [27]. ILP was also ineffective in the treatment of sarcoma [28]. Therefore, other chemotherapeutic agents such as dacarbazine (DTIC), actinomycin-D, thiotepa, mitomycin-C, doxorubicin, cisplatin, and carboplatin were explored in the ILP setting. These agents were ineffective, the duration of the response too short, or the local toxicity too high and therefore abounded in the perfusion treatment [29–32].

Another approach was investigated by Eilber, University of California, Los Angeles (UCLA), in the 1980s: the induction treatment of intra-arterial chemotherapy, including adriamycin, in combination with preoperative radiation [33]. Although the treatment was effective with low local recurrence rates and high limb salvage rates, the short- and long-term-related morbidity was too high, even after various modifications of the protocol with respect to the applied radiation doses [33, 34]. Today, this kind of treatment approach is hardly ever used anymore.

There was a renewed interest in ILP in the early 1990s when Lejeune and Lienard added tumor necrosis factor-α (TNF-α) to melphalan (TM-ILP) in the treatment of locally advanced STS of the limbs. This treatment approach resulted in an extremely high tumor response and limb salvage rates with acceptable local and systemic toxicity [35]. TM-ILP in the limb salvage treatment of locally advanced STS of the limbs had four major advantages: (1) hyperthermia caused increased blood flow, (2) "first-pass" effect of TNF-α resulted in a disrupture of the tumor vascularity, (3) locally high dosage of cytostatic agents with no systemic toxicity, and (4) increased permeability of the cell membrane with an increased drug uptake inducing hemorrhagic necrosis [36]. This treatment approach was explored in various institutes in Europe in an effective and efficient manner under the two principal investigators, Lejeune and Eggermont [37–40]. Tumor necrosis factor-alpha (TNF-α, Beromun®, Boehringer Ingelheim International GmbH, Ingelheim am Rhein, Germany) was registered in 1999 by the European Medicines Evaluation Agency (EMEA) for the therapeutic extremity perfusion of locally advanced soft tissue sarcoma and melanoma. In contrast to Europe, Beromun® was not registered by the FDA [41]. Today, ILP with Beromun® is offered in 36 institutions worldwide.

This chapter describes the isolated limb perfusion technique with TNF-α and melphalan (TM-ILP) and the current results achieved with TM-ILP in the treatment of primarily irresectable, locally advanced STS of the limbs, recent development in new applications of this kind of treatment modality, and future directions.

28.3 Perfusion Technique

ILP is an invasive, major surgical procedure performed under general anesthesia. The lower limb might be perfused at three different levels (iliac, inguinal, or popliteal level) and the upper limb at two levels (the axillary or brachial level) (Fig. 28.1).

Isolation of a limb is achieved by ligation of collateral vessels and clamping and cannulation of the major artery and vein after systemic heparinization of the patient with heparin 3.3 mg/kg BW. The 14–16 F catheters are connected to the oxygenated extracorporeal circuit. An Esmarch bandage is twisted around the root

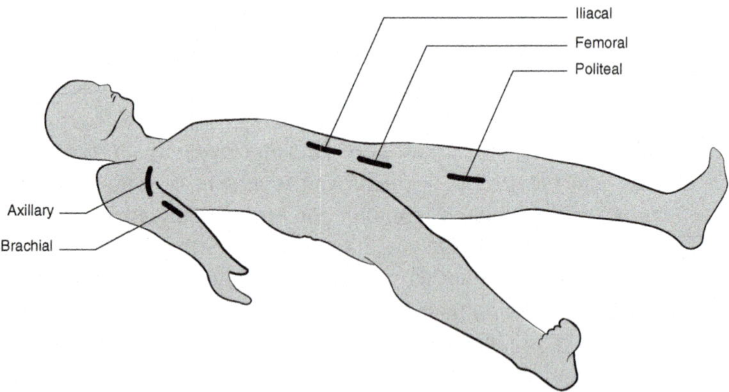

Fig. 28.1 Various perfusion levels on the upper and lower limbs

of the limb and fixed around an inserted pin in the head of the humerus (axillary perfusions) or iliac crest (iliac perfusions) or, in case of brachial or popliteal perfusions, the application of an inflating tourniquet (300–400 mmHg) is used. The extremity is wrapped in a heating blanket to maintain optimal temperature, continuously monitored with thermistors in subcutaneous tissue and muscle tissue. The leakage of the limb to the systemic circulation is monitored with radiolabeled 131-I human serum albumin with a precordial scintillation probe [24]. The day before surgery, the thyroid is saturated through oral administration of iodine.

Pressure-regulated perfusion is performed under mild hyperthermia (38–40 °C) with the use of an extracorporeal circuit with a membrane oxygenator, gas mixture of air/oxygen, and heat exchanger at flow rate of approximately 35–40 ml/L limb volume/min. The perfusate consists of 250 ml of Isodex in saline 0.9 %, 250 ml of white-cell-reduced (filtered) packed red cells, 30 ml of 8.4 % $NaHCO_3$, and 0.5 ml of 5,000 IU/ml heparin. When the temperature in the subcutaneous tissue of the limb is 38 °C and the pH of the perfusate is between 7.2 and 7.35, cytostatic agents are injected in the perfusion circuit or (slowly) into the arterial line. Duration of the perfusion is 60–90 min. Adjustment of flow rates and the tourniquet may be necessary if the leakage of the perfusion circuit into the systemic circulation does exceed 10 %. At the end of the perfusion, the extremity is washed out with 3–6 L saline and filled, if indicated, with one unit red blood cell concentrate. Catheters are removed and vessels repaired. It is in general not necessary to neutralize heparin with protamine sulfate. A closed fasciotomy is performed to prevent a compartment syndrome [42]. Systemic toxicity is related to the leakage and can be managed with IV fluids, appropriate use of vasopressors, and/or antiphlogistics with or without short stay at the intensive care unit. Local toxicity is graded according to Wieberdink (Table 28.1) and is in general mild and mostly related to an excessive high local temperature of the perfused limb, rather than the used drugs [26]. For additional technical information regarding the perfusion technique, refer to the surgical handbooks and detailed technical publications (Fig. 28.2) [23–26, 42, 43].

In the near future, small perfusion equipment might allow ILP in a noninvasive manner by minimal invasive intervention radiology techniques, especially for sarcomas located distal to the limbs where a pneumotourniquet can be used for vessel occlusion.

Table 28.1 Wieberdink's acute regional toxicity grading system

Grade I	No reaction
Grade II	Slight erythema or edema
Grade III	Considerable erythema or edema with some blistering; slightlydisturbed motility permissible
Grade IV	Extensive epidermolysis or obvious damage to the deep tissues,causing definite functional disturbances; threatening or manifestcompartmental syndrome
Grade V	Reaction that may necessitate amputation

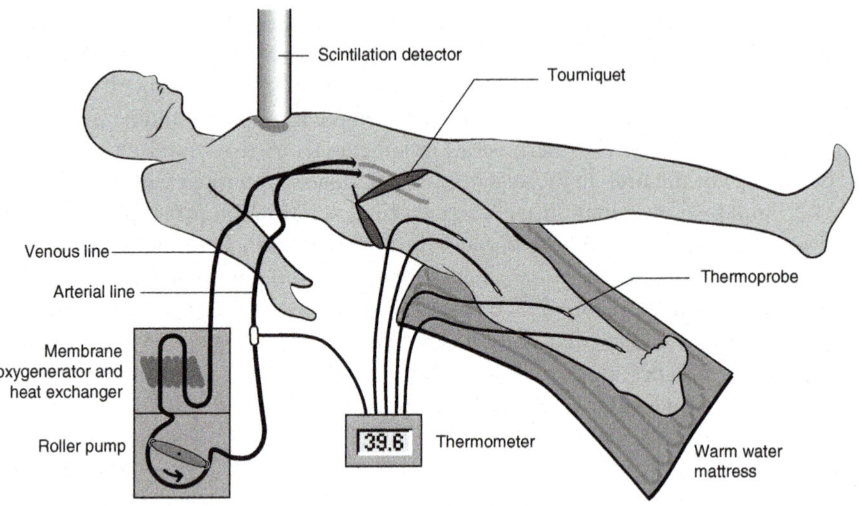

Fig. 28.2 Isolated regional perfusion

28.4 Perfusion Agents TNF-α and Melphalan

Regional concentrations of chemotherapeutic agents are 15–25 times higher in ILP than those reached after systemic administration [44]. For TNF-α, 10–50-fold higher doses than the maximum intravenous dosage can be administered with ILP [45].

TNF-α causes "selective destruction of the tumor vasculature" and facilitates drug penetration in the tumor due to intratumoral vessel permeability [37]. The addition of TNF-α to the perfusate has led to a four- to fivefold increased uptake of melphalan by the tumor [46]. A clinical dose finding study for TNF-α was never performed, although Fraker showed in a dose-escalation study that higher TNF-α doses up to 6 mg of TNF did not increase the response rate [47]. Some studies showed excellent results with lower TNF-α doses, even for a TNF-α dose of 125 μg [48, 49].

According to EMEA, TM-ILP is only applied in dedicated centers with experience in treatment of STS and ILP, since TM-ILP can be accomplished by severe systemic toxicity, e.g., "systemic inflammatory response syndrome" (SIRS). TNF-α (Beromun) is registered at a total dose of 3 mg for upper limb ILP and 4 mg for lower limb ILP [41].

After the registration of Beromun®, Bonvalot and Lejeune performed a phase II dose-reduction trial with 0.5–4 mg TNF-α and melphalan in soft tissue sarcomas. At the range of TNF-α doses tested, there was no dose effect detected for the objective tumor response. Systemic toxicity was significantly correlated with higher TNF-α doses [50]. Low-dose TNF-α and doxorubicin ILP have similar response and limb salvage rates but no major advantage to the combination of TNF-α and melphalan [51].

During recent years, some modifications of the clinical TM-ILP program were applied at the UMCG, to reduce the cardiovascular "instability," and based on the previous described studies with lower doses of TNF-α [49, 50]. The first modification was in 2001 when the overall perfusion time was shortened from 90 to 60 min to reduce the overall "leakage" to the systemic circulation. In 2003, a TNF-α dose reduction was introduced. Since 2003, TM-ILP are perfusions at the UMCG performed at 39–40 °C with reduced TNF-α dosage and overall perfusion time. The currently used dosage of melphalan (Alkeran®, GlaxoSmithKline Pharmaceuticals, Research Triangle Park, NC) is based on limb volume, 10 mg/l lower limb volume and 13 mg/l upper limb volume, and the dosage TNF-α (Beromun®, Boehringer Ingelheim International GmbH, Ingelheim am Rhein, Germany) is related to the perfusion levels, 1 mg TNF-α for the upper limb and 1–2 mg TNF-α for the lower limb. TNF-α is directly injected in the arterial perfusion line. TNF-α concentrations remain stable during perfusion and 15 min perfusion seems appropriate. After 15 min, melphalan is slowly injected into the arterial line and circulates for 45 min. There is a rapid uptake of melphalan, and almost all uptake of melphalan occurs within the first 30 min [52]. The overall perfusion time is therefore reduced from 90 to 60 min [53]. Lower doses of TNF-α are not advised for the risk of loss of activity [49, 50, 53]. True hyperthermia (>40 °C) should not be used in combination with TM-ILP because of its regional toxicity to normal tissues. The reduced overall perfusion time and extensive "washout" led to a decrease in cardiovascular "instability" of the anesthetized patient without reducing the therapeutic efficacy [53]. Today the iliac perfused TM-ILP patients stay for 24 h at the intensive care unit and the other TM-ILP patients for 24 h at the recovery room due to the reduced overall perfusion time, and the extensive washout SIRS is hardly seen anymore after TM-ILP [53, 54].

28.5 Measuring Noninvasive Tumor Response

In the early days, pre- and post-perfusion angiographies (6 weeks) were performed to assess the response of treatment. An angiographic response was defined as a complete disappearance of tumor vascularity and tumor stain (normal angiography) and no response as persistence of tumor vascularity and tumor stain (abnormal angiography). The histological score of tumor response to TM-ILP was complete response (I), partial response (90 % necrosis) (II), partial response (50 % necrosis) (III), and no change (IV). Scores I and II were considered as responders and scores III and IV as nonresponders. There is indeed a significant correlation between angiography and pathological classification ($P < 0.001$) of the sarcomas treated by perfusion [55]. Angiogenetic vessels are "destroyed," while the quiescent vessels are undestroyed. This is caused by a specific deactivation of an integrin only expressed in angionetic vessels within tumors [56]. Assessing tumor response by angiography or MRA is today only performed in nonresponders who could benefit from a second TM-ILP.

The literature, with respect to the role of PET in the treatment and therapeutic evaluation of STS, showed that there is no indication to use FDG-PET, tyrosine PET, or FLT-PET in the diagnostic and standard (perfusion) treatment evaluation of sarcomas [7, 57–59]. IMRT treatment of STS might reduce radiation effectiveness and reduction of radiation toxicity to normal tissue [60]. A new application of FDG-PET might be the PET-CT-guided IMRT treatment of STS patients.

28.6 TM-ILP Results

28.6.1 Overall Results

The worldwide experience in TNF-based perfusions is limited to 36 centers, and only 10 centers have over 20 years TM-ILP experience. The achieved results published in the literature are limited to a few European cancer centers from the Netherlands, Germany, France, Italy, Belgium, Switzerland, and Israel. A large proportion of TM-ILP publications are "duplications" of previous publications, including a larger number of TM-ILP patients with overall the same conclusions; TM-ILP is a safe limb-saving treatment modality [53, 54].

In the early days, publications focused on the amount of therapy-induced necrosis described as complete response (CR), partial response (PR), or no change or progressive disease (NC/PD). More important are the achieved short- and long-term limb salvage rates, the short- and long-term treatment-related morbidity, as well as disease-specific survival. An overview of the results in extremity perfusion for STS is presented in Table 28.2 from multicenter and single-center studies with various cytostatic agents, response rates, limb salvage rates, local recurrence rates, 5-year survival rates, and specific study remarks. Low clinical response rates have been reported for non-TNF-α-based perfusions. For more detailed information, refer to the original papers; references are mentioned in the table.

The local resection is performed 6–12 weeks after the TM-ILP. The surgical resection margin is defined as an R0 resection (microscopic negative), R1 (microscopic positive), or R2 (macroscopic positive). Based on the resection margin, patients receive adjuvant radiation. Radiation increased significantly the local tumor control ($P<0.05$) without increasing the local treatment morbidity in primarily irresectable extremity sarcomas treated with a TM-ILP [95]. TM-ILP is feasible in patients with recurrent sarcomas who were previous irradiated [88, 109].

Overall, at the UMCG, a limb salvage rate of 89 % is achieved with TM-ILP, figures in the literature ranging from 64 % to 100 %, and a local recurrence rate of 11 %, ranging in the literature from 11 to 42; see Table 28.2. Overall the risk for distant failures in the literature for the patients treated with TM-ILP from 25 % to 44 % varies [38, 54, 101].

There are a few series published in the literature with low doses of TNF, and these are summarized in Table 28.3. Dose reduction might lead to lower pathological responses (CR/PR) without increasing local recurrence rate and disease-specific and overall survival [53]. The level of isolation is a prognostic factor for leakage.

Table 28.2 Overview results in extremity perfusion for sarcoma

Author	Year	Study	Cytostatics	N	CR %	PR %	NC %	LS %	LR %	5-year survival %	Remarks
Krementz et al. [61]	1977	Single	M/Act-D/HN2	17	0	35	65	NS	NS	NS	Historical
Muchmore et al. [62]	1985	Single	M/Act-D/NH2/ various	51	6	12	82	NS	NS	NS	Historical
Stehlin et al. [63]	1984	Single	M/Act-D	65	NS	NS	NS	94	NS	73	Historical
Lehti et al. [64]	1986	Single	M/Act-D	64	NS	NS	NS	100	11	67	Feasibility EBRT
Krementz [65]	1986	Single	M/Act-D	56	NS	NS	NS	100	21	65	Historical
Hoekstra et al. [28]	1987	Single	M	14	NS	NS	NS	100	7	69	Historical
Pommier et al. [30]	1988	Single	Cisplatin	17	0	18	82	NS	NS	NS	Cisplatin
Di Filippo et al. [66]	1988	Single	M/Act-D	55	NS	NS	NS	78	24	48	Historical
Klaase et al. [29]	1989	Single	Dox/M	13	7	0	93	61	0–24	44–77	Doxorubicin
Kettelhack et al. [67]	1991	Single	M/Act-D	9	NS	NS	NS	78	33	66	Historical
Eggermont [68]	1993	Single	TNF/M _ IFN	20	55	40	5	90	NS	NS	TNF-α
Hill et al. [48]	1993	Single	TNF/M	8	100	0	0	64	NS	NS	Low-dose TNF-α
Fletcher et al. [69]	1994	Single	Cisplatin	75	NS	NS	NS	NS	7	100–48	Largest cisplatin study
Rossi et al. [70]	1994	Single	Dox	23	NS	74	26	91	27	48	Doxorubicin
van Ginkel et al. [32]	1996	Single	Cisplatin	4	NS	NS	NS	NS	NS	NS	Cisplatin
Eggermont et al. [38]	1996	Multi	TNF/M _ IFN	55	18	64	18	84	13	NS	First multicenter
Eggermont et al. [39]	1996	Multi	TNF/M _ IFN	186	18	57	25	82	11	NS	Beromun_ registration
Santinami et al. [71]	1996	Single	TNF/M	10	70	20	10	89	NS	NS	None

(continued)

Table 28.2 (continued)

Author	Year	Study	Cytostatics	N	CR %	PR %	NC %	LS %	LR %	5-year survival %	Remarks
Rossi et al. [72]	1996	Single	TNF þ Dox	18	NS	NS	NS	81	10	NS	None
Gutman et al. [73]	1997	Single	TNF/M _ IFN	35	37	54	9	85	0/31	NS	None
Olieman et al. [55]	1997	Single	TNF/M	25	40	52	8	NS	NS	NS	Angiographic response
Olieman et al. [74]	1998	Single	TNF/M _ IFN	34	35	59	6	85	14	60	Feasibility EBRT
Olieman et al. [75]	1998	Single	TNF/M _ IFN	9	44	33	23	89	22	0	Palliative treatment
Lev-Chelouche et al. [76]	1999	Single	TNF/M _ IFN	5	20	80	0	80	NS	NS	Kaposi sarcoma
Lev-Chelouche et al. [77]	1999	Single	TNF/M _ IFN	6	33	50	17	100	33	NS	Desmoid
Lev-Chelouche et al. [78]	1999	Single	TNF/M _ IFN	13	38	54	8	85	38	NS	Multifocal
Eggermont et al. [40]	1999	Multi	TNF/M _ IFN	246	28	47	25	76	NS	NS	Definition irresectability
Rossi et al. [79]	1999	Single	TNF þ Dox	20	26	64	10	84	10	64	None
Lejeune et al. [80]	2000	Single	TNF/M _ IFN	22	18	64	18	77	14	86	None
Daryanani et al. [31]	2000	Single	Carboplatin	4	NS	NS	NS	100	NS	NS	Carboplatin
Hohenberger et al. [81]	2001	Single	TNF/M _ IFN	55	NS	NS	NS	84	NS	NS	None
Lans et al. [82]	2002	Single	TNF/M _ IFN	16	56	31	13	80	NS	NS	Lymphangiosarcoma
Noorda et al. [83]	2003	Single	TNF/M _ IFN	49	8	55	37	57	13	48	None
van Etten et al. [84]	2003	Single	TNF/M _ IFN	29	38	38	24	76	NS	NS	Elderly patients >75 years of age
Di Filippo et al. [85]	2003	Single	Dox _ TNF	NS	22	55	23	77	7	69	Phase I and II study Dox and Dox þ TNF
Feig et al. [86]	2004	Single	Dox	14	0	0	100	25	NS	NS	Doxorubicin
Rossi et al. [51]	2005	Single	TNF/Dox	21	5	57	38	71	19	57	TNF-α þ doxorubicin

Grunhagen et al. [49]	2005	Single	TNF/M _ IFN	240	24	50	26	82	NS	±45	Largest single center
Grunhagen et al. [49]	2005	Single	TNF/M _ IFN	48	38	31	29	85	NS	36	Dose reduction
Bonvalot et al. [50]	2005	Single	TNF/M	100	36	29	35	77	24	NS	Dose reduction
Grunhagen et al. [87]	2005	Single	TNF/M _ IFN	12	17	58	25	100	17	NS	Desmoid
Lans et al. [88]	2005	Single	TNF/M _ IFN	26	20	50	30	65	27/45	40	Previous irradiated recurrences
Grunhagen et al. [89]	2005	Single	TNF/M _ IFN	64	42	45	13	82	45	39	Multifocal/recurrent sarcoma
Grunhagen et al. [90]	2006	Single	TNF/M _ IFN	217	18	51	31	75	26	49	Prognostic factor
Grunhagen et al. [91]	2006	Single	TNF/M _ IFN	37	16	68	16	92	NS	NS	Palliative treatment
Schlag and Tunn [92]	2006	Single	TNF/M _ IFN	125	19	53	28	81	18	NS	None
Hayes et al. [93]	2006	Single	TNF/M	18	NS	NS	NS	NS	NS	NS	None
Thijssens et al. [94]	2006	Single	TNF/M	39	NS	NS	NS	NS	NS	NS	Quality of life
Thijssens et al. [95]	2006	Single	TNF/M	64	NS	NS	NS	89	NS	61	Value adjuvant RT
van Ginkel et al. [96]	2007	Single	TNF/M _ IFN	73	25	69	6	60	NS	70 %	70 % Long-term LS outcome
Hoven-Gondrie et al. [97]	2007	Single	TNF/M _ IFN	32	NS	NS	NS	NS	NS	NS	Vascular morbidity
Pennacchioli et al. [98]	2007	Single	M or Doxo with or without TNF-α	88	32	59	8	83	27	NS	Melphalan or Doxo with or without TNF-α
Cherix et al. [99]	2008	Single	TNF/M	51	25	41	28	76	35	44	Long-term results

(continued)

Table 28.2 (continued)

Author	Year	Study	Cytostatics	N	CR %	PR %	NC %	LS %	LR %	5-year survival %	Remarks
Hoven-Gondrie et al. [100]	2008	Single	TNF/M	73	NS	NS	NS	NS	NS	NS	Long-term effects according to LENT-SOMA
Bonvalot et al. [101]	2009	Single	TNF/M	100	19	39	42	87	14	NS	None
Di Fillippo et al. [102]	2009	Single	TNF_Doxo	75	34	48	18	85	21	62	TNF and Doxo
Nachmany et al. [103]	2009	Single	TNF/M	42	17	36	47		42	NS	High- vs. low-dose TNF-α
Lasithiotakis et al. [104]	2010	Multi	TNF/M	6	17	50	33	100	NS	NS	None
Wray et al. [105]	2011	Multi	TNF/M	17	6	64	30	41	NS	NS	Phase II trial: comparison
			Doxo	10	0	0	100	20	NS	NS	of two regimens
Grabellus et al. [106]	2011	Single	TNF/M	53	NS	NS	NS	NS	11	NS	Histologic response
Deroose et al. [54]	2011	Single	TNF/M	208	18	53	29	81	30	42	Long-term results largest single center
Hoven-Gondrie [53]	2011	Single	TNF/M	102	22	55	23	77	15	NS	TNF dose reduction
Deroose et al. [107]	2011	Single	TNF/M	122	4	66	29	89	21	NS	Role of adjuvant RT
Deroose et al. [108]	2012	Single	TNF/M	29	33	38	29	NS	32	52	ILP for distal part limb
Seinen et al. [116]	2012	Single	TNF/M	72	NS	NS	NS	NS	NS	NS	Treatment-related fractures
Seinen et al. [117]	2012	Single	TNF/M	88	17	55	28	NS	11	NS	Local recurrence after ILP

Act-D dactinomycin-D, *DOX* doxorubicin, *EBRT* external beam radiotherapy, *IFN* interferon-g, *LR* local recurrence, *LS* limb salvage, *M* melphalan, *Multi* multicenter, *NC* no change, *HN2* mechlorethamine (nitrogen mustard), *NS* not stated, *Ref* reference, *Single* single center Extremity perfusion for sarcoma 813

Table 28.3 Overview of published clinical dose-reduction studies

References	N	Dose TNF (mg)	Median FU (months)	Clin. Resp. (%)	Path. Resp. (CR/PR) (%)	LS (%)	LR (%)	OS (%)	DFS (%)	LRFS (%)	DMFS (%)
Bonvalot et al. [50]	100		24				27[a]	82[a]	49[a]	NA	NA
	25	0.5		68	43	88					
	25	1		56	62	80					
	25	2		72	67	88					
	25	3–4		64	64	92					
Grunhagen et al. [49]	240		NA								
	192	3–4		74	NA	NA	NA	47[b]	NA	59[b]	50[b]
	48	<3–4		69	NA	85	NA	36[b]	NA	44[b]	45[b]
Bonvalot et al. [101]	100	1	27	79	58	87	18[c]	89[c]	NA	NA	67[c]
Nachmany et al. [103]	43			NA				NA	NA	NA	NA
	26	3–4	58[d]		65	76	38				
	17	1	30[d]		31	53	46				
Hoven-Gondrie [53]	102		76[e]	NA	76[f]	77	15	56[g]	NA	85[b]	52[b]

TNF tumor necrosis factor-alpha, *FU* follow-up, *Clin. Resp.* clinical response, *Path. Resp.* pathological response, *CR/PR* complete response/partial response, *LS* limb survival, *LR* local recurrence, *OS* overall survival, *DFS* Disease-free survival, *LRFS* local recurrence-free survival, *DMFS* distant metastasis-free survival, *NA* not available

[a]Two-year rates

[b]Five-year rates

[c]Three-year rates

[d]Mean FU

[e]Only for patients alive after FU

[f]In case of no resection clinical response was used

[g]Five-year disease-specific survival (DSS) was used

A complete isolation is more difficult to achieve at the iliac and femoral level in contrast to the axillary or popliteal level [24, 25]. Since iliac/femoral perfusions have always a certain amount of leakage, the dose reduction together with the increased washout lowered the risk for the occurrence of SIRS. Changes in TM-ILP, e.g., reduction of TNF-α dose and overall perfusion time, have not compromised the outcome, limb salvage rate or local recurrence rate [53]. TM-ILP can also be used for multifocal primary sarcomas (Stewart-Treves syndrome, Kaposi sarcoma, epithelioid sarcoma) [89].

The management of locally advanced soft tissue sarcoma of the extremities of patients who present with regional and/or distant disease at the time of diagnosis remains an unsolved problem, since there is still no effective systemic therapy [14]. Palliative perfusion in metastatic extremity sarcoma is an excellent procedure to provide local tumor control and limb salvage, e.g., alleviation of pain, and to avoid ablative surgery for the short survival of these STS patients. Based on the life expectancy and the patient's performance index, a palliative TM-ILP is discussed with the patient, family, and caregivers. If decided to perform a palliative perfusion, delayed resection of the tumor and even adjuvant radiation is indicated to ensure adequate local tumor control, even in complete responders [75, 91]. Since the overall survival is limited, a tailored treatment is more and more offered to STS patients with synchronous disease. Radiation ± systemic treatment, with or without a clinical trial, is a good alternative for an invasive and intensive TM-ILP.

Based on the achieved results obtained with TM-ILP, the non-TNF-α-based perfusions are no longer performed in Europe in the limb salvage treatment for locally advanced extremity soft tissue sarcomas. The overall survival after TM-ILP is equivalent to amputation [40]. With the TNF-α and melphalan perfusions (TM-ILP), a short-term limb salvage of 80–90 % is achieved and a 10-year limb salvage rate of 60 % with acceptable local and negligible systemic toxicity [53, 54]. On the other hand, the treatment is intensive. Twenty percent of the TM-ILP cancer survivors experienced a posttraumatic stress syndrome (PTSS) [94].

28.6.2 Complications

Patient's comorbidity, local disease, and previous treatment are important risk factors for TM-ILP treatment-related complications. Complications encountered during ITM-LP might be caused by the surgical and/or perfusion procedure: (1) acute toxic reactions of the perfused tissues (muscle, nerves, vessels, skin), (2) systemic toxicity due to leakage, and (3) long-term perfusion and treatment-related morbidity.

Systemic leakage during a TNF perfusion might result in a characteristic SIRS: hypotension and respiratory failure. There is minor leakage (<10 %) in almost 90 % of the TM-ILP patients, and SIRS is hardly encountered [53, 54, 110, 111].

Regional toxicity is graded according to Wieberdink (Table 28.1), and a slight edema exists during the first 48 h, the limb is warm and uncomfortable, and edema resolves within 1–2 weeks. During the following weeks, the redness becomes darker; there is some blistering of the palm of the hand or sole of the foot, inhibition of hair growth, neuralgia, and temporary loss of nails; and the limb will "recover" in several weeks. Regional toxicity is moderate and not different from ILP with melphalan alone [112].

An effective perfusion might result in a complete disappearance of the tumor; on the other hand, an effective perfusion might lead to an increase of tumor volume due to tumor necrosis and liquification and even result in skin necrosis with tumor perforation which might result in an amputation, since resection and plastic surgical reconstruction are no longer a treatment option. Late morbidity can be caused by local recurrence, reduced functional morbidity due to fibrosis, pathological fractures, and critical leg ischemia. In the latter, objective measurements show a time-related decrease of ankle-brachial index (ABI) and femoral pulsatility index (PI) in the perfused extremity [97].

Since half of the TM-ILP patients became cancer survivors, treatment-related complications will become an increasingly important concern. TNF-α and melphalan will give no short- and long-term complications. The vast majority of complications, wound healing disturbances, fibrosis, edema, and functional impairment are caused by the extensive surgical resections and the applied radiation treatment [12, 113, 114]. Two-thirds of the TM-ILP patients experienced serious late toxic effects such as edema, fibrosis, limited mobility, impaired wound healing, and, less commonly, vascular disturbances, pain, bony fractures, and secondary tumors [53, 96, 100, 115, 116]. In a recent study performed at the UMCG, an overall risk of a treatment-related fracture (TAF) at 10 years of 17 % was found, and even every fourth patient with a sarcoma of the thigh developed after TM-ILP a TAF. Elderly patients (>65 years) and patients in whom a periosteal stripping was performed were at higher risk to develop a TAF. In only 11 % of the TAF patients, union was achieved. The treatment of TAF is intramedullary nailing or an endoprosthesis [116]. The new radiation technique with IMRT can possible decrease the incidence of these late complications.

In the initial series of 78 TM-ILP patients treated at the UMCG, 17 patients (23 %) had another primary neoplasm (OPN): 8 before the STS diagnosis (47 %), 1 synchronously, 1 between 2 other OPNs, and 7 patients developed an OPN after the TM-ILP treatment (41 %) [115].

28.6.3 Limb Function

Overall the limb salvage rates vary between 20 % and 100 % (Table 28.2). The four major reasons for amputation after TM-ILP are (1) insufficient tumor response to TM-ILP, (2) extensive induced tumor necrosis hampering local resection, (3) impaired wound healing, and/or (4) tumor recurrence.

An anterolateral fasciotomy prevents the risk of a compartment syndrome with neuropraxia of the peroneal nerve [41]. Lymphedema and pain can also be extremely invalidating. Limitations in the ankle joint mobility after ILP have previously been described for melanoma patients in 25–40 % of the patients [118, 119]. These limitations are much less reported in sarcoma patients [100]. Nevertheless, the largest TM-ILP series from Rotterdam showed a general functional impairment of 17 % [54]. The LENT-SOMA scoring system evaluates uniformly all long-term local toxic effects and showed that after TM-ILP two-thirds of the patients experienced serious late toxic effects [100].

28.6.4 Local Recurrence

The incidence of local recurrence after ILP treatment for locally advanced sarcomas varies in the literature from 11 % to 45 % as shown in Table 28.3 and is related to five factors: (1) tumor size, grade, and anatomical location, (2) single vs. multifocal disease, (3) primary vs. recurrent disease, (4) the use of adjuvant radiation, and finally (5) the experience of the ILP STS team. The recurrence rate after TM-ILP in one of the largest single-center series from Groningen (11 %) is equivalent with the current published recurrence rates after STS treatment with pre- or postoperative radiotherapy of 7–8 % [12]. Adjuvant radiation might reduce the risk of local recurrence in TM-ILP-treated patients [95, 107]. There is no correlation, e.g., increased risk, for systemic disease after a local recurrence in TM-ILP patients [54].

28.6.5 Systemic Progression

These patients are at risk to develop systemic disease, which is encountered in 40–50 % of the TM-ILP patients and not different from conventional STS treatment. After the development of systemic disease, the median survival is in general short, but all patients should be offered, after multidisciplinary consultation, a tailored treatment, e.g., surgery, radiation, and/or systemic treatment, to prolong overall survival and quality of life.

28.7 Future Directions

Over 50 years, the technique of extremity perfusion is explored in the limb salvage treatment of locally advanced, recurrent, and multifocal sarcomas. The "discovery" of TNF-α in combination with melphalan was a real breakthrough in the treatment of primary irresectable extremity STS outside the USA, since TNF-α (Beromun®) is not registered there.

TM-ILP is the current most optimal limb-saving treatment for these tumors with low-dose TNF-α and melphalan, followed 6 weeks later by surgical resection and, if indicated, 4–6 weeks later 50–70 Gy adjuvant radiation treatment. The TM-ILP is an intensive treatment with a 10-year limb salvage rate of 60 %. This treatment regimen also has disadvantages: (1) potential regrowth of initial "killed tumor cells" after TM-ILP before surgical resection is applied, (2) the delivery of high-dose postoperative radiation on a large surgical field, (3) serious short- and long-term treatment-related morbidity caused by extensive surgical resection and a large radiation treatment field, and (4) overall treatment time of ± 21 weeks. It is therefore of the utmost importance to reduce the treatment-related morbidity and overall treatment time.

Development of new treatment strategies in extremity perfusion, better perfusion, or infusion equipment might further improve the outcome of ILP treatment. TM-ILP should be combined with more precise preoperative radiation treatment followed directly by surgical resection to increase the treatment effectiveness and reduce overall treatment time. New innovations in STS diagnostic imaging, PET-CT, or PET-MRI are available and make a more precise preoperative IMRT planning possible with smaller radiation fields and lower radiation dose to reduce treatment-related morbidity.

ILP is an invasive, technical demanding, and time-consuming procedure, and therefore, John Thompson developed the technique of isolated limb infusion (ILI) [120]. There is some limited experience with the noninvasive technique of ILI in the treatment of locally advanced limb sarcoma since it allows also repeated infusions. Isolated limb infusion with melphalan, 7.5 mg/L limb volume for lower extremity and 10 mg/L limb volume for upper extremity, with a maximum total dose of 100 mg for lower extremity and 50 mg for upper extremity. Actinomycin-D, 100 µg/L limb volume, provides an attractive alternative therapy for regional disease control and limb preservation in patients with limb-threatening soft tissue malignant neoplasms. Short-term response rates appear encouraging, yet durability of response is unknown [121].

As long as we have no specific drug targeting therapy for the various sarcomas, we have to rely on Europe on TM-ILP for the limb salvage treatment of locally advanced STS, which can overcome 90 % of the "indicated amputations" for STS. For centers in the USA, ILI might possibly be a good alternative, when more long-term data will become available.

The use of molecular imaging technology might provide noninvasive tumor response information and is already applied in ILP [7, 57–59]. In sarcoma surgery, the resection margins are intraoperatively defined by the pathologist at the time of resection on frozen section analysis of the tumor margins with often sampling errors. Near-infrared (NIR) imaging agents might provide more insight in the resections of tumor tissue and were recently successfully used clinically in the treatment of ovarian cancer [122]. The technique could also identify residual disease after intraoperative detection and removal of microscopic residual sarcoma in a mouse model [123]. This new molecular imaging technology and the development of handheld intraoperative molecular imaging devices will further improve the outcome of surgical resections of locally advanced sarcoma treatment by an induction treatment of ILP and preoperative radiation.

References

1. http://www.iknl.nl.
2. American Cancer Society: cancer facts and figures 2012. http://www.cancer.org/Research/CancerFactsFigures/index.
3. Nijhuis PH, Schaapveld M, Otter R, Molenaar WM, van der Graaf WT, Hoekstra HJ. Epidemiological aspects of soft tissue sarcomas (STS) – consequences for the design of clinical STS trials. Eur J Cancer. 1999;35:1705–10.
4. Fletcher CDM, Unni K, Mertens F, editors. World Health Organization classification of tumours. Pathology and genetics. Tumours of soft tissue and bone. Lyon: IARC Press; 2002.
5. Trojani M, Contesso G, Coindre JM, et al. Soft tissue sarcomas of adults: study of pathological prognostic variables and definition of histopathological grading system. Int J Cancer. 1984;33:37–42.
6. Panicek DM, Gatsonis C, Rosenthal DI, Seeger LL, Huvos AG, Moore SG, Caudry DJ, Palmer WE, McNeil BJ. CT and MR imaging in the local staging of primary malignant musculoskeletal neoplasms: report of the Radiology Diagnostic Oncology Group. Radiology. 1997;202:237–46.
7. Bastiaannet E, Groen H, Jager PL, Cobben DC, van der Graaf WT, Vaalburg W, Hoekstra HJ. The value of FDG-PET in the detection, grading and response to therapy of soft tissue and bone sarcomas; a systematic review and meta-analysis. Cancer Treat Rev. 2004;30: 83–101.

8. Yang JC, Chang AE, Baker AR, et al. Randomized prospective study of the benefit of adjuvant radiation therapy in the treatment of soft tissue sarcomas of the extremity. J Clin Oncol. 1998;16:197–203.

9. Ham SJ, van der Graaf WT, Pras E, Molenaar WM, van den Berg E, Hoekstra HJ. Soft tissue sarcoma of the extremities. A multimodality diagnostic and therapeutic approach. Cancer Treat Rev. 1998;24:373–91.

10. Singer S, Demetri GD, Baldini EH, Fletcher CD. Management of soft-tissue sarcomas: an overview and update. Lancet Oncol. 2000;1:75–85.

11. Alektiar KM, Brennan MF, Singer S. Local control comparison of adjuvant brachytherapy to intensity-modulated radiotherapy in primary high-grade sarcoma of the extremity. Cancer. 2011;117:3229–34.

12. O'Sullivan B, Davis AM, Turcotte R, et al. Preoperative versus postoperative radiotherapy in soft-tissue sarcoma of the limbs: a randomised trial. Lancet. 2002;359:2235–41.

13. Davis AM, O'Sullivan B, Turcotte R, et al. Late radiation morbidity following randomization to preoperative versus postoperative radiotherapy in extremity soft tissue sarcoma. Radiother Oncol. 2005;75:48–53.

14. Adjuvant chemotherapy for localised resectable soft-tissue sarcoma of adults: meta-analysis of individual data. Sarcoma Meta-analysis Collaboration. Lancet. 1997;350(9092):1647–54.

15. Dematteo RP, Ballman KV, Antonescu CR, et al. Adjuvant imatinib mesylate after resection of localised, primary gastrointestinal stromal tumour: a randomised, double-blind, placebo-controlled trial. Lancet. 2009;373:1097–104.

16. http://www.cancer.gov/cancertopics/factsheet/Therapy/targeted.

17. Schöffski P, Ray-Coquard IL, Cioffi A, et al. Activity of eribulin mesylate in patients with soft-tissue sarcoma: a phase 2 study in four independent histological subtypes. Lancet Oncol. 2011;12:1045–52.

18. Klopp C, Alford TC, Bateman J, Berry GN, Winship T. Fractionated intra-arterial cancer chemotherapy with methyl bis-amine hydrochloride; a preliminary report. Ann Surg. 1950;132:811–32.

19. Creech OJ, Krementz ET, Ryan RF, Winblad JN. Chemotherapy of cancer. Regional perfusion utilizing an extracorporeal circuit. Ann Surg. 1958;148:616–32.

20. Krementz ET, Carter RD, Sutherland CM, Muchmore JH, Ryan RF, Creech Jr O. Regional chemotherapy for melanoma: a 35 year experience. Ann Surg. 1994;220:520–35.

21. Lebrun J, Smets W. Regional perfusion by extracorporeal circulation. Surgical technique permitting the administration of anti-cancer chemotherapeutic agents in massive doses. Acta Chir Belg. 1961;60:368–405.

22. Cavaliere R, Ciocatto EC, Giovanella BC, Heidelberger C, Johnson RO, Margottini M, et al. Selective heat sensitivity of cancer cells. Biochemical and clinical studies. Cancer. 1967;20:1351–81.

23. Fontijne WP, Mook PH, Schraffordt Koops H, Oldhoff J, Wildevuur CR. Improved tissue perfusion during pressure regulated hyperthermic regional isolated perfusion. A clinical study. Cancer. 1985;55:1455–61.

24. Daryanani D, Komdeur R, Ter Veen J, Nijhuis PH, Piers DA, Hoekstra HJ. Continuous leakage measurement during hyperthermic isolated limb perfusion. Ann Surg Oncol. 2001;8:566–72.

25. van Ginkel RJ, Limburg PC, Piers DA, Koops HS, Hoekstra HJ. Value of continuous leakage monitoring with radioactive iodine-131-labeled human serum albumin during hyperthermic isolated limb perfusion with tumor necrosis factor-alpha and melphalan. Ann Surg Oncol. 2002;9:355–63.

26. Wieberdink J, Benckhuysen C, Braat RP, et al. Dosimetry in isolated perfusion of the limbs by assessment of perfused tissue volume and grading of toxic tissue reactions. Eur J Cancer Clin Oncol. 1992;18:905–10.

27. Schraffordt Koops H, Vaglini M, Suciu S, et al. Prophylactic isolated limb perfusion for localized, high-risk limb melanoma: results of a multicenter randomized phase III trial. J Clin Oncol. 1998;16:2906–12.

28. Hoekstra HJ, Schraffordt Koops H, Molenaar WM, Oldhoff J. Results of isolated regional perfusion in the treatment of malignant soft tissue tumours of the extremities. Cancer. 1987;60:1703–7.

29. Klaase JM, Kroon BBR, Benckhuijsen C, van Geel AN, Albus-Lutter CE, Wieberdink J. Results of regional isolation perfusion with cytostatics in patients with soft tissue tumours of the extremities. Cancer. 1989;64:616–21.

30. Pommier RF, Moseley HS, Cohen J, Huang CS, Townsend R. Fletcher WS Pharmacokinetics, toxicity, and short-term results of cisplatin hyperthermic isolated limb perfusion for soft-tissue sarcoma and melanoma of the extremities. Am J Surg. 1988;155:667–71.

31. Daryanani D, de Vries EG, Guchelaar HJ, van Weerden TW, Hoekstra HJ. Hyperthermic isolated regional perfusion of the limb with carboplatin. Eur J Surg Oncol. 2000;26: 792–7.

32. van Ginkel RJ, Schrafford Koops H, de Vries EG, Molenaar WM, Uges DR, Hoekstra HJ. Hyperthermic isolated limb perfusion with cisplatin in four patients with sarcomas of soft tissue and bone. Eur J Surg Oncol. 1996;22:528–31.

33. Eilber FC, Rosen G, Eckardt J, Forscher C, Nelson SD, Selch M, Dorey F, Eilber FR. Treatment-induced pathologic necrosis: a predictor of local recurrence and survival in patients receiving neoadjuvant therapy for high-grade extremity soft tissue sarcomas. J Clin Oncol. 2001;19:3203–9.

34. Nijhuis PH, Pras E, Sleijfer DT, Molenaar WM, Shraffordt Koops H, Hoekstra HJ. Long-term results of preoperative intra-arterial doxorubicin combined with neoadjuvant radiotherapy, followed by extensive surgical resection for locally advanced soft tissue sarcomas of the extremities. Radiother Oncol. 1999;51:15–9.

35. Lienard D, Ewalenko P, Delmotte JJ, Renard N, Lejeune FJ. High-dose recombinant tumor necrosis factor alpha in combination with interferon gamma and melphalan in isolation perfusion of the limbs for melanoma and sarcoma. J Clin Oncol. 1992;10:52–60.

36. Eggermont AM, de Wilt JH, ten Hagen TL. Current uses of isolated limb perfusion in the clinic and a model system for new strategies. Lancet Oncol. 2003;4:429–37.

37. van Horssen R, Ten Hagen TL, Eggermont AM. TNF-alpha in cancer treatment: molecular insights, antitumor effects, and clinical utility. Oncologist. 2006;11:397–408.

38. Eggermont AM, Schrafford Koops H, Lienard D, Kroon BB, van Geel AN, Hoekstra HJ, Lejeune FJ. Isolated limb perfusion with high-dose tumor necrosis factor-alpha in combination with interferon-gamma and melphalan for nonresectable extremity soft tissue sarcomas: a multicenter trial. J Clin Oncol. 1996;14:2653–65.

39. Eggermont AM, Schrafford Koops H, Klausner JM, et al. Isolated limb perfusion with tumor necrosis factor and melphalan for limb salvage in 186 patients with locally advanced soft tissue extremity sarcomas. The cumulative multicenter European experience. Ann Surg. 1996;224:756–64.

40. Eggermont AM, Schrafford Koops H, Klausner JM, et al. Limb salvage by isolated perfusion with tumor necrosis factor alpha and melphalan for locally advanced extremity soft tissue sarcomas: result of 270 perfusions in 247 patients. Proc ASCO. 1999;11:497.

41. http://www.ema.europa.eu.

42. Schrafford Koops H. Prevention of neural and muscular lesions during hyperthermic regional perfusion. Surg Gynecol Obstet. 1972;135:401–3.

43. Hoekstra HJ. Isolated limb perfusion. In: Audisio RA, editor. Atlas of surgical procedures in surgical oncology with critical, evidence-based commentary notes. Singapore: World Scientific Publishing; 2010. p. 259–65.

44. Guchelaar HJ, Hoekstra HJ, de Vries EG, Uges DR, Oosterhuis JW, Schrafford KH. Cisplatin and platinum pharmacokinetics during hyperthermic isolated limb perfusion for human tumours of the extremities. Br J Cancer. 1992;65:898–902.

45. Asher A, Mulé JJ, Reichert CM, Shiloni E, Rosenberg SA. Studies on the anti-tumor efficacy of systemically administered recombinant tumor necrosis factor against several murine tumors in vivo. J Immunol. 1987;138:963–74.

46. De Wilt JH, Manusama ER, van Tiel ST, van IJken MG, ten Hagen TL, Eggermont AM. Prerequisites for effective isolated limb perfusion using tumour necrosis factor alpha and melphalan in rats. Br J Cancer. 1999;80:161–6.
47. Fraker DL, Alexander HR, Andrich M, Rosenberg SA. Treatment of patients with melanoma of the extremity using hyperthermic isolated limb perfusion with melphalan, tumor necrosis factor, and interferon gamma: results of a tumor necrosis factor dose-escalation study. J Clin Oncol. 1996;14:479–89.
48. Hill S, Fawcett WJ, Sheldon J, Soni N, Williams T, Thomas JM. Low-dose tumour necrosis factor alpha and melphalan in hyperthermic isolated limb perfusion. Br J Surg. 1993;80:995–7.
49. Grunhagen DJ, de Wilt JH, van Geel AN, Graveland WJ, Verhoef C, Eggermont AM. TNF dose reduction in isolated limb perfusion. Eur J Surg Oncol. 2005;31:1011–9.
50. Bonvalot S, Laplanche A, Lejeune F, Stoeckle E, Le Péchoux C, Vanel D, Terrier P, Lumbroso J, Ricard M, Antoni G, Cavalcanti A, Robert C, Lassau N, Blay JY, Le Cesne A. Limb salvage with isolated perfusion for soft tissue sarcoma: could less TNF-alpha be better? Ann Oncol. 2005;16:1061–8.
51. Rossi CR, Mocellin S, Pilati P, Foletto M, Campana L, Quintieri L, De Salvo GL, Lise M. Hyperthermic isolated perfusion with low-dose tumor necrosis factor alpha and doxorubicin for the treatment of limb-threatening soft tissue sarcomas. Ann Surg Oncol. 2005;12:398–405.
52. Scott RN, Kerr DJ, Blackie R, Hughes J, Burnside G, MacKie RM, Byrne DS, McKay AJ. The pharmacokinetic advantages of isolated limb perfusion with melphalan for malignant melanoma. Br J Cancer. 1992;66:159–66.
53. Hoven-Gondrie ML, Bastiaannet E, van Ginkel RJ, Suurmeijer AJ, Hoekstra HJ. TNF dose reduction and shortening of duration of isolated limb perfusion for locally advanced soft tissue sarcoma of the extremities is safe and effective in terms of long-term patient outcome. J Surg Oncol. 2011;103:648–55.
54. Deroose JP, Eggermont AM, van Geel AN, et al. Long-term results of tumor necrosis factor alpha- and melphalan-based isolated limb perfusion in locally advanced extremity soft tissue sarcomas. J Clin Oncol. 2011;29:4036–44.
55. Olieman AF, van Ginkel RJ, Hoekstra HJ, Mooyaart EL, Molenaar WM, Schraffordt Koops H. Angiographic response of locally advanced soft-tissue sarcoma following hyperthermic isolated limb perfusion with tumor necrosis factor. Ann Surg Oncol. 1997;4:64–9.
56. Rüegg C, Yilmaz A, Bieler G, Bamat J, Chaubert P, Lejeune FJ. Evidence for the involvement of endothelial cell integrin alphaVbeta3 in the disruption of the tumor vasculature induced by TNF and IFN-gamma. Nat Med. 1998;4:408–14.
57. van Ginkel RJ, Hoekstra HJ, Pruim J, Nieweg OE, Molenaar WM, Paans AM, Willemsen AT, Vaalburg W, Koops HS. FDG-PET to evaluate response to hyperthermic isolated limb perfusion for locally advanced soft-tissue sarcoma. J Nucl Med. 1996;37:984–90.
58. van Ginkel RJ, Kole AC, Nieweg OE, Molenaar WM, Pruim J, Koops HS, Vaalburg W, Hoekstra HJ. L-[1-11C]-tyrosine PET to evaluate response to hyperthermic isolated limb perfusion for locally advanced soft-tissue sarcoma and skin cancer. J Nucl Med. 1999;40:262–7.
59. Been LB, Suurmeijer AJ, Elsinga PH, Jager PL, van Ginkel RJ, Hoekstra HJ. 18F-fluorodeoxythymidine PET for evaluating the response to hyperthermic isolated limb perfusion for locally advanced soft-tissue sarcomas. J Nucl Med. 2007;48:367–72.
60. Alektiar KM, Hong L, Brennan MF, Della-Biancia C, Singer S. Intensity modulated radiation therapy for primary soft tissue sarcoma of the extremity:preliminary results. Int J Radiat Oncol Biol Phys. 2007;68:458–64.
61. Krement ET, Carter RD, Sutherland CM, et al. Chemotherapy of sarcomas of the limb by regional perfusion. Ann Surg. 1977;185:555–64.
62. Muchmore JH, Carter RD, Krementz ET. Regional perfusion for malignant melanoma and soft tissue sarcoma: a review. Cancer Invest. 1985;3:129–43.
63. Stehlin Jr JS, Giovanella BC, Gutierrez AE, et al. 15 years' experience with hyperthermic perfusion for treatment of soft tissue sarcoma and malignant melanoma of the extremities. Front Radiat Ther Oncol. 1984;18:1977–82.

64. Lehti PM, Moseley HS, Janoff K, et al. Improved survival for soft tissue sarcoma of the extremities by regional hyperthermic perfusion, local excision and radiation therapy. Surg Gynecol Obstet. 1986;162:149–52.
65. Krementz ET. Lucy Wortham James lecture. Regional perfusion. Current sophistication, what next? Cancer. 1986;57:416–32.
66. Di Filippo F, Calabrò AM, Cavallari A, et al. The role of hyperthermic perfusion as a first step in the treatment of soft tissue sarcoma of the extremities. World J Surg. 1988;12:332–9.
67. Kettelhack C, Kraus T, Hupp T, et al. Hyperthermic limb perfusion for malignant melanoma and soft tissue sarcoma. Eur J Surg Oncol. 1990;16:370–5.
68. Eggermont AM. Treatment of irresectable soft tissue sarcomas of the limbs by isolation perfusion with high dose TNF-α in combination with γ-interferon and melphalan. In: Fiers W, Buurman WA, editors. Tumor necrosis factor: molecular and cellular biology and clinical relevance. Basel: Karger Publishers; 1993. p. 239–43.
69. Fletcher WS, Pommier RF, Woltering EA, et al. Pharmacokinetics and results of dose escalation in cisplatin hyperthermic isolation limb perfusion. Ann Surg Oncol. 1994;1:236–43.
70. Rossi CR, Vecchiato A, Foletto M, et al. Phase II study on neoadjuvant hyperthermic-antiblastic perfusion with doxorubicin in patients with intermediate or high grade limb sarcomas. Cancer. 1994;73:2140–6.
71. Santinami M, Deraco M, Azzarelli A, et al. Treatment of recurrent sarcoma of the extremities by isolated limb perfusion using tumor necrosis factor alpha and melphalan. Tumori. 1996;82:579–84.
72. Rossi CR, Foletto M, Alessio S, et al. Limb-sparing treatment for soft tissue sarcomas: influence of prognostic factors. J Surg Oncol. 1996;63:3–8.
73. Gutman M, Inbar M, Lev-Shlush D, et al. High dose tumor necrosis factor-alpha and melphalan administered via isolated limb perfusion for advanced limb soft tissue sarcoma results in a >90% response rate and limb preservation. Cancer. 1997;79:1129–37.
74. Olieman AF, Pras E, van Ginkel RJ, et al. Feasibility and efficacy of external beam radiotherapy after hyperthermic isolated limb perfusion with TNF-alpha and melphalan for limb-saving treatment in locally advanced extremity soft-tissue sarcoma. Int J Radiat Oncol Biol Phys. 1998;40:807–14.
75. Olieman AF, van Ginkel RJ, Molenaar WM, et al. Hyperthermic isolated limb perfusion with tumour necrosis factor-alpha and melphalan as palliative limb-saving treatment in patients with locally advanced soft-tissue sarcomas of the extremities with regional or distant metastases. Is it worthwhile? Arch Orthop Trauma Surg. 1998;118:70–4.
76. Lev-Chelouche D, Abu-Abeid S, Merimsky O, et al. Isolated limb perfusion with high-dose tumor necrosis factor alpha and melphalan for Kaposi sarcoma. Arch Surg. 1999;134:177–80.
77. Lev-Chelouche D, Abu-Abeid S, Nakache R, et al. Limb desmoid tumors: a possible role for isolated limb perfusion with tumor necrosis factor-alpha and melphalan. Surgery. 1999;126:963–7.
78. Lev-Chelouche D, Abu-Abeid S, Kollander Y, Meller I, Isakov J, Merimsky O, Klausner JM, Gutman M. Multifocal soft tissue sarcoma: limb salvage following hyperthermic isolated limb perfusion with high-dose tumor necrosis factor and melphalan. J Surg Oncol. 1999;70:185–9.
79. Rossi CR, Foletto M, Di Filippo F, et al. Soft tissue limb sarcomas: Italian clinical trials with hyperthermic antiblastic perfusion. Cancer. 1999;86:1742–9.
80. Lejeune FJ, Pujol N, Liénard D, et al. Limb salvage by neoadjuvant isolated perfusion with TNF-alpha and melphalan for non-resectable soft tissue sarcoma of the extremities. Eur J Surg Oncol. 2000;26:669–78.
81. Hohenberger P, Kettelhack C, Hermann A, et al. Functional outcome after preoperative isolated limb perfusion with rhTNF-alpha/melphalan for high grade extremity sarcoma. Eur J Cancer. 2001;37:S34–5.
82. Lans TE, de Wilt JH, van Geel AN, et al. Isolated limb perfusion with tumor necrosis factor and melphalan for nonresectable Stewart-Treves lymphangiosarcoma. Ann Surg Oncol. 2002;9:1004–9.

83. Noorda EM, Vrouenraets BC, Nieweg OE, et al. Isolated limb perfusion with tumor necrosis factor-alpha and melphalan for patients with unresectable soft tissue sarcoma of the extremities. Cancer. 2003;98:1483–90.
84. van Etten B, van Geel AN, de Wilt JH, et al. Fifty tumor necrosis factor-based isolated limb perfusions for limb salvage in patients older than 75 years with limb-threatening soft tissue sarcomas and other extremity tumors. Ann Surg Oncol. 2003;10:32–7.
85. Di Filippo F, Garinei R, Anzà M, et al. Doxorubicin in isolation limb perfusion in the treatment of advanced limb soft tissue sarcoma. J Exp Clin Cancer Res. 2003;22 Suppl 4:81–7.
86. Feig BW, Ross MI, Hunt KK. A prospective evaluation of isolated limb perfusion with doxorubicin in patients with unresectable extremity sarcomas. Ann Surg Oncol. 2004;11(Suppl):S80 [abstract 98].
87. Grunhagen DJ, de Wilt JH, Verhoef C, et al. TNF-based isolated limb perfusion in unresectable extremity desmoid tumours. Eur J Surg Oncol. 2005;31:912–6.
88. Lans TE, Grünhagen DJ, de Wilt JH, van Geel AN, Eggermont AM. Isolated limb perfusions with tumor necrosis factor and melphalan for locally recurrent soft tissue sarcoma in previously irradiated limbs. Ann Surg Oncol. 2005;12:406–11.
89. Grunhagen DJ, Brunstein F, Graveland WJ, et al. Isolated limb perfusion with tumor necrosis factor and melphalan prevents amputation in patients with multiple sarcomas in arm or leg. Ann Surg Oncol. 2005;12:473–9.
90. Grunhagen DJ, de Wilt JH, Graveland WJ, et al. Outcome and prognostic factor analysis of 217 consecutive isolated limb perfusions with tumor necrosis factor-alpha and melphalan for limb threatening soft tissue sarcoma. Cancer. 2006;106:1776–84.
91. Grunhagen DJ, de Wilt JH, Graveland WJ, et al. The palliative value of tumor necrosis factor alpha-based isolated limb perfusion in patients with metastatic sarcoma and melanoma. Cancer. 2006;106:156–62.
92. Schlag PM, Tunn PU. Isolated limb perfusion with tumor necrosis factor-alpha and melphalan. Dtsch Arztebl. 2007;104:2268–73.
93. Hayes AJ, Neuhaus SJ, Clark MA, Thomas JM. Isolated limb perfusion with melphalan and tumor necrosis factor alpha for advanced melanoma and soft-tissue sarcoma. Ann Surg Oncol. 2007;14:230–8.
94. Thijssens KM, Hoekstra-Weebers JE, van Ginkel RJ, Hoekstra HJ. Quality of life after hyperthermic isolated limb perfusion for locally advanced extremity soft tissue sarcoma. Ann Surg Oncol. 2006;13:864–71.
95. Thijssens KM, van Ginkel RJ, Pras E, Suurmeijer AJ, Hoekstra HJ. Isolated limb perfusion with tumor necrosis factor alpha and melphalan for locally advanced soft tissue sarcoma: the value of adjuvant radiotherapy. Ann Surg Oncol. 2006;13:518–24.
96. van Ginkel RJ, Thijssens KM, Pras E, van der Graaf WT, Suurmeijer AJ, Hoekstra HJ. Isolated limb perfusion with tumor necrosis factor alpha and melphalan for locally advanced soft tissue sarcoma: three time periods at risk for amputation. Ann Surg Oncol. 2007;14:1499–506.
97. Hoven-Gondrie ML, Thijssens KM, Van den Dungen JJ, Loonstra J, van Ginkel RJ, Hoekstra HJ. Long-term locoregional vascular morbidity after isolated limb perfusion and external-beam radiotherapy for soft tissue sarcoma of the extremity. Ann Surg Oncol. 2007;14:2105–12.
98. Pennacchioli E, Deraco M, Mariani L, et al. Advanced extremity soft tissue sarcoma: prognostic effect of isolated limb perfusion in a series of 88 patients treated at a single institution. Ann Surg Oncol. 2007;14:553–9.
99. Cherix S, Speiser M, Matter M, et al. Isolated limb perfusion with tumor necrosis factor and melphalan for non-resectable soft tissue sarcomas:long-term results on efficacy and limb salvage in a selected group of patients. J Surg Oncol. 2008;98:148–55.
100. Hoven-Gondrie ML, Thijssens KM, Geertzen JH, Pras E, van Ginkel RJ, Hoekstra HJ. Isolated limb perfusion and external beam radiotherapy for soft tissue sarcomas of the extremity: long-term effects on normal tissue according to the LENT-SOMA scoring system. Ann Surg Oncol. 2008;15:1502–10.

101. Bonvalot S, Rimareix F, Causeret S, Le Péchoux C, Boulet B, Terrier P, Le Cesne A, Muret J. Hyperthermic isolated limb perfusion in locally advanced soft tissue sarcoma and progressive desmoid-type fibromatosis with TNF 1 mg and melphalan (T1-M HILP) is safe and efficient. Ann Surg Oncol. 2009;16:3350–7.
102. Di Filippo F, Giacomini P, Rossi CR, Santinami M, Garinei R, Anzà M. Hyperthermic isolated perfusion with tumor necrosis factor-alpha and doxorubicin for the treatment of limb-threatening soft tissue sarcoma: the experience of the Italian Society of Integrated Locoregional Treatment in Oncology (SITILO). In Vivo. 2009;23:363–7.
103. Nachmany I, Subhi A, Meller I, Gutman M, Lahat G, Merimsky O, Klausner JM. Efficacy of high vs low dose TNF-isolated limb perfusion for locally advanced soft tissue sarcoma. Eur J Surg Oncol. 2009;35:209–14.
104. Lasithiotakis K, Economou G, Gogas H, Ioannou C, Perisynakis K, Filis D, Kastana O, Bafaloukos D, Decatris M, Catodritis N, Frangia K, Papadakis G, Magarakis M, Tsoutsos D, Chrysos E, Chalkiadakis G, Zoras O. Hyperthermic isolated limb perfusion for recurrent melanomas and soft tissue sarcomas: feasibility and reproducibility in a multi-institutional Hellenic collaborative study. Oncol Rep. 2010;23:1077–83.
105. Wray CJ, Benjamin RS, Hunt KK, Cormier JN, Ross MI, Feig BW. Isolated limb perfusion for unresectable extremity sarcoma: results of 2 single-institution phase 2 trials. Cancer. 2011;117:3235–41.
106. Grabellus F, Kraft C, Sheu-Grabellus SY, Bauer S, Podleska LE, Lauenstein TC, Pöttgen C, Konik MJ, Schmid KW, Taeger G. Tumor vascularization and histopathologic regression of soft tissue sarcomas treated with isolated limb perfusion with TNF-α and melphalan. J Surg Oncol. 2011;103:371–9.
107. Deroose JP, Burger JW, van Geel AN, den Bakker MA, de Jong JS, Eggermont AM, Verhoef C. Radiotherapy for soft tissue sarcomas after isolated limb perfusion and surgical resection: essential for local control in all patients? Ann Surg Oncol. 2011;18:321–7.
108. Deroose JP, van Geel AN, Burger JW, Eggermont AM, Verhoef C. Isolated limb perfusion with TNF-alpha and melphalan for distal parts of the limb in soft tissue sarcoma patients. J Surg Oncol. 2012;105:563–9.
109. van Ginkel RJ, Hoekstra HJ, Eggermont AM, Pras E, Schraffordt Koops H. Isolated limb perfusion of an irradiated foot with tumor necrosis factor, interferon, and melphalan. Arch Surg. 1996;131:672–4.
110. Zwaveling JH, Maring JK, Clarke FL, van Ginkel RJ, Limburg PC, Hoekstra HJ, Schraffordt Koops H, Girbes AR. High plasma tumor necrosis factor (TNF)-alpha concentrations and a sepsis-like syndrome in patients undergoing hyperthermic isolated limb perfusion with recombinant TNF-alpha, interferon-gamma, and melphalan. Crit Care Med. 1996;24:765–70.
111. Vrouenraets BC, Kroon BB, Ogilvie AC, van Geel AN, Nieweg OE, Swaak AJ, Eggermont AM. Absence of severe systemic toxicity after leakage-controlled isolated limb perfusion with tumor necrosis factor-alpha and melphalan. Ann Surg Oncol. 1999;6:405–12.
112. Vrouenraets BC, Eggermont AM, Hart AA, Klaase JM, van Geel AN, Nieweg OE, Kroon BB. Regional toxicity after isolated limb perfusion with melphalan and tumour necrosis factor-alpha versus toxicity after melphalan alone. Eur J Surg Oncol. 2001;27:390–5.
113. Cannon CP, Ballo MT, Zagars GK, et al. Complications of combined modality treatment of primary lower extremity soft-tissue sarcomas. Cancer. 2006;107:2455–61.
114. Friedmann D, Wunder JS, Ferguson P, et al. Incidence and severity of lymphoedema following limb salvage of extremity soft tissue sarcoma. Sarcoma. 2011;2011:289673. Epub 2011.
115. http://dissertations.ub.rug.nl/FILES/faculties/medicine/2006/k.m.j.thijssens/19423_Thijssens.pdf.
116. Seinen JM, Jutte PC, van Ginkel RJ, Pras E, Hoekstra HJ. Treatment associated fractures after multimodality treatment with isolated limb perfusion of soft tissue sarcomas; what to do? 2012; submitted.

117.	Seinen JM, van Ginkel RJ, Hoekstra HJ. How to deal with local limb failure after limb sparing treatment with isolated perfusion with TNFα and Melphalan and delayed surgery for soft tissue sarcoma patients? 2012; submitted.
118.	in't Vrouenraets BC, Veld GJ, Nieweg OE, van Slooten GW, van Dongen JA, Kroon BB. Long-term functional morbidity after mild hyperthermic isolated limb perfusion with melphalan. Eur J Surg Oncol. 1999;25:503–8.
119.	Van Geel AN, van Wijk J, Wieberdink J. Functional morbidity after regional isolated perfusion of the limb for melanoma. Cancer. 1989;63:1092–6.
120.	Thompson JF, Kam PC. Isolated limb infusion for melanoma: a simple but effective alternative to isolated limb perfusion. Surg Oncol. 2004;88:1–3.
121.	Turaga KK, Beasley GM, Kane 3rd JM, et al. Limb preservation with isolated limb infusion for locally advanced nonmelanoma cutaneous and soft-tissue malignant neoplasms. Arch Surg. 2011;146:870–5.
122.	Van Dam GM, Themelis G, Crane LM, et al. Intraoperative tumor-specific imaging in ovarian cancer by folate receptor-a targeting: first in-human results. Nat Med. 2011;17:1315–9.
123.	Mito JK, Ferrer JM, Brigman BE, et al. Intraoperative detection and removal of microscopic residual sarcoma using wide-field imaging. Cancer. 2012;118:5320–30.

Induction Chemotherapy in Treatment of Sarcomas

29

Frederick O. Stephens[†]

The most appropriate place of induction chemotherapy in management of large and aggressive sarcomas remains controversial [1–3]. Early studies showed very encouraging results when intra-arterial infusion chemotherapy was administered as induction treatment continuously for up to 5 or 6 weeks. Results were encouraging for both soft tissue sarcomas and osteosarcomas [4–21].

To achieve an advantage by intra-arterial delivery, the sarcoma must be fully contained in tissue supplied by one or more arteries that can be effectively cannulated and infused. However there were two significant problems in the early experience using regional chemotherapy. First, the numbers of patients treated were not sufficient for randomised studies to be conducted. Second, this management required the services of skilled and experienced medical and nursing staff to be readily available, day or night, for up to 6 weeks in case of the need to readjust the catheter placement or the doses of agents administered otherwise mistakes will be made [22–25].

After some years of surgically inserting intra-arterial catheters, a radiological technique of catheter insertion was developed [9, 11]. Though effective this treatment was expensive in terms of 'inpatient' hospital costs [25] (Fig. 29.1).

In some cases another indication of tumour response to regional chemotherapy can be seen by drawing lines around the palpable tumour periphery at weekly intervals as shown in Fig. 29.2.

CAT scans can also give a good indication of tumour response to chemotherapy in some patients. The CAT scans in Fig. 29.3 show a malignant fibrous histiosarcoma in a thigh before commencing intra-arterial chemotherapy (Fig. 29.3a) and after 3 weeks of continuous chemotherapy when the mass was distinctly smaller (Fig. 29.3b).

[†]Author was deceased at the time of publication

F.O. Stephens
The University of Sydney, Inkerman Street 16, 2088, Mosman, Sydney, NSW, Australia
e-mail: fredstephens@optusnet.com.au

© Springer-Verlag Berlin Heidelberg 2016
K.R. Aigner, F.O. Stephens (eds.), *Induction Chemotherapy,*
DOI 10.1007/978-3-319-28773-7_29

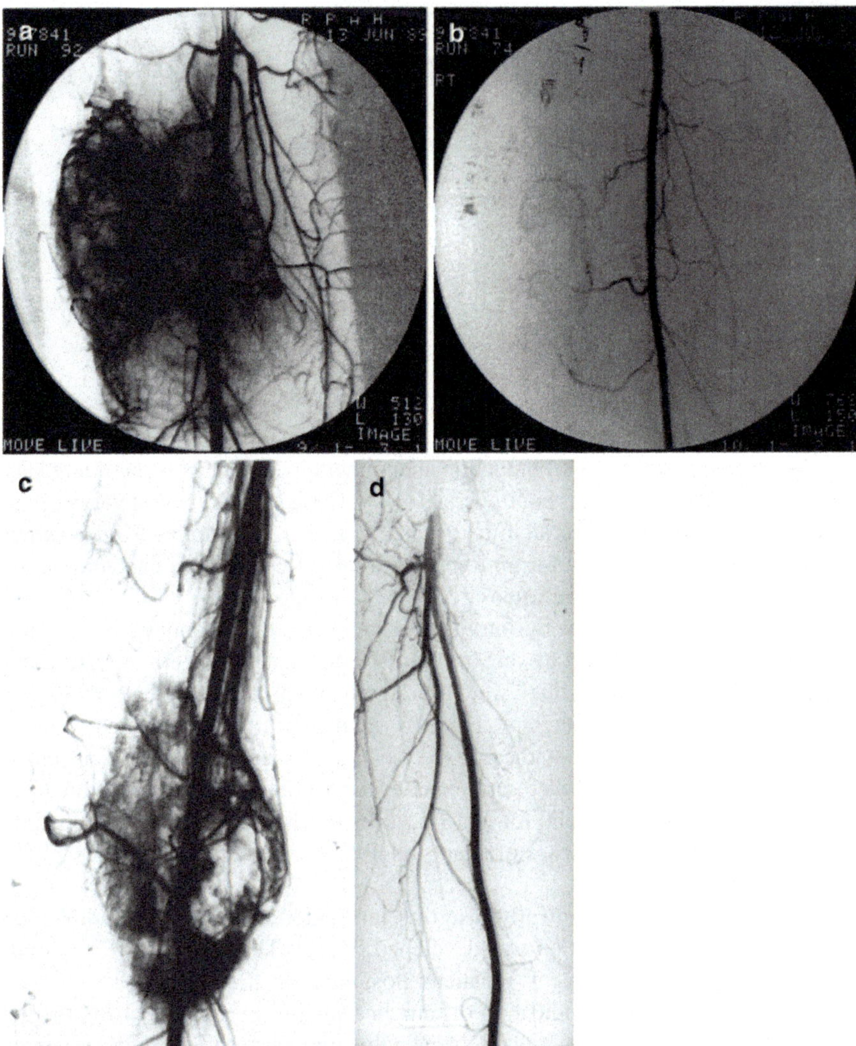

Fig. 29.1 The angiograms show just two of several limb sarcomas treated initially by intra-arterial induction chemotherapy in the Sydney unit. The illustrations (**a, b**) show the vascularity of a large synoviosarcoma of popliteal fossa before and after 4 weeks of chemotherapy infusion into the femoral artery. The illustrations (**c, d**) show a similar tumour vascularity blush before and after 3 weeks intra-arterial chemotherapy infusion given as induction treatment of this malignant fibrous histiocytoma. These reduced cancers were then easily resected without the limb amputations that had originally been proposed. Both patients remained well and without evidence of cancer for the 10 years of follow-up

Effective regional delivery can be managed safely only by experienced clinicians with appropriate equipment. This will reduce risk of mistakes that could be made by these more exacting techniques of delivery [25]. Similar results can be achieved using systemic chemotherapy but the doses required will inevitably cause greater systemic toxicity.

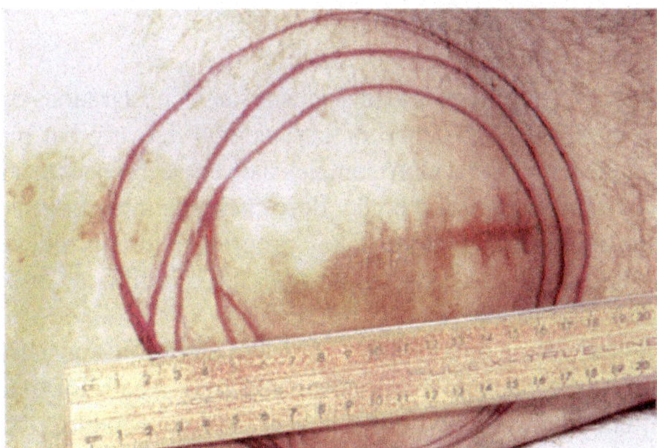

Fig. 29.2 The *circles* around this liposarcoma were drawn at weekly intervals after commencing intra-arterial chemotherapy. Three weeks after completion of chemotherapy, the residual small necrotic mass was excised. The patient was followed-up for 10 years without evidence of residual tumour. The regimen used was adriamycin 20 mg, actinomycin D 0.5 mg and vincristine 0.5 mg on alternate days with oral hydroxyurea 1 g and cyclophosphamide 50 mg on day 4. For 6 months, systemic adjuvant chemotherapy was given postoperatively

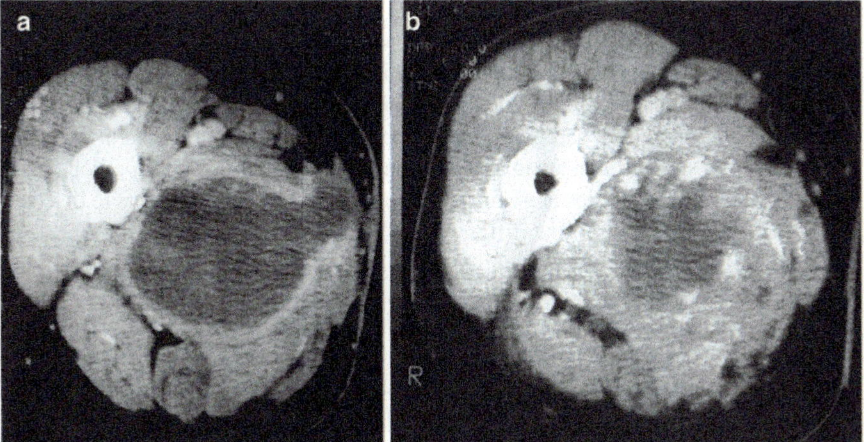

Fig. 29.3 CTs (CAT Scans) (**a**) before and (**b**) after 3 weeks of continuous intra-arterial infusion chemotherapy for a large soft tissue sarcoma of mid thigh

29.1 Radiotherapy

Radiotherapy alone is not so effective in treating any sarcoma as is a combination of radiotherapy and chemotherapy [3].

29.2 Closed Circuit Techniques

Some sarcomas show a poor response to standard safe concentrations of chemotherapy delivered either by standard systemic or intra-arterial delivery but may be made to respond more significantly by the more complex delivery techniques that achieve tumour exposure to more concentrated and higher dose chemotherapy for a short period [26].

Thus short-term closed circuit perfusion programs were introduced. Closed circuit techniques also avoid the need and cost of close continuous in-patient supervision and care for some weeks [27–31].

These results have been encouraging but for such highly specialised techniques highly skilled surgical staff and facilities are required. Again for treatment of large numbers of patients, the costs of such facilities are considerable.

29.3 Systemic Chemotherapy

Induction chemotherapy by systemic delivery is most appropriate in treating sarcomas without a single artery or limited arteries of supply or when the cancers are not contained in a single body cavity. Systemic delivery is also more appropriate when technical skills and facilities for regional delivery are not available or when the patient's general health, poor cooperation or long-term prognosis precludes the additional complexity of regional delivery.

This third and more universally available technique option is to administer most appropriate chemotherapeutic agents by systemic infusion prior to administering radiotherapy and/or surgical resection of the diminished tumour. Such treatment regimens are particularly appropriate for sarcomas that are not confined to a limb or are in sites with multiple arterial supplies that are not readily cannulated, such as the retroperitoneum.

Many randomised studies are being conducted worldwide in attempts to discover most effective regimens to treat different histological sarcoma types and especially sarcomas, the blood supply of which cannot be isolated or cannulated. The major problem with systemic chemotherapy is to determine the most effective combinations of agents used without unacceptable systemic toxicity [3, 32–35].

29.4 Principles and Practice of Induction Chemotherapy

In summary it has been established that chemotherapy alone is unlikely to totally eradicate malignant cells in a large or aggressive sarcomas, but in most cases, initial *induction chemotherapy* will induce changes in tumour size and aggressive characteristics prior to subsequent management. The residual partly or wholly damaged or necrotic primary tumour can then often be eradicated by operative surgery or radiation therapy or by a combination of both radiotherapy and surgery.

It is because at presentation the tumour has a good blood supply, uncompromised by previous radiotherapy or surgery, that chemotherapy, being carried to the tumour in the bloodstream, has a greater therapeutic potential in initially treating such locally advanced tumours. Chemotherapy is much less likely to be effective if the tumour blood supply had been compromised by previous operative surgery or irradiation-induced vascular damage [23]. The most effective combinations and schedules of systemic induction chemotherapy are currently the subject of several studies.

29.5 Other Options

The more complex techniques of hyperthermia with isolated perfusion, stop flow infusion, closed circuit perfusion, chemo-filtration infusion and closed circuit infusion are aimed at achieving even greater localised initial tissue concentrations of chemotherapy than simple intra-arterial infusion. These more complex techniques are described elsewhere in this book but should remain the subject of ongoing studies in highly specialised units.

The limitation to dose and concentration of safe chemotherapy given by systemic administration is the risk of systemic side effects, especially bone marrow suppression.

29.6 Choice of Treatment Options

Certain conditions are necessary for intra-arterial chemotherapy to be justified. These include:

(a) The primary tumour must be supplied by blood vessels (usually one or two) that can be safely cannulated so allowing the greatest potential impact of dose and concentration of the chemotherapy to be delivered by direct infusion into the artery or arteries of supply. Unless the whole tumour periphery is effectively infused, the desired impact on the whole tumour mass will not be achieved.

With some agents (e.g. methotrexate used to treat some osteosarcomas in young people), an effective and adequate local and systemic tumoricidal dose can be safely given by the more simple means of intravenous delivery. There would be no need to deliver such dosage by a more complex intra-arterial delivery system [36].

(b) Administration of regional chemotherapy requires time, effort, expense, special facilities and experienced staff.

29.7 Precautions in the Use of Regional Chemotherapy

Some people have used intra-arterial chemotherapy without first learning the importance of keeping a close vigil to be sure the cannula stays in the correct position and does not stream or slip into an artery supplying blood to another tissue not containing the cancer.

The need for very close and diligent supervision otherwise mistakes will be made is illustrated in Fig. 29.4. The damage done to normal tissues in this patient's

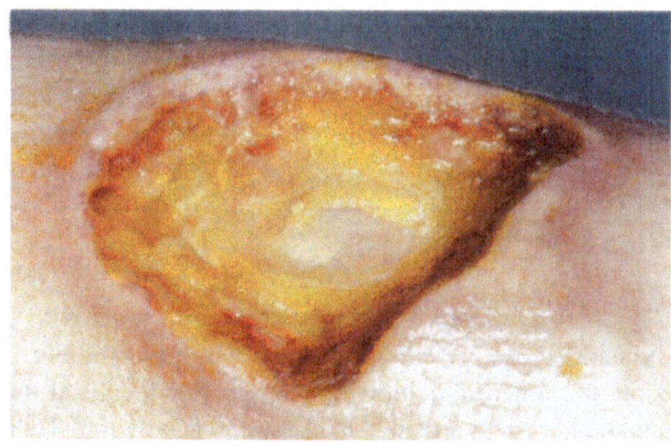

Fig. 29.4 A deep necrotic ulcer developed in this patient's thigh because it had not been noticed the intra-arterial infusion catheter had moved in its position thus causing streaming of the chemotherapy into healthy tissues rather than into the cancer

thigh was because it had not been noticed that the chemotherapy had been flowing into a branch of the artery into which it had previously been placed. A red blush had appeared in the skin of this patient's thigh, but the significance of this was not understood. Disulphan blue or patent-blue dye injected into the infusion cannula at an early stage would have confirmed that the cannula position needed adjustment before serious tissue damage had occurred.

Without the services of well-trained and experienced nurses to constantly watch for such errors, intra-arterial infusions of chemotherapy can cause such problems. This is an example of why intra-arterial chemotherapy is not practised in some cancer clinics without these facilities [22–25].

References

1. Benjamen RS, Chawla SP, Carrasco CH, et al. Preoperative chemotherapy for osteosarcoma with intravenous adriamycin and intra-arterial cisplatinum. Ann Oncol. 1992;3 Suppl 2:53–6.
2. Eilber FR, Giulano AE, Huth JF, et al. Intravenous (IV) vs. intraarterial (IA) adriamycin, 2800r radiation and surgical resection for extremity soft-tissue sarcomas: a randomized prospective trial. Proc Am Soc Clin Oncol. 1990;9:309.
3. Pisters PWT, O'Sullivan B, Maki RG. Evidence-based recommendations for local therapy for soft tissue sarcomas. J Clin Oncol. 2007;25:1003–8.
4. Stephens FO. CRAB chemotherapy. Med J Aust. 1976;2:41–6.
5. Stephens FO, Crea P, Harker GJS, Lonergan DM. Intra-arterial infusion chemotherapy in salvage of limbs involved with advanced neoplasms. ANZ J Surg. 1980;50:387–92.
6. Stephens FO, Harker GJS, Crea P. The intra-arterial infusion of chemotherapeutic agents as "basal" treatment of cancer: evidence of increased drug activity in regionally infused tissues. ANZ J Surg. 1980;50:597–602.
7. Stephens FO, Stevens MM, McCarthy SW, Johnson N, Packham NA, Richie JD. Treatment of advanced and inaccessible sarcomas with continuous intra-arterial chemotherapy prior to definitive surgery or radiotherapy – a possible alternative to amputation or disabling radical surgery. ANZ J Surg. 1987;57:435–40.
8. Stephens FO, Marsden W, Tattersall MHN. Experience in avoiding amputation or mutilating surgery by the management of large and aggressive sarcomas with intra-arterial chemotherapy followed by radiotherapy and/or surgery. Proceedings of the 3rd international conference on advances in regional cancer therapy, University of Ulm, Ulm; September 1987.

9. Stephens FO, Tattersall MNH, Marsden W, Waugh RC, Green D, McCarthy SW. Regional chemotherapy with the use of cisplatin and doxorubicin as primary treatment for advanced sarcomas in shoulder, pelvis and thigh. Cancer. 1987;60:724–35.

10. Stephens FO. The influence of intra-arterial chemotherapy on local control of bone sarcoma. In: Yamamuro T, editor. New developments for limb salvage in musculo-skeletal tumours. Tokyo: Springer; 1989. p. 193–8.

11. Marsden FW, Stephens FO, Tattersall MHN, McCarthy SW, Waugh R. The influence of intra-arterial chemotherapy on local control of bone sarcoma. In: Yamamoto T, editor. New developments for limb salvage in musculo-skeletal tumours. Tokyo: Springer; 1989. p. 193–8.

12. Marsden FW, Stephens FO, McCarthy SW, Ferrari SM. IIB osteosarcoma: current management, local control and survival statistics – experience in Australia. Clin Orthop Relat Res. 1991;(270):113–19.

13. Stephens FO. Developments in surgical oncology: induction (neo-adjuvant) chemotherapy – the state of the art. Clin Oncol. 1990;2:168–72.

14. Stephens FO, Marsden W, Tattersall MHN. Regional induction chemotherapy followed by radiotherapy and/or surgery in management of large and aggressive sarcomas in shoulder, pelvis and limbs. In: Jakesz R, Rainer H, editors. Progress in regional cancer therapy. Berlin: Springer; 1990. p. 160–7.

15. Stephens FO, Marsden FW, Storey DW, Thompson JF, McCarthy WH, Renwick SB, et al. Developments in surgical oncology – past, present and future trends. Med J Aust. 1991;155:803–7.

16. Stephens FO, Marsden W. Intra-arterial induction (neo-adjuvant) chemotherapy with limb salvage surgery in management of patients with locally advanced sarcomas in pelvis, buttocks, shoulders and limbs. Proceedings of the 3rd international congress on neo-adjuvant chemotherapy, Paris; 1991.

17. Soulen MC, Weissmann JR, Sullivan KL, et al. Intraarterial chemotherapy with limb-sparing resection of large soft-tissue sarcomas of the extremities. J Vasc Interv Radiol. 1992;3:659–63.

18. Pennington DG, Marsden FW, Stephens FO. Fibrosarcoma of metacarpal treated by combined therapy and immediate reconstruction with vascularised bone graft. J Hand Surg Am. 1991;16(5):877–81.

19. Mccarthy SW, Marsden FW, Stephens FO. Intra-arterial induction chemotherapy as initial management of patients with large and aggressive sarcomas. Reg Cancer Treat. 1993;6:155–6.

20. Stephens FO. Induction [neo-adjuvant] chemotherapy systemic and arterial delivery techniques and their clinical applications. ANZ J Surg. 1995;65:699–707.

21. Stephens FO. Induction [neo-adjuvant] chemotherapy: the place and techniques of using chemotherapy to downgrade aggressive or advanced localised cancers to make them potentially more curable by surgery and/or radiotherapy. Eur J Surg Oncol. 2001;27(7):627–88.

22. Bezwade HP, Granick MS, Long CD, et al. Soft-tissue complications of intra-arterial chemotherapy for extremity sarcomas. Ann Plast Surg. 1998;40:382–7.

23. Stephens FO. Intra-arterial perfusion of the chemotherapeutic agents methotrexate and "Epodyl" in patients with advanced localised carcinomata recurrent after radiotherapy. ANZ J Surg. 1970;39:371–9.

24. Stephens FO, Aigner KR. Basics of oncology. Dordrecht: Springer; 2009.

25. Davis AM, O'Sullivan B, Bell RS, et al. Function and health status outcomes in a randomised trial comparing preoperative and postoperative radiotherapy in extremity soft tissue sarcoma. J Clin Oncol. 2002;20(22):4472–7.

26. Eggermont AM, Shraffordt Koops H, Klausner JM, et al. Isolated limb perfusion with tumor necrosis factor and melphalan for limb salvage in 186 patients with locally advanced soft tissue extremity sarcomas. The cumulative multicenter European experience. Ann Surg. 1996;224:756–65.

27. Eggermont AMM, Schraffordt Koops H, Liénard D, et al. Isolated limb perfusion with high-dose tumor necrosis factor-α in combination with interferon-χ and melphalan for nonresectable extremity soft tissue sarcomas: a multicenter trial. J Clin Oncol. 1996;14:2653–65.

28. Bonvalot S, Laplanche A, Lejeune F, et al. Limb salvage with isolated perfusion for soft tissue sarcoma: could less TNF-α be better? Ann Oncol. 2005;16:1061–8.
29. Cherix S, Speiser M, Matter M, et al. Isolated limb perfusion with tumor necrosis factor and melphalan for non-resectable soft tissue sarcomas: long-term results on efficacy and limb salvage in a selected group of patients. J Surg Oncol. 2008;98:148–55.
30. Grünhagen DJ, de Wilt JHW, van Geel AN, et al. TNF dose reduction in isolated limb perfusion. Eur J Surg Oncol. 2005;31:1011–9.
31. Hohenberger P, Wysocki WM. Neoadjuvant treatment of locally advanced soft tissue sarcoma of the limbs: which treatment to choose? Oncologist. 2008;13:175–86.
32. Le Cesne A, Judson I, Crowther D, et al. Randomized phase III study comparing conventional dose doxorubicin plus ifosfamide versus high dose doxorubicin plus ifosfamide plus rhGMCSF in advanced soft tissue sarcomas: 2000. J Clin Oncol. 2000;18(14):2676–84.
33. Milano A, Apice GG, Ferrari E, et al. New emerging drugs in soft tissue sarcoma. Crit Rev Oncol Hematol. 2006;59:74–84.
34. Eilber FC, Tap WD, Nelson SD, et al. Advances in chemotherapy for patients with extremity soft tissue sarcoma. Orthop Clin N Am. 2006;37:15–22.
35. Lewis SJ, Wunder JS, Couture J, et al. Soft tissue sarcomas involving the pelvis. J Surg Oncol. 2001;77:8–14.
36. Jaffe N. Osteosarcoma: review of the past, impact on the future. The American experience. Cancer Treat Res. 2009;152:239–62.

Isolation Perfusion Systems: Lungs

30

Jeroen Maria Hendriks, Willem den Hengst, and Paul Emile Van Schil

Several techniques of isolated lung perfusion are described since 1958 [1], including single-lung perfusion [2–9] and total lung perfusion with extracorporeal circuits [10], and also hyperthermic conditions as high as 44.4 °C for 2 h were studied [11, 12]. Nowadays, a single-lung perfusion is most frequently used, and differences between reported techniques are related to the perfusion circuit (with or without oxygenator), to the patient population (operable versus inoperable), to the drugs that are used within the circuit, and whether it is combined with surgical resection or not.

The technique of isolated lung perfusion that is used at the Antwerp University Hospital is described in our report of the phase-I dose-escalating trial [3] and is combined with a complete metastasectomy. It was shown by Schröder et al. that a complete metastasectomy with subsequent isolated lung perfusion during one operation was feasible and technically safe without an increase in mortality or morbidity [8], and therefore it became our approach of choice. The procedure is performed through a muscle-sparing thoracotomy unless a posterolateral thoracotomy is needed for anatomical reasons. In case of bilateral disease, staged thoracotomies are planned with an interval of 4–8 weeks. This interval allows adequate observation of (sub)acute toxicity while leaving time for the patient to recover. Once the thoracic cage is entered, all nodules are palpated and their anatomic localization is documented before starting isolated lung perfusion. In case no preoperative histologic diagnosis is present, frozen section of one of the tumor nodules is performed to obtain pathological confirmation of metastatic disease. If frozen section is negative for pulmonary metastases, further analysis is done of other nodules until metastatic disease is confirmed. Next, the main pulmonary artery and both pulmonary veins are isolated. The pericardium is opened to clamp the pulmonary artery and veins centrally. The patient is systemically anticoagulated with intravenous heparin up to

J.M. Hendriks • W. den Hengst • P.E. Van Schil (✉)
Department of Thoracic and Vascular Surgery, Antwerp University Hospital, Edegem, Belgium
e-mail: paul.van.schil@uza.be

© Springer-Verlag Berlin Heidelberg 2016
K.R. Aigner, F.O. Stephens (eds.), *Induction Chemotherapy,*
DOI 10.1007/978-3-319-28773-7_30

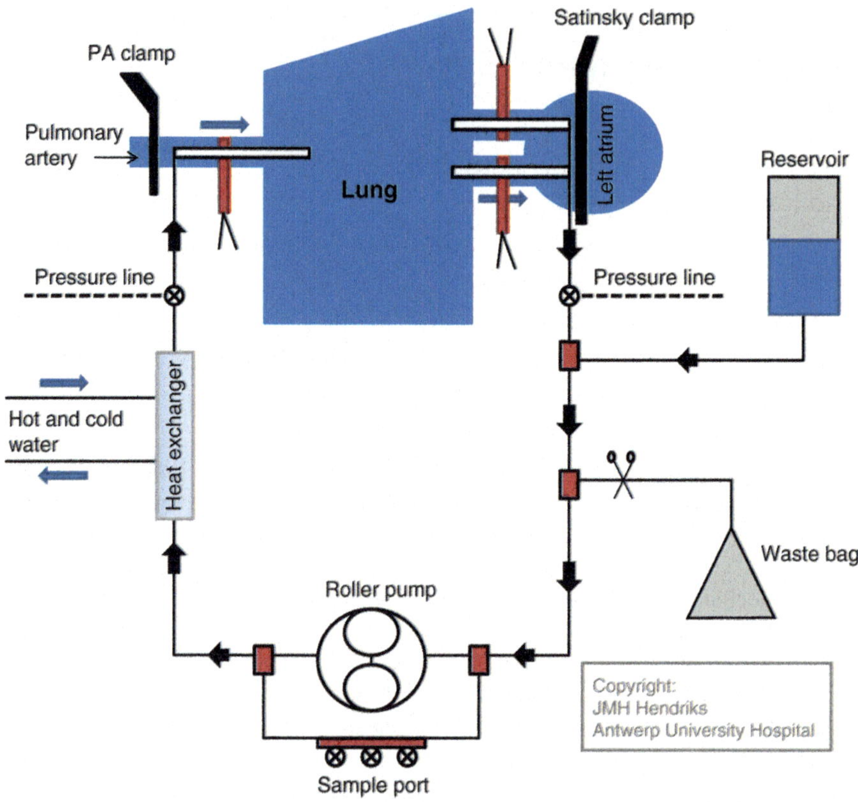

Fig. 30.1 Circuit of isolated lung perfusion (note that no oxygenator is incorporated into the circuit) (Copyright: JMH Hendriks Antwerb University Hospital)

an activated clotting time (ACT) of above 200 s. The pulmonary artery and veins are cannulated by standard techniques (Figs. 30.1, 30.2, and 30.3), and the main bronchus is snared in order to occlude bronchial arterial blood flow. The cannulas are connected to a perfusion circuit (Fig. 30.1) with a small priming volume (approximately 1 L), which only consists of a centrifugal pump, a heat exchanger, and special extracorporeal circuit tubings. No filter is incorporated. This way we try to avoid a washout of the chemotherapeutic agent. The perfusion is carried out for a period of 30 min in case of isolated lung perfusion with melphalan. The flow rate is calculated preoperatively (based on the weight and length of the patient) but adjusted to a mean pulmonary artery pressure below 30 mm of mercury to avoid pulmonary edema. After stabilization of temperature and flow, and without signs of leakage (loss of priming volume out of the circuit), melphalan is injected into the circuit as a bolus through the pulmonary artery line. Detection of leakage with radioactive tracers during isolated lung perfusion was not performed in our institution so far, but is advised when using more aggressive agents like tumor necrosis factor which can be life-threatening even with minimal leaks [6]. During perfusion, the lungs are ventilated

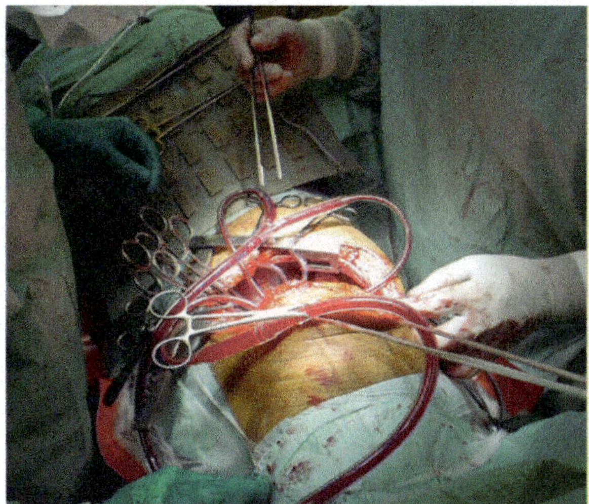

Fig. 30.2 View of the operative field (left muscle-sparing thoracotomy)

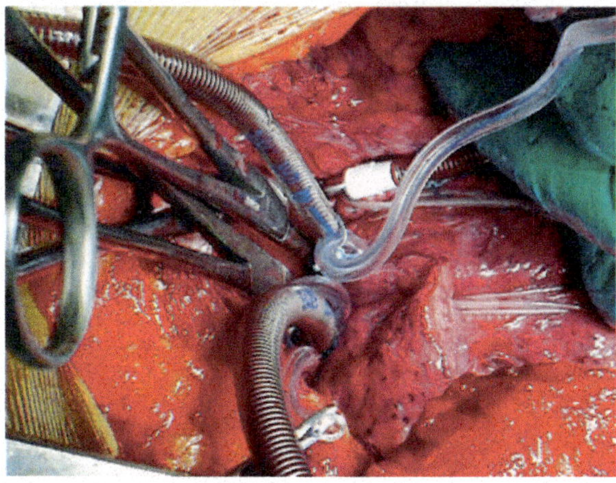

Fig. 30.3 Cannulas are placed in the pulmonary artery and both pulmonary veins

to ensure homogeneous distribution of the chemotherapeutic agent in the lung. After 30 min of perfusion, melphalan is washed out of the lung with a total of three times the priming volume. At the end of the washing period, the cannulas are removed, the arteriotomy and the venotomies repaired, and the clamps removed after de-airing, restoring blood flow to the lung. After correcting the ACT, a complete metastasectomy is performed. Schröder et al. recommended to perform surgery before isolated lung perfusion based on their experience with four patients. They had difficulty to identify metastatic nodules due to the edematous lung tissue after isolated lung perfusion [8]. In our experience, we choose to identify and record all metastatic disease before cannulating the pulmonary artery and veins. Next, isolated lung perfusion is performed before metastasectomy in order to have a homogenous perfusion of the drug throughout the lung since resection of nodules and staple lines can disturb this. In addition, less bleeding will occur at the sites of resection because heparin is corrected with protamine before a resection is performed.

References

1. Creech O, Krementz ET, Ryan RF, Winblad JN. Chemotherapy of cancer: regional perfusion utilizing an extracorporeal circuit. Ann Surg. 1958;148:616–32.
2. Burt ME, Liu D, Abolhoda A, et al. Isolated lung perfusion for patients with unresectable metastases from sarcoma: a phase I trial. Ann Thorac Surg. 2000;69:1542–9.
3. Hendriks JM, Grootenboers MJ, Schramel FM, et al. Isolated lung perfusion with melphalan for resectable lung metastases: a phase I clinical trial. Ann Thorac Surg. 2004;78:1919–27.
4. Johnston MR, Minchin R, Shull JH, et al. Isolated lung perfusion with adriamycin. A preclinical study. Cancer. 1983;53:404–9.
5. Johnston MR, Christensen CW, Minchin RF, et al. Isolated total lung perfusion as a means to deliver organ-specific chemotherapy: long-term studies in animals. Surgery. 1985;98:35–44.
6. Pass HI, Mew DJ, Kranda KC, Temeck BK, Donington JS, Rosenberg SA. Isolated lung perfusion with tumor necrosis factor for pulmonary metastases. Ann Thorac Surg. 1996;61:1609–17.
7. Ratto GB, Toma S, Civalleri D, et al. Isolated lung perfusion with platinum in the treatment of pulmonary metastases from soft tissue sarcomas. J Thorac Cardiovasc Surg. 1996;112:614–22.
8. Schröder C, Fisher S, Pieck AC, et al. Technique and results of hyperthermic isolated lung perfusion with high-doses of cisplatin for the treatment of surgically relapsing or unresectable lung sarcoma metastasis. Eur J Cardiothorac Surg. 2002;22:41–6.
9. Schrump DS, Zhai S, Nguyen DM, et al. Pharmacokinetics of paclitaxel administered by hyperthermic retrograde isolated lung perfusion techniques. J Thorac Cardiovasc Surg. 2002;123:686–94.
10. Johnston MR, Minchin RF, Dawson CA. Lung perfusion with chemotherapy in patients with unresectable metastatic sarcoma to the lung or diffuse bronchioloalveolar carcinoma. J Thorac Cardiovasc Surg. 1995;110:368–73.
11. Cowen M, Mulvin D, Howard R, et al. Lung tolerance to hyperthermia by in vivo perfusion. Eur J Cardiothorac Surg. 1992;6:167–73.
12. Rickaby D, Fehring J, Johnston M, et al. Tolerance of the isolated perfused lung to hyperthermia. J Thorac Cardiovasc Surg. 1991;101:732–9.

Paul Emile Van Schil, Willem den Hengst,
and Jeroen Maria Hendriks

31.1   Introduction

For selected cases, surgical resection of lung metastases is a widely accepted procedure but due to local and distant recurrences, reported 5-year survival rates are only 30–40 %. Main prognostic factors are histological type and complete resection. A better survival is reported in patients with a single metastasis who have a disease-free survival of more than 3 years [1]. Reoperations are feasible, but often patients become inoperable due to insufficient pulmonary reserve and new treatment modalities are looked for [2]. The maximal dose of intravenous chemotherapy is limited due to systemic side effects, mainly haematological. As isolated limb and liver perfusion, isolated lung perfusion (ILuP) has the advantage of selectively delivering an agent into the lung while diverting the venous effluent. Other techniques to deliver high-dose locoregional chemotherapy in the lung are also investigated, and these include chemo-embolization, embolic trapping of loaded particles in the pulmonary circulation and pulmonary artery infusion where a cytostatic drug is injected in the pulmonary artery without control of the venous effluent. This is mostly performed with a balloon catheter inflated in the pulmonary artery, so-called blood flow occlusion, right after the injection of the chemotherapeutic agent. In this way, the pulmonary circulation is temporarily arrested to allow a better uptake of the injected drug in the lung parenchyma.

In this review, surgical resection for lung metastases is discussed, followed by a summary of clinical studies performed until now with the intent to deliver high-dose chemotherapy to the lung parenchyma.

P.E. Van Schil (✉) • W. den Hengst • J.M. Hendriks
Department of Thoracic and Vascular Surgery, Antwerp University Hospital,
Antwerp, Belgium
e-mail: paul.van.schil@uza.be

© Springer-Verlag Berlin Heidelberg 2016
K.R. Aigner, F.O. Stephens (eds.), *Induction Chemotherapy*,
DOI 10.1007/978-3-319-28773-7_31

31.2 Surgery for Pulmonary Metastases

Due to their filtering capacity for the entire circulation, the lung and liver are common sites for malignant spread. Two distinct patterns of haematogenous metastases exist, the portal and caval type. The portal type mainly metastasises to the liver and the caval type to the lungs. Among patients with metastatic cancer, 20–30 % will have secondary spread to the lung according to necropsy series.

In 1786, John Hunter reported the first case in history of pulmonary metastases. The primary cancer was a malignant tumour of the femur, and the patient died of widespread pulmonary deposits only 7 weeks after the leg had been amputated. It took about 141 years before the first successful resection of a true pulmonary metastasis was performed by Divis in 1927 [3]. A well-known case was reported in 1939 by Barney and Churchill who removed a solitary lung mass by lobectomy which proved to be a metastasis from a renal cell carcinoma [4]. The patient subsequently had a nephrectomy for the primary tumour and survived for over 20 years without any evidence of recurrence.

Although no prospective randomised trials are available which demonstrate a survival benefit, surgical resection is a widely accepted treatment for certain pulmonary metastases. Retrospective studies are in favour of surgical resection for some lung metastases. An aggressive approach in carefully selected patients is indicated after careful evaluation by an interdisciplinary oncological team consisting of oncologists, thoracic surgeons and radiotherapists.

The specific criteria for pulmonary metastasectomy, as originally described by Ehrenhaft and colleagues nearly 40 years ago, have changed little despite the availability of chemotherapy and radiation therapy as alternative therapeutic options [5]. These criteria include radical treatment of the primary tumour, absence of extrathoracic metastases and low operative risk and the fact that complete resection can be performed and no alternative treatment is available with a better outcome. Ongoing discussions in the surgical treatment of pulmonary metastases focus on the preoperative imaging of lung metastases, the optimal surgical approach including video-assisted thoracoscopic surgery (VATS), the role of adjuvant therapy and the maximum number of resectable lesions and reoperation for recurrences.

Preoperative imaging by chest CT misses between 21 and 36 % of all the malignant nodules present inside the lung. The only way to discover those is by thoracotomy and digital palpation [6–8]. VATS is therefore mostly indicated for diagnosis but can be utilised for definitive treatment when only one small peripheral lesion is present on chest CT [9, 10]. However, if there is any doubt or the peroperative findings do not represent the preoperative imaging, conversion is indicated. In case of surgical resection, a systematic nodal dissection is advocated as for primary lung cancer [11]. Approximately 20 % of patients will also have lymph node involvement which heralds a poor prognosis [12].

Other than chemotherapy for pulmonary metastatic tumours of the testicle, breast cancer and germ cell cancer, surgical resection is still the primary treatment for metastatic disease if a complete resection is possible [13]. In germ cell tumours, resection of lung metastases and lymph nodes has an adjuvant role after chemotherapy, to confirm complete pathological remission and to remove any mature teratoma that may cause obstructive symptoms [14]. In patients with prior breast cancer, resection of metastatic disease is a valid therapeutic option and offers a real chance of cure in case of a new primary lung cancer [15, 16]. Patients who may benefit from pulmonary metastasectomy are those with various types of head and neck cancer, tumours of endocrine origin, colorectal cancer, renal cell cancer and sarcoma [17–21]. This is specially true for squamous cell carcinoma of the head and neck region, where a new lung nodule may represent a primary lung cancer instead of a lung metastasis.

An additional problem with these chemotherapy-resistant tumours is the high frequency of secondary pulmonary recurrences, probably due to micrometastases present in the lung at the time of pulmonary resection, resulting in a high recurrence rate and low long-term survival [1, 22].

Results of an international registry of 5,206 cases of lung metastasectomy operated from 1991 to 1995 were reported in 1997 by U. Pastorino [1]. This is the largest reported series on surgical resection of pulmonary metastases. Complete resection was possible in 88 % of cases. Overall mortality was 1 %. Mean follow-up was 46 months. In case of complete resection, median survival time (MST) was 35 months and for incomplete resection only 15 months. Metastases to hilar or mediastinal lymph nodes were present in 5 % of cases, indicating a poor prognosis. After a second metastasectomy, a 10-year survival of 29 % was obtained.

A multivariate analysis was performed on patients who underwent a complete resection. Significant prognostic factors were primary tumour type, disease-free interval and number of metastases [1].

What are the technical limitations of thoracic surgery? Resection of pulmonary metastases by pneumonectomy or beyond pneumonectomy is exceptional. However, in carefully selected patients, extensive resections might be successfully performed with an operative mortality less than 5 % and a 5-year survival rate of 20 % following complete resection [23]. In our own series reported in 2001, eight patients underwent a primary or completion pneumonectomy indicating the limit of our surgical possibilities [22]. These extensive operations may be offered to selected patients with isolated primary or recurrent pulmonary metastases, sufficient pulmonary reserve and prognostic favourable primary tumours as colorectal and renal cell carcinoma.

As shown by the International Registry and also in our own series, most patients who underwent resection of lung metastases from primary carcinomas or sarcomas will have recurrent disease inside the chest [1, 22]. For this reason, combined modality therapies including surgery and chemotherapy are currently evaluated to obtain a better local control and improve overall survival. Methods to deliver high-dose locoregional chemotherapy will be further discussed in this review.

31.3 High-Dose Locoregional Chemotherapy: Rationale and Historical Review

The poor results of surgical resection of pulmonary metastases from certain tumours combined with intravenous chemotherapy are probably due to genetic drug resistance and the inability to achieve effective drug concentrations within the tumour mass, the so-called first-order targeting [24, 25]. This implies that better chemotherapeutic agents and more efficient drug delivery as an adjuvant to surgery are needed. Specific biophysical methods to improve drug targeting in lung parenchyma include embolic trapping (chemo-embolization), regional infusion in the pulmonary artery without control of the venous effluent and ILuP in which the lung is completely separated from the systemic circulation [25].

These are all promising techniques for the treatment of tumours metastatic to the lungs which do not respond to conventional systemic chemotherapy [24]. ILuP has the advantage of both selectively delivering an agent and diverting the venous effluent. This allows a drug to be delivered in a higher dose, while drug levels in critical organs that are relatively sensitive to the drug are kept low enough to avoid severe complications. An additional advantage is the prevention or delay of loss of active drug through metabolism.

Creech was the first to report a method of pulmonary perfusion in 1959 [26]. He perfused both lungs simultaneously with divided circuits for systemic and pulmonary circulations. Krementz, a co-author of the paper of 1959, commented in 1986 that four patients had undergone lung perfusion of which one experienced an impressive clinical response but two others died postoperatively. It was the first clinical report of lung perfusion for the treatment of cancer [27]. In 1983, Johnston put the basis for further clinical and experimental studies by showing ILuP to be a reproducible and safe technique [28, 29]. He determined a dosage of Adriamycin (doxorubicin) without apparent systemic toxicity in a dog model, without any control of the bronchial arterial circulation. This can be explained by experimental, autopsy and clinical studies which show that a significant portion of both pulmonary and metastatic tumour vasculature is fed by the pulmonary circulation. On the other hand, bronchial artery infusion is the desired route in primary bronchogenic carcinoma. Milne also showed that primary lung tumours are predominantly vascularised by the bronchial arteries, whereas in lung metastases, the pulmonary artery is predominant: 48 % of all lung metastases receive their nutrition from the pulmonary artery only, 16 % from bronchial arteries only and 36 % have a dual vascularisation [30]. Mochizuki et al. evaluated vascular supply pattern through first-pass dynamic CT in differentiating solitary pulmonary nodules [31]. Based on the final diagnosis, they concluded that a pulmonary artery pattern was a good indicator of metastatic lung tumours or inflammatory nodules in contrast with the aortic supply pattern which was a better indicator of primary bronchogenic carcinoma.

Toxicity after ILuP, as documented by Johnston, was closely related to drug uptake in the lung and concentration of the drug in the perfusate [29]. Lactate dehydrogenase levels in perfusate and postperfusate serum indicating cell necrosis showed dose-dependent increases. These dose-dependent relations were also found by Baciewicz at a lower dose [32]. This could be explained by the use of mild hyperthermia (39 °C) which may increase doxorubicin uptake into the perfused lung tissue.

A second step forward was the development of a surgical procedure by Johnston that allowed both lungs to be perfused simultaneously. As lung metastases may present bilaterally, the advantage of total lung perfusion is obvious [33].

These initial reports stimulated further experimental and clinical research in ILuP and related methods to deliver high-dose chemotherapy to the lung parenchyma. Our current clinical technique of ILuP is described in Chap. 25.

31.4 Recent Clinical Studies of High-Dose Locoregional Chemotherapy

In the clinical setting, a small number of phase I trials and only one phase II trial have been completed until now [7, 34–48].

31.4.1 Pulmonary Artery Perfusion with Blood Flow Occlusion

Blades et al. were the first to report pulmonary artery perfusion with blood flow occlusion in 1958 [34]. With this technique, a balloon catheter provides local lung perfusion by endovascular means. Balloon insufflation blocks the pulmonary circulation, allowing the chemotherapeutic agent to diffuse into the lung tissue. A second clinical report about this technique was published in 1981 by Karakousis et al. [35]. They performed 56 selective lobar perfusions in 7 patients with Adriamycin. They used this technique in patients with metastatic soft tissue sarcomas who had intrapulmonary recurrence under systemic chemotherapy. Adriamycin was used in small doses of 10–20 mg. One pneumothorax and three infiltrates that resolved without intervention were detected. During this study, only one partial responder was found. After this trial, no other clinical studies evaluating this method have been reported. However, with the increasing abilities to perform endovascular techniques, and the promising results in some animal studies, there is a renewed interest for this non-invasive repeatable type of treatment [49–53].

31.4.2 Chemo-embolization (Embolic Trapping)

The technique of transpulmonary chemo-embolization was applied by Vogl and colleagues in 52 patients with 106 unresectable lung metastases [48]. Microspheres combined with mitomycin C were injected by a pulmonary artery catheter with balloon protection. There were no complications. Regression was observed in 16 patients, stable disease in 11 and progressive disease in 25. Further phase I studies are necessary to determine the maximum tolerated dose (MTD) and precise toxicity of this procedure.

31.4.3 Isolated Lung Perfusion (ILuP)

The group of Johnston performed a pilot clinical trial of ILuP based on the insight gained in their previous experimental studies. The trial consisted of four patients with unresectable metastatic sarcoma to the lung and four patients with diffuse bronchioloalveolar carcinoma [41]. There were no intraoperative complications. No objective clinical responses were seen and all patients died of progressive disease 23–151 days after perfusion. However, this study demonstrated that the complex procedure of ILuP was well tolerated and reproducible [41].

Most agents tested in laboratory settings were subsequently investigated in human phase I trials. As it is difficult to extrapolate results of animal studies into a clinical setting, most protocols in patients study the feasibility of ILuP in resectable or unresectable lung metastases and determine dose-limiting toxicity (DLT) and MTD of the chemotherapeutic agent used in ILuP. Incremental dosages are used, and MTD is defined as one dose level below DLT. Clinical studies from 1995 on are summarised in Table 31.1 [7, 36, 38, 40–45].

31.4.3.1 Doxorubicin

In the pilot study by Johnston et al., four patients with pulmonary metastatic sarcoma and four patients with diffuse bronchioloalveolar carcinoma were treated with doxorubicin and cisplatin via ILuP [41]. Six patients were perfused with doxorubicin and two with cisplatin. The latter are discussed further under the heading cisplatin.

Single left lung perfusion was performed in three patients and total lung perfusion in five patients. Perfusion time ranged from 45 to 60 min at ambient or normothermic temperatures, except for one patient who underwent perfusion at moderate hyperthermia of 40 °C.

Pulmonary perfusate drug concentrations increased with higher doxorubicin dosages. Drug tissue levels also tended to increase with higher doses with only minimal systemic leakage.

No intraoperative complications occurred but there was one postoperative complication. This patient developed pneumonia with subsequent sternal dehiscence. The pneumonia responded to antibiotics and the sternal non-union was treated conservatively as it was asymptomatic [41]. None of the eight patients had a partial or complete response to the regional chemotherapy and all died of progressive disease 23–151 days after lung perfusion.

Burt et al. described their results of ILuP with doxorubicin after extensive laboratory research [36]. Eight patients with inoperable lung metastases from sarcoma underwent single-lung perfusion in a phase I protocol. Intrapulmonary concentrations of doxorubicin correlated with the dose given, while systemic levels were minimal or undetectable. However, tumour levels were lower compared to lung levels. The MTD in this study was defined at 40 mg/m^2 of doxorubicin since an important chemical pneumonitis developed in one patient at a dose of 80 mg/m^2. On postoperative lung scanning, no ventilation or perfusion was present at the perfused lung in this patient. No perioperative deaths were encountered. There were no partial or complete responses. One patient had stabilisation of disease in the perfused lung, whereas the lesions in the untreated lung progressed markedly. In the seven patients perfused with 40 mg/m^2 or less of doxorubicin, there was a significant decrease in the forced expiratory volume in 1 s and a trend towards a significant decrease in diffusing capacity [36].

Table 31.1 Human isolated lung perfusion studies from 1995 on

Year	Authors	Ref.	Drug	n	Lung temp. (°C)	Perfusion time (min)	Resectable metastases	MTD
1995	Johnston et al.	[41]	Doxorubicin/cisplatin	8	NA	45–60	No	NA
1996	Pass et al.	[42]	TNF-α + γ-interferon	15	38–39.5	90	No	6 mg
1996	Ratto et al.	[44]	Cisplatin	6	37	60	Yes	200 mg/m²[a]
2000	Burt et al.	[36]	Doxorubicin	8	37	20	No	40 mg/m²
2002	Putnam	[43]	Doxorubicin	16	37	NA	No	60 mg/m²
2002	Schröder et al.	[45]	Cisplatin	4	41	21–40	Both	70 mg/m²[a]
2004	Hendriks et al.	[40]	Melphalan	16[b]	37,42	30	Yes	45 mg – 42 °C[c]
2014	Den Hengst et al.	[7]	Melphalan	50	37	30	Yes	NA[d]

MTD maximum tolerated dose, *n* number of patients, *min* minutes, *NA* not available, *Ref.* reference, *TNF* tumour necrosis factor

[a]Fixed dose

[b]21 procedures (five bilateral)

[c]In an extension trial [38], safe MTD was found to be 45 mg at 37 °C (see text)

[d]Phase II clinical trial using MTD defined by Hendriks et al. [40] and the subsequent extension trial [38]

Putnam and co-workers presented their phase I study of isolated single-lung perfusion of doxorubicin in 16 patients with unresectable pulmonary metastatic disease and also in sarcoma patients [43]. Systemic levels were minimal or undetectable, while two patients developed a grade 4 pulmonary toxicity at a dose of 75 mg/m^2, therefore defining the MTD at 60 mg/m^2 of doxorubicin in this study. Overall operative mortality was 18.8 %. One patient died of a paradoxical tumour embolus, one of drug-related lung injury and one of pneumonia 3 weeks postoperatively. Early morbidity was noted in three patients and consisted of prolonged chest tube drainage more than 7 days, persistent air leak longer than 7 days and grade 4 lung injury. Late toxicity included a decrease in forced expiratory volume in 1 s, forced vital capacity and a decrease in ventilation and perfusion in the treated lung. Only one major response occurred. MST was 19.1 months in this study [43].

31.4.3.2 Tumour Necrosis Factor Alpha (TNF-α) and γ-Interferon

Results of ILuP with TNF-α were published by Pass et al. in 1996, which is the only clinical study with TNF-α [42]. Twenty patients were registered for this phase I trial but five patients did not have lung perfusion: three underwent resection of their metastases, one procedure was aborted for mechanical reasons and one because of extraparenchymal pleural involvement. In the remaining 15 patients, 16 lung perfusions were performed – 6 on the left and 10 on the right side. One patient had staged bilateral perfusions. Pulmonary metastases were from soft tissue sarcoma, melanoma, Ewing's sarcoma, adenoid cystic carcinoma, renal cell carcinoma and colon adenocarcinoma. Lung perfusion was performed for 90 min with increasing doses of TNF-α and γ-interferon at moderate hyperthermia. No deaths occurred and no significant systemic changes in systemic blood pressure or cardiac output were observed. Isolation of the lung was complete in ten patients with 0 % leak. There were no operative deaths. Mean hospitalisation time was 9 days. Three patients had a short-term partial response with progressive disease occurring after 6–9 months [42].

31.4.3.3 Cisplatin

In the study by Johnston et al., two patients were treated with cisplatin [41]. One patient with diffuse bronchioloalveolar carcinoma was treated with a dose of 14 µg/mL in normothermic conditions, and the other patient with metastatic chondrosarcoma was given 20 µg/mL with moderate hyperthermia. In both of them, total lung perfusion was done during cardiopulmonary bypass. Perfusion times were 50 and 60 min, respectively. Metastasectomy was not undertaken. One patient developed a pneumonia and subsequently empyema 4 days later. He required reintubation and died after 81 days [41].

Ratto et al. used the bimodality treatment of ILuP and resection in six patients with lung metastases from soft tissue sarcomas [44]. Major end points were feasibility, toxicity and distribution of cisplatin in normal and neoplastic tissues. Cisplatin was perfused at a fixed, high dose of 200 mg/m^2 for 60 min; so, DLT could not be determined in this study. Lung perfusion temperature ranged from 37 to 37.5 °C. Mean pulmonary artery pressure was kept below 35 mmHg. No patient died during or after the procedure. Two patients developed interstitial and alveolar lung oedema after 48 h, for which one patient required prolonged respiratory support. No systemic toxicity was noted. Total cisplatin concentration in the lung exceeded more than 40 times systemic plasma concentrations. There was no difference in cisplatin lung and tumour concentration. No histological damage of lung specimens was observed. Decline in ventilatory function 10 or 30 days after the ILuP procedure was significant for forced vital capacity, forced expiratory volume in 1 s and carbon monoxide diffusion capacity, although reassessments in two patients after 12 months showed further improvement [44]. After a median follow-up of 13 months, four patients were alive without any evidence of disease. One patient died of extrapulmonary metastases 11 months after the operation and the sixth patient had both local and distant recurrences 9 months after perfusion.

Schröder et al. conducted a pilot study in four patients with unilateral ($n=2$) and bilateral ($n=2$) sarcoma metastases confined to a lobe or entire lung [45]. Metastasectomy was performed, followed by ILuP with cisplatin at an in-flow temperature of 41 °C. Eligibility included at least four previous surgical metastasectomies, controlled primary site and no other effective treatment options in contrast to Ratto's study [44]. Cisplatin was given at a fixed dose of only 70 mg/m^2 for about 30 min at 41 °C. Systemic cisplatin plasma levels were low. Throughout the ILuP, there was no evidence of drug-related systemic toxicity. Postoperatively, all patients developed transient pulmonary toxicity presenting as non-cardiogenic lung oedema. After a mean follow-up of 12 months, three patients were alive and disease-free and one patient died of cerebral metastases after 13 months without pulmonary recurrence at post-mortem examination.

It is difficult to make some general remarks based on so few studies with small groups of heterogeneous patients treated with cisplatin. Furthermore, above-mentioned investigations differed profoundly in some aspects. For instance, Johnston's patients were not treated with metastasectomy and Schröder and Ratto were investigating two different groups of patients: those with resectable pulmonary metastases and those without any treatment options left, making any conclusions fragile, especially on survival data [41, 44, 45].

31.4.3.4 Melphalan

Regarding melphalan, only one phase I study was performed to determine the MTD in clinical ILuP [40]. In an initial study, 21 procedures were performed in 16 patients with resectable lung metastases. The primary tumour was colorectal in seven patients, renal in 5, sarcoma in 3 and salivary gland in 1. ILuP was performed unilaterally in 11 patients and staged bilaterally in 5. All procedures were performed without technical difficulties. Operative mortality was 0 %, and no systemic toxicity was encountered. The MTD was found to be 45 mg at 42 °C. However, in an extension trial of this study, more toxicity was observed with a perfusion temperature of 42 °C [38]. So, a safe MTD should be set at 45 mg of melphalan at 37 °C. Pharmacokinetic studies in this trial showed a significant correlation between perfused melphalan dose, perfusate area under the concentration-time curve and lung tissue melphalan concentrations [39, 46]. However, there was no correlation between melphalan dose and tumour tissue concentrations. The peak concentration and area under the curve of melphalan were 250- and tenfold higher than in the systemic circulation, respectively [39]. Long-term 5-year overall survival in this trial was 54.8 ± 10.6 % and median disease-free survival 19 months (95 % confidence interval 4.4–33.6) [37]. This phase I trial was followed by a phase II trial including a total of 50 patients with resectable lung metastases from colorectal carcinoma, osteosarcoma and soft tissue sarcoma [7]. Perfusion was performed with the MTD defined in the phase I trial, namely, 45 mg melphalan at a perfusion temperature of 37 °C. Lung function data suggested no long-term pulmonary toxicity of the ILuP procedure. Postoperative comorbidity was comparable with a regular thoracotomy with lung metastasectomy. When comparing quality of life after lung metastasectomy by thoracotomy with a thoracotomy which combines lung metastasectomy with ILuP, no difference was found [54]. These results show that ILuP in combination with lung metastasectomy is a safe procedure. After a median follow-up of 24 months, the 3-year OS was 57 ± 9 % with a 3-year DFS of 36 ± 8 %, which is comparable to the literature [7]. During follow-up, 30 patients had recurrent disease of which only seven had their first recurrence in the treated lung meaning a reduction to 23 % instead of the 44–66 % as mentioned in the literature [1]. Currently an extension trial is running to include another 50 patients to support these results.

31.5 High-Dose Locoregional Chemotherapy: Conclusions

After extensive experimental research performed in many laboratories over the world, ILuP now has become a mature clinical technique. In summary of the clinical studies, ILuP procedures are generally well tolerated, reproducible and significant drug levels are obtained in pulmonary metastases and lymph nodes without systemic toxicity offer a valid clinical model for further investigation of combined chemotherapy and surgery in patients with pulmonary metastases [46]. At the present time, only one phase II trial has been completed suggesting an improved local control with comparable OS and DFS, without additional long-term toxicity or worse quality of life. An extension trial is currently running to gather more data. These results need to be confirmed in the future in a randomised trial comparing regular thoracotomy with lung metastasectomy against thoracotomy with lung metastasectomy combined with ILuP.

To obtain a better international cooperation and exchange of experimental and clinical data, a research group on ILuP was created within the European Association for Cardio-Thoracic Surgery (EACTS) with a yearly meeting during the annual congress.

Alternative strategies for ILuP are also developed. Experimental data on less invasive procedures as pulmonary artery infusion and chemo-embolization are accumulating. These techniques can be applied by a percutaneously inserted pulmonary artery catheter making repetitive application possible. In this way, these promising techniques can be used as induction or adjuvant treatment, not only for lung metastases but also for primary bronchogenic carcinoma.

Hopefully in the near future, these new developments in locoregional high-dose chemotherapy, combined with surgical resection, will provide a better outcome in our patients treated for lung metastases.

References

1. Pastorino U, Buyse M, Friedel G, et al. Long-term results of lung metastasectomy: prognostic analyses based on 5206 cases. The International Registry of Lung Metastases. J Thorac Cardiovasc Surg. 1997;113(1):37–49.
2. Van Schil PE. Surgical treatment for pulmonary metastases. Acta Clin Belg. 2002;57(6): 333–9.
3. Divis G. Ein beitrag zur operativen behandlung der lungengeschwülste. Acta Chir Scand. 1927;62:329–41.
4. Barney JD, Churchill E. Adenocarcinoma of the kidney with metastasis to the lung cured by nephrectomy and lobectomy. J Urol. 1939;42:269–76.
5. Ehrenhaft JL, Lawrence MS, Sensenig DM. Pulmonary resections for metastatic lesions. AMA Arch Surg. 1958;77(4):606–12.
6. Althagafi K, Alashgar O, Almaghrab H, Nasralla A, Ahmed M, Alshehri A, et al. Missed pulmonary metastases. Asian Cardiovasc Thorac Ann. 2014;22:183–6.
7. Den Hengst WA, Hendriks JM, Balduyck B, Rodrigus I, Vermorken JB, Lardon F, et al. Phase II multicenter clinical trial of pulmonary metastasectomy and isolated lung perfusion with melphalan in patients with resectable lung metastases. J Thorac Oncol. 2014;9(10):1547–53.
8. Kayton ML, Huvos AG, Casher J, Abramson SJ, Rosen NS, Wexler LH, et al. Computed tomographic scan of the chest underestimates the number of metastatic lesions in osteosarcoma. J Pediatr Surg. 2006;41(1):200–6.
9. Mutsaerts EL, Zoetmulder FA, Meijer S, Baas P, Hart AA, Rutgers EJ. Outcome of thoracoscopic pulmonary metastasectomy evaluated by confirmatory thoracotomy. Ann Thorac Surg. 2001;72(1):230–3.
10. Van Schil P, Van MJ, Vanmaele R, Eyskens E. Role of thoracoscopy (VATS) in pleural and pulmonary pathology. Acta Chir Belg. 1996;96(1):23–7.
11. Pfannschmidt J, Klode J, Muley T, Dienemann H, Hoffmann H. Nodal involvement at the time of pulmonary metastasectomy: experiences in 245 patients. Ann Thorac Surg. 2006;81(2): 448–54.
12. Veronesi G, Petrella F, Leo F, Solli P, Maissoneuve P, Galetta D, et al. Prognostic role of lymph node involvement in lung metastasectomy. J Thorac Cardiovasc Surg. 2007;133(4):967–72.
13. Sternberg DI, Sonett JR. Surgical therapy of lung metastases. Semin Oncol. 2007;34(3): 186–96.
14. Liu D, Abolhoda A, Burt ME, Martini N, Bains MS, Downey RJ, et al. Pulmonary metastasectomy for testicular germ cell tumors: a 28-year experience. Ann Thorac Surg. 1998;66(5): 1709–14.
15. Friedel G, Pastorino U, Ginsberg RJ, Goldstraw P, Johnston M, Pass H, et al. Results of lung metastasectomy from breast cancer: prognostic criteria on the basis of 467 cases of the International Registry of Lung Metastases. Eur J Cardiothorac Surg. 2002;22(3):335–44.
16. Lanzo LA, Natarajan G, Roth JA, Putnam JB. Long-term survival after resection of pulmonary metastases from carcinoma of the breast. Ann Thorac Surg. 1982;54:244–7.
17. Beattie EJ, Harvey JC, Marcove R, Martini N. Results of multiple pulmonary resections for metastatic osteogenic sarcoma after two decades. J Surg Oncol. 1991;46(3):154–5.
18. Putnam JB. Secondary tumors of the lung. In: Shields TW, LoCicero III J, Penn RB, editors. General thoracic surgery. Philadelphia: Lippincott, Williams & Wilkins; 2000. p. 1555–91.
19. Regnard JF, Grunenwald D, Spaggiari L, Girard P, Elias D, Ducreux M, et al. Surgical treatment of hepatic and pulmonary metastases from colorectal cancers. Ann Thorac Surg. 1998; 66(1):214–8.

20. Robinson BJ, Rice TW, Strong SA, Rybicki LA, Blackstone EH. Is resection of pulmonary and hepatic metastases warranted in patients with colorectal cancer? J Thorac Cardiovasc Surg. 1999;117(1):66–75.
21. van Geel AN, Pastorino U, Jauch KW, Judson IR, Van Coevorden F, Buesa JM, et al. Surgical treatment of lung metastases: the European Organization for Research and Treatment of Cancer-Soft Tissue and Bone Sarcoma Group study of 255 patients. Cancer. 1996;77(4): 675–82.
22. Hendriks JM, Romijn S, van Putte BP, Eyskens E, Vermorken JB, Van ME, et al. Long-term results of surgical resection of lung metastases. Acta Chir Belg. 2001;101(6):267–72.
23. Koong HN, Pastorino U, Ginsberg RJ. Is there a role for pneumonectomy in pulmonary metastases? International Registry of Lung Metastases. Ann Thorac Surg. 1999;68(6):2039–43.
24. Hendriks JM, van Putte BP, Grootenboers M, van Boven WJ, Schramel F, Van Schil PE. Isolated lung perfusion for pulmonary metastases. Thorac Surg Clin. 2006;16(2):185–98, vii.
25. Ranney DF. Drug targeting to the lungs. Biochem Pharmacol. 1986;35(7):1063–9.
26. Creech Jr O, Krementz ET, Ryan RF, Reemtsma K, Winblad JN. Experiences with isolation-perfusion technics in the treatment of cancer. Ann Surg. 1959;149(5):627–40.
27. Krementz ET. Lucy Wortham James lecture. Regional perfusion. Current sophistication, what next? Cancer. 1986;57(3):416–32.
28. Johnston MR. The origin and history of isolated lung perfusion. In: Van Schil P, editor. Lung metastases and isolated lung perfusion. New York: Nova; 2007. p. 95–114.
29. Johnston MR, Minchin R, Shull JH, Thenot JP, McManus BM, Terrill R, et al. Isolated lung perfusion with adriamycin. A preclinical study. Cancer. 1983;52(3):404–9.
30. Milne EN. Pulmonary metastases: vascular supply and diagnosis. Int J Radiat Oncol Biol Phys. 1976;1(7–8):739–42.
31. Mochizuki A, Kurihara Y, Yokote K, Nakajima Y, Osada H. Discrimination of solitary pulmonary nodules based on vascular supply patterns with firstpass dynamic CT. Lung Cancer. 2000;29 suppl 1:242 (abstract 824).
32. Baciewicz Jr FA, Arredondo M, Chaudhuri B, Crist KA, Basilius D, Bandyopadhyah S, et al. Pharmacokinetics and toxicity of isolated perfusion of lung with doxorubicin. J Surg Res. 1991;50(2):124–8.
33. Johnston MR, Christensen CW, Minchin RF, Rickaby DA, Linehan JH, Schuller HM, et al. Isolated total lung perfusion as a means to deliver organ-specific chemotherapy: long-term studies in animals. Surgery. 1985;98(1):35–44.
34. Blades B, Hall ER. Preliminary observations on the injection of potentially carcinolytic drugs into the pulmonary artery with temporary occlusion of the blood supply of the lung. Am Surg. 1958;24(7):492–4.
35. Karakousis CP, Park HC, Sharma SD, Kanter P. Regional chemotherapy via the pulmonary artery for pulmonary metastases. J Surg Oncol. 1981;18(3):249–55.
36. Burt ME, Liu D, Abolhoda A, Ross HM, Kaneda Y, Jara E, et al. Isolated lung perfusion for patients with unresectable metastases from sarcoma: a phase I trial. Ann Thorac Surg. 2000;69(5):1542–9.
37. Den Hengst WA, van Putte BP, Hendriks JM, Stockman B, van Boven WJ, Weyler J, et al. Long-term survival of a phase I clinical trial of isolated lung perfusion with melphalan for resectable lung metastases. Eur J Cardiothorac Surg. 2010;38(5):621–7.
38. Grootenboers MJ, Schramel FM, van Boven WJ, van Putte BP, Hendriks JM, Van Schil PE. Re-evaluation of toxicity and long-term follow-up of isolated lung perfusion with melphalan in patients with resectable pulmonary metastases: a phase I and extension trial. Ann Thorac Surg. 2007;83(3):1235–6.
39. Grootenboers MJ, Hendriks JM, van Boven WJ, Knibbe CA, Van Putte B, Stockman B, et al. Pharmacokinetics of isolated lung perfusion with melphalan for resectable pulmonary metastases, a phase I and extension trial. J Surg Oncol. 2007;96(7):583–9.
40. Hendriks JM, Grootenboers MJ, Schramel FM, van Boven WJ, Stockman B, Seldenrijk CA, et al. Isolated lung perfusion with melphalan for resectable lung metastases: a phase I clinical trial. Ann Thorac Surg. 2004;78(6):1919–26.

41. Johnston MR, Minchen RF, Dawson CA. Lung perfusion with chemotherapy in patients with unresectable metastatic sarcoma to the lung or diffuse bronchioloalveolar carcinoma. J Thorac Cardiovasc Surg. 1995;110(2):368–73.
42. Pass HI, Mew DJ, Kranda KC, Temeck BK, Donington JS, Rosenberg SA. Isolated lung perfusion with tumor necrosis factor for pulmonary metastases. Ann Thorac Surg. 1996;61(6): 1609–17.
43. Putnam Jr JB. New and evolving treatment methods for pulmonary metastases. Semin Thorac Cardiovasc Surg. 2002;14(1):49–56.
44. Ratto GB, Toma S, Civalleri D, Passerone GC, Esposito M, Zaccheo D, et al. Isolated lung perfusion with platinum in the treatment of pulmonary metastases from soft tissue sarcomas. J Thorac Cardiovasc Surg. 1996;112(3):614–22.
45. Schroder C, Fisher S, Pieck AC, Muller A, Jaehde U, Kirchner H, et al. Technique and results of hyperthermic (41 degrees C) isolated lung perfusion with high-doses of cisplatin for the treatment of surgically relapsing or unresectable lung sarcoma metastasis. Eur J Cardiothorac Surg. 2002;22(1):41–6.
46. Van Schil P, Grootenboers M. Clinical studies. In: Van Schil P, editor. Lung metastases and isolated lung perfusion. New York: Nova; 2007. p. 213–8.
47. Van Schil PE, Hendriks JM, van Putte BP, Stockman BA, Lauwers PR, Ten Broecke PW, et al. Isolated lung perfusion and related techniques for the treatment of pulmonary metastases. Eur J Cardiothorac Surg. 2008;33(3):487–96.
48. Vogl TJ, Lehnert T, Zangos S, Eichler K, Hammerstingl R, Korkusuz H, et al. Transpulmonary chemoembolization (TPCE) as a treatment for unresectable lung metastases. Eur Radiol. 2008;18(11):2449–55.
49. Den Hengst WA, Hendriks JM, Van Hoof T, Heytens K, Guetens G, De BG, et al. Selective pulmonary artery perfusion with melphalan is equal to isolated lung perfusion but superior to intravenous melphalan for the treatment of sarcoma lung metastases in a rodent model. Eur J Cardiothorac Surg. 2012;42(2):341–7.
50. Demmy TL, Wagner-Mann C, Allen A. Isolated lung chemotherapeutic infusions for treatment of pulmonary metastases: a pilot study. J Biomed Sci. 2002;9(4):334–8.
51. van Putte BP, Hendriks JM, Romijn S, Pauwels B, De BG, Guetens G, et al. Pharmacokinetics after pulmonary artery perfusion with gemcitabine. Ann Thorac Surg. 2003;76(4):1036–40.
52. Brown DB, Ma MK, Battafarano RJ, Naidu S, Pluim D, Zamboni WC, et al. Endovascular lung perfusion using high-dose cisplatin: uptake and DNA adduct formation in an animal model. Oncol Rep. 2004;11(1):237–43.
53. van Putte BP, Grootenboers M, van Boven WJ, van Oosterhout M, Pasterkamp G, Folkerts G, et al. Selective pulmonary artery perfusion for the treatment of primary lung cancer: improved drug exposure of the lung. Lung Cancer. 2009;65(2):208–13.
54. Balduyck B, Van Thielen J, Cogen A, Den Hengst W, Hendriks J, Lauwers P, et al. Quality of life after pulmonary metastasectomy: a prospective study comparing isolated lung perfusion with standard metastasectomy. J Thorac Oncol. 2012;7(10):1567–673.

Isolated Thoracic Perfusion with Chemofiltration (ITP-F) for Advanced and Pretreated Non-small-cell Lung Cancer

Karl Reinhard Aigner and Emir Selak

Lung cancer is the most frequent cause of death from malignancy in men. About 500,000 patients in the northern hemisphere per year and more than 1,000,000 patients worldwide die from lung cancer every year. Non-small-cell lung cancer accounts for about 80 % of all patients with lung cancer. At the time of diagnosis, most patients already have advanced disease, only some 30 % are still operable, and in those, 1-year life expectancy is about 43 %. The majority of patients are unsuitable for radical surgery or radiotherapy. Life expectancy with current first-line platinum-based doublets with or without additional drug combinations or targeted drugs remains unchanged at about 8–10 months. An impressive change of median overall survival has not yet been achieved, only some minor changes of prolongation of progression-free survival (PFS) of a few months. Extended survival time by a few months was achieved with dose-intense or prolonged chemotherapy but was associated with unacceptable toxicity [1–4] and a negative impact on the patient's quality of life.

In an attempt to extend survival time, improve quality of life, and administer a therapy that is less expensive than therapies already available, we initiated a technique that generates high local drug exposure by means of segmental vascular isolation of the chest and simultaneously reduces or avoids toxic side effects by extracorporeal purification of blood.

K.R. Aigner, MD (✉) • E. Selak
Department of Surgical Oncology, Medias Klinikum GmbH & Co KG,
Krankenhausstrasse 3a, Burghausen 84489, Germany
e-mail: info@prof-aigner.de; prof-aigner@medias-klinikum.de

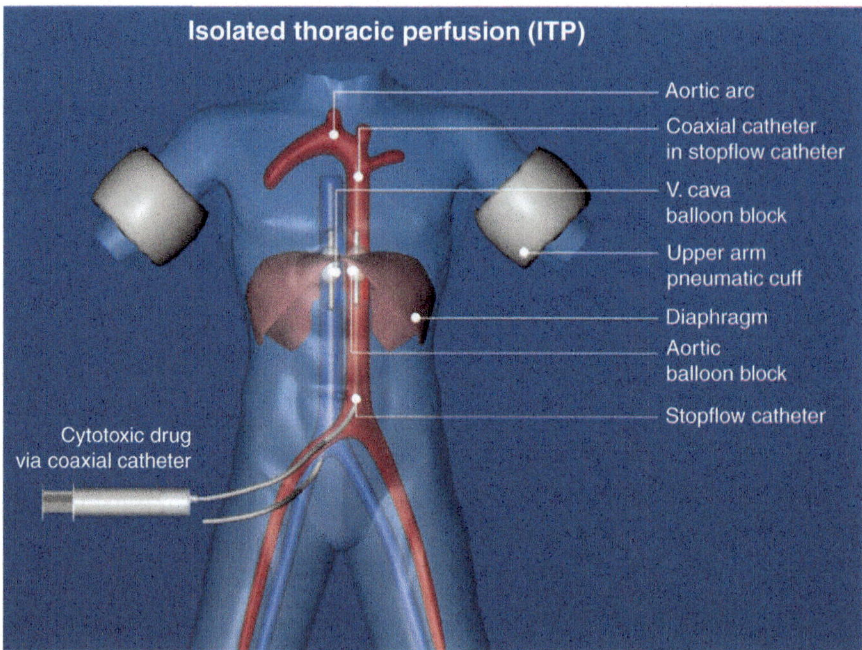

Fig. 32.1 Scheme of isolated thoracic perfusion

32.1 Technique of Isolated Thoracic Perfusion with Chemofiltration

For isolated thoracic perfusion with chemofiltration (ITP-F), under general anesthesia, an arterial and venous stop-flow-three-channel balloon catheter is inserted through femoral access, and the aorta and vena cava are blocked just below the diaphragm (Fig. 32.1). By means of two additional pneumatic cuffs around the upper arms, the isolation of the head-neck-chest area is completed. Chemotherapeutics are injected with high pressure against the aortic blood stream through the coaxial channel that exits at the tip of the aortic catheter. The drug can equally well be injected through the coaxial channel of the vena cava balloon catheter. After a 15 min exposure time, all blocks are released, and through the larger channels in both stop-flow catheters, the arteriovenous chemofiltration is maintained over a median of 40 min at a maximal flow rate of 500 mL/min. This substantially reduces the systemic drug exposure by detoxification. It also prevents major toxicity caused by vascular leakages into the systemic blood circuit (Fig. 32.2).

At the end of chemofiltration, both catheters are removed and the femoral vessels repaired with running sutures.

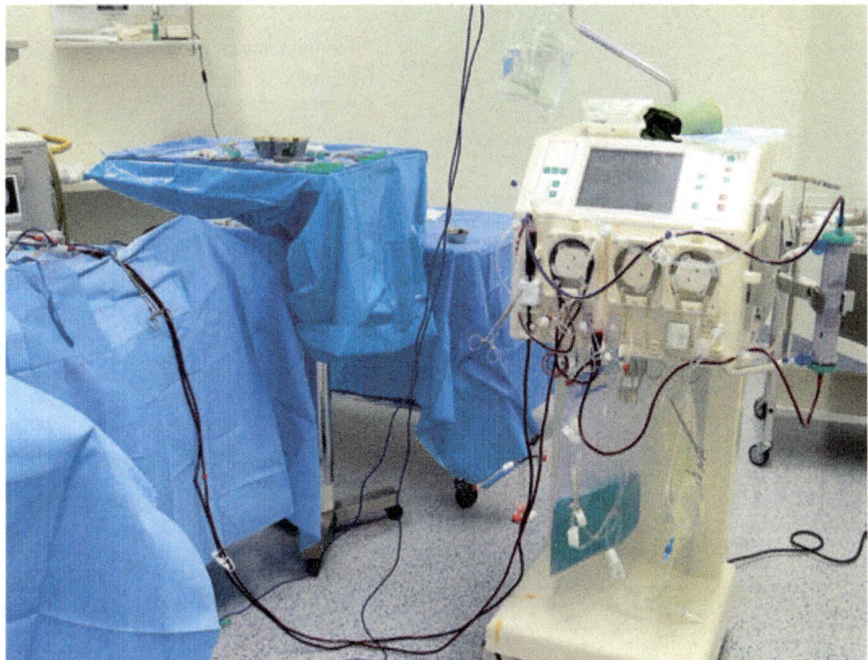

Fig. 32.2 Chemofiltration

32.2 Pharmacokinetics and Pharmacodynamics

In treating lung cancer, there are two aspects of how to create higher drug exposure as compared with systemic chemotherapy. First is the application of an isolated perfusion circuit showing how to generate maximum drug concentration at the target area taking benefit of the "first-pass uptake." The second is the manipulation of the arterial blood flow and infusion time.

First, with isolated circuit perfusion, there is the increase of drug levels and drug concentration in a closed system by reduction of the circulating blood volume. In a theoretical model, a volume reduction to one-third or one-fourth of the primary volume will increase the drug concentration by a factor of 3 or 4. Figure 32.3 shows the difference of mitomycin plasma levels when the same total dose of 20 mg is administered as an intravenous systemic bolus as compared to intra-aortic bolus infusion. The therapy had been performed in the same patient first as systemic chemotherapy, then as isolated thoracic perfusion (Fig. 32.3). The drug levels in the isolated circuit are, in accordance with the reduced blood volumes, three to four times higher than in the entire systemic system. The advantage is reduced to twice the concentration at 6 min postinjection, most likely because of increased tissue uptake due to higher first-pass concentration, and equalizes with systemic drug

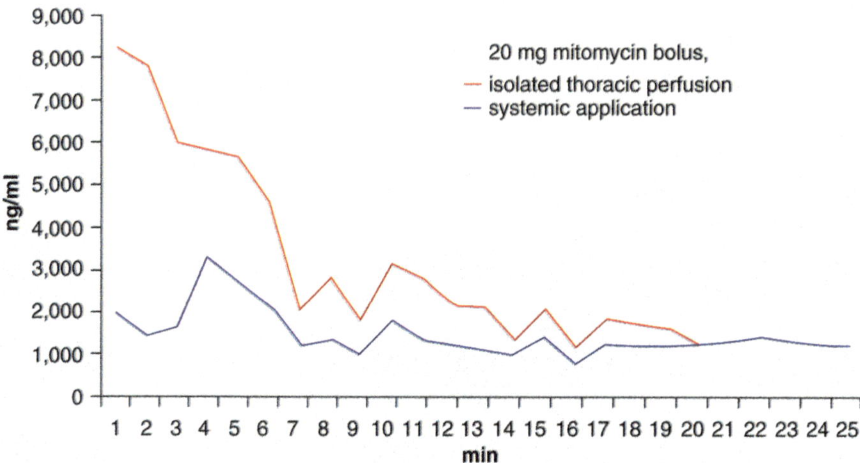

Fig. 32.3 Mitomycin plasma levels in isolated thoracic perfusion with chemofiltration versus intravenous application

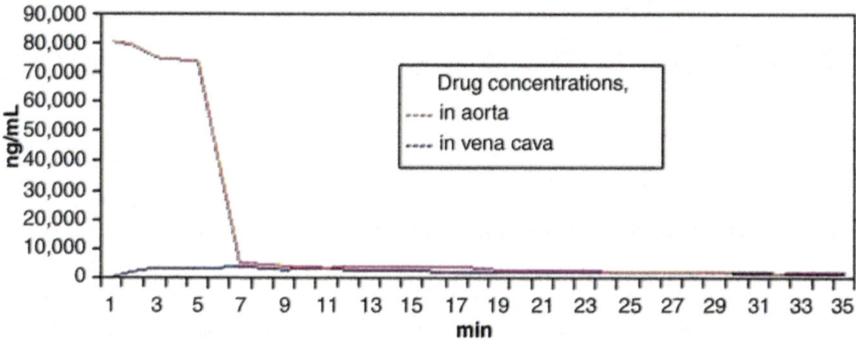

Fig. 32.4 Intra-aortic pulsatile infusion of 80 mg of cisplatin

levels after 20 min. Chemofiltration had been started at 15 min, after releasing the venous and arterial blocks of the isolated system.

A manual pulsatile jet injection through the coaxial channel of the stop-flow catheter generates first-pass peak concentrations of cis-platinum of about 75,000–80,000 ng/mL in the aorta, while venous concentrations taken in samples from the vena cava are equivalent to those in the reduced volume model and range between 1000 and 3000 ng/mL maximally. This translates into a 20- to maximally 80-fold advantage of the intra-aortic application in terms of first-pass effect (Fig. 32.4).

32.3 Patients and Methods

Sixty-four patients with non-small-cell lung cancer, 84 % in progression after systemic platin-based chemotherapy or radiochemotherapy were assigned for isolated thoracic perfusion and chemofiltration [5]. Nineteen patients were in UICC stage III and 45 patients in UICC stage IV.

Table 32.1 Response rates after four cycles of isolated thoracic perfusion

CR (complete remission)	8 %	Total 64 %
PR (partial remission)	56 %	
SD (stable disease)	28 %	
PD (progression)	8 %	

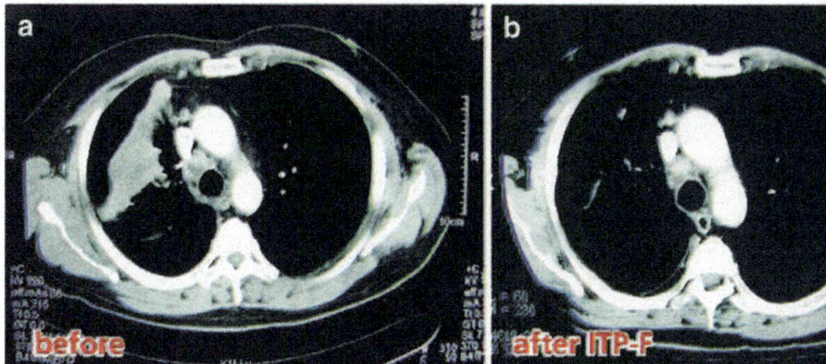

Fig. 32.5 (**a**) CT scan before isolated thoracic perfusion with chemofiltration. (**b**) CT scan 4 weeks after isolated thoracic perfusion with chemofiltration

The treatment consisted of four cycles of isolated thoracic perfusion at 4-week intervals each. A three-drug combination of cisplatin, adriamycin, and mitomycin was administered as a pulsatile jet-bolus through the central channel of the arterial balloon catheter against the aortic blood stream. Infusion time was 3–5 min. Standard dosage in a 70 kg patient was 100 mg cisplatin, 50 mg adriamycin, and 20–30 mg mitomycin. Chemotherapeutics were administered into reduced blood volumes of the chest area, amounting to one-third to one-fourth of the total body blood volume. Thus, the achieved drug concentrations due to lower blood volume are increased adequately. Drug exposure time, such as total isolation of the hypoxic lower hemibody was 15 min. Average chemofiltration time was 40 min. For follow-up control, a CT scan was performed after the first, the third, and the last therapy. In cases showing no concrete response within 4 weeks after the first treatment, the administered drug combination was changed, mostly according to chemosensitivity testing. In cases showing no visible or clinical response after two courses of regional chemotherapy with different drug combinations, the treatment was discontinued. In cases showing continuous response as, for example, stepwise tumor shrinkage and improvement of respiratory parameters, the therapy was usually continued for up to four cycles, but in a few selected cases up to six cycles. One patient had resection of a responding tumor that before therapy had infiltrated the chest wall.

32.4   Results

Quality of response was noted mainly as partial remission in 56 % of the patients. Possibly because of advanced stage IV cancers with mostly bulky tumors, the rate of complete remissions in CT scan was only 8 % (Table 32.1). The overall response rate (CR and PR) was 64 % with 28 % stable disease and 8 % progressive disease. Five patients had complete remissions (8 %). This was already noted after the first or second isolated thoracic perfusion (Fig. 32.5a, b).

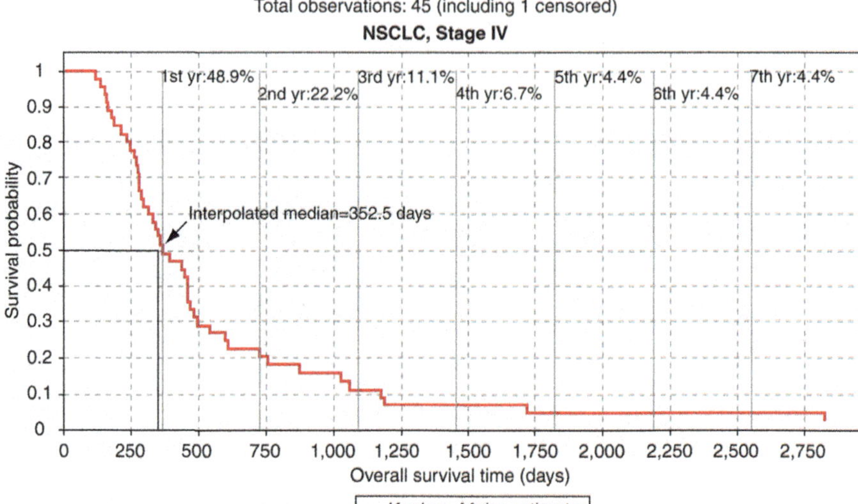

Fig. 32.6 Kaplan-Meier survival estimate $n=45$ NSCLC stage IV patients

Table 32.2 Survival ITP-F versus cancer data base (AJCC) NSCLC stage IV

Survival years	1	2	3	4	5
ITP-F	48.9 %	22.2 %	11.1 %	6.7 %	4.4 %
AJCC	16.9 %	5.8 %	3.1 %	2.1 %	1.6 %

Overall survival was one of the endpoints of the study. In UICC Stage IV patients, 1-year survival was 48.9 %, 2-year survival 22.2 %, and 3-year survival 11.1 % (Fig. 32.6). A comparison of these survival data with the American Joint Committee on Cancer (AJCC) data [6] is shown in Table 32.2.

32.5 Side Effects

Hematological toxicity was low and did not exceed WHO Grade I or II. Nausea and vomiting rarely occurred. A few patients reported slight nausea. This had a clear correlation to the rate and intensity of chemofiltration. It had been observed in a former study that patients who had perfusion without chemofiltration had side effects comparable to those after systemic chemotherapy and an inpatient stay in the hospital of 10–12 days postoperatively, whereas patients who had prior chemofiltration had almost no side effects at all and were discharged on the third to fifth postoperative day.

Because of simultaneous chemotherapy of the chest, head, and neck area, more than 95 % of the patients receiving isolated thoracic perfusion suffer hair loss despite the application of a cool cap. A transient symptom is facial edema (Fig. 32.7a, b)

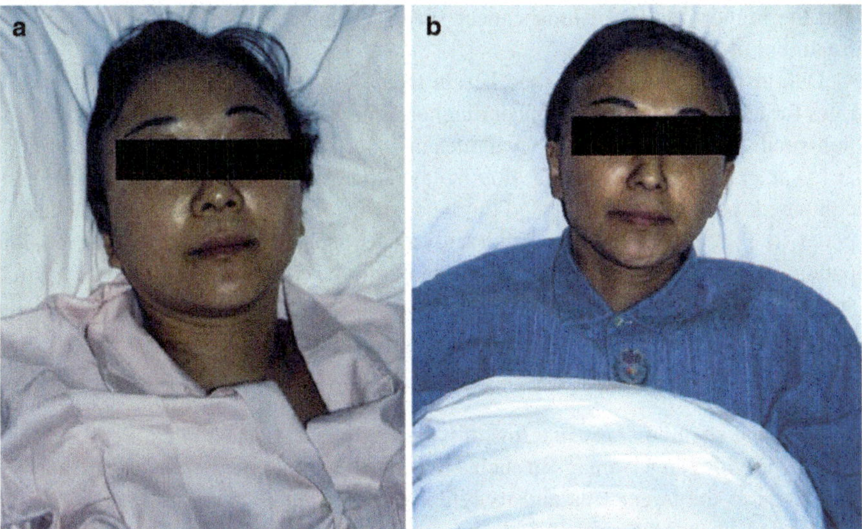

Fig. 32.7 (**a**) Facial edema directly after isolated thoracic perfusion. (**b**) Facial edema 2 days after isolated thoracic perfusion

which is due to the high drug concentrations and drug exposure. It remains between 2 and 3 days and has no significant effect on the patient's quality of life or well-being. Patients with prior borderline respiratory function may need additional oxygen due to slight interstitial edema on the first two or three postoperative days. In most cases, respiratory parameters are improved by the fourth or fifth postoperative day.

Fatigue has not been observed, except in cases where isolated thoracic perfusion has led to immediate tumor necrosis within the first postoperative days. Major toxicity grade 4 or febrile neutropenia has not occurred. Toxicity from 15 min hypoxia was mainly reflected in terms of transient slight elevation of liver enzymes and serum creatinine. Permanent kidney or liver damage has not been found.

32.6   Discussion

It has been shown in this study that an increase in local drug exposure translates into an increase in response rate and overall survival. Quality of life, which was the second important endpoint of the study, could be improved impressively by means of chemofiltration, which reduces the residual drug in the systemic blood circuit. Therefore, there were no undue treatment-associated side effects, which are commonly noted after dose-intense therapies, which predominantly only reveal improvements in PFS, not being accompanied by improvements in quality of life. Considering overall survival, so far there has been no substantial progress with systemic chemotherapy. Nearly all improvements in survival have been achieved in localized cancer cases. And those gains in survival are more or less the result of advances in treatment, such as better surgical techniques in general, and the higher quality of lung cancer surgery related to better imaging and pre-treatment planning [6].

Data from the study published herein were compared with the relative survival rates for non-small-cell lung cancer diagnosed in the USA in 1992 and 1993 [7]. For non-small-cell lung cancer, survival rates in 44,410 patients in stage IV were 16.9 % at 1 year, compared with 48.9 % after isolated thoracic perfusion, 5.8 % after 2 years compared to 22.2 % after isolated thoracic perfusion, and 3.1 % after 3 years compared to 11.1 % after isolated thoracic perfusion. Of course, more than 44,000 patients, representing an overall trend, can hardly be compared with 64 patients in a small study; however, those 44,000 patients indeed represent reliable data which do not change significantly despite all therapeutic endeavors [3, 4, 8–16].

Conclusion

Regional chemotherapy in terms of isolated thoracic perfusion with chemofiltration provides an advantage in such a way that dose-intense therapy can be administered to the target area and its lymphatic pathways which are predominantly invaded by cancer, without causing collateral toxicity to the entire organism. Chemofiltration plays the predominant role in this concept [17–20]. Due to isolation perfusion combined with chemofiltration, tumors can be treated more effectively without the deleterious effects of systemic treatment on the patient's quality of life.

Another important item is drug exposure. It has been shown that short-term bolus infusions induce high drug uptake in tumor tissues which consequently enhances the tumoricidal effect. Residual drug in the systemic blood pool is reduced or eliminated by subsequent chemofiltration.

A clear trend toward regional chemotherapy is obvious since patients with a poor life expectancy in progression after radiochemotherapy or chemotherapy clearly had a benefit from isolated thoracic perfusion. Taking into account that a patient with non-small-cell lung cancer at the time of diagnosis has a 1-year life expectancy of ±43 % and, after being in progression after intensive pretreatment with surgery, chemotherapy, and radiotherapy, and a definitely reduced performance and a life expectancy of a few weeks, again has a 46 % chance to survive 1 year, it can be concluded that isolated thoracic perfusion is effective. Nevertheless, these data should be confirmed in a controlled phase III study, comparing conventional therapy in UICC stage IV patients with no therapy and regional chemotherapy focusing on the primary endpoints, overall survival, and quality of life.

References

1. Ando M, Okamoto I, Yamamoto N, Takeda K, Tamura K, Seto T, et al. Predictive factors for interstitial lung disease, antitumor response, and survival in non-small-cell lung cancer patients treated with gefinitib. J Clin Oncol. 2006;24:2549–56.
2. Hapani S, Chu D, Wu S. Risk of gastrointestinal perforation in patients with cancer treated with bevacizumab: a meta-analysis. Lancet Oncol. 2009;10:559–68.

3. Non-small Cell Lung Cancer Collaborative Group. Chemotherapy in non-small cell lung cancer: a meta-analysis using updated data on individual patients from 52 randomized clinical trials. BMJ. 1995;311:899–909.
4. Soon YY, Stockler MR, Askie LM, Boyer MJ. Duration of chemotherapy for advanced non-small-cell lung cancer: a systematic review and meta-analysis of randomized trials. J Clin Oncol. 2009;27:3277–83.
5. Aigner KR, Selak E. Isolated thoracic perfusion as induction chemotherapy for non-small-cell lung cancer. Submitted for publication.
6. Woodward RM, Brown ML, Stewart ST, Cronin KA, Cutler DM. The value of medical interventions for lung cancer in the elderly. Results from SEER-CMHSF. doi: 10.1002/cncr.23058. Published online 22 Oct 2007 in Wiley InterScience (www.interscience.wiley.com).
7. American Joint Committee on Cancer (AJCC). In: Frederick LG, David LP, Irvin DF, April GF, Charles MB, Daniel GH, Monica M, editors. Cancer staging handbook. 6th ed. New York: Springer; 2002. p. 191–202.
8. Fidias PM, Dakhil SR, Lyss AP, et al. Phase III study of immediate compared with delayed docetaxel after front-line therapy with gemcitabine plus carboplatin in advanced non-small-cell lung cancer. J Clin Oncol. 2009;27:591–8.
9. Johnson DH, Fehrenbacher L, Novotny WF, Herbst Roy S, Nemunaitis JJ, Jablons DM, et al. Randomized phase II trial comparing bevacizumab plus carboplatin and paclitaxel with carboplatin and paclitaxel alone in previously untreated locally advanced or metastatic non-small-cell lung cancer. J Clin Oncol. 2004;22:2184–91.
10. Mok TSK, Wu YL, Yu CJ, Zhou C, Chen YM, Zhang L, et al. Randomized, placebo-controlled, phase II study of sequential erlotinib and chemotherapy as first-line treatment for advanced non-small-cell lung cancer. J Clin Oncol. 2009;27:5080–7.
11. Hanna N, Bunn Jr PA, Langer C, et al. Randomized phase III trial comparing irinotecan/cisplatin with etoposide/cisplatin in patients with previously untreated extensive-stage disease small-cell-lung cancer. J Clin Oncol. 2006;24:2038–43.
12. Niho S, Kubota K, Goto K, Yoh K, Ohmatsu H, Kakinuma R, et al. First-line single agent treatment with gefitinib in patients with advanced non-small-cell lung cancer: a phase II study. J Clin Oncol. 2006;24:64–9.
13. Riely GJ, Rizvi NA, Kris MG, Milton DT, Solit DB, Rosen N, et al. Randomized phase II study of pulse erlotinib before or after carboplatin and paclitaxel in current or former smokers with advanced non-small-cell lung cancer. J Clin Oncol. 2009;27:264–70.
14. Scagliotti GV, Parikh P, von Pawel J, et al. Phase III study comparing cisplatin plus gemcitabine with cisplatin plus pemetrexed in chemotherapy-naive patients with advanced-stage non-small-cell lung cancer. J Clin Oncol. 2008;26:3543–51.
15. Socinski MA, Stinchcombe TE. Duration of first line chemotherapy in advanced non-small cell lung cancer: less is more in the era of effective subsequent therapies. J Clin Oncol. 2007;25:5155–7.
16. Stinchcombe TE, Socinski MA. Treatment paradigms for advanced stage non-small cell lung cancer in the era of multiple lines of therapy. J Thorac Oncol. 2009;4:243–50.
17. Aigner KR, Müller H, Walter H, et al. Drug filtration in high-dose regional chemotherapy. Contrib Oncol. 1988;29:261–80.
18. Aigner KR, Tonn JC, Hechtel R, Seuffer R. Die intraarterielle zytostatikatherapie mit venöser filtration im halboffenen system. Onkologie. 1983;6(2):2–4.
19. Muchmore JH, Aigner KR, Beg MH. Regional chemotherapy for advanced intraabdominal and pelvic cancer. In: Cohen AM, Winawer SJ, Friedman MA, Günderson LL, editors. Cancer of the colon, rectum and anus. New York: McGraw-Hill; 1995. p. 881–9.
20. Tonn JC. Die portocavale hämofiltration bei der isolierten perfusion der leber. Beitr Onkol. 1985;21:108–16.

Toxicity Profiles with Systemic Versus Regional Chemotherapy

Karl Reinhard Aigner and Nina Knapp

33.1 Introduction

In chemotherapy of malignant tumors, the principle of dose-response applies in most clinical approaches. Dose-intensified therapy usually results in higher response rates and an extension of progression-free intervals and in some cases to a prolongation of overall survival time – but also to more severe side effects. The same applies both to a continuation of adjuvant chemotherapy after remission or stable disease and for new combination therapies [1] with new substances. The endeavor to improve progression-free intervals and survival times with intensified therapeutic efforts or new substances often fails due to increasing and no longer tolerable toxicity.

Toxicity constitutes the limiting factor, often forcing the patient to reduce the dosage or even to discontinue treatment. This in turn leads to a decrease in the expected progression-free survival and even overall survival, which means the potential benefit of any new therapy is relativized [2]. As such, any possible gain in survival time is canceled out by the increased toxicity or toxicity-related discontinuations of treatment.

The importance of quality of life in the treatment of tumors has continuously increased over the last 20 years. Guidelines for measuring quality of life (Quality of Life Scales, QOLS) were first created in the 1970s and 1980s by the American psychologist John Flanagan [3, 4]. In 1993, the Quality of Life Department (QLD) was formed at the EORTC Data Center and very rapidly gained in importance and international recognition [5]. For every type of tumor, there is an appropriately designed questionnaire, in which the possible problems and complications characteristic of tumors and treatment can be investigated. As a result, there are prospective statements about tumors in terms of the therapeutic results to be expected as well as the side effects.

K.R. Aigner (✉) • N. Knapp
Department of Surgical Oncology, Medias Klinikum GmbH & Co KG,
Krankenhausstrasse 3a, Burghausen 84489, Germany
e-mail: info@prof-aigner.de; prof-aigner@medias-klinikum.de

© Springer-Verlag Berlin Heidelberg 2016
K.R. Aigner, F.O. Stephens (eds.), *Induction Chemotherapy*,
DOI 10.1007/978-3-319-28773-7_33

A meta-analysis of EORTC studies in relation to quality of life during and after treatment of various tumors has shown that quality of life constitutes a prognostic factor during therapy. In evaluating the prognosis, the prospective estimate of survival should even be included in relation to tumor localization, existing distant metastasis, and intended treatment procedures, in order to acquire a more reliable picture of the expected prognosis; this is because patients with a better quality of life during therapy live longer [6]. As such, this casts a different light on the side effects to be "expected" or "avoided." If it is possible to achieve a reduction in the tumor or metastases with as few side effects as possible, it should be possible to achieve a prolongation of life in two respects – as a result of the tumor reduction and the improved quality of life.

33.2   Regional Chemotherapy

The purpose of regional chemotherapy is effective locally segmental therapy while reducing or completely preventing systemic side effects. Two basic techniques are used here:

1. Arterial infusion or chemoembolization via angiocatheters placed using the Seldinger technique or arterial port catheters implanted. Both access routes can be applied for the arterial infusion of carotids, the subclavian artery, mammary artery, hepatic artery, the celiac artery, the femoral artery, the iliac artery, and the abdominal aorta.
2. Isolated perfusion in the closed circuit of a life support machine or as a short-term hypoxic infusion over 15 min. In addition to the traditional isolated limb perfusion with melanomas and sarcomas use is also made of isolated pelvic perfusion with tumors or metastases in the lesser pelvis, isolated abdominal perfusion with extensive peritoneal carcinosis, and isolated thoracic perfusion with tumors of the lung, pleura, mediastinum, and thoracic wall [7–10].

33.3   Chemofiltration

Immediately after therapy, the existing high systemic cytotoxic levels are reduced through the arterial and venous catheters used for isolated perfusion via capillary filters with a high flow rate [9], where subjective side effects in the vast majority of cases are greatly minimized and may be completely prevented in individual cases. Objective side effects in the form of bone marrow suppression occur in an extenuated form, so that under normal conditions the substitution of blood components or infection prophylaxis due to bone marrow suppression is not required.

33.4   Material and Methods

Patients in tumor progression or with regional metastasis following systemic chemotherapy were given locoregional chemotherapy. Side effect parameters, about which patients report primarily and which impair their quality of life significantly, were scrutinized in the questionnaire as "after systemic" and "after regional" chemotherapy.

One hundred patients were included in the study as a result, whose tumors or metastases were in progression after systemic chemotherapy or had not given a primary response. These mainly involved malignancies in the head and neck area, non-small-cell lung cancers, lung metastases of various primary tumors, thoracic wall recurrences of breast cancer, liver metastases of various primary tumors, the platinum-refractory, and advanced ovarian cancer and tumors in the pelvic area, such as soft tissue sarcomas, advanced cervical cancer, and anal cancer.

33.5   Regional Therapies

With tumors in the head and neck area, treatment was by angiographically placed carotid artery catheters or implanted carotid artery Jet Port all-round catheters. These therapies were conducted either in arterial short-term infusions on 4 days or arterial infusion under isolated thoracic perfusion conditions [7]. Bronchial cancers or thoracic wall recurrences were treated with isolated thoracic perfusion and aortal short-term infusion. Liver metastases were subject to fractionated chemoembolization on four consecutive days. If metastases on the liver hilum or diffuse peritoneal metastasis persisted, therapy consisted of isolated abdominal perfusion in accordance with the perfusion technique with platinum-refractory ovarian cancer. When restricted to malignancies of the pelvis, the pelvis was subject to isolated perfusion. All perfusion procedures were combined with consecutive chemofiltration to reduce the imminent but also cumulative toxicity.

33.6   Questionnaires on Quality of Life (QoL)

The questions to patients were related to the most obvious symptoms that they complained of after chemotherapy. These are

- Nausea and vomiting
- Hair loss
- Diarrhea
- Mucosal changes
- Fatigue
- Exhaustion
- Weight loss
- Loss of appetite
- Hand-foot syndrome was not included because it was never observed after regional chemotherapy.

For each of the listed side effects, the patient rated the perceived intensity of the side effect at increasing levels from 1 ("very mild") to 6 ("very strong"). In the following charts, the levels of side effects after regional chemotherapy are shown respectively in blue columns, with those of systemic chemotherapy in red columns.

33.7   Results

Nausea and vomiting occurred after regional chemotherapy mainly in a very mild form, whereas after systemic chemotherapy, the highest frequency was found in the largest level of severity 6 (Fig. 33.1).

Number of patients
Systemic
Regional
Intensity of toxicity level

Hair loss occurred after regional chemotherapy very rarely, and, if so, only after isolated thoracic perfusion, when despite a cold cap, the hair loss could not be prevented. The focus after systemic chemotherapy is clearly on the highest severity level of 6 (Fig. 33.2).

Diarrhea occurred after both treatment methods. The differences are not very remarkable, although a slight increase in higher levels of severity was recorded after systemic chemotherapy compared with regional chemotherapy (Fig. 33.3).

Mucosal changes occurred after regional chemotherapy mainly at the mild level 1, where the trend after systemic chemotherapy is increasingly toward the higher levels of severity (Fig. 33.4).

Fatigue and an increased need for sleep are along with exhaustion one of the most obvious symptoms of therapy-related toxicity. Even after regional

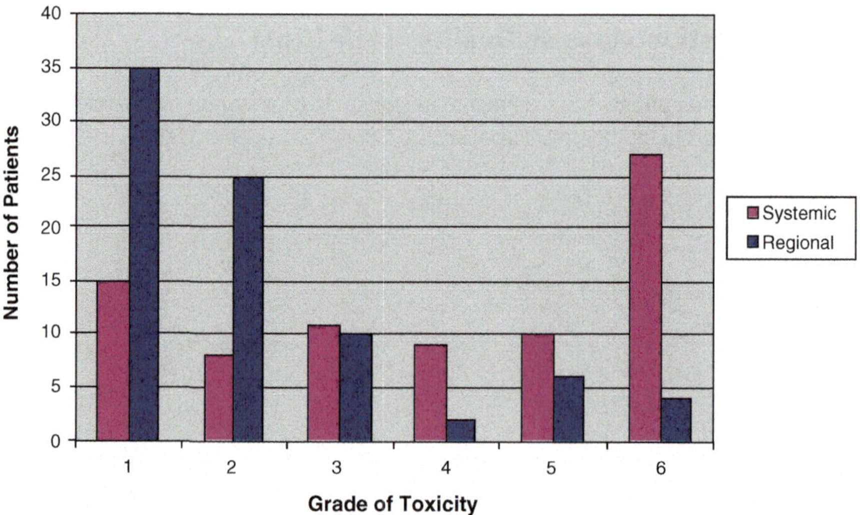

Fig. 33.1 Nausea/vomiting

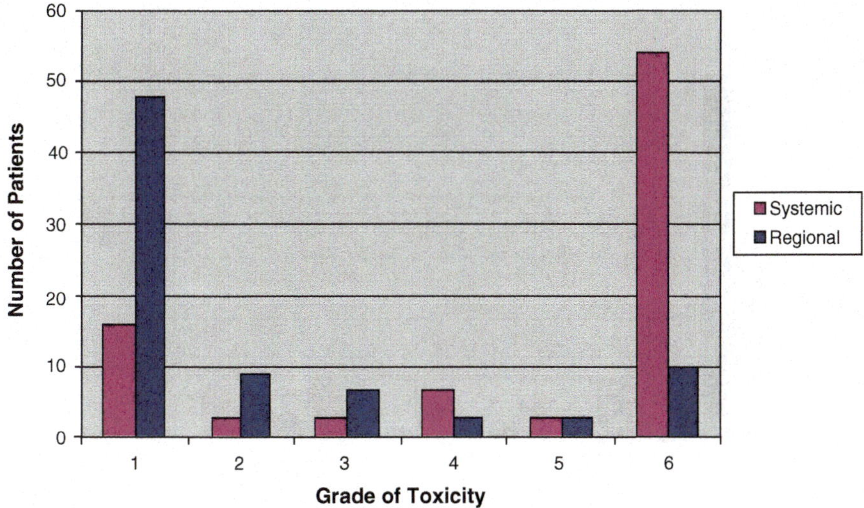

Fig. 33.2 Hair loss

chemotherapy – just after isolated perfusion procedures – patients report no insignificant fatigue at severity levels 2 and 3. Systemic chemotherapy is rated here clearly, however, with a maximum on severity levels 5 and 6 (Fig. 33.5).

Exhaustion runs parallel to fatigue with the maximum point after regional chemotherapy among the milder levels of side effects and a clear maximum in the higher side effects range after systemic chemotherapy (Fig. 33.6).

Weight loss is observed both after regional as well as systemic chemotherapy, but here again results are more favorable for regional chemotherapy (Fig. 33.7).

Loss of appetite is reported following regional chemotherapy especially at severity levels 1 and 2, while levels 3 and 4 are also considerable. After systemic chemotherapy, the maximum point is in turn at levels 5 and 6 (Fig. 33.8).

A summation of toxicity profiles after systemic chemotherapy in comparison with regional is presented in Fig. 33.9. A summation of all the symptoms (I–VIII) results in a very clear picture of the side effects of both treatment methods. The side effects during and after regional chemotherapy attain their maximum at the mild severity level 1 with a consecutively decreasing tendency to severity level 6, whereas during and after systemic chemotherapy (pink columns), the same patients report an increasing tendency in side effects from low severity level 2 to the proportionately most frequent severity level 6.

Patient collective

Systemic

Regional

Intensity of toxicity level

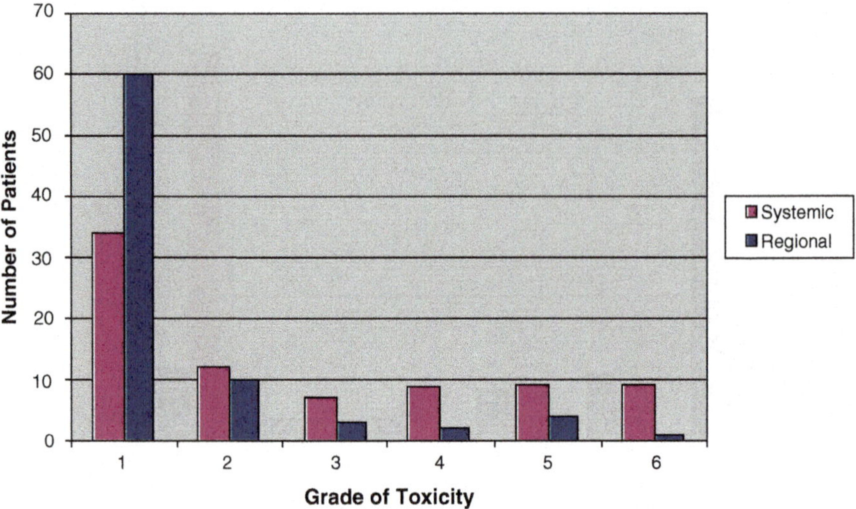

Fig. 33.3 Diarrhea

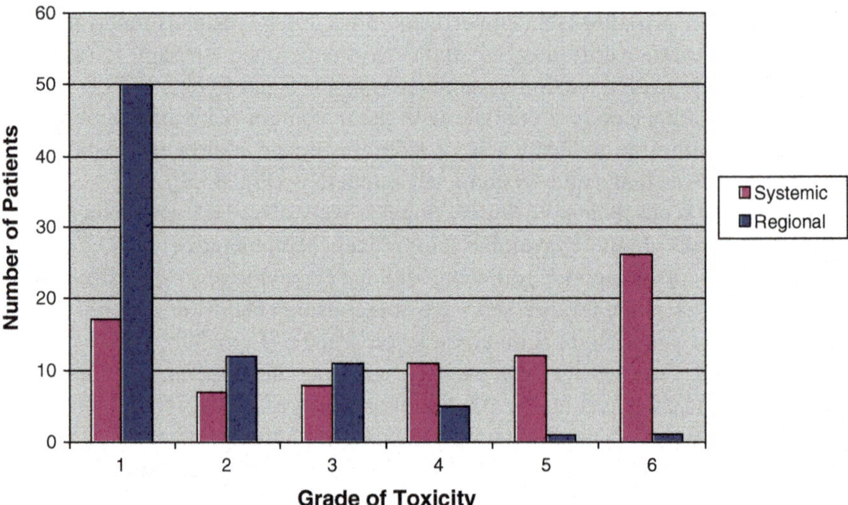

Fig. 33.4 Mucosal changes

33.8 Discussion

Treatments of malignant diseases can be very stressful. This applies to mutilating interventions after extensive tumor resections, especially in the head and neck area but also on extremities and in breast surgery. It relates to the very stressful toxicity after high-dose systemic chemotherapy as well as permanent late damages that have

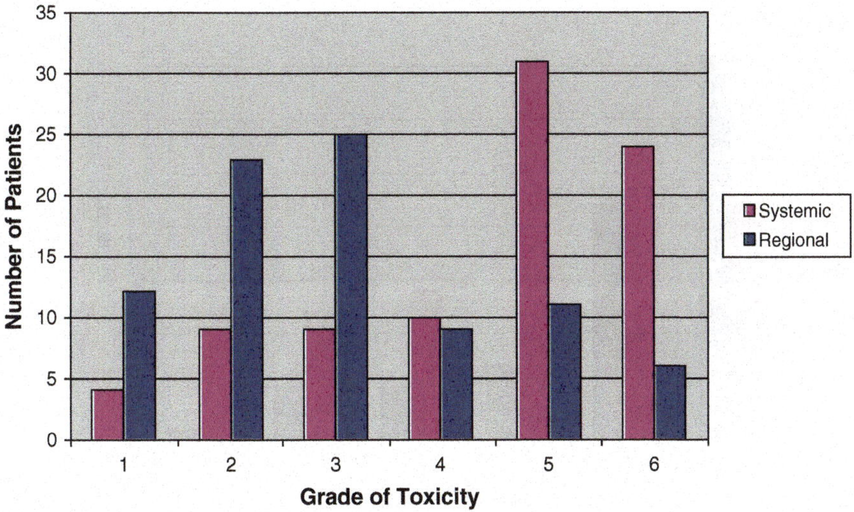

Fig. 33.5 Fatigue

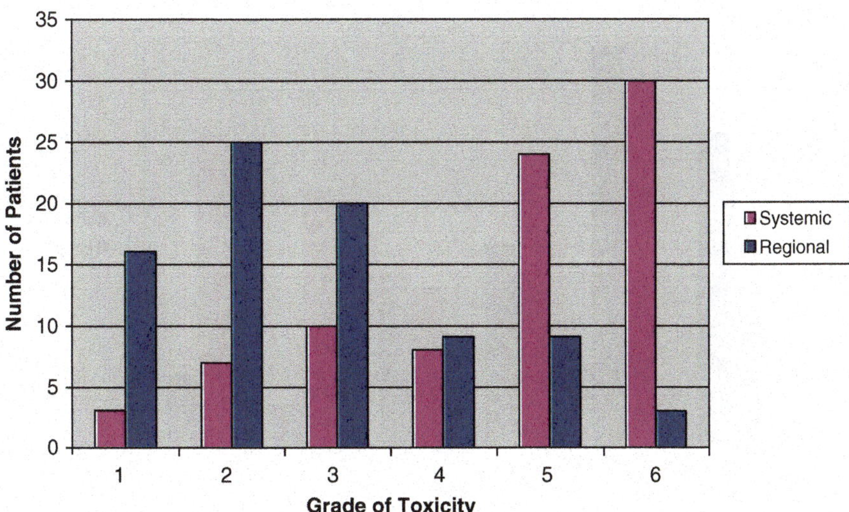

Fig. 33.6 Exhaustion

a severe adverse effect on quality of life after radiotherapy. The proportionality between reasonable toxicity and an achievable clinical result should always be maintained. If toxicity increases at the expense of a clinically irrelevant improvement in the treatment outcome, this proportionality is no longer maintained. If instead of impressive tumor remissions, the elimination of tumor pain or significant life extensions, clinically "evidence-based" alternate parameters are chosen to justify stressful treatments, this proportionality and clinical relevance is no longer

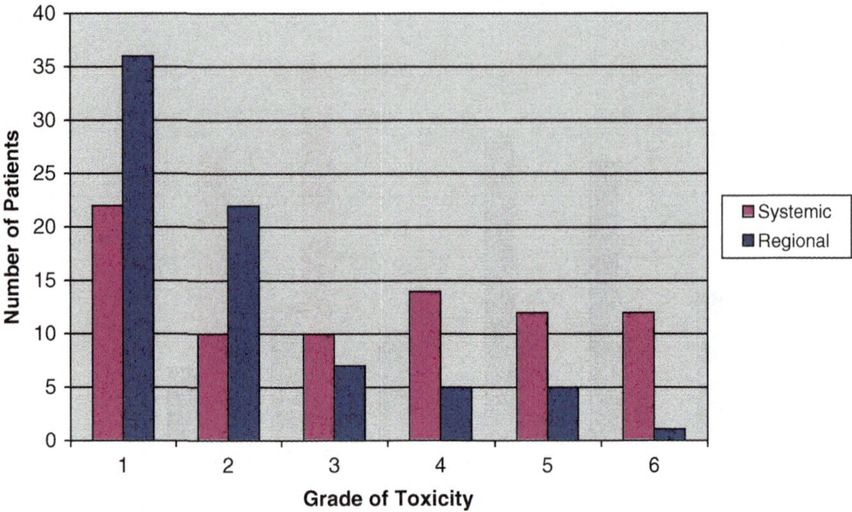

Fig. 33.7 Weight loss

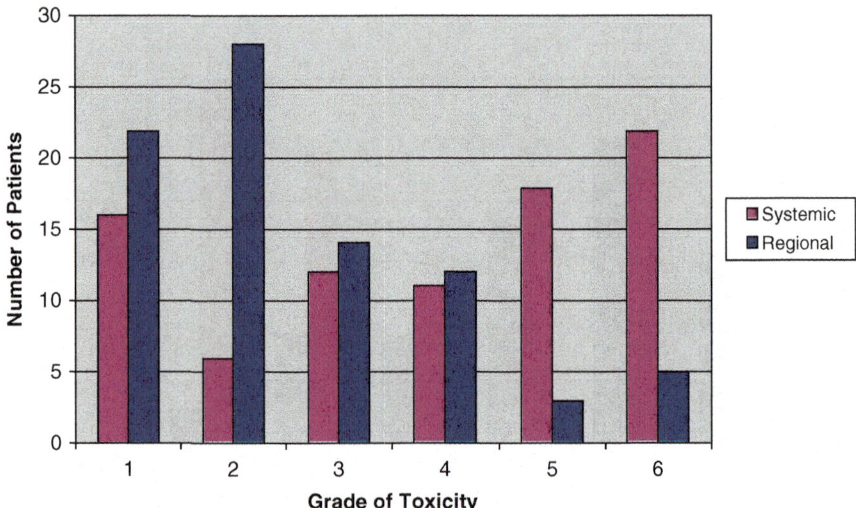

Fig. 33.8 Loss of appetite

ensured [11], and the question of critical evaluation of quality of life is raised. This already occurred in the mid-1970s, when the American psychologist John Flanagan began to produce measurable parameters to determine quality of life [3, 4]. With the establishment of the Quality of Life Department in 1993, the EORTC unleashed a huge growing movement and developed detailed questionnaires for all types of tumors and their specific treatments, even though they were very stressful but

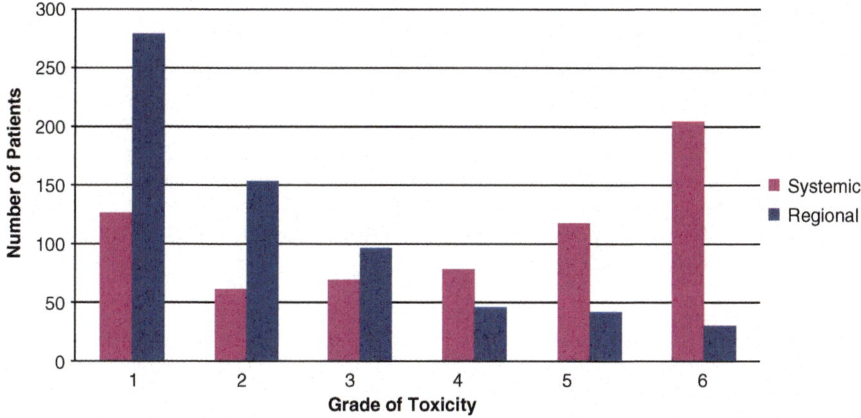

Fig. 33.9 Overall toxicity profiles after systemic versus regional chemotherapy

evidence based. These questionnaires at a very high scientific standard gained rapidly in importance internationally were also translated into other languages and adopted in other countries. This is without doubt a great advance in the control of escalating toxic treatment measures. But if a therapy is recognized as a guideline therapy, its toxicity is more or less noted as an inevitable result of it.

Of crucial importance in the assessment of side effects is the question of who reports them. The comment, "The therapy was very well tolerated" is very common and easy to express. But it also raises the question – is the patient saying this or his therapist? In a study by Petersen [12] on quality of life in palliative treatment, patients and doctors were each asked the same questions (EORTC QLQ – C30) to determine quality of life. The results turned out to be completely different and were not comparable at all. Patients rated their quality of life worse than their doctors did. The conclusion drawn from this was that doctors may make a biased assessment and this is the reason patients need to be interviewed. If the self-assessment of the situation is obtained not from the patient himself but only based on clinical findings, there is a risk of trivializing toxicity perceived by the patient as subjectively unacceptable and regarding it as justifiable.

In this study, patients who had received both types of chemotherapy – systemic and regional – were asked objectively about their state of health. The questions were divided roughly into six levels of severity. They were not asked about many symptoms but only the most common ones, where those considered the most important were those the patients complained about most in the interview. These are especially fatigue, exhaustion, nausea and hair loss. Hand-foot syndrome, which is felt to be very stressful, was not investigated, as it never occurs with regional chemotherapy. If it is true, as published by the Quality of Life Department of the EORTC in *Lancet Oncology* [6], that quality of life is a prognostic parameter for survival time, then regional chemotherapy would have to have the effect of prolonging life based merely on the improvement in quality of life.

References

1. Rugo HS, Barry WT, Moreno-Aspitia A, et al. CALGB 40502/NCCTG N063H: randomized phase III trial of weekly paclitaxel (P) compared to weekly nanoparticle albumin bound nab-paclitaxel (NP) or ixabepilone (Ix) with or without bevacizumab (B) as first-line therapy for locally recurrent or metastatic breast cancer (MBC). Program and abstracts of the American Society of Clinical Oncology Annual Meeting and Exposition; 1–5 June 2012; Chicago. Abstract CRA1002.
2. Miller KD. Can efficacy be derailed by toxicity? Posted online 07/02/2012. www.medscape.com/viewarticle/766488_print.
3. Flanagan JC. A research approach to improving our quality of life. Am Psychol. 1978;33:138–47.
4. Flanagan JC. Measurement of the quality of life: current state of the art. Arch Phys Med Rehabil. 1982;63:56–9.
5. EORTC quality of life. Glossary. http://groups.eortc.be/qol/glossary.
6. Quinten C, Coens C, Mauer M, et al. Baseline quality of life as a prognostic indicator of survival: a meta-analysis of individual patient data from EORTC clinical trials. Lancet Oncol. 2009;10:865–71.
7. Aigner KR, Selak E. Isolated thoracic perfusion with carotid artery infusion for advanced and chemoresistant tumors of the parotid gland. In: Aigner KR, Stephens FO, editors. Induction chemotherapy. Berlin: Springer Press; 2011. p. 119–25.
8. Aigner KR, Jansa J. Induction chemotherapy for cervical cancer. In: Aigner KR, Stephens FO, editors. Induction chemotherapy. Berlin: Springer Press; 2011. p. 261–5.
9. Aigner KR, Gailhofer S. Regional chemotherapy for recurrent platin refractory ovarian cancer. In: Aigner KR, Stephens FO, editors. Induction chemotherapy. Berlin: Springer Press; 2011. p. 183–93.
10. Aigner KR, Selak E. Isolated thoracic perfusion with chemofiltration (ITP-F) for advanced and pre-treated non-small-cell lung cancer. In: Aigner KR, Stephens FO, editors. Induction chemotherapy. Berlin: Springer Press; 2011. p. 321–9.
11. Aigner KR, Stephens FO. Guidelines and evidence-based medicine – evidence of what? EJCMO 2012. Published online. http://www.slm-oncology.com/Guidelines_and_Evidence_Based_Medicine_Evidence_of_What_,1,272.html.
12. Petersen MA, Larsen H, Pedersen L, et al. Assessing health-related quality of life in palliative care: comparing patient and physician assessments. Eur J Cancer. 2006;42:1159–66.

Printed by Printforce, the Netherlands